Novel Anticancer Strategies

Novel Anticancer Strategies

Editor

Hassan Bousbaa

MDPI • Basel • Beijing • Wuhan • Barcelona • Belgrade • Manchester • Tokyo • Cluj • Tianjin

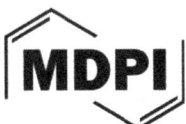

Editor
Hassan Bousbaa
UNIPRO–Oral Pathology and
Rehabilitation Research Unit
CESPU
Gandra PRD
Portugal

Editorial Office
MDPI
St. Alban-Anlage 66
4052 Basel, Switzerland

This is a reprint of articles from the Special Issue published online in the open access journal *Pharmaceutics* (ISSN 1999-4923) (available at: www.mdpi.com/journal/pharmaceutics/special_issues/novel_anticancer).

For citation purposes, cite each article independently as indicated on the article page online and as indicated below:

LastName, A.A.; LastName, B.B.; LastName, C.C. Article Title. *Journal Name* **Year**, *Volume Number*, Page Range.

ISBN 978-3-0365-7031-0 (Hbk)
ISBN 978-3-0365-7030-3 (PDF)

© 2023 by the authors. Articles in this book are Open Access and distributed under the Creative Commons Attribution (CC BY) license, which allows users to download, copy and build upon published articles, as long as the author and publisher are properly credited, which ensures maximum dissemination and a wider impact of our publications.

The book as a whole is distributed by MDPI under the terms and conditions of the Creative Commons license CC BY-NC-ND.

Contents

About the Editor vii

Hassan Bousbaa
Novel Anticancer Strategies
Reprinted from: *Pharmaceutics* **2021**, *13*, 275, doi:10.3390/pharmaceutics13020275 1

Khaled AbouAitah and Witold Lojkowski
Delivery of Natural Agents by Means of Mesoporous Silica Nanospheres as a Promising Anticancer Strategy
Reprinted from: *Pharmaceutics* **2021**, *13*, 143, doi:10.3390/pharmaceutics13020143 5

Sibusiso Alven and Blessing Atim Aderibigbe
The Therapeutic Efficacy of Dendrimer and Micelle Formulations for Breast Cancer Treatment
Reprinted from: *Pharmaceutics* **2020**, *12*, 1212, doi:10.3390/pharmaceutics12121212 57

Ik Sup Jin, Min Jeong Jo, Chun-Woong Park, Youn Bok Chung, Jin-Seok Kim and Dae Hwan Shin
Physicochemical, Pharmacokinetic, and Toxicity Evaluation of Soluplus® Polymeric Micelles Encapsulating Fenbendazole
Reprinted from: *Pharmaceutics* **2020**, *12*, 1000, doi:10.3390/pharmaceutics12101000 107

Sathishbabu Paranthaman, Meghana Goravinahalli Shivananjegowda, Manohar Mahadev, Afrasim Moin, Shivakumar Hagalavadi Nanjappa and Nandakumar Dalavaikodihalli Nanjaiyah et al.
Nanodelivery Systems Targeting Epidermal Growth Factor Receptors for Glioma Management
Reprinted from: *Pharmaceutics* **2020**, *12*, 1198, doi:10.3390/pharmaceutics12121198 123

Yongwhan Choi, Hyounkoo Han, Sangmin Jeon, Hong Yeol Yoon, Hyuncheol Kim and Ick Chan Kwon et al.
Deep Tumor Penetration of Doxorubicin-Loaded Glycol Chitosan Nanoparticles Using High-Intensity Focused Ultrasound
Reprinted from: *Pharmaceutics* **2020**, *12*, 974, doi:10.3390/pharmaceutics12100974 153

Ragnhild Haugse, Anika Langer, Elisa Thodesen Murvold, Daniela Elena Costea, Bjørn Tore Gjertsen and Odd Helge Gilja et al.
Low-Intensity Sonoporation-Induced Intracellular Signalling of Pancreatic Cancer Cells, Fibroblasts and Endothelial Cells
Reprinted from: *Pharmaceutics* **2020**, *12*, 1058, doi:10.3390/pharmaceutics12111058 169

Bárbara Pinto, Ana C. Henriques, Patrícia M. A. Silva and Hassan Bousbaa
Three-Dimensional Spheroids as In Vitro Preclinical Models for Cancer Research
Reprinted from: *Pharmaceutics* **2020**, *12*, 1186, doi:10.3390/pharmaceutics12121186 187

Laia Hernandez-Oller, Joaquin Seras-Franzoso, Fernanda Andrade, Diana Rafael, Ibane Abasolo and Petra Gener et al.
Extracellular Vesicles as Drug Delivery Systems in Cancer
Reprinted from: *Pharmaceutics* **2020**, *12*, 1146, doi:10.3390/pharmaceutics12121146 225

Jaeduk Park, Hyuk Lee, Yu Seok Youn, Kyung Taek Oh and Eun Seong Lee
Tumor-Homing pH-Sensitive Extracellular Vesicles for Targeting Heterogeneous Tumors
Reprinted from: *Pharmaceutics* **2020**, *12*, 372, doi:10.3390/pharmaceutics12040372 245

Levente E. Dókus, Eszter Lajkó, Ivan Ranelović, Diána Mező, Gitta Schlosser and László Kőhidai et al.
Phage Display-Based Homing Peptide-Daunomycin Conjugates for Selective Drug Targeting to PANC-1 Pancreatic Cancer
Reprinted from: *Pharmaceutics* **2020**, *12*, 576, doi:10.3390/pharmaceutics12060576 261

Ayman Abouzayed, Hanna Tano, Ábel Nagy, Sara S. Rinne, Fadya Wadeea and Sharmishtaa Kumar et al.
Preclinical Evaluation of the GRPR-Targeting Antagonist RM26 Conjugated to the Albumin-Binding Domain for GRPR-Targeting Therapy of Cancer
Reprinted from: *Pharmaceutics* **2020**, *12*, 977, doi:10.3390/pharmaceutics12100977 281

Adriana G. Quiroz-Reyes, Jose F. Islas, Paulina Delgado-Gonzalez, Hector Franco-Villarreal and Elsa N. Garza-Treviño
Therapeutic Approaches for Metastases from Colorectal Cancer and Pancreatic Ductal Carcinoma
Reprinted from: *Pharmaceutics* **2021**, *13*, 103, doi:10.3390/pharmaceutics13010103 299

Joseph J. Noh, Myeong-Seon Kim, Young-Jae Cho, Soo-Young Jeong, Yoo-Young Lee and Ji-Yoon Ryu et al.
Anti-Cancer Activity of As_4O_6 and its Efficacy in a Series of Patient-Derived Xenografts for Human Cervical Cancer
Reprinted from: *Pharmaceutics* **2020**, *12*, 987, doi:10.3390/pharmaceutics12100987 323

Guillaume Sicard, Clément Paris, Sarah Giacometti, Anne Rodallec, Joseph Ciccolini and Palma Rocchi et al.
Enhanced Antisense Oligonucleotide Delivery Using Cationic Liposomes Grafted with Trastuzumab: A Proof-of-Concept Study in Prostate Cancer
Reprinted from: *Pharmaceutics* **2020**, *12*, 1166, doi:10.3390/pharmaceutics12121166 337

Guillaume Sicard, Frédéric Fina, Raphaelle Fanciullino, Fabrice Barlesi and Joseph Ciccolini
Like a Rolling Stone: Sting-Cgas Pathway and Cell-Free DNA as Biomarkers for Combinatorial Immunotherapy
Reprinted from: *Pharmaceutics* **2020**, *12*, 758, doi:10.3390/pharmaceutics12080758 353

Jong Hyuk Byun, In-Soo Yoon, Yong Dam Jeong, Sungchan Kim and Il Hyo Jung
A Tumor-Immune Interaction Model for Synergistic Combinations of Anti PD-L1 and Ionizing Irradiation Treatment
Reprinted from: *Pharmaceutics* **2020**, *12*, 830, doi:10.3390/pharmaceutics12090830 369

About the Editor

Hassan Bousbaa

Hassan Bousbaa is a cancer researcher at the Oral Pathology and Rehabilitation Research Unit (UNIPRO) and associate professor of cellular and molecular biology at the Instituto Universitário de Ciências da Saúde—CESPU. Research interests include targeted anticancer therapy; targeting mitosis for cancer therapy; antimitotic agents; biological evaluation of natural and synthetic compounds; and cancer biomarkers. He is acting as a Section Editor of the *Pharmaceutics* journal.

Editorial
Novel Anticancer Strategies

Hassan Bousbaa

CESPU, Instituto de Investigação e Formação Avançada Em Ciências e Tecnologias da Saúde, Instituto Universitário de Ciências da Saúde, 4585-116 Gandra PRD, Portugal; hassan.bousbaa@iucs.cespu.pt

Cancer incidence and mortality continue to increase rapidly worldwide. Owing to the dynamic, rapid, and adaptive nature of cancer progression, side effects and resistance associated with the existing therapies provide continuous and challenging exercises for searching for additional drugs and drug delivery strategies with the goal of offering more effective therapeutic options. Therefore, novel therapeutic strategies are constantly needed in order to overcome the drawbacks associated with the strategies in use in the clinic. This Special Issue (https://www.mdpi.com/journal/pharmaceutics/special_issues/novel_anticancer (accessed on 11 February 2021)) is dedicated to innovative research on the development and validation of novel anticancer approaches, hopefully with relevant clinical value in the near future. In this sense, we have received interesting contributions, in the form of original works and reviews, that cover innovative drug delivery systems, improvement of the efficacy of approved anticancer agents, and validation of new anticancer drugs.

Nanoparticles are 1 to 100 nm sized materials and are grouped into different classes according to their properties, shapes, or sizes. They have a wide range of applications in modern medicine, namely, as carriers for drug and gene delivery into tumors. Due to their unique proprieties, mesoporous silica nanoparticles (MSNs) have deserved increasing interest in nanoparticle-mediated drug delivery research. MSNs are chemically stable with good biocompatibility, which, when adequately tailored, can provide large surface area and pore volume for high loading capacity, as well as selective and controlled delivery of therapeutic agents. Particularly interesting is the effective delivery potential of MSNs of poorly soluble anticancer agents, namely, prodrugs derived from different natural origins, as reviewed by Abouaitah and Lojkowski [1].

Dendrimers and polymeric micelles are other promising drug delivery systems. Dendrimers are regularly hyperbranched and mainly 3D macromolecules. They are nano-sized radially symmetric molecules with a well-defined, homogeneous, and monodisperse structure. These characteristics make dendrimers a good choice for the delivery of anticancer drugs. Polymeric micelles are formed by the spontaneous arrangement of amphiphilic block copolymers in aqueous solutions. Their hydrophobic core–hydrophilic shell architecture facilitates the loading of hydrophobic drugs into the core, providing a main to improve the solubility of anticancer drugs. Alven and Aderibigbe summarize the application and outcomes of dendrimers and micelles loaded with different known anticancer agents using in vitro and in vivo models of breast cancer [2]. Jin et al. report the use of Soluplus polymeric micelles to encapsulate the veterinary anthelmintic fenbendazole (FEN), also known for its anticancer efficacy, in order to overcome its low solubility problem [3]. They observed that micellar formulation exhibited superior bioavailability compared with that of free FEN, with no severe toxicity, as revealed by in vivo toxicity assay, thereby paving the way for preclinical and clinical safety and efficacy trials on FEN-loaded Soluplus micelles.

Nanotechnology could be a promising solution to overcome delivery and resistance concerns of currently available chemotherapeutics against glioblastoma, one of the most aggressive types of cancer. Low drug solubility, blood–brain barrier penetration, and drug–target residence time are major issues in translating in vitro potency to in vivo efficacy for glioblastoma treatment. In their review, Paranthaman et al. describe the molecular basis of glioblastoma, emphasizing the role of receptor tyrosine kinases (RTKs) and small molecules under clinical trials, and provide an updated research literature and future guidelines on epidermal growth factor receptor (EGFR)-RTK inhibitors-based nanodelivery systems [4].

Deep tumor penetration of drug-loaded nanoparticles can be compromised by a dense extracellular matrix (ECM), thereby limiting their therapeutic efficacy. To overcome this issue, Choi et al. used high-intensity focused ultrasound (HIFU) technology to improve the tumor penetration of doxorubicin (DOX)-loaded glycol chitosan nanoparticles (CNPs) [5]. The treatment of ECM-rich tumor-bearing mice with HIFU resulted in an increased accumulation of DOX-CNPs at targeted tumor tissues via deep tumor penetration, through HIFU-mediated dense ECM destruction, providing a means to increase deep penetration into heterogeneous tumors with dense ECM structures. In another study, Haugse et al. analyzed the mechanism behind the use of ultrasound and microbubbles—known as sonoporation—in improving the efficacy of chemotherapy [6]. They observed that sonoporation was associated with an immediate transient activation of MAP kinases (p38, ERK1/2) and an increase in phosphorylation of ribosomal protein S6 together with dephosphorylation of 4E-BP1, a stress response resembling cellular responses to electroporation and pore-forming toxins. Their data also suggest that cells in the tumor microenvironment may be relevant for sonoporation efficacy, which could be exploited therapeutically. However, such analysis should be performed on heterotypic 3D cultures so as to recapitulate the patient tumor architecture and the heterogeneity of cell types and cell–cell interactions [7].

A natural solution for drug delivery is provided by extracellular vesicles (EVs), which are lipid-bound vesicles secreted by cells into the extracellular space, with key roles in intercellular communication. EVs include microvesicles, exosomes, and apoptotic bodies, whose content consists of lipids, nucleic acids, and proteins. Although their isolation and analysis methods still suffer from a lack of standardization, EVs have unique features that are relevant for drug delivery and are expected to overcome the inefficiency, cytotoxicity, and/or immunogenicity associated with synthetic delivery systems, as reviewed by Hernandez-Oller et al. [8]. Park et al. report the use of tumor-homing pH-sensitive EV blends made from tumor-specific EVs, extracted from two different tumor cell types, and pH-sensitive HDEA (3-(diethylamino)propylamine). These EVs were loaded with hyaluronic acid grafted with HDEA and doxorubicin (DOX, as a model antitumor drug) [9]. HDEA/DOX-anchored EVs were able to target the two different parent tumor cells owing to the EVs' homing ability. The pH-sensitive disruption of EVs, owing to DEAP (3-(diethylamino)propylamine) molecules, promoted DOX release, resulting in the effective killing of the heterogeneous parent tumor cells. The finding highlights the potential of EV blends as effective targeted therapies for various tumor cells.

Specific addressing of tumor cells while sparing healthy tissues is currently a major desire in cancer therapy. Tumor-specific binding agents can be conjugated to an anticancer drug to guide the drug to the targeted the tumor. Dókus et al. developed peptide-based drug conjugates against pancreatic cancer cells (PANC-1) [10]. They used the SKAAKN hexapeptide, derived from the previously reported CKAAKN sequence by the substitution of Cys to Ser, in conjugates containing daunomycin (Dau). One conjugate exhibited significant tumor growth inhibition on PANC-1 tumor-bearing mice with negligible side effects, highlighting the promising potential of peptide-based drug delivery systems for pancreatic cancer treatment. Due to their rapid blood clearance, repeated administration of peptide-based therapeutic agents may be necessary. Abouzayed et al. report a successful conjugation of the gastrin-releasing peptide receptor (GRPR) antagonist RM26 and an albumin-binding domain. The conjugate retained GRPR targeting in vivo and, due to binding to albumin, resulted in an increased residence time in blood and in tumors, while retaining specificity and its antagonistic function against GRPR [11]. Although its use for radionuclide therapy is precluded due to undesirable elevated activity uptake in kidneys, the approach deserves further optimization.

Cancer recurrence arises from the incomplete eradication of tumor cells after chemo- and radiotherapy, being one of the major reasons for the failure of cancer treatment strategies. Cancer stem cells (CSCs) are believed to be one of the important drivers of cancer relapse. CSCs are characterized by self-renewal capacity and differentiation potential. Various cancers include a small population of CSCs that confer them metastasis, heterogeneity, drug and radiation resistance, and tumor relapse. In this sense, Quiroz-Reyes et al. provide a comprehensive review on conventional and novel developments in cancer therapeutics for liver, lung, and pancreatic metastasis, with a focus on CSCs as a valuable target to eradicate tumor relapse [12]. Further targeting of CSCs and cancer resistance, using EVs as natural drug delivery systems, is also reviewed by Hernandez-Oller et al. [8].

Arsenic derivatives have been shown to exert anticancer effects, namely, by inducing apoptosis, providing a new alternative to classical chemotherapeutics and radiotherapy. For instance, arsenic trioxide (As_2O_3, Trisenox) has been approved for the treatment of acute promyelocytic leukemia. Noh et al. report the anticancer effects of tetraarsenic hexoxide (TAO, As_4O_6) in a series of patient-derived xenograft (PDX) mouse models of cervical cancer [13]. They showed that TAO induced significant anticancer effect in PDXs with primary cancers, and when combined with cisplatin, PDXs with recurrent cancers were also significantly inhibited. This highlights the potential usefulness of TAO for cervical cancer treatment.

A major obstacle in translating discoveries from preclinical research (bench) into human applications for cancer therapy (bed) resides in the fact that preclinical models do not mimic the real tumor microenvironment. For instance, 2D monolayer cell cultures have reduced cell–cell contacts and lack interactions with a surrounding extracellular framework in three dimensions. In this sense, 3D tumor models, by recapitulating relevant properties of tumor microenvironment interactions, promise to bridge the gap between 2D cell culture and in vivo experiments, and advance our current understanding of cancer. Pinto et al. provide a concise and useful review of the current techniques used to prepare and analyze in vitro 3D spheroids, and discuss the significance of 3D cultures in drug resistance for the evaluation of the therapeutic efficacy of nanomedicines [7]. Using in vitro 2D and 3D spheroid models, Sicard et al. conducted a pilot study to demonstrate that antiproliferative efficacy against prostate cancer (PCa) can be achieved by encapsulating antisense oligonucleotide (ASO) into liposomes to silence TCTP [14]. Interestingly, the most promising efficacy on 3D spheroids was achieved with immunoliposomes targeting Her2, provided that incubation time was long enough, despite a low expression of Her2 in PCa cells.

Cancer immunotherapy (IT) has brought a new hope to cancer patients. The use of immune checkpoint inhibitors has led to a net improvement of survival and quality of life, when compared with standard therapies. However, its use is restricted to very limited cancer types. To extend its use to a larger number of cancers, immune checkpoint inhibitors are being combined with standard therapeutic strategies. However, due to immunomodulating features, an optimal time window to combine immune checkpoint inhibitors with other drugs needs to be defined in order to achieve maximum efficacy while controlling toxicities. Sicard et al. describe the putative biomarkers that could help define this window, with a special focus on circulating tumor DNA whose detection indicates that the STING–cGAS pathway is activated by the immune checkpoint inhibitors [15]. Still in the field of IT, Byun et al. modeled the tumor-immune interactions occurring during combined IT and ionizing irradiation therapy, and suggest that the ratio of PD-1 to PD-L1 in T cells could be considered in combination therapy [16].

In summary, persistence in developing novel anticancer strategies is inevitable to face the adaptive nature of cancer progression. New anticancer drugs are always welcome as alternatives to circumvent side effects and resistance to existing drugs. It is noteworthy that the use of preclinical models that mimic the real tumor microenvironment is important to speed up the translation of research from lab to clinic. Further efforts are also needed to maximize the efficacy of existing drugs, either by chemical modifications or by specific targeting to the desired tumor. Approaches that provide deep penetration of nancarriers into heterogeneous tumors with dense ECM structures bear tremendous potential to improve the efficacy of chemotherapy. The contributions published in this Special Issue are examples of progress towards the achievement of such objectives.

Conflicts of Interest: The author declares no conflict of interest.

References

1. Abouaitah, K.; Lojkowski, W. Delivery of natural agents by means of mesoporous silica nanospheres as a promising anticancer strategy. *Pharmaceutics* **2021**, *13*, 143. [CrossRef] [PubMed]
2. Alven, S.; Aderibigbe, B.A. The therapeutic efficacy of dendrimer and micelle formulations for breast cancer treatment. *Pharmaceutics* **2020**, *12*, 1212. [CrossRef] [PubMed]
3. Jin, I.S.; Jo, M.J.; Park, C.W.; Chung, Y.B.; Kim, J.S.; Shin, D.H. Physicochemical, pharmacokinetic, and toxicity evaluation of soluplus® polymeric micelles encapsulating fenbendazole. *Pharmaceutics* **2020**, *12*, 1000. [CrossRef] [PubMed]
4. Paranthaman, S.; Shivananjegowda, M.G.; Mahadev, M.; Moin, A.; Nanjappa, S.H.; Nanjaiyah, N.; Chidambaram, S.B.; Gowda, D.V. Nanodelivery systems targeting epidermal growth factor receptors for glioma management. *Pharmaceutics* **2020**, *12*, 1198. [CrossRef] [PubMed]
5. Choi, Y.; Han, H.; Jeon, S.; Yoon, H.Y.; Kim, H.; Kwon, I.C.; Kim, K. Deep tumor penetration of doxorubicin-loaded glycol chitosan nanoparticles using high-intensity focused ultrasound. *Pharmaceutics* **2020**, *12*, 974. [CrossRef] [PubMed]
6. Haugse, R.; Langer, A.; Murvold, E.T.; Costea, D.E.; Gjertsen, B.T.; Gilja, O.H.; Kotopoulis, S.; de Garibay, G.R.; McCormack, E. Low-intensity sonoporation-induced intracellular signalling of pancreatic cancer cells, fibroblasts and endothelial cells. *Pharmaceutics* **2020**, *12*, 1058. [CrossRef] [PubMed]
7. Pinto, B.; Henriques, A.C.; Silva, P.M.A.; Bousbaa, H. Three-dimensional spheroids as in vitro preclinical models for cancer research. *Pharmaceutics* **2020**, *12*, 1186. [CrossRef] [PubMed]
8. Hernandez-Oller, L.; Seras-Franzoso, J.; Andrade, F.; Rafael, D.; Abasolo, I.; Gener, P.; Schwartz, S. Extracellular vesicles as drug delivery systems in cancer. *Pharmaceutics* **2020**, *12*, 1146. [CrossRef] [PubMed]
9. Park, J.; Lee, H.; Youn, Y.S.; Oh, K.T.; Lee, E.S. Tumor-homing ph-sensitive extracellular vesicles for targeting heterogeneous tumors. *Pharmaceutics* **2020**, *12*, 372. [CrossRef] [PubMed]
10. Dókus, L.E.; Lajkó, E.; Ranđelović, I.; Mező, D.; Schlosser, G.; Kőhidai, L.; Tóvári, J.; Mező, G. Phage display-based homing peptide-daunomycin conjugates for selective drug targeting to panc-1 pancreatic cancer. *Pharmaceutics* **2020**, *12*, 576. [CrossRef] [PubMed]
11. Abouzayed, A.; Tano, H.; Nagy, Á.; Rinne, S.S.; Wadeea, F.; Kumar, S.; Westerlund, K.; Tolmachev, V.; Karlström, A.E.; Orlova, A. Preclinical evaluation of the grpr-targeting antagonist rm26 conjugated to the albumin-binding domain for grpr-targeting therapy of cancer. *Pharmaceutics* **2020**, *12*, 977. [CrossRef] [PubMed]
12. Quiroz-Reyes, A.G.; Islas, J.F.; Delgado-Gonzalez, P.; Franco-Villarreal, H.; Garza-Treviño, E.N. Therapeutic approaches for metastases from colorectal cancer and pancreatic ductal carcinoma. *Pharmaceutics* **2021**, *13*, 103. [CrossRef] [PubMed]
13. Noh, J.J.; Kim, M.S.; Cho, Y.J.; Jeong, S.Y.; Lee, Y.Y.; Ryu, J.Y.; Choi, J.J.; Bae, I.; Wu, Z.; Kim, B.G.; et al. Anti-cancer activity of as4o6 and its efficacy in a series of patient-derived xenografts for human cervical cancer. *Pharmaceutics* **2020**, *12*, 987. [CrossRef] [PubMed]
14. Sicard, G.; Paris, C.; Giacometti, S.; Rodallec, A.; Ciccolini, J.; Rocchi, P.; Fanciullino, R. Enhanced antisense oligonucleotide delivery using cationic liposomes grafted with trastuzumab: A proof-of-concept study in prostate cancer. *Pharmaceutics* **2020**, *12*, 1166. [CrossRef] [PubMed]
15. Sicard, G.; Fina, F.; Fanciullino, R.; Barlesi, F.; Ciccolini, J. Like a rolling stone: Sting-cGAS pathway and cell-free DNA as biomarkers for combinatorial immunotherapy. *Pharmaceutics* **2020**, *12*, 758. [CrossRef] [PubMed]
16. Byun, J.H.; Yoon, I.S.; Jeong, Y.D.; Kim, S.; Jung, I.H. A tumor-immune interaction model for synergistic combinations of anti pd-l1 and ionizing irradiation treatment. *Pharmaceutics* **2020**, *12*, 830. [CrossRef] [PubMed]

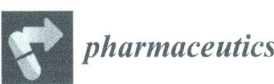

Review

Delivery of Natural Agents by Means of Mesoporous Silica Nanospheres as a Promising Anticancer Strategy

Khaled AbouAitah [1,2,*] and Witold Lojkowski [1,*]

1. Laboratory of Nanostructures and Nanomedicine, Institute of High Pressure Physics, Polish Academy of Sciences, Sokolowska 29/37, 01-142 Warsaw, Poland
2. Medicinal and Aromatic Plants Research Department, Pharmaceutical and Drug Industries Research Division, National Research Centre (NRC), 33 El-Behouth St., Dokki 12622, Giza, Egypt
* Correspondence: k.abouaitah@labnano.pl (K.A.); w.lojkowski@labnano.pl (W.L.); Tel.: +48-22-888-0429 or +48-22-632-4302 (K.A. & W.L.); Fax: +48-22-632-4218 (K.A. & W.L.)

Abstract: Natural prodrugs derived from different natural origins (e.g., medicinal plants, microbes, animals) have a long history in traditional medicine. They exhibit a broad range of pharmacological activities, including anticancer effects in vitro and in vivo. They have potential as safe, cost-effective treatments with few side effects, but are lacking in solubility, bioavailability, specific targeting and have short half-lives. These are barriers to clinical application. Nanomedicine has the potential to offer solutions to circumvent these limitations and allow the use of natural pro-drugs in cancer therapy. Mesoporous silica nanoparticles (MSNs) of various morphology have attracted considerable attention in the search for targeted drug delivery systems. MSNs are characterized by chemical stability, easy synthesis and functionalization, large surface area, tunable pore sizes and volumes, good biocompatibility, controlled drug release under different conditions, and high drug-loading capacity, enabling multifunctional purposes. In vivo pre-clinical evaluations, a significant majority of results indicate the safety profile of MSNs if they are synthesized in an optimized way. Here, we present an overview of synthesis methods, possible surface functionalization, cellular uptake, biodistribution, toxicity, loading strategies, delivery designs with controlled release, and cancer targeting and discuss the future of anticancer nanotechnology-based natural prodrug delivery systems.

Keywords: mesoporous silica nanoparticles; controlled release; drug delivery systems; anticancer natural prodrugs; natural products; cancer targeting; nanoformulations/nanomedicine applications

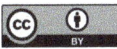

1. Introduction

In 2001, Vallet-Regi et al. [1] introduced a mesoporous silica material called MCM-41 that can be used as a drug carrier. The nanostructure (e.g., pore size) of MCM-41 can be optimized using different surfactants. Since then, many efforts and attempts have been made to synthesize versatile mesoporous silica nanoparticles (MSNs) with different nanostructures and morphologies to meet the demand for pharmaceutical and medical applications. The history of the synthesis of mesoporous silica materials dates back to 1992, when they were discovered by the Mobile Oil Corporation [2]. Silica is one of the most abundant minerals in the Earth's crust and is also found in the food chain and the human body [3]. As a biomaterial, silica is extensively used in many applications such as dentistry, orthopedics, and dermatology. MSNs have a characteristic mesoporous nanostructure that offers many advantages for medical applications in disease diagnosis and therapy [4]. The unique features include easy synthesis, the possibility of various surface modifications, the ability to obtain a tunable particle size, uniform pore size, high surface area to pore volume, good biocompatibility, and chemical stability [5–9]. In addition, easy functionalization to achieve magnetic, fluorescent, and photothermal properties increases the chance of using MSNs in bioimaging. MSN nanostructures can provide excellent nanoplatforms to fabricate smart drug delivery systems (DDSs) with a high drug loading capacity and stimuli-responsive drug release effect compared to other nanocarriers [6,10]. Several nanocarriers have been used to deliver and control drug release, including niosomes, liposomes, dendrimers, lipid nanoparticles, and polymeric nanoparticles, but most of them have low stability and need external stabilization during synthesis. In contrast, MSNs have a strong Si-O bond that makes them stable (chemically and mechanically) to external responses in the surrounding environment [11–13]. It is generally accepted that encapsulation of drugs or therapeutic agents into MSNs can enhance their therapeutic activity, solubility, and bioavailability, as indicated by many studies [14–20].

A consequence of these advantages is that MSNs have gained much attention and popularity in DDSs during the last few decades for the delivery of cargo to specific sites in the organism. A large number of in vivo studies indicate the high biocompatibility/safety profile and low toxicity of MSNs if they are synthesized using an optimized way [21–23]. A careful optimization process is needed because many details of the nanostructure of engineered MSNs, i.e., size, shape, surface, presence of surfactant, and other factors like dose, administration route affect the safety profile. According to many animal studies, the toxicity of MSNs can be diminished by optimizing the synthesis parameters and surface modification, resulting in safe nanoparticles [24,25].

The administration route is an important characteristic for constructing any DDS. MSNs can be applied via different routes, including oral and intravenous injection [26–30]. Many choices in the development of pharmaceutical formulations depend on the target tissues and organs in the human body. An important advantage of DDS-based MSNs is that the amorphous forms of silica and silicates are generally recognized as safe materials for use as oral delivery ingredients (up to 1500 mg per day) according to the US Food and Drug Administration and the European Food Safety Authority [27]. MSNs are promising materials because they exhibit low toxicity levels in animals when applied, i.e., orally, injection [31].

The global market for nanomedicine accounts for 5% when novel nanomedicines translated from the lab to the clinics are concerned [32]. Recently, the first clinical trial in humans was conducted with oral delivery of fenofibrate formulation based on the ordered mesoporous silica [33].

Despite these promising results for nanotechnology application in building DDSs, most research for targeted cancer therapy has been focused on drugs and therapeutic molecules of a synthetic nature. Combating cancers with synthetic drugs is an established therapy, however, progress in this area of medicine is slow and the treatments are frequently associated with undesirable effects: side effects and also insufficient patient compliance. For this reason, extensive research is carried out to apply natural prodrugs (known also as natural products and natural agents) in anticancer therapies.

Nature is a huge source of therapeutic substances, which can be derived from plants, microbes, and animals. Natural medicines account for 60% of anticancer agents used in clinical applications [34]. For example, vincristine, taxanes, and camptothecin are used in the treatment and prevention of cancer. There are still hundreds of promising new active natural anticancer agents to be discovered and renewed for cancer therapy [35–37]. The main advantages to using and developing natural prodrugs are that they offer safe, cost-effective, and have versatile pharmacological properties [38]. The main limitations for their use in cancer therapy are their poor water solubility, low bioavailability, short half-life, and non-specific targeting.

Nanotechnology offers many ways to overcome these obstacles [39–44]. Natural pro-drugs can be embedded into MSNs, which can serve as effective nanocarriers for the delivery of anticancer natural prodrugs to target cancers. In this review, we present an overview of synthesis methods, surface functionalization, as well as biodistribution, biocompatibility, toxicity, biological performance. Additionally, drug loading and release strategies, and active targeting approaches for MSNs will be addressed. We also discuss delivery and controlled release systems for selected prodrugs using MSNs.

Available data provide considerable evidence that MSNs allow the limitations associated with prodrugs, such as poor water solubility, poor bioavailability, and low specific targeting ability, to be overcome. Compared to organic delivery systems (e.g., lipid nanoparticles, polymeric nanoparticles) [45,46], the delivery of natural prodrugs by means of MSNs allows high drug loading and permits multifunctional delivery or co-delivery systems. Generally, MSNs allow long-term release compared to organic nanoparticles. This is because the prodrugs are trapped inside nano-pores. In the case of encapsulation of prodrugs into organic nanoparticles, fast degradation of the organic substance leads to quick prodrug release. The MSN-based nanomedicine technology is mature enough to be extended to thousands of prodrugs not yet investigated in clinical applications.

To the best of our knowledge, this is the first review considering MSNs as delivery systems for anticancer natural prodrugs. The need for such a review is a consequence of rapid development in the field. This review may help researchers accelerate research and development of this important field of nanomedicine and, ultimately, clinical applications.

2. Synthesis of Mesoporous Silica Nanostructures

Numerous synthesis methods have been developed to obtain MSNs with different morphological, structural, and pore geometry. Particular attention was paid to the production of biocompatible MSNs for medicine. Figure 1 presents the number of scientific publications (research articles, review articles, and book chapters) as an indicator of the growth in MSN synthesis methods due to their emergence as nanostructures for various promising applications.

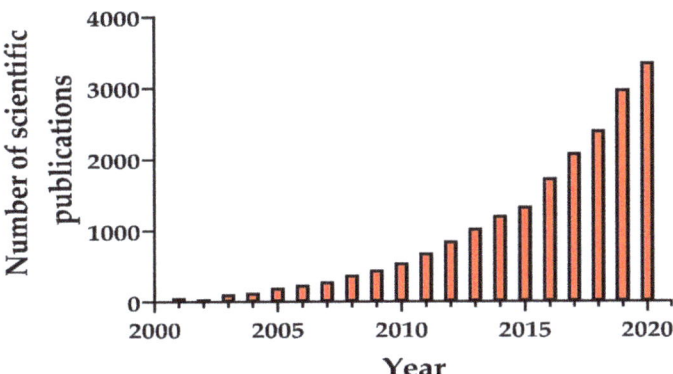

Figure 1. Number of scientific publications (research papers, reviews, book chapters) during the period 2001–2020 found by entering key words "mesoporous silica nanoparticles and synthesis". The search was performed in ScienceDirect 10 September 2020.

2.1. Discovery, Synthesis, and Properties of MSNs

Porous materials (natural or artificial) are characterized by the presence of pores, including cavities, channels, or interstices. The properties of these materials vary depending on the characteristics of their pores: size, arrangement/structure, shape, porosity, and chemical composition. They have been extensively studied in different areas, including water purification, gas separation, catalysts, energy storage, adsorbents, electronics, engineering, tissue engineering, and drug delivery systems, among others [47]. Depending on the predominant pore size, the International Union of Pure and Applied Chemistry (IUPAC) classifies porous materials into three categories as shown in Table 1 [48,49].

Table 1. Classification of porous materials by pore size.

Type of Porosity	Size (nm)
Microporous	<2
Mesoporous	2–50
Macroporous	>50

The history of MSN materials dates back to the early 1990s, when the Kuroda group at Waseda University and researchers from the Mobil Company discovered Mobil crystalline materials (MCMs), nanoparticles with a hexagonal porous structure [2]. In 1992 with the discovery of MCM-41, a material prepared using the cooperative assembly of surfactant with silicates, a breakthrough in the area of ordered mesoporous structures and their successful preparation occurred [50,51]. In addition, an ionic template, such as cetyltrimethylammonium bromide (CTAB), could be employed as a structure-directing agent to produce MCM-41 and MCM-48 with pore sizes of 2 to 10 nm [50,51]. MCM-41 has a hexagonal pore shape and MCM-84 has a cubic pore shape. For DDSs purpose, MCM-41 is considered to be one of the most widely explored materials. The synthesis mechanism for MCM-41 is shown in Figure 2 and electron microscope images in Figure 3.

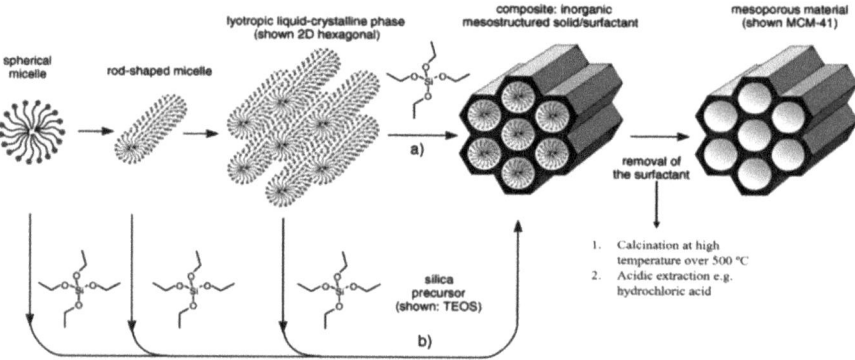

Figure 2. The formation mechanism for mesoporous materials by structure-directing agents. (**a**) True liquid–crystal template mechanism. (**b**) Cooperative liquid–crystal template mechanism. Reproduced with permission from [52], WILEY-VCH Verlag GmbH and Co. KGaA, 2006.

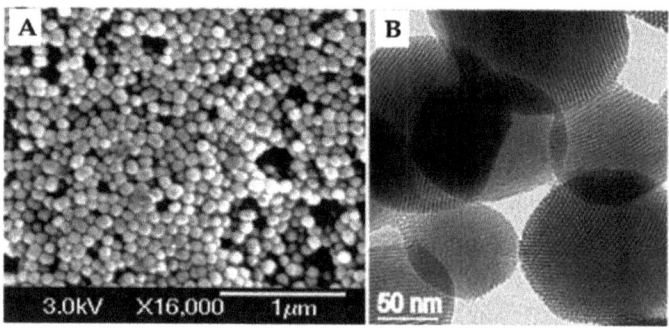

Figure 3. (**A**) Scanning electron microscopy (SEM) and (**B**) transmission electron microscopy (TEM) of MCM-41 material. Reproduced with permission from [23], Wiley-VCH Verlag GmbH and Co. KGaA, 2010.

In 1996, another kind of MSN was discovered that has a non-ordered pore structure, named KIT-1 (Korea Advanced Institute of Science and Technology Number 1) [53]. The KIT family currently has many members, such as KIT-6, which has a hexagonal arrangement of pores [54], and KIT-5, which has a cubic ordered structure [55]. In 1998, the SBA-15 type (pore size 4–6 nm) MSNs introduced by Santa Barbara Amorphous (SBA), which have a hexagonal or cubic pore structure, were developed by means of nonionic surfactants in acidic conditions [56]. The cubic SBA-11, 3D hexagonal SBA-12, hexagonal SBA-15, and SBA-16 are mainly prepared based on non-ionic triblock copolymers, such as alkyl poly(ethylene oxide) (PEO) oligomeric surfactants and poly(alkylene oxide) block copolymers [10]. The typical synthesis of SBA-15 is dependent on tetramethyl-orthosilicate (TMOS) or tetraethyl-orthosilicate (TEOS) as the silica precursor reacting with a series of block-copolymer surfactants as structure-directing agents. The MCM and SBA materials are recognized as the first generation of hexagonally ordered pore structures and are the common MSNs used in research. A variety of strategies have been designed to attain tunable pore sizes (from less than 2 nm up to 30 nm). In this scenario, the adjustments are made depending on the surfactant template's properties [57], pore swelling agents, such as mesitylene [50], or hydrothermal treatments [58].

Importantly, in 2010, high surface-area silica nanospheres with a fibrous morphology and non-ordered pore structure were discovered by a research group of the Catalysis Center at King Abdullah University of Science and Technology (KAUST Catalysis Center, KCC) [59]. This material, KCC-1, features a high surface area due to the presence of dendrimeric silica fibers and their respective channels, making KCC-1 a first-of-its-kind material. It is a spherical particle with 3D tomography, a uniform size ranging from 250 nm to 500 nm, high surface area, and large pore size in a non-ordered structure (Figure 4). Synthesis of KCC-1 [59] was accomplished by a microwave-assisted, templated, solvothermal strategy using cetylpyridinium bromide (CPB) or cetyltrimethylammonium bromide (CTAB) as a surfactant (template), 1-pentanol as a co-surfactant, TEOS as the silica source, urea (catalyst-hydrolyzing agent), and a mixture of the cyclohexane solvent and water (as the reaction solvent). The chemicals were introduced to the reaction system stepwise with mixing and microwave-assisted heating applied (in a closed vessel >1200 °C) for a predetermined time for the reaction. Finally, the solution was filtered or centrifuged, washed, and the obtained material calcinated at high temperature (>550 °C). Many research groups changed the surface of substances used in the synthesis in addition to the parameters. For example, Bayal et al. [60] showed that changing the concentrations of urea, surfactant (CTAB instead of CPB), or solvent (1-pentanol), the reaction time, or temperature can result in various particle sizes, fiber densities, surface areas, and pore volumes for KCC-1. Such easy manipulation and controlled synthesis of this material make KCC-1 a good solution for versatile applications in the environment, energy, biology, medicine, and other fields [42,43,61–68]. KCC-1 could be recommended for different small or large drug/therapeutic agents, possibly for any design and pathological disorder due to KCC-1 s unique physicochemical features. Our research team is among the first to study KCC-1 for DDSs [42,43,68,69], and we think that research on KCC-1 will increase soon. In the literature, there are references to "spherical wrinkled mesoporous silica" (WMS) [70–72] and KCC-1 is known also "dendritic fibrous nano-silica" (DFNS) [73]. They were all obtained based on changing the synthesis conditions and parameters of the original synthesis method for KCC-1 particles.

Unlimited opportunities exist for the synthesis of MSNs in pure, doped, composite, and modified forms by employing different templates (soft and hard), conditions, and methods [74].

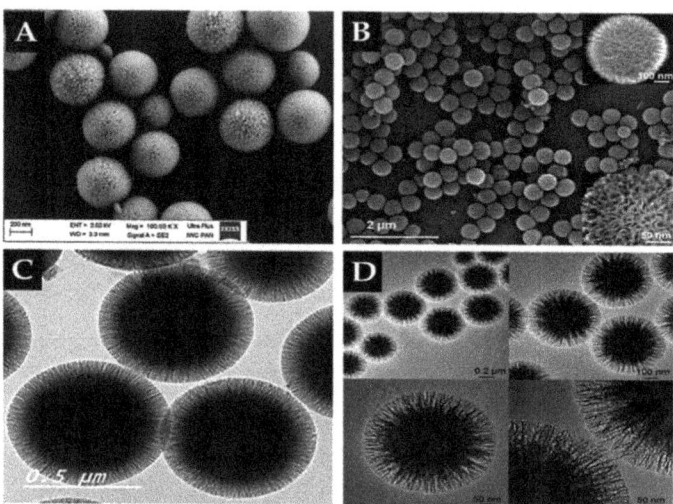

Figure 4. Electron microscope images of prepared KCC-1 material. (**A,B**) Scanning electron microscopy (SEM). (**C,D**) Transmission electron microscopy (TEM). Note, the dendritic fibrous 3D mesopore structure is clearly seen by SEM in B. A and C reproduced from [42,43], Impact Journals, 2018 and MDPI, 2020. B and D reproduced with permission from [59], WILEY-VCH Verlag GmbH and Co. KGaA, 2010.

Due to the unique properties of the KCC-1 family, they offer a wide range of possible applications. It seems that KCC-1 has comparable potential as the commonly used members of the MCM and SBA families, as well as Stober silica, solid silica discovered before all the families [73]. Table 2 presents the major physicochemical properties for fibrous KCC-1, MCM-41, SBA-15, and others. Below, we highlight the common and promising families that could be favored for drug delivery and medical applications. Numerous interesting review articles have been published on MSN synthesis strategies and applications that we recommend for further reading [10,22,32,73,75–83].

Table 2. The physicochemical properties of the most common mesoporous silica nanoparticles (MSNs) synthesized by various approaches.

Type	BET-Specific Surface Area ($m^2\ g^{-1}$)	Pore Volume ($cm^3\ g^{-1}$)	Pore Size (nm)	Mechanical Stability (Mpa)	Hydrothermal Stability (°C) (time/h)	Thermal Stability (°C)	Particle Size	Pore Structure	Morphology/Structure
MCM-41	≥1000	0.7–1.2	1.5–10	86	50	707	~100–200 or microns	Ordered hexagonal	Almost spherical
SBA-15	700–1000	0.75–1.15	5–8	260	100	600	microns	Ordered hexagonal	Rods
KCC-1/DFNS/WMS	~450–1250	0.54–2.18	3–40	216	100	950 or over	50–1100	Disordered	Spherical
Stober silica	~10–350	0.017–0.217	1.2–5.9	NA	NA	NA	20–3000	NA	Solid spheres
KIT					NA	NA	Few microns		
Others	~290–1160	0.85–0.95	~2–10	NA	NA	NA	Few nanometers to microns	Varied	porous

Note: The above-mentioned characteristics of these materials can be controlled and can vary (more or less) from these values. Reproduced with permission from [75], Wiley-VCH Verlag GmbH and Co. KGaA, 2017. NA = not available.

2.2. Surface Modification of MSNs for Drug Delivery

The keystone in the development of DDSs is to functionalize their surface [84,85] to increase their drug loading and release, leading to high therapeutic effects. The surface chemistry modulates the interaction of MSNs with the surrounding media. The MSNs have a high density of silanol groups (Si-OH) on their surface, allowing surface modification by various organic functionalities (e.g., silanes, polymers, proteins, and targeting moieties). Thus, MSNs can load various drugs with high capacity and release them in a sustained or controlled manner. A variety of functional groups can be used, such as amine, carboxylate, phosphonate, polyethylene glycol, octadecyl, thiol, carboxylic acid, and octadecyl groups. To introduce functional groups on the surface of MSNs, covalent bonding and electrostatic interactions are generally used [86]. The common approach to modify MSNs is to use organic silane groups via direct covalent attachment by means of co-condensation or post-synthetic grafting.

The co-condensation method is referred to as a one-pot synthesis method [87,88] as presented in Figure 5A. The desired functional group of silanes, such as 3-aminopropyl-triethoxysilane (APTES "NH_2") is added during the sol-gel synthesis process together with the silica source (e.g., TEOS). Next, the template is removed (Figure 5A) [52,87,89]. To remove the surfactant template, an extractive method using alcoholic/acidic solution under reflux can be used [90]. Removing the template anchors the organic residue covalently to the porous walls of the MSNs. This approach has the advantages of easy preparation, more homogeneous distribution of organic units, and high drug loading [52,83]. Despite these advantages, disadvantages are a potential change in the mesoscopic order, disordering the porosity and reducing the pore diameter, pore volume, and specific surface areas [52].

A post-synthetic approach refers to the subsequent modification of the inner/outer surface of MSNs by covalent and electrostatic interactions. The modification is usually achieved after surfactant removal from MSNs (Figure 5B). The most remarkable advantages of this approach are selective functionalization (either external or internal surfaces) and retention of the mesostructure of MSNs during synthesis. The major disadvantages include reduced pore size and non-homogeneous distribution of functional groups into/onto pores [52,91,92].

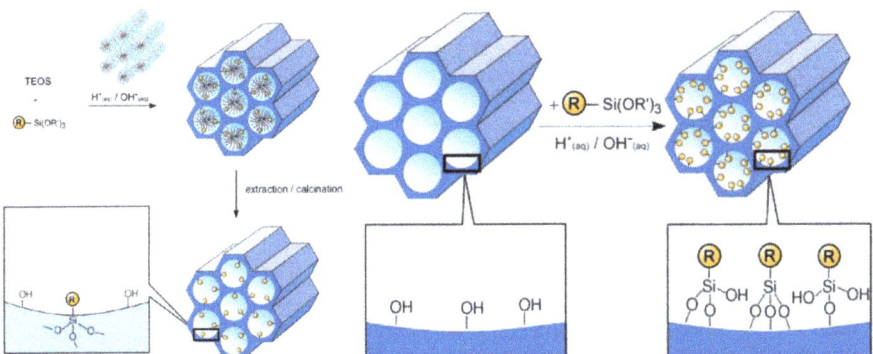

Figure 5. A schematic presentation of the organic functionalization methods for mesoporous silica materials. (**A**) Co-condensation method and (**B**) grafting method. Reproduced with permission from [52], WILEY-VCH Verlag GmbH and Co. KGaA, 2006.

2.3. The Biological Performance of MSNs
2.3.1. Cellular Uptake

Any nanocarriers have to cross the cell membrane boundary to enter cells, allowing the therapeutic effects of the delivered drugs. The internalization of nanoparticles carrying therapeutic agents into cells represents the initial step in successful drug delivery [93,94].

The acting mechanisms and surface chemistry of nanocarriers are the major parameters in designing a preferred DDS for any pathological disease [78]. Nanoparticles mainly access the cell interior via simple diffusion or translocation as an energy-dependent process [95]. The most common mechanism of their internalization is the energy-dependent endocytosis, which allows the uptake of nanoparticles and submicron particles from an extracellular environment to the cell plasma membrane [96]. The mechanisms can generally be classified into phagocytosis, pinocytosis, micropinocytosis, receptor-mediated endocytosis, clathrin-mediated endocytosis, caveolin-mediated endocytosis, and others (e.g., Arf-6, Rho-A or IL2Rb-dependent pathway, flotillin, or CDC42 (CLIC/GEEC)-dependent endocytosis) [93]. The intracellular uptake and trafficking mechanisms by which nanoparticles are internalized in cells vary broadly depending on many factors, including size, shape, charge, and surface modification. Therefore, these factors should be taken into consideration in constructing DDSs.

Size of MSNs

Particle size determines the intracellular uptake of MSNs (Figure 6) [97]. It is generally accepted that particles with the smaller size of 50 nm can internalize into cells via non-phagocytosis [98]. Nanoparticles up to 150 and 200 nm in size are internalized by pinocytosis, such as clathrin-mediated endocytosis and caveolin-mediated endocytosis, respectively [99,100]. In contrast, particles from 250 nm to 3 µm in size can internalize the cells by macropinocytosis and phagocytosis [101]. It is also accepted that the microparticles are efficiently taken up through phagocytosis but the process depends also on other parameters, such as geometry, surface charges, and functional groups of microparticles [102]. Particles with sizes ranging from 30 to 50 nm internalize also efficiently via receptor-mediated endocytosis [103]. Despite extensive investigations exploring the relationship between particle size and uptake pathways, the results are inconsistent [101,104–106]. The main reason for such contradictions can be attributed to the complexity of control of structural parameters, such as shape and surface charges. For successful internalization, particles should avoid degradation (within endosomal/lysosomal vesicles) and release their cargo in the cytoplasm [107]. Therefore, particle size is important in tailoring DDSs. It is also important for their intersections with the reticulo-endothelial system (RES), which is responsible for elimination of nanoparticles from the body, and prolong the circulation time in the blood. In this context, several studies have shown that increasing the particle size increases clearance from the body, reducing the therapeutic impact [108–112].

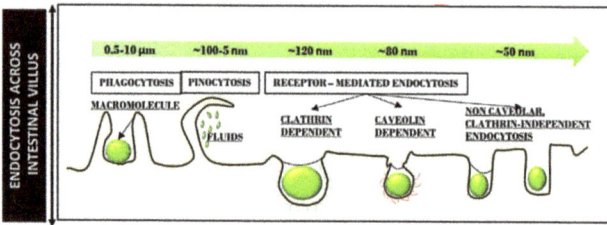

Figure 6. Different endocytosis pathways across the intestinal villus for particles of different sizes. Reproduced with permission from [97], Elsevier Inc., 2020.

Lu et al. [103] investigated the impact of various sizes (30, 50, 110, 170 nm) of MSNs on cellular uptake by HeLa cancer cells using MSNs labeled with fluorescein isothiocyanate (FITC) green fluorescence (MSN-FITC) and confocal laser scanning microscopy. They found that the MSNs were internalized as non-uniform green-fluorescent aggregates in the perinuclear region, and no MSNs penetrated the nucleus (Figure 7). Quantifying the internalization of MSNs, they concluded that the cellular uptake is highly particle size-dependent, observing the order 50 > 30 > 110 > 280 > 170 nm (Figure 8). Haddick et al. [113] demonstrated that MSNs with a size of 160 nm had the fastest cellular internalization in

T24 bladder cancer cells through receptor-mediated cellular internalization compared to 60, 80, 100, and 130 nm, leading to the highest level of gene knock-down for antitumoral effects. Yang et al. [114] tested different sizes of rod-shaped SBA-15 (from 80 to 200 nm) and spherical MCM-41 particles, as well as their intracellular uptake in human osteosarcoma cancer cells (KHOS). They found that the cellular uptake efficiency depends on the particle size and shape.

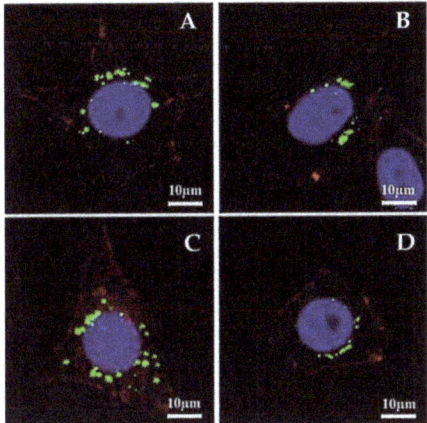

Figure 7. Confocal laser microscopy images of HeLa cells after incubation with different sizes of MSNs labeled with fluorescein isothiocyanate (FITC) green fluorescence (MSN-FITC) (100 µg mL^{-1}, green) for 5 h at 37 °C. (**A**) 170 nm, (**B**) 110 nm, (**C**) 50 nm, and (**D**) 30 nm. The cell skeleton was stained with rhodamine-phalloidin (red), and the cell nucleus with 4′,6-diamidino-2-phenylindole (DAPI; blue). Reproduced with permission from [103], WILEY-VCH Verlag GmbH and Co. KGaA, 2009.

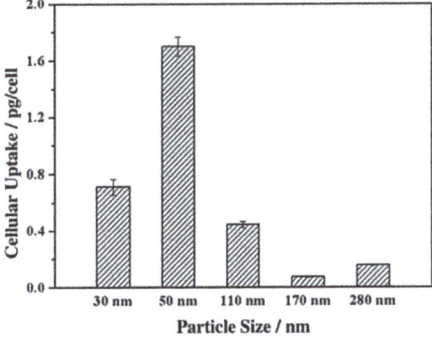

Figure 8. Cellular uptake of FITC-MSN-x based on nanoparticle size. Reproduced with permission from [103], WILEY-VCH Verlag GmbH and Co. KGaA, 2009.

Surface Charges of MSNs

Another critical factor influencing the cellular uptake of nanoparticles is the surface charge. MSNs are characterized by silanol groups permitting to add different functional groups, modifying their surface to be either cationic or anionic [115]. Most cells have a negatively charged cell membrane, enhancing the uptake of positively charged nanoparticles. Several studies have shown that positively charged nanoparticles internalize with higher uptake than neutral and negatively charged nanoparticles [116–119]. Furthermore, neutral nanoparticles usually have lower cellular uptake compared to negatively charged nanoparticles [98,120]. As a result of the internalization of nanoparticles by cells, their interaction with the cell membrane can occur by means of gelation of membranes (with negatively charged nanoparticles) or fluidity of membranes (with positively charged nanoparticles) [121,122]. On the one hand, the positively charged nanoparticles mainly enter cells via micropinocytosis; on the other hand, the negatively charged nanoparticles always enter cells by clathrin- or caveolae-independent endocytosis [123].

Positively charged MSNs generally exhibit higher endocytosis efficiency compared to negatively charged MSNs due to the higher affinity for the negatively charged cell membranes. Jambhrunkar et al. [124] prepared MCM-41 with negative and positive charges for delivering curcumin. They found that the positively charged MCM-41-NH_2 had more efficient uptake in the human squamous cell carcinoma cell line (SCC25) than negatively charged particles. Baghirov et al. [125] studied spherical and rod-shaped MSNs that were either non-modified or modified with a poly(ethylene glycol)-poly(ethylene imine) (PEG-PEI) block copolymer in in vitro models of the blood–brain barrier. The results showed that the modified MSN-PEG-PEI particles exhibited robust uptake in RBE4 rat brain endothelial cells and Madin–Darby canine kidney epithelial cells. Our group performed a comprehensive study of cellular uptake using two types of MSNs: KCC-1 and MCM-41 (non-modified, positive charges with -NH_2, and folic acid ligands) [42]. The FA-conjugated MSNs exhibited higher cellular uptake than MSNs-NH_2 and non-modified MSNs.

Morphological Structures of MSNs

The morphological structures (i.e., different shapes) play an important role in the cellular uptake and trafficking of nanoparticles into cells or organs. Trewyn et al. [126] studied the impact of different MSN shapes on cellular uptake in vitro, finding that a tubular structure achieves more efficient uptake by both cancer and normal cells than those of spherical morphology. Huang et al. [127] investigated the effect of three differently shaped particles on non-specific cellular uptake by human melanoma (A375) cells. Their results proved that particles with a larger aspect ratio are efficiently internalized by cells in large amounts at faster rates. Another study tested the core–shell MSNs with spherical or rod-like shapes for cellular uptake, showing that a rod shape results in more internalization by cells than a spherical shape [128] It is generally accepted that this effect could be due to the larger contact area of the rod than a sphere, permitting high favored internalization of nanoparticles in cell membranes [116,128] Furthermore, rod-shaped MSNs exhibit superior intracellular uptake compared to spherical MSNs [129]. The shape of the nanoparticles can allow a specific mechanism of intracellular uptake. In this context, Hao et al. [130] reported that the spherical particles are taken up by cells via clathrin-mediated endocytosis, whereas the rod-shaped particles enter cells through caveolae-mediated endocytosis.

Other Features of MSNs

One significant characteristic of any nanocarrier delivery system is hydrophobicity. Nanoparticles that have a hydrophobic nature exhibit a higher affinity for interacting with the cell membrane than those with a hydrophilic nature, contributing to improved cellular uptake [94].

2.3.2. Biocompatibility and Biodistribution of MSNs

Any DDSs introduced into clinical investigations should exhibit biocompatibility with body tissues and organs. The biocompatibility is dependent on many MSN characteristics, such as size, shape, surface functionality, porosity, route of administration, and structure (Figure 9) [131].

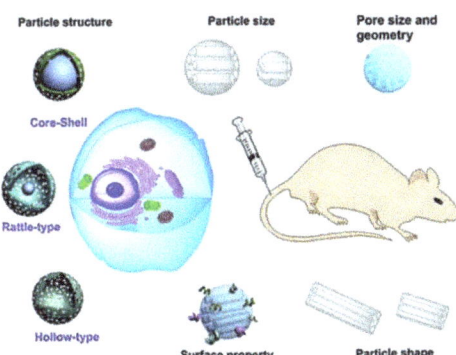

Figure 9. Schematic illustration of the biocompatibility and biotranslocation of MSNs and the main physical–chemical characteristics. These highly influence the cellular uptake, intracellular translocation, and cytotoxicity on the in vitro level, and the biodistribution, biodegradation, excretion, and toxicity on the in vivo level. Reproduced with permission from [131], WILEY-VCH Verlag GmbH and Co. KGaA, 2012.

Most animal studies indicate the high biocompatibility and safety of MSNs [31,132,133]. The degree of biocompatibility of MSNs can vary according to many factors such as synthesis conditions, suitable structural features, and appropriate route at the right dosage [8,133–137]. As with other nanomaterials, for future translation to clinical applications, the safety aspects of MSNs should be considered carefully for each type [133]. Below, we present some studies highlighting the biocompatibility of MSNs in vitro and in vivo. Park et al. [138] investigated the biodistribution and biocompatibility of MSNs intravenously injected into mice at 20 mg/kg. The histopathological examination showed no significant toxicity compared to the control group. Their studies also indicated that MSNs are mostly cleared from the liver, spleen, heart, kidneys, brain, and lungs after 4 weeks. Hudson et al. [139] examined the biocompatibility of non-modified MSNs with particle sizes of ~150 (pores about 3 nm), 800 nm (pores about 7 nm), and ~4 µm (pores about 16 nm) at different does/concentrations. In vitro results in mesothelial cells showed that the cytotoxicity depends on the concentration; increasing concentration increases cytotoxicity towards cells. For in vivo studies, mcice were injected (intra-peritoneal, intra-peritoneal, and subcutaneous) at single dose of 30 mg/mL per mouse. The biocompatibility of MSNs in vivo depends on the dose and the route of administration. The subcutaneous injection of MSNs in rats indicates good biocompatibility, whereas intraperitoneal and intravenous injections at very high dose ~1.2 g/kg is lethal for mice due to toxicity or distress necessitating euthanasia, but at dose of ~40 mg/kg is safe. This severe systemic toxicity can be mitigated by further surface modification of the MSNs. Lu et al. [23] evaluated various doses of MSNs intravenously injected in mice (twice per week) for 14 days, they concluded that dose at 50 mg/kg is well tolerated in mice, no toxicity, no apparent abnormalities on the histopathological level or lesions were observed. They also revealed that this dose is adequate for the pharmacological application in cancer therapy.

Huang et al. [30] evaluated the biocompatibility of differently shaped and PEGylated MSNs (Figures 10–12), measuring various blood and serum biochemical indicators 24 h and 18 days after injection of MSNs at a dose of 20 mg/kg. All hematology markers were within normal ranges without any considerable toxicity, showing excellent biocompatibility. The results indicated that these particles do not influence liver function, and other parameters were also in the normal range. Concerning the quantitative determination of biodistribution and clearance, approximately 80% of MSNs are trapped in RES of the liver, spleen, and lung after 2 h of administration. Comparing the Si contents of different organs (at 2 h, 24 h, and 7 days), the Si content obviously decreased over time, indicating the possible degradation and clearance of MSNs from the liver, spleen, lung, and kidney. Moreover, the circulation time of MSNs in blood shows that long rod MSN (NLR) has a longer blood circulation time than short rod MSN (NSR), and the effect of surface modification by PEGylation is partially dependent on the shape.

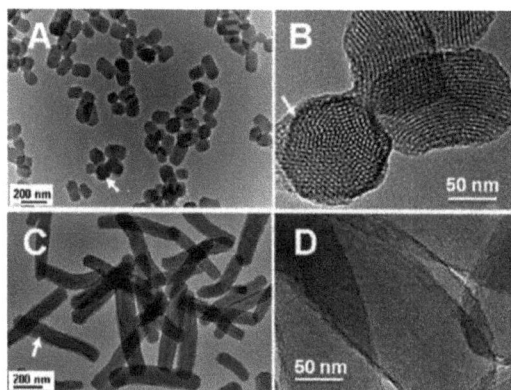

Figure 10. Characterization of short rod MSN labeled with FITC (NSRFITC) and long rod MSN labeled FITC (NLRFITC). (**A**) TEM image of NSRFITC. (**B**) TEM image showing the mesostructure of NSRFITC. (**C**) TEM image of NLRFITC. (**D**) TEM image showing the mesostructure of NLRFITC. Arrows denote FITC embedded in a particle. Reproduced with permission from [30], American Chemical Society, 2011.

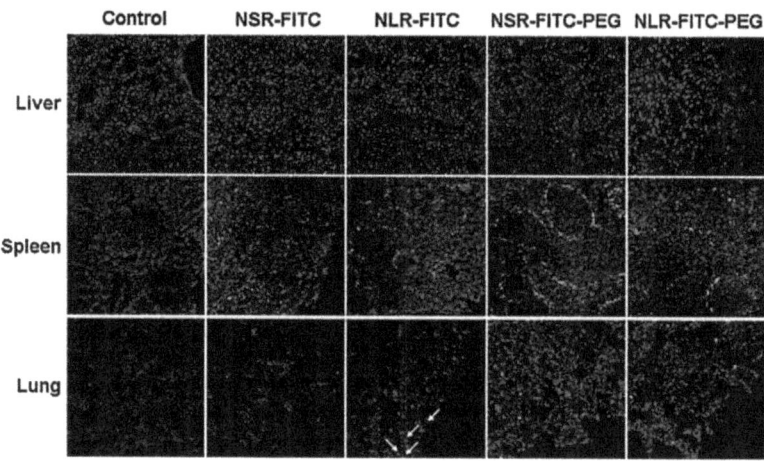

Figure 11. Biodistribution of differently shaped and poly(ethylene glycol) (PEG)ylated MSNFITC in liver, spleen, and lung observed by confocal microscopy 2 h after intravenous injection. Arrows denote NLRFITC distribution in the lung. Reproduced with permission from [30], American Chemical Society, 2011.

Yildirim et al. [140] evaluated the interactions of MSNs with different surface functional groups (ionic, polar, neutral, and hydrophobic) on blood parameters (hemolytic activity, thrombogenicity, and adsorption of blood proteins) to understand their biocompatibility. They concluded that the blood compatibility of MSNs positively improves with surface functional groups. Table 3 shows some data reported on the biocompatibility, biodistribution, and clearance of MSNs in vitro and in vivo.

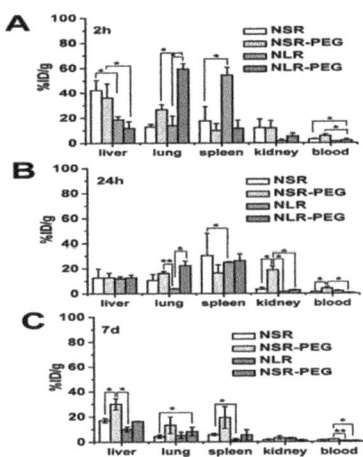

Figure 12. Quantitative analysis of differently shaped and PEGylated MSNs in organs and blood by ICPOES. Relative Si contents in liver, spleen, and kidney at (**A**) 2 h, (**B**) 24 h, and (**C**) 7 d post-injection. Data are the mean ± SD from three separate experiments. * $p < 0.05$; ** $p < 0.01$ for the comparison of Si contents of differently shaped and PEGylated MSNs in organs and blood. Reproduced with permission from [30], American Chemical Society, 2011.

Table 3. The biocompatibility, biodistribution, and clearance of MSNs with different shapes, sizes, and surface modifications in vitro or in vivo (injection or oral administration).

MSNs	Study	Biocompatibility	Biodistribution in Organs	References
MSNs (150 to 4000 nm)	Subcutaneous injection Intravenous injections	Good biocompatibility on histological level Death or euthanasia	NA	[139]
Bare, functionalized, polyethylene glycol or hyaluronic acid	In vitro	Biocompatible; do not induce ROS/RNS production; no changes in mitochondrial membrane potential or cell cycle	NA	[141]
MSNs and PEGylated MSNs	Tail vein injection in mice	All treated mice survive well for 1 month after being injected with all MSN and PEG–MSN No pathological abnormality on gross and microscopic histological examinations	Mainly located in liver and spleen; minority in lung, kidney, and heart	[142]
MSNs and solid silica nanoparticles	Lateral tail vein in mice	NA	Liver and spleen due to reticulo-endothelial system; increased accumulation in the lungs due to amine modification; degraded and excreted by urinary and hepatobiliary routes	[143]
MSNs with different shapes	Oral administration in mice	No abnormalities in liver, lung, heart, and spleen; kidneys show particle shape-dependent tissue damage	Liver, lung, spleen, kidney, and intestine Rapidly excreted from feces, and some fraction excreted renally	[144]
MSNs (spheres and rod)	Oral administration in mice	Long-rod MSNs have longer blood circulation than short-rod and spheres	Mainly found in liver and kidney; renal excretion-spherical MSNs cleared faster than rod MSNs	[145]

Table 3. *Cont.*

MSNs	Study	Biocompatibility	Biodistribution in Organs	References
Multifunctional MSNs	Tail vein injection in mice	Good biocompatibility with low toxicity	Mainly found in liver and spleen Excreted in urine and feces	[21]
Magnetic-doped MSNs	In vitro and in vivo (mouse)	Good biocompatibility	NA	[146]
Biomimetic MSNs	In vitro and in vivo	Biocompatible and no obvious toxicity	Tendency to be biodistributed in brain	[147]
MSNs with different sizes	Intravenous injection in mice	Incidence and severity of inflammatory response was obtained with large size; no abnormal changes obtained for small size	Spleen and liver; clearance in urine and bile depending on size	[148]
MSNs	In vitro and in vivo	No toxicity	Liver and spleen; clearance from urine	[82]

2.3.3. Toxicity of MSNs

For preclinical and further clinical investigations, nanocarriers should be optimized to avoid undesirable characteristics (e.g., toxicity, side effects, non-specific interactions) and to allow good biological performance [131]. As one of the most abundant materials on Earth, silica (or silicon dioxide) in crystalline form can be found in nature as sand or quartz [149]. In contrast, the amorphous form is present in biological materials, including plants, cells, microbes (e.g., bacteria), vertebrates, and invertebrates [150]. Silica is also endogenous to human tissues, such as cartilage and bone [151]. Several efforts are underway to identify the toxicity of both the crystalline and amorphous forms of silica in different methods of application [10]. Crystalline silica mainly results in toxicity as a result of breathing fine crystalline powders created by the extraction of stone materials in soil [86]. Because it is found in vegetables, whole grains, and seafood, silica is a considerable part of the human diet (approximately 20–50 mg silicon/day for Western populations and reaching 200 mg/day for people whose diet is mainly plant-based as in China and India) [152]. Furthermore, after ingestion of silica, it circulates in the blood plasma and is absorbed in the form of silicic acid; up to 41% of silicic acid is excreted in the urine [153]. Silica nanomaterials are hydrolytically unstable and dissolve into the soluble form of silicic acid ($Si(OH)_4$, pKa 9.6) [152]. This can occur through three different processes: hydration, hydrolysis, and ion-exchange [154]. A schematic representation of silica degradation is shown in Figure 13 [155]. Silicic acid has good bioavailability, contributing many health benefits, such as maintaining bone health [154,156,157]. The FDA has approved silica as "generally recognized as safe" for use in food additives and pharmaceutical products [86,155]. Silica nanoparticles have also been approved by the FDA for cancer imaging in clinical trials [158] and MSNs being developed with high potential for DDSs in clinical investigations [159].

The biosafety of engineered MSNs has been confirmed by several studies. As shown in the literature, MSNs have insignificant toxicity, and the degree of toxicity is identified as low from in vivo studies. Additionally, even such insignificant toxicity can be reduced with the optimization of the synthesis process. However, a few reported data [160–163] provide contrary reports. The plausible reason for this is that there are many factors affecting the biocompatibility and safety of MSNs (e.g., shape, size, surface functional groups, physicochemical properties). For example, the method of removing the surfactant/template after MSNs synthesis (by calcination or by refluxing) influences the final cytotoxicity [139]. According to a number of in vivo experiments, a coherent message regarding the toxicity of MSNs is that that the toxicity depends on the dose/concentration used. For example, Hudson et al. [139] investigated the toxicity for MSNs (single dose) in vivo, they evaluated various doses and administration routes. They concluded that a very high dose (1.2 g/kg) is lethal for mice compared to the half dose which is well-tolerated and safe when applied by intraperitoneal or intravenous injection. Liu et al. [164] studied the single and repeated dose of MSNs via intravenous administration in mice. In the single-dose toxicity investigations, they found that the LD50 is higher than 1000 mg/kg. They also demonstrated that the groups that received low doses of MSNs did not show any behavioral, hematology, and pathological changes, whereas the groups that received high doses (1280 mg/kg) did not survive. In the repeated dose toxicity experiments, the mice groups were given continuously for 14 days followed by observation for a month. The results display that no mortality and no remarkable changes (in pathology or blood parameters) were detected. They also reported that the treatment of MSNs at daily doses (80 mg/kg) for 14 days is safe without any adverse effects in animals. Fu et al. [29] evaluated toxicity of MSNs (110 nm) in ICR mice treated by different routes: hypodermic, intramuscular, intravenous injections, and oral administration. They found that the oral route is well tolerated in mice even when increased to 5000 mg/kg compared to the intravenous route which shows the least threshold. As such results and others available from literature generated evidence to show that MSNs are well tolerated and safe in animals by various routes of administrations, i.e., oral, and intravenous injections [29,133,164,165]. However, there is no doubt that optimized production of MSNs and the final nanoformulation can achieve good biocompatibility and safe nanoparticles for treating diseases. Table 4 lists some studies that have explored the toxicity of MSNs and their delivery systems. For more reading concerning the toxicity and biosafety of MSNs, there are several extensive reviews [10,137,151,166–168]. The toxicity of any material/object, including MSNs, in a given environment is dependent on the dose [168]. As reviewed by Croissant et al. [168], there are mainly two mechanisms governing the toxicity of MSNs on the cellular level [88]. The first mechanism is surface silanolates that lead to membranolysis after the electrostatic interactions between MSNs and phospholipids of the cell membrane occur [169]. The second mechanism is reactive oxygen species (ROS) generation, which leads to cell death (by necrosis or apoptosis) by means of membranolysis [170]. Reducing the possible toxicity and improving the biosafety of MSNs can be achieved by optimizing the synthesis properties of MSNs for drug delivery and biomedical applications.

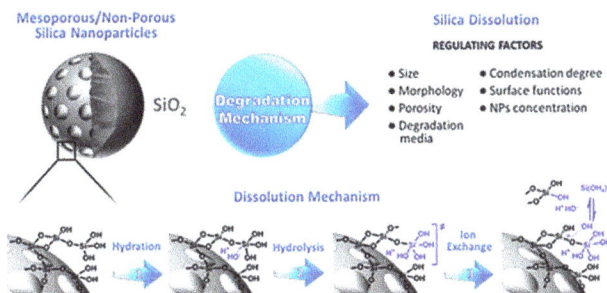

Figure 13. Schematic representation of the intact and degraded structures of silica material nanoparticles with the mechanisms and regulating factors underlying degradation. Reproduced from [155], WILEY-VCH Verlag GmbH and Co. KGaA, 2017.

Table 4. The toxicity and biosafety of MSNs of various size, shape, surface modification, and route of administration in in vivo studies.

MSNs	Dose	Route of Administration	Period	Toxicity	References
MSNs of 110 nm	Repeated dose at 20, 40, and 80 mg/kg	Intravenous injection in mice	14 days	No death; LD50 of single dose = 1000 mg/kg	[164]
MSNs of 150 nm, 800 nm, and 4 μm	Different doses at single dose	Different routes in rats	3 months	Toxicity depends on route of administration. An amount of 40 mg/kg is safe	[139]

Table 4. Cont.

MSNs	Dose	Route of Administration	Period	Toxicity	References
MSNs	40 mg/kg in CD-1 mice	Intravenous injection in mice/rats	14 days	Safe for I.V. administration	[171]
MSNs with aspect ratios of 1, 1.75, and 5	40 mg/kg	Oral administration	14 days	Safe and no changes observed	[144]
MSNs: different sizes and surface modified	Single dose at 25 mg/kg	Lateral tail vein injection	7 days	No clinical toxicity based on histological evaluations; blood biocompatibility	[82]
Functionalized Fe3O4@MSN-PEG and non-modified PEG	40 mg/kg	Intravenous injections in mice	4 days	Non-MSN-PEG caused toxicity to liver, kidney, and spleen tissues; modified PEG nanoparticles showed no toxicity	[172,173]
MSNs and silymarin loaded-MSNs	250 mg/kg	Oral administration in rats	22 days	No evident toxicity in rats	[174]
MSNs	Single dose at 10, 25, and 50 mg/kg	Intraperitoneal application in mice	7 days	No death; almost all tested parameters in liver within normal range	[175]
MSNs of 110 nm	50 mg/kg	Intravenous, hypodermic, intramuscular injection and oral administration in mice	7 days	Caused inflammatory response around the injection sites after intramuscular and hypodermic injection; some toxicity to liver depending on route of application	[29]
MSNs and colloidal silica nanoparticles	2, 20, and 50 mg/kg/day	Intraperitoneal injection in mice	4 weeks	No overt sign of clinical toxicity; some damage to systemic immunity of spleen	[176]
MSNs with different sizes with no surface modification	Single dose	Intravenous administration in female and male BALB/c mice	1 year	No significant changes in body weight, blood cell count, or plasma biomarker indices; no significant changes in post necropsy examination of internal organs and organ-to-body weight ratio; significant liver inflammation and aggregates of histiocytes with neutrophils within the spleen; no chronic toxicity observed	[28]

3. Drug Loading and Release Strategies

3.1. Drug Loading Strategies

A unique feature of MSNs (e.g., large pore volume, high surface, pores, stability) makes them one of the most common nanocarriers exploited for drug delivery with a high drug loading capacity for a variety of drugs. Generally, drugs or therapeutic molecules can be loaded into MSNs with or without pore-capping. In the first technique without pore-capping, hydrophobic or hydrophilic therapeutic agents directly load MSNs with covalent or noncovalent bonding or electrostatic interactions. Loading of drugs or therapeutic agents into the mesopore network of MSNs delivers them to target tissues while simultaneously saving them from undesirable factors found in the surrounding environment (e.g., enzymatic degradation in the body) [9]. To load a suitable amount of drug, MSNs are immersed in the desired stock solution of the drug or therapeutic agent under stirring/shaking, during which the drug loading is highly driven by the concentration gradient, the competition between drug (adsorbate) and MSNs (adsorbent), adsorbate and solvent, and adsorbent and solvent [177,178]. As such, a loading process has been reported with a variety of drugs, such as camptothecin (hydrophobic anticancer molecule) [90], doxorubicin (Dox) hydrochloride [179], curcumin [69], quercetin [68], 5-fluorouracil (5-

FU) [180], erythromycin [181], alendronate [182], silymarin [183], and paclitaxel (PTX) [184]. Importantly, the degree of drug loading can be maximized by choosing the desired solvent for the drug, modifying the MSN surface, and adjusting the loading parameters (e.g., time, temperature) [10,86,185].

In the second strategy with capping as the "gatekeeper" for the pore openings of MSNs [168], the first stage is to engineer the outer surface of MSNs via many techniques: molecular or supramolecular functionalization, capping with nanoparticles, and coating with polymer, protein, or lipid. This approach can control the release and delivery of therapeutic agents. In the molecular or supramolecular approach, caps are mainly rotaxanes, pseudorotaxanes, and others consisting of a long chain-like molecule that is threaded via a cyclic molecule [186]. Under certain conditions (e.g., pH, redox), the cyclic molecule can attract rotaxane (to one end of it), with the presence of a stimulus allowing it to slide to the other end. By attaching the thread near the pore opening on MSNs, the sliding cyclic molecule blocks the pore when it is near the particle or opens if it slides away. The idea of nanoparticles as gatekeepers was pioneered by Lin and co-workers [187–190] with many nanoparticles, such as iron oxide nanoparticles and gold nanoparticles. These small nanoparticles can graft on top of MSNs loaded with cargos through chemical bonding upon cleavage of the chemical bonds linking the nanoparticles with MSNs. Consequently, under certain conditions (pH, redox), external stimuli can trigger the release of cargos in a controlled manner. Next, in the coating strategy, different types of biomaterials, such as polymer, proteins, and lipids, can be introduced onto the surface of MSNs loaded with drugs. Drug release can occur upon degradation of these biomaterials or changing the surrounding environment stimuli, either external or internal [191–193]. Table 5 lists some examples of reported studies on prodrug loading in MSNs and their loading capacity. Table 6 provides the different loading strategies and their relationship to stimulate release under various conditions for MSNs, showing the connection between loading and release effects.

Table 5. Loading capacity for natural prodrugs into MSNs established as recent drug delivery systems for natural medicinal substances.

MSN Type	Surface Modification	Natural Cargo	Loading Content (%)	References
MSNs	Aptamer-functionalized	Curcumin	3.4	[194]
MSNs	Amine-functionalized and chitosan-coated	Gallic acid	Up to 58	[195]
KIT-6	Guanidine-functionalized and PEGylated	Curcumin	50	[196]
KIT-6 and KIL-2	Amino-modified	Curcumin	5–28	[197]
MSNs	Non-modified	Essential oils (lemongrass and clove)	29–36	[198]
MSNs	siRNA, folic acid functionalized	Myricetin	36	[199]
MSNs	Amino-modified	Ursolic acid	22	[200]
MSNs	Non-modified	Curcumin and chrysin	11–14	[201]
MSNs	Non-modified and copolymer-grafted MSNs	Quercetin	3–9.5	[202]
MSNs	Non-modified, amino-functionalized, folic acid-functionalized	Umbelliferone	12–19	[203]
KCC-1 and MCM-41	Folic acid-functionalized	Quercetin, curcumin, colchicine	2–29	[42]
KCC-1	Phosphonate-functionalized	Colchicine	3.5	[43]
MSNs	Non-modified	Thymoquinone	~7.5	[44]
MSNs	Non-modified	Harmine	~45	[204]

Table 6. Different loading strategies and their relationships to stimuli release under various conditions for MSNs.

Strategy	Nano System Design	Release	References
Molecular or supramolecular	MSNs-rotaxane	Diffusion under pH	[205,206]
	Pseudorotaxane	Diffusion under redox, pH	[207–209]
	Cleavable molecular bridges	Diffusion under plasmonic heating, two-photon irradiation	[210,211]
	Molecular nanovalves	Diffusion under plasmonic heating, various stimuli	[210,212]
Nanoparticles as gatekeepers	Iron oxide nanoparticles	Diffusion under redox, pH	[188,213]
	Cadmium sulfide nanoparticles	Diffusion under redox	[190]
	Gold nanoparticles	Diffusion under pH	[214]
	Zinc nanoparticles	Diffusion under pH	[215]
	Calcium carbonate nanoparticles	Diffusion under pH	[216]
Coatings	Polymer coating	Diffusion under pH	[44]
	Proteins coating	Diffusion under pH	[193]
	Lipid coating	Diffusion under different conditions	[217]

3.2. Drug Delivery Strategies

In this section, we provide a summary of delivery strategies that have been developed to treat cancer. This topic is well discussed in several reports for MSN delivery systems, and the readers are referred to these selected reviews [15,32,79,168,218–221]. Open pores on MSNs, the so-called cavities due to their porous structure, are not only used to load therapeutic agents, but also allow them to diffuse out in the surrounding solution. Closing these pores loaded with therapeutic agents is an essential step to avoid their premature release into the blood vessels, protecting from several side effects because of non-specific release [221]. Much effort has been made in controlled delivery systems with the stimulated or responsive release of therapeutic agents under certain conditions. Two major common strategies for delivering drugs have been reported by internal stimuli release (typical of the treated pathology), such as pH, redox potential, and enzymes, or by external stimuli (remotely applied by the clinician), such as magnetic fields, ultrasound, and light (Figure 14) [32].

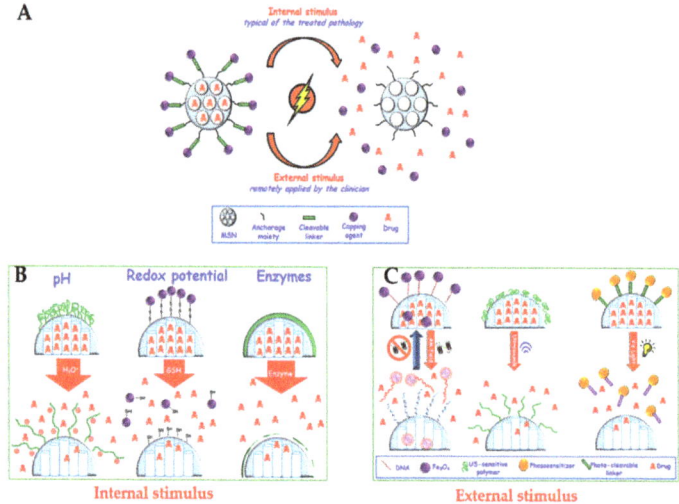

Figure 14. (**A**) Schematic representation of stimuli-responsive release of drugs from MSNs. (**B**) Internal stimuli-responsive release. (**C**) External stimuli-responsive release. Reproduced from [81], MDPI, 2017.

3.2.1. Internal Stimuli-Responsive Drug Release from MSNs

pH-Responsive Release

Cancer is well-known for its acidic tumor microenvironment with a lower pH than healthy cells/tissues. Consequently, pH-sensitive release is one of the approaches used in cancer nanomedicines. The most investigated pH-responsive delivery systems for anticancer therapeutic drugs have been inspired by applying diverse techniques and vary according to the loading strategies. In this section, we focus on some examples of recent studies published for natural anticancer prodrugs with pH-sensitive release. Nasab et al. [222] fabricated MSNs (MCM-41) capped with chitosan polymer and subsequently loaded with curcumin. This pH-responsive design depends on the degradation of chitosan, allowing high curcumin release at a low pH of 5.5 and resulting in low release at normal physiological pH (7.4). This is favorable for killing U87MG glioblastoma cancer cells. Mishra et al. [223] synthesized MSNs (SBA-15), followed by folic acid functionalization and further loading with quercetin and acid-labile magnetic nanoparticles (Figure 15). The system was investigated in vitro and in vivo in HCT-116 human colorectal carcinoma cells. The results showed that quercetin release was a pH-dependent effect, increasing with decreasing pH. Eventually, the system exhibits promising chemo-theranostic effects for managing colon carcinoma. In this context, Rashidi et al. [224] reported that the release of gallic acid (GA) from MSNs strongly depends on the pH levels of the release media. Furthermore, a pH-sensitive delivery system for ursolic acid prodrug was synthesized by incorporating an acid-sensitive linkage between the drug and MSNs [200]. This sustained release of ursolic acid enhances the anticancer effects against hepatocellular carcinoma cancer. A pH-responsive release of evodiamine and berberine was also achieved by loading them into lipid-coated MSNs [225]. In another strategy using Fe3O4 nanoparticles as gatekeepers, artemisinin is initially loaded into the inner space of hollow MSNs and Fe3O4 capped onto the pore outlets through acid-labile acetal linkers. The results proved that the system is stable under neutral conditions at pH 7.4 (no release), but it releases the prodrug upon exposure to the acidic lysosomal compartment (pH 3.8–5.0). The acetal linkers can be hydrolyzed under acidic conditions. This delivery system has an efficient and desirable anticancer action [226].

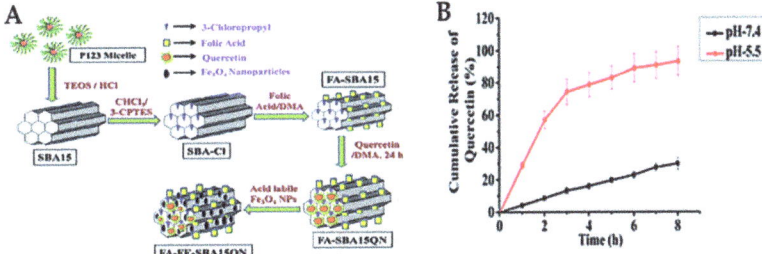

Figure 15. (A) Schematic representation of the delivery design for quercetin "FA-FE-SBA15QN". (B) The release kinetics of quercetin from FA-FE-SBA15QN at different pH (7.4 and 5.5). The values are represented as the mean ± SEM. Reproduced with permission from [223], The Royal Society of Chemistry, 2020. This article is licensed under a Creative Commons Attribution-Non-commercial 3.0 Unported License.

Redox-Responsive Release

The delivery systems that consider redox-sensitive release are popular in cancer-targeted therapy. They take advantage of intracellular conditions and rely specifically on the presence of glutathione (GSH) with a high level of expression in cancer cells compared to normal cells [227]. For example, Lin et al. [228] prepared pH and redox dual-stage responsive release of curcumin with Dox through specific cleavable PEGylation and hydrogel coating (crosslinked by disulfide bonds). The used MSNs were loaded with Dox, whereas the curcumin was encapsulated in a hydrogel coating. The results indicated that dual-responsive release by means of GSH and pH allows efficient and specific cancer targeting (Figure 16). In another example, Xu et al. [229] developed a stimuli-responsive delivery for curcumin gatekeepers based on MSNs characterized by large pores (named LP). In this design, curcumin is anchored to the surface of LP using thiol-ene as the click chemistry approach, followed by a coating of the pluronic polymer (F127) on the surface by means of self-assembly. The release studies proved that curcumin exhibits a redox-responsive release depending on the absence or presence of GSH at different pH levels.

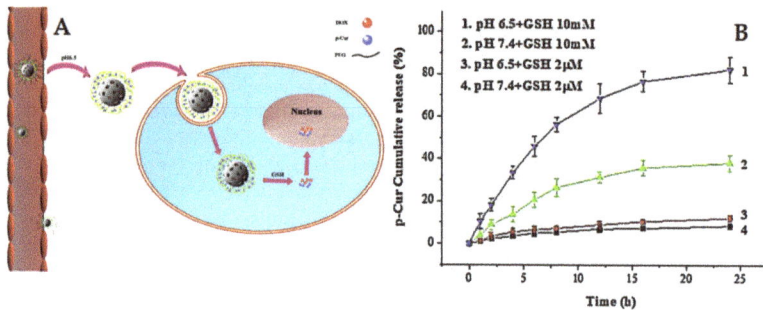

Figure 16. (**A**) Illustration of the dual-response release of p-Cur and Dox co-delivery. (**B**) In vitro release profiles of Cur from MSN/SP/bPEG at 37 °C. Error bars indicate standard deviation. Reproduced with permission from [228], Elsevier B.V, 2019.

Enzyme-Responsive Release

In the human body, many chemicals and enzymes are inherently expressed during pathological conditions, including cancers, which are explored to trigger drug release from numerous MSN types [10]. A delivery system tailored for anticancer treatment with enzyme-responsive release, in which matrix metalloproteinase (MMP) substrate peptide containing PLGLAR, which is sensitive to MMPs, is immobilized onto amine-modified MSNs and further capped with bovine serum albumin by covalent bonding. The results revealed that the nanoplatform delivery exhibits enzyme-triggered release of drug and efficiently inhibits tumor growth in vivo. MMP enzyme-trigger release of cisplatin-based MSNs was reported by Vaghasiya [230]. The system constructed by coating collagen on the surface of drug-loaded MSNs eventually results in sensitive enzyme release.

3.2.2. External Stimuli-Responsive Drug Release from MSNs
Responsive Release Using Magnetic Fields

This approach is largely employed for responsive release due to the magnetic guidance by a permanent magnetic field and locally increases the internal temperature by changing the magnetic field potential [32]. The delivery systems concerning this method widely use magnetic nanoparticles (superparamagnetic iron oxide-SPIONs) 5–10 nm in size as a core and mesoporous silica shell permitting drug loading and release [231]. Regarding natural prodrugs, the nano platform developed by Janus MSNs consists of magnetic nanoparticles to achieve magnetic targeting and delivery of berberine. This system produces a sustained release and exerts extraordinarily site-specific internalization into hepatocellular carcinoma cells, facilitating a high antitumor effect against liver cancer due to an external magnetic field [232]. Another very recent example is Asgari et al. [233] developing a novel in situ encapsulation delivery for curcumin consisting of magnetite-silica core-shell nanocomposites. The system could be effective for clinical application by means of magnetic hyperthermia therapy. In addition, nanoparticles of DNA-capped magnetic mesoporous silica composite exhibit temperature-dependent release of Dox and magnetic hyperthermia effects against cancer [234].

Responsive Release of Drugs Using Light

As a non-invasive and spatiotemporal strategy, different wavelengths of ultraviolet, visible, or near-infrared light can be employed to trigger and control drugs from MSNs. The main advantages are easy application by the clinician and focalization to the target tissue [235–237].

Kuang et al. [238] developed a curcumin delivery system by means of photodynamic therapy, achieving PEGylated MSNs loaded with curcumin (Figure 17). The results demonstrated that the developed system, "MSN-PEG@Cur", exhibits efficient endocytosis into cells and the release of curcumin. As a photodynamic therapy, it promptly generates ROS upon irradiation, allowing effective treatment for cancer. In another example, Li et al. [239] preloaded berberine into folic acid-modified Janus gold MSNs. The in vitro and in vivo results demonstrated that the delivery system verifies sustained release dependent on light and an efficient anti-tumor effect with good biosafety for normal tissue. Feng et al. [225] fabricated a dual delivery platform for evodiamine and berberine loaded into lipid-coated MSNs with thermo-sensitive release. Their results suggest that the temperature-responsive release is promising for both hydrophobic and hydrophilic drugs. Using an important natural prodrug of capsaicin, the main ingredient in red or hot chili pepper, Yu et al. [240] reported a novel design of NIR-triggered plasmonic nanodot-capped MSNs for inhibiting metastasis of human papillary thyroid carcinoma. The nanoplatform consisting of gold nanodot-capped MSNs loaded the prodrug. The results depicted that the delivery of capsaicin by the developed nanoformulation exhibited strong cytotoxicity against the FTC-133 and B-CPAP cell lines compared to free capsaicin.

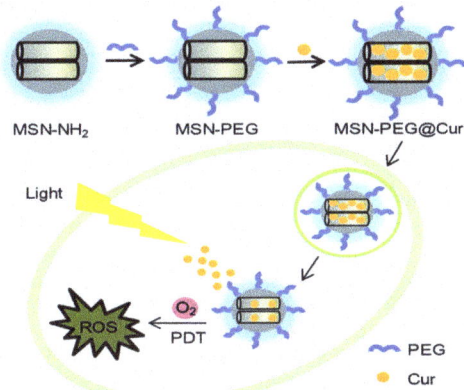

Figure 17. The preparation process for MSN-PEG@Cur and schematic representation of the intracellular photodynamic therapy (PDT) process after endocytosis of MSN-PEG@Cur. Reproduced with permission from [238], The Royal Society of Chemistry, 2020. This article is licensed under a Creative Commons Attribution-Non-commercial 3.0 Unported License.

Responsive Release of Drugs by Ultrasound

Ultrasound is considered an interesting and efficient approach to trigger the release of drugs from MSNs. The main advantages include deep penetration of living tissues without causing damage, and it is non-invasive and can be concentrated to the desired tissue [32,241]. In this approach, drugs can be released from pores of MSNs due to the thermal effect of ultrasound radiation on chemical bonds and thermosensitive polymers while closing in the absence of a radiation effect [242–244]. An example is MSNs modified with amine groups covered by sodium alginate polymer and subsequently loaded with a model cargo (rhodamine B) [245]. The results indicated that rhodamine B releases based on changing the ultrasound potential (ultrasound on–off responsiveness).

4. Selective Targeting Strategies for Cancer

One of the hottest areas in delivery systems is the delivery of drugs or therapeutic agents directly to specific tissues where the desired therapy is required. The main goal of nanomedicine application for cancers is avoiding the expected side effects from drugs and damaging the healthy cells surrounding the tumor site [21,246]. Two routes have been used depending on nano-particulate delivery for cancers, passive and active selective targeting.

Passive targeting was first postulated by Matsumura and Maeda in 1986 [247]. Nanoparticles can accumulate in tumor tissue by the enhanced permeability and retention (EPR) effect. They hypothesized that the localization of macromolecules and particles of certain sizes differ, which is attributed to the tumor microenvironment, the relatively slow elimination rate, and poor lymphatic drainage. Particle size, surface charge, or hydrophobicity can be mediated by the so-called EPR effect, or passive targeting [248,249] (Figure 18). Passive targeting is due to abnormalities in tumor blood vessels, which have wide interendothelial junctions with pores (700 nm). Injected nanoparticles travel through the bloodstream and accumulate in the tumor interstitium because of this characteristic of tumor vessels [247,249]. The nanoparticles already located in the tumor would remain there because of the ineffective lymphatic drainage with the fast growth of the tumor tissue [221]. However, the EPR effect is often not efficient enough to selectively deliver and reduce the side effects of anticancer drugs [250].

Active targeting is used to enhance the ability of a nanoparticle delivery platform carrying drugs to be taken up and bind to cancer cells via specific receptors on their surfaces compared to normal cells [251]. It is well known that some tumor cells overexpress certain receptors on their surface. Thus, nano-delivery systems functionalized with various ligands permit a high affinity for receptors facilitating specific retention and uptake by cancer cells. Thus, the role of targeting ligands is to allow the nanocarriers to selectively enter the cancerous cells, but not normal cells. This not only reduces the administration dosage, but also diminishes toxic side effects of drugs during circulation [252]. Many ligands have been investigated to functionalize/decorate nano-delivery systems based on MSNs for selectively targeting cancers (Figure 18). These include antibodies, proteins, peptides, aptamers, small molecules, and saccharides [221]. For example, transferrin [237], folic acid [42], epidermal growth factor (EGF) [253], methotrexate [254], RGD-type peptide [255], anti-HER2/neu [256], hyaluronic acid [257], and mannose [258].

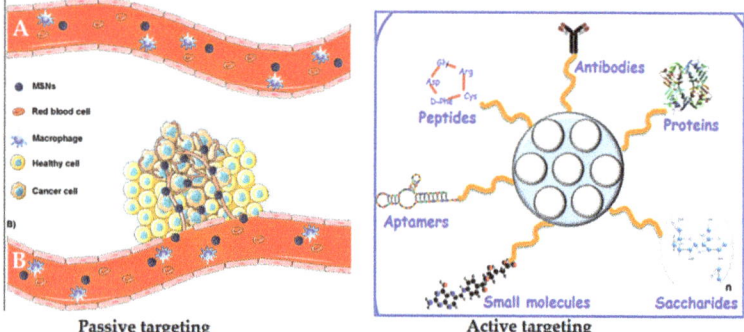

Figure 18. Schematic representation of the enhanced permeability and retention (EPR) effect (lift side). (**A**) Normal blood vessels (no fenestrations), showing that MSNs remain in the bloodstream. (**B**) Tumor tissues (defective blood vessels present) showing that MSNs leak out through the endothelial gap–gap and eventually accumulate in the tumor. On the right is a schematic depiction of active targeting with a variety of possibilities depending on the MSNs. Reproduced from [32,259], MDPI, 2020.

As an example, Kundu et al. [203] designed targeted delivery for umbelliferone prodrug, with the system consisting of umbelliferone loaded in MSNs and capped with a pH-sensitive poly acrylic acid and further grafted with folic acid on the surface. The delivery with folic acid conjugation increases the anticancer potential of umbelliferone against breast cancer cells. In another example, Yinxue et al. [199] investigated myricetin prodrug (Myr)-loaded MSNs combined with multidrug resistance protein (MRP-1) siRNA and the surface modified with folic acid to treat non-small cell lung cancer (NSCLC). In vivo fluorescence demonstrated that folic acid-conjugated MSNs with Myr and MRP-1 nanoparticles could specifically accumulate at tumor sites. Compared to free Myr and MSNs combined with MRP-1/Myr nanoparticles, folic acid-conjugated MSNs loaded with Myr and MRP-1 nanoparticles could more effectively suppress tumor growth with few side effects. Overall, a folic acid-conjugated nanoparticle system could provide a novel and effective platform for the treatment of NSCLC. We also reported a targeted delivery system consisting of folic acid conjugated to amine-modified MSNs (KCC-1 and MCM-41) and subsequently loaded with various prodrugs (curcumin, colchicine, and quercetin) [42]. The nanoformulation containing curcumin exhibited the highest anticancer activity against liver cancer cells through apoptosis via caspase-3, H_2O_2, c-MET, and MCL-1 (Figure 19). Table 7 lists some other examples of targeted delivery systems for anticancer natural prodrugs.

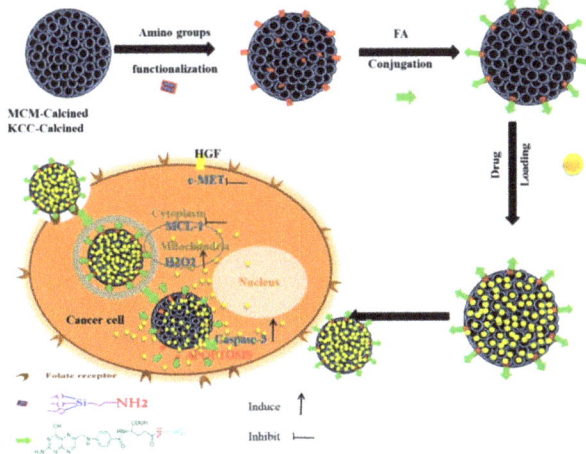

Figure 19. Schematic representation of the preparation, internalization, and anticancer mechanism of action of the prepared nanosystem in human liver carcinoma (HepG2) cells. This schematic shows the prodrug release into cancer cells and the main anticancer action for inducing apoptosis via activation of caspase-3 for killing HepG2 cancer cells proposed by assistance from important signaling pathways (c-MET, MCL-1, and H_2O_2). Reproduced from [42], Impact Journals, 2018.

Table 7. Some examples of targeted delivery systems for anticancer natural prodrugs using MSNs.

Prodrug	Ligand Used	Cancer Type	In Vitro/In Vivo	References
Berberine	FA	Liver cancer	In vitro and in vivo	[239]
Colchicine	FA	Colon cancer cells	In vitro	[43]
Curcumin	FA	Liver cancer cells	In vitro	[42]
Curcumin	FA	Breast cancer cells	In vitro and in vivo	[260]
Curcumin	FA	Breast cancer cells	In vitro	[261]

Table 7. Cont.

Prodrug	Ligand Used	Cancer Type	In Vitro/In Vivo	References
Quercetin and doxorubicin co-delivery	HA	Gastric carcinoma	In vivo	[262]
ZD6474 and epigallocatechin gallate	EGFR, VEGFR2, and Akt	Tamoxifen-resistant breast cancer.	In vitro and in vivo	[263]
Topotecan and quercetin co-delivery	Arginine-glycine-aspartic acid (cRGD) peptide	Triple negative breast cancer and multi-drug resistant breast cancer cells (MCF-7)	In vitro	[264]
Quercetin	FA	Breast cancer cells	In vitro	[265]
Epigallocatechin-3-gallate	Peptide	Breast cancer	In vivo	[266]
Anti-miRNA21 and resveratrol co-delivery	HA	Gastric carcinoma	In vitro and in vivo	[267]
Thymoquinone	Whey protein, Arabic gum, or chitosan–stearic acid	Brain cancers	In vitro	[44]
Quercetin	R5 peptide	Colon cancer	In vitro	[268]

FA = folic acid, HA = hyaluronic acid.

5. Motivation towards Natural Anticancer Agents

Nature is a great source of thousands of chemical substances/compounds generally considered natural products, as well as natural prodrugs if they are used for treating diseases [269,270]. Natural products (of natural origin) and herbal medicines have been used in traditional and modern medicine to treat cancer, and account for nearly 60% of pharmaceutical drugs [271–279]. Natural prodrugs provide medical effects against cancers as either chemotherapeutics or chemopreventive drugs. Regarding chemotherapeutics, anticancer natural prodrugs have been utilized for various cancer treatments and are becoming rising stars in the field of drug discovery for their contributions [280]. Some available drugs used in clinical applications for cancer patients diagnosed with different cancers are derived from plants, including vincristine, vinblastine, topotecan, and taxol [281]. There are also some examples of anticancer drugs originating from microbes, including Dox, daunorubicin, and bleomycin. Regarding cancer prevention, there are numerous natural substances (e.g., in fruits and vegetables) that have also been applied in cancer prevention along with human health enhancement with no detectable side effects [282]. To achieve cancer prevention goals, by completely preventing or delaying cancer, the main strategies that can be used, such as maintenance (healthy lifestyle), avoidance (exposure to toxicants/carcinogens), and dietary consumption (chemopreventive substances to drugs) [283]. There is no doubt that prevention leads to better management and treatment of tumor growth and the risk for developing metastases, secondary tumors, and recurrence [283]. Eliminating cancer, decreasing metastasis, reducing reappearance, and improving patient survival are key to curing cancers [284].

Among the main natural sources, plants are a considerable domain for supplying a variety of natural products with diverse chemical structures with a wide range of health benefits. The natural products are the main secondary metabolites produced by plants and can be classified into four major classes: phenolics and polyphenolics, terpenes, nitrogen-containing alkaloids, and sulfur-containing compounds (Figure 20) [285–287].

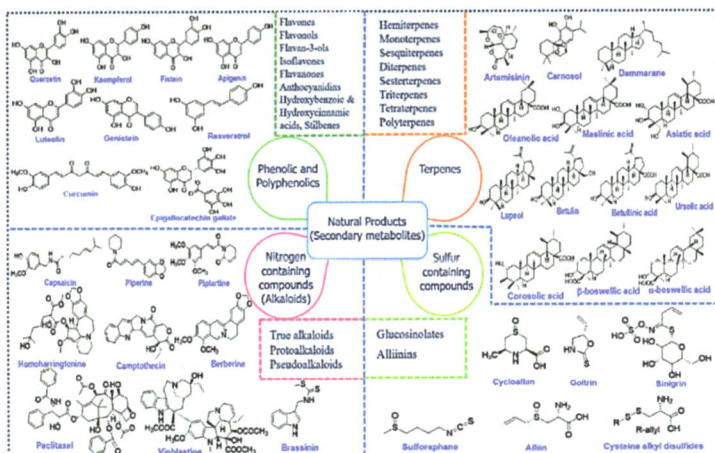

Figure 20. Chemical structures of various classes of natural compounds (prodrugs). Reproduced with permission from [285], Elsevier Ltd., 2019.

In recent years, attention has been focused on solving the problems associated with natural prodrug substances to increase their use in cancers and other pathological disorders. As an advanced strategy, nanotechnology application in medicine, called nanomedicine, is a promising approach being developed to overcome the limitations of natural prodrugs and improve their efficiency in cancer therapy. The advent of nanomedicine for cancer therapy occurred recently, and the rate of its progress and transformation in cancer treatments has also been rapid [285]. This technology can solve the major drawbacks of natural anticancer prodrugs, including low aqueous solubility, low bioavailability, multidrug resistance, and non-specific targeting. The developed nanoformulations for delivery of natural anticancer prodrugs are intentionally being explored with several classes of prodrugs based on various organic and inorganic nanocarriers [285,288–298]. By reviewing in vitro and in vivo cancer models in the literature, it seems that nanoplatforms for delivering anticancer natural prodrugs have potentially improved the therapeutic activity, specific targeting, solubility, and bioavailability, and reduced side effects. The better patient response and survival are accompanied by possible enhancement of the pharmacological impacts and clinical outcome. Below, we discuss the delivery systems that have been established for select anticancer natural prodrugs employing MSNs.

5.1. Curcumin

Curcumin (1,7-bis(4-hydroxy-3-methoxyphenyl)-1,6-heptadiene-3,5-dione) is a natural hydrophobic polyphenol compound, and is the major constituent derived from turmeric rhizome (*Curcuma longa* L.). Turmeric is a well-known spice in the kitchen and has a long history in traditional medicine for a wide range of diseases. Curcumin has numerous pharmacological activities, including anticancer, antiviral, antioxidant, anti-inflammatory, wound healing, and antimicrobial, among others [299–315].

Despite these potential pharmacological activities, the pharmacokinetics of curcumin show inherently poor solubility and bioavailability because of the limited absorption, rapid metabolism, and quick systematic elimination [316–319]. To take advantage of the medical actions of curcumin and improve the inherent limitations, versatile nanoplatform delivery systems have been constructed and studied, including MSNs. Concerning MSNs for curcumin delivery contribution, MSN-based nanosystems show great promise for combating cancers and will be seen soon in clinical stages.

Ma'mani and co-workers [196] fabricated guanidine-functionalized PEGylated KIT-6 MSNs 60–70 nm in size for delivery of curcumin to breast cancer cells. The system exhibited pH-sustained release of curcumin with long-term anticancer efficacy in human breast cancer cells (MCF-7 human breast adenocarcinoma cells, 4T1 mouse breast cancer cells, and MCF10A human mammary epithelial cells). A similar trend was observed for MSNs, namely MSU-2 and MCM-41 loaded with curcumin showing significant anticancer effects against different cancer cells (A549 human lung carcinoma cells, MCF-7 human breast cancer cells, and B16F10 mouse melanoma cells) compared to pure curcumin [320]. In further investigations, they found that the plausible mechanism contributing to anticancer effects is the generation of intracellular ROS and the induction of apoptosis. Lin et al. [228] tailored a co-delivery system of Dox loaded into MSNs as the core and curcumin loaded into the polymeric coating shell. The results indicate the long duration of blood circulation due to the PEG shell, GSH-sensitive release effect for drugs, and high cellular uptake resulting in synergistic anticancer effects through enhanced apoptosis of Hela cells. As an interesting nanoplatform, the fabricated lipid bilayer-coated curcumin-based MSNs unveiled a controllable and highly biocompatible theranostic nanosystem for cancer delivery [321]. Another recent strategy for building a delivery system for curcumin is by loading the prodrug into amino-MSNs using APTES silanes (KIL-2 and KIT-6), then coated by polyelectrolyte polymer complex by means of the layer-by-layer technique [197]. Based on the comparative data from this study, the nanoformulation exerts an anticancer effect on human cell lines, namely HL-60, EJ, and HEK-293, compared to free curcumin, demonstrating the promising delivery of prodrug with a sustained release effect. Considering active cancer-targeting designs, our group constructed selective targeted anticancer delivery of curcumin using MSNs (KCC-1-NH2-FA-CUR and MCM-41-NH2-FA-CUR) showing selective targeting of liver cancer cells (HepG2). The killing mechanism was found to be apoptosis [42]. The aspartic acid-functionalized PEGylated MSN-graphene oxide loaded with curcumin exhibited pH-sensitive release and excellent killing of breast cancer cells (MCF-7) [322]. With the occurrence of drug resistance in come cancers, silver-decorated SBA-15 (as metal-doped nanocomposites) coated with melanin-like polydopamine was used to deliver curcumin [323]. They found that the utilization of a nanoplatform containing curcumin enhances anticancer efficiency against select cancer cells (HeLa and taxol-resistant NSCLC (A549/TAX) compared to free curcumin.

To verify the antitumor action against breast cancer in vivo, Gao et al. investigated PEGylated lipid bilayer-coated MSNs for a dual-delivery of PTX and curcumin with prolonged release to determine their pharmacokinetic properties, uptake, subcellular localization, biodistribution and tumor site targeting, and effectiveness [324]. The delivery system could significantly increase the anti-tumor effect either by intravenous or intratumoral administration compared to free drug. The nanoplatform effectively led to the accumulation of the nanoformulation carrying drugs in the tumor site, resulting in highly efficient therapeutic effects in breast cancer. As such evidence of utilization of curcumin for co-delivery systems is important for further improvements and reducing side effects and drug resistance in cancers, which is the main issue for conventional cancer therapy. Sun et al. [325] conducted a study of cancer targeting by means of folic acid and PEI-modified-MSNs for curcumin; they concluded that the system exhibits sustained release (pH-sensitive delivery), which is suitable for antineoplastic drugs. Several studies have reported the delivery of curcumin in different cancers in vitro or in vivo (Table 8).

Table 8. Delivery designs for curcumin in cancer (in vitro/in vivo studies) based on mesoporous silica nanoparticles (MSNs).

Delivery Design	Trigger Release Effect	Cancer Type	Anticancer Mechanism	References
CUR-loaded MSNs incorporated into poly-ε-caprolactone/gelatin (PCL/GEL) hybrid	Sustained release	Human adipose-derived stem cells (hADSCs)	Down-regulation of p16INK4A; up-regulation of hTERT	[326]
SBA-15 doped with silver nanoparticles, coated melanin-like polydopamine, and loaded CUR	pH-sensitive release	Human cervical cancer cells (HeLa) and taxol-resistant non-small cell lung cells (A549/TAX)	NA	[323]
Co-delivery: spiropyran- and fluorinated silane-modified MSNs, loaded doxorubicin and CUR	pH-responsive release	In vivo: HepG2-xenografted mice	NA	[327]
Hollow MSNs, loaded CUR	pH-triggered release	NA	NA	[328]
Co-delivery: PEGylated lipid bilayer coated MSNs, loaded paclitaxel and CUR	Sustained release	In vivo: breast	NA	[324]
Targeted delivery with folic acid-modified MSNs	pH-triggered release	NA	NA	[325]
CUR loaded MSNs	NA	Hepatocellular carcinoma cells (HepG2, liver)	NA	[329]
MSNs functionalized with PEI and loaded CUR	NA	Breast cancers: MCF-7 and MCF-7R cells	Apoptosis: activation of caspase-9, -6, -12, PARP, CHOP, and PTEN; downregulation of survival protein Akt1; downregulation of ER resident protein: IRE1α, PERK, and GRP78	[330]
Targeted delivery: folic acid-conjugated amine-modified MSNs (KCC-1 and MCM-41), loaded CUR	NA	Human hepatocellular carcinoma cells (HepG2) and HeLa cancer cells	Apoptosis: by specific signaling molecular pathways (caspase-3, H2O2, c-MET, and MCL-1)	[42]
Targeted delivery: MSN-modified hyaluronan (HA) or polyethyleneimine-folic acid and loaded CUR	Redox-responsive	Breast cancer cell line (MDA-MB-231). In vivo: mouse xenograft model.	NA	[260]
Targeted delivery: gold nanoparticles immobilized on folic acid-conjugated dendritic MSNs, coated reduced graphene oxide nanosheets, loaded CUR	pH-sensitive and photothermal potency	Human cancer cell lines (MCF-7, human breast carcinoma cells and A549, human lung carcinoma cells)	NA	[261]
Aspartic acid functionalized PEGylated MSNs contained graphene oxide nanohybrid loaded CUR	pH-responsive	Breast cancer MCF-7 cells	NA	[322]
Targeted delivery: folic acid-modified MSNs, loaded CUR	pH-sensitive	Breast cancer MCF-7 cell	NA	[331]
Glycyrrhetinic acid-functionalized MSNs, loaded CUR	NA	Liver hepatocellular carcinoma (HepG2) cells	NA	[332]
Polyethylenimine-modified curcumin-loaded MCM-41	pH-sensitive	Breast cancer MCF-7 cells	NA	[333]
MCM-41 capped by chitosan natural polymer	pH-sensitive	Glioblastoma cancer cell line (U87MG)	NA	[222]
Carboxymethyl cellulose-grafted mesoporous silica hybrid nanogels	NA	Human breast cancer cell line (MDA-MB-231)	NA	[334]
Targeted delivery: CUR-loaded and calcium-doped dendritic MSNs modified with folic acid	pH-responsive	Human breast cancer cells (MCF-7); in vivo animal	Apoptosis: increasing intracellular ROS generation; decreasing mitochondrial membrane potential; enhancing cell cycle retardation at G2/M phase	[335]
Amine-functionalized KIT-6, MSU-2, and MCM-41; loaded CUR	NA	Cancer cells	Apoptosis: generation of intracellular ROS; downregulation of poly-ADP ribose polymerase (PARP) enzyme	[336]
MCM-41 modified, different functionalities, and loaded CUR	Sustained release	Human squamous cell carcinoma cell line (SCC25)	Apoptosis	[124]
KCC-1 and MCM-41 amino-modified and loaded CURC	pH-responsive	NA	NA	[69]

NA = Not applicable, CUR = curcumin.

5.2. Quercetin

Quercetin is a dietary flavonoid compound derived from plants (e.g., medicinal plants, vegetable, fruits). It is a 3,3′,4′,5,7-pentahydroxyflvanone named by the International Union of Pure and Applied Chemistry (IUPAC) [337]. Quercetin has unique biological properties that play an important role in mental/physical performance, as well as reducing infection risk [338]. It has shown numerous pharmacological actions, including anti-oxidant, anti-microbial, anti-diabetic, anti-inflammatory, anti-cancer, anti-Alzheimer, psychostimulant, mitochondrial biogenesis stimulant, lipid peroxidation inhibitor, platelet aggregation inhibitor, and capillary permeability inhibitor, among others [339–348]. The dietary intake of quercetin varies in many countries. The estimated intake dosage of flavonoid (quercetin accounts for nearly 75%) ranges from 50–800 mg/day according to the consumption of fruits, vegetables, tea, and herbals [349]. In addition, quercetin is safe with a single dose of up to 4000 mg orally and up to 100 mg via intravenous administration [350]. Quercetin is an excellent free radical scavenging antioxidant [344] and is considered one of the most effective antioxidants [351]. Consequently, quercetin exhibits promising effects against cancer [339,352] in vitro and in vivo [353–360]. Nevertheless, its potential impacts in clinical applications are drastically limited due to its poor solubility, low bioavailability, and instability [361]. According to the pharmacokinetics of quercetin in humans, only ~2% is bioavailable (from single dose) with an absorption rate of 3 to 17% (from 100 mg applied in individual healthy persons) [337]. The factors affecting oral bioavailability are low absorption, extensive metabolism, and/or rapid elimination, in addition to low solubility and non-selective targeting of cancers. Several nanoplatform delivery systems focus on overcoming these challenges to introduce quercetin into clinical applications soon for cancer [362–368].

The use of MSNs to develop new delivery systems for quercetin against cancers has attracted many research groups. Liu et al. [369] fabricated a system for dual delivery of PTX and quercetin into MSNs to overcome multidrug resistance in breast cancer. The nanosystem exhibited CD44 receptor-mediated active targeting for MCF-7/ADR cells. At the same time, the addition of quercetin with PTX significantly improves the sensitivity of MCF-7/ADR cells to PTX, providing a solution to multidrug resistance in breast cancer. Huang et al. [370] designed a novel nanoformulation consisting of quercetin-loaded MSNs coating cancer cell membranes for enhanced tumor targeting and radiotherapy. In vitro and in vivo investigations revealed that the system has many advantages, including excellent tumor targeting ability and efficient inhibition of tumor growth. The platform fulfills innovative ideas for targeting cancer and improving therapy. In another attempt, polydopamine-coated hollow MSNs combining Dox hydrochloride with quercetin efficiently overcame multidrug resistance in taxol and Dox double-resistant human colorectal cancer cells (HCT-8/TAX cells) [371]. Fang et al. [262] developed a hyaluronic acid-modified MSNs that co-deliver quercetin and Dox to enhance the efficacy of chemotherapy for gastric carcinoma. They found that the system enables stability, sustained release, and selective killing effects. An in vivo study disclosed that the co-delivery significantly enhances the anticancer efficacy compared to a single drug, showing the importance of quercetin in clinical application. In this context, Murugan et al. [264] loaded topotecan into the pores of MSNs, followed by poly(acrylic acid)-chitosan as an outer layer to further conjugate quercetin, and then grafting with arginine-glycine-aspartic acid (cRGD) peptide on the surface as targeting ligands for cancers. The system released the drugs as a function of pH and uptake occurred through integrin receptor-mediated endocytosis, enabling efficient anti-tumor effects in multidrug resistant breast cancer cells and animal studies. As far as active targeting and bioavailability are concerned, MSNs conjugated with folic acid and loaded with quercetin exhibit higher cellular uptake and more quercetin bioavailability in breast cancer cells, as well as an enhanced antitumor effect through apoptosis [265]. These studies demonstrate the prospective application of quercetin in cancers by means of single or co-delivery, facilitating efficient targeting and antitumor effects, creating new possibilities for clinical applications.

5.3. Resveratrol

Resveratrol (RSV, 3,5,4′-trihydroxy-trans-stilbene) is a natural polystilbene and non-flavonoid polyphenol. As a phytoestrogen compound, RSV is present in a wide range of plants and is abundant in extracts from the grape skin and other fruits and vegetables. RSV has been reported to exert multiple pharmacological effects, including anti-inflammatory, anti-viral, anti-microbial, anti-Alzheimer, anticancer, cardioprotective, neuroprotective, and immunomodulatory actions [372–386]. Concerning the anticancer effects on the preclinical level, RSV has also been reported to possess important antitumor actions in several preclinical animal models [387–398]. The clinical prospective of RSV has also been evaluated in a few clinical trials. The first clinical trial by Nguyen et al. [399] indicated that the freeze-dried grape powder (containing RSV) effectively inhibits colon cancer in patients. In addition, Patel et al. [374] showed that a daily dose of RSV at 0.5 or 1.0 g produces sufficient anticarcinogenic effects in colorectal cancer. Furthermore, Howells et al. [400] demonstrated that RSV given at micronized formulation with 5.0 g daily for 14 days in patients with colorectal cancer and hepatic metastases prevented malignancies by increasing apoptosis.

Despite promising preclinical (in vitro and in vivo) and prospective clinical results as an anticancer agent, RSV still has many challenges due to the pharmacokinetics, metabolism, bioavailability, and toxicity in cancer patients [374,401]. These associated properties prevent translation into more clinical trials and human benefits. In addition, RSV has shown poor bioavailability due to its quick extensive metabolism, and large doses (up to 5 g/day) should be applied to provide anticancer therapeutic activity [402]. Such high doses result in adverse effects (e.g., diarrhea, nausea, and abdominal pain with >1 g/day) [402]. As the poor bioavailability limits the RSV activity, there are various approaches for overwhelming the bioavailability, including co-delivery with piperine prodrug [403], micronized powders [403], and nanoplatform delivery [404–407]. Application of nanomedicine can improve the stability and bioavailability, and minimize side effects of RSV, which is making RSV a prospective candidate for treating many diseases, including cancers.

Few investigations in recent years have used MSNs for the delivery of RSV. Chaudhary et al. [408] loaded RSV into MSN-modified phosphonate or MSN-modified amine to improve the anti-proliferative activity and sensitization of drug-resistant prostate cancer. The RSV is released as a function of pH, and the phosphonate-modified nanoparticles effectively kill cancer cells better than amine-modified nanoparticles. Hu et al. [267] constructed a dual delivery system for anti-miR21 and RSV using MSNs conjugated with hyaluronic acid to target gastric carcinoma through overexpression of the CD44 receptor on cell membranes. They found that this nanoformulation has a superior anticancer effect due to synergistic effects specifically delivered by combining anti-miR21 and RSV in gastric cancer cells. Furthermore, Summerlin et al. [409] encapsulated RSV in colloidal MCM-48 and found that the nanoformulation enhances saturated solubility (∼95%) and release effect compared to pure RSV. The nanoformulation also possesses a higher killing ability for HT-29 and LS147T colon cancer cells compared to pure RSV by mediating the PARP and cIAP1 pathways.

5.4. Berberine

Berberine is an isoquinoline alkaloid found in a handful of plants widely used in botanical medical practice, such as *Hydrastis canadensis* (Goldenseal), *Berberis aquifolium* (Oregon grape), *Berberis vulgaris* (Barberry), and *Coptis chinensis* (Chinese Goldthread) [410,411]. Versatile pharmacological activities have been reported for berberine, including anti-viral, anti-microbial, anticancer, anti-diabetic, anti-diarrhea, and anti-inflammatory, and treatment for congestive heart failure, cardiac arrhythmia, and hypertension. Recently, berberine extract or pure compound has gained much attention in the newly published research and is among the top pharmaceutical supplements on shelves [412]. The preclinical evidence from huge studies reveals the capability of berberine to treat many diseases [411,413–419]. Thus, berberine is clinically studied for many diseases, such as diabetes [410,420–423]. Particular attention has been given to berberine in cancers, so it is expected to be one of the most common natural compounds under the scope of extensive clinical investigations of cancers [424]. The main challenges in translating berberine to the clinical application are low solubility, poor aqueous solubility, slight absorption, and low bioavailability. There are some strategies to deal with these limitations, such as producing berberine hydrochloride to increase its solubility. Another approach is encapsulating berberine into nanocarriers for nanoplatform delivery [425–427].

Berberine loaded into folic acid-conjugated gold-MSNs shows superb anticancer effects, good biosafety, and protection of normal tissue in vitro and in vivo for chemo-radiotherapy of liver cancer [239]. Another conformation obtained by Feng et al. [225] showed that MSNs based on dual delivery of hydrophobic prodrugs with berberine and evodiamine through thermo/pH-responsiveness improves antitumor effects in vitro and in vivo. Other results propose that the berberine-loaded Janus nanocarriers (MSNs containing iron oxide) driven by a magnetic field provide an effective and safe approach against hepatocellular carcinoma [232]. As with other drugs, berberine can be released depending on different conditions; by disulfide bond linking, berberine releases from MSNs under glutathione conditions upon breakage of the disulfide bond, promoting the anticancer action against liver cancer [428].

5.5. Thymoquinone

Thymoquinone (TQ, 2-methyl-5-isopropyl-1,4-benzoquinone), a monoterpene diketone compound, is the main active component in essential oil (volatile oil) of *Nigella sativa* L. (known as black seed or black cumin). TQ was isolated for the first time in 1963 [429] and exhibits various pharmacological activities in vitro and in preclinical investigations. The most reported activities are anticancer, antioxidant, anti-microbial, neuroprotective, anti-inflammatory, anti-microbial, and anti-diabetic [430–440]. A considerable amount of available data from preclinical studies encourage the translation of TQ into clinical settings. There is no doubt of the promising anticancer effects of TQ, but the lack of bioavailability and pharmacokinetic parameters delay the use of TQ in clinical applications. The main issues are low bioavailability, solubility, biodistribution in the body, rapid metabolism, and excretion [441–443]. In recent years, several strategies have been investigated to improve these limitations, such as the development of novel analogs [444], use of different routes (e.g., oral, intraperitoneal, intravenous), and nano-delivery systems [296,445,446].

Few delivery systems have been designed for TQ based on MSNs. The TQ-loaded MSNs produce more anticancer effects against MCF-7 and HeLa cells than pure TQ [447]. In addition, both TQ-loaded MSNs and pure TQ exert their anticancer activity by means of ROS-mediated apoptosis. To enhance the targeting ability towards glioma cells, we fabricated core–shell nanoformulations [44], with the core consisting of MSNs loaded with TQ and the shell consisting of whey protein–Arabic gum or chitosan–stearic acid complex. Interestingly, TQ releases as a function of pH and induces selective killing of cancer cells compared to normal cells. Furthermore, the core–shell nanoformulations significantly kill glioma cancer cells via apoptosis-mediated pathways due to caspase-3 activation, cytochrome c triggers, and cell cycle arrest at G2/M signaling. In this sense, the efficient anticancer effects against brain cancers can be attributed to the distribution of TQ-loaded MSNs [448]. The study showed that encapsulating TQ in MSNs improves delivery to some brain areas, including the cortex, thalamus, hypothalamus, and midbrain, but reduces its delivery to the cerebellum compared to pure TQ. The results also indicated that neither free TQ nor MSN-TQ reaches the hippocampus. Thus, MSNs potentially target TQ to certain brain areas.

5.6. Gallic Acid

GA (3,4,5-trihydroxybenzoic acid) is one of the most abundant phenolic acids present in plants (e.g., fruits and medicinal plants). GA can be isolated from different plants of *Quercus* spp. and has extensive applications in the food and pharmaceutical industries [449]. The therapeutic uses include antimicrobial [450], anticancer, gastrointestinal disease, cardiovascular disease, metabolic disease, neuropsychological disease, and other miscellaneous diseases [449,451–455]. GA has a potential antioxidant action modulated by various signaling pathways (e.g., inflammatory cytokines, and enzymatic and nonenzymatic antioxidants) that lead to its therapeutic effects [453]. However, as with many prodrugs, limitations still exist for clinical use of GA and to confirm its therapeutic outcomes. Several nanostructures have been used to fabricate delivery systems to solve these limitations and achieve effectiveness to translate GA into clinical investigations [456–460].

Only a few studies have been reported on MSN nanosystems for GA. MSNs functionalized with amino acid and coated with chitosan exhibit a high loading capacity of ~20–38%, leading to better killing potency of MCF-7cells than pure GA [195]. GA is an unstable molecule under specific pH; by encapsulating it in MSNs, the release of GA can be controlled by media with different pH and released in the presence of higher antioxidant activity [224]. With respect to the anticancer effect, incorporation of GA into MSNs by means of covalent bonding increases its activity against HeLa and KB cells, with a killing efficiency of up to 67% [461]. Thus, GA-loaded MSNs easily internalize into Caco-2 cells, releasing GA to enhance cytotoxic effects against colon cancer [462].

5.7. Essential Oils

Among the plant natural prodrugs, the essential oils (also known as volatile oils) have particular importance in many sectors (e.g., pharmaceutical, cosmetic, agricultural, and food) [463,464]. With a long history in many cultures, essential oils can be used for different purposes [465]. For example, Ancient Egyptians used essential oils as early as 4500 BC for cosmetics and ointments [466]. They made a mixture of many herbals containing essential oils (e.g., aniseed, cedar, onion, myrrh, grapes, etc.) as preparations in perfume or medicine. In recent years, the most important use of essential oils has been aromatherapy due to their curative effects [467]. Essential oils are complex mixtures of volatile compounds found especially in aromatic plants, such as clary sage (*Salvia sclarea* L.), eucalyptus (*Eucalyptus globulus* Labill.), geranium (*Pelargonium graveolens* L.), lavender (*Lavandula officinalis* Chaix), lemon (*Citrus limon* L.), peppermint (*Mentha piperita* L.), roman chamomile (*Anthemis nobilis* L.), rosemary (*Rosmarinus officinalis* L.), basil (*Ocimum basilicum*), rosemary (*Rosmarinus officinalis*), and ginger (*Zingiber officinale*). The essential oils are obtained from plant sources by several methods, such as hydrodistillation, steam distillation, cold pressing, solvent extraction, microwave-assisted processing, and carbon dioxide extraction. Concerning their chemical composition, essential oils were originally characterized as monoterpene and sesquiterpene hydrocarbons together with their oxygenated derivatives, besides the aliphatic aldehydes, alcohols, and ester structures [466]. Due to the chemical compositions of essential oils with versatile compounds that possess many roles and modes of action in various pharmacological entities and therapeutics, including anticancer, cardiovascular disease treatment, anti-bacterial, anti-viral, anti-oxidants, analgesics, and antidiabetics [468,469]. The main applications are enhanced transdermal drug delivery due to their skin penetration, and aroma and massage therapy [470]. Essential oil compounds have been reported to have potential anticancer effects in vitro and in animal models [471–477]. However, essential oils generally have low stability, high volatility, and a high risk of deterioration by exposure to direct heat, humidity, light, or oxygen [478]. Nanoformulations are a recent strategy being developed for essential oils and their constituents to solve these problems [463,479–482].

To the best of our knowledge, no anticancer nanoformulations have been designed for essential oils and their constituents. MSNs are efficient particles for the high loading of essential oil substances. Melendez-Rodriguez et al. demonstrated that eugenol, an important component in various essential oils of herbs, is efficiently encapsulated in pores of MSNs up to 50 wt.%. by means of vapor adsorption [483]. Ebadollahi et al. [484] reported that the loading of essential oils of thymus species into MCM-41 increases their stability and persistence up to 20 days. Furthermore, Janatova et al. [485] demonstrated that different encapsulated essential oil components in MCM-41 provide long-term effects through controlled release compared to the same pure substances. In addition, Jobdeedamrong et al. [486] showed that the release of essential oils (peppermint, thyme, cinnamon, and clove oil) is controlled by loading them into MSN-functionalized particles and grafting them with hyaluronic acid. Confirmation of delayed volatilization was reported for lavender oil loaded into MSNs [487]. Jin et al. [488] showed that MCM-41 modified nanoparticles enable high loading of pepper fragrant along with bactericidal activities against different microbes. Thus, the incorporation of essential oils from different herbs could be used effectively for infectious diseases [489,490] and treating biofilm [491].

5.8. Other Natural Products

Artemisinin is a sesquiterpene lactone derived from *Artemisia annua*. It is used as an antimalarial for treating multi-drug-resistant strains of falciparum malaria. It has also shown promising anticancer effects [492]. Artemisinin loaded into pores of hollow MSNs and capped with Fe3O4 nanoparticles act as gatekeepers [226]. The system shows a pH-dependent release effect, with stable release achieved at pH 7.4 and higher artemisinin release at low pH (3.8–5.0). This system exhibits excellent anticancer efficacy. Another multifunctional nanocarrier, Fe3O4@C/Ag@mSiO2 loaded with a high amount of artemisinin, allows pH-stimuli release and more killing of HeLa cancer cells compared to free artemisinin [493].

Some natural prodrugs are toxic compounds, and this toxicity prevents them from being used to treat cancers. An important example is colchicine, a natural alkaloid derived mainly from *Colchicum automnale*. It has long been used clinically to treat gout and familial Mediterranean fever. Colchicine is an important antimitotic prodrug and efficiently kills cancer cells [494], but the major challenge to its use is its toxicity. Earlier, Cauda et al. reported a one-step fabrication of colchicine-loaded in lipid bilayer-coated MSNs, making the system more stable and leading to effective microtubule depolymerization upon cell uptake [495]. We also loaded colchicine into folic acid-conjugated MCM-41 and KCC-1 for anticancer and antioxidant effects, obtaining higher anticancer effects than with free colchicine [42]. Very recently, we developed a novel DDS for colchicine. The system consisted of KCC-1-functionalized with phosphonate groups and loaded with colchicine, and subsequently coated with folic acid chitosan–glycine complex (MSNsPCOL/CG-FA) [43]. This nanoformulation revealed enhanced selective killing towards cancer cells compared to free colchicine in this order: colon cancer (HCT116) > liver cancer (HepG2) > prostate cancer (PC3). As its cytotoxicity is a major concern, the system is also promising because it exhibits low cytotoxicity (4%) compared to free colchicine (~60%) in normal BJ1 cells. The main mechanism of action was studied in detail for HCT116 cells, indicating primarily intrinsic apoptosis as a result of enhanced antimitotic effects with a contribution of genetic regulation by MALAT 1 and mir-205 and immunotherapy effects by Ang-2 protein and PD-1.

Loading glabridin, a prodrug compound obtained from the root extract of *Glycyrrhiza glabra*, on MSNs leads to remarkable improvement in its saturation solubility and dissolution velocity [496]. In this context, loading of breviscapine in MSNs significantly improves the solubility and bioavailability [17]. In addition, Ibrahim et al. [183] concluded that incorporating silymarin in MSNs within a lyophilized tablet remarkably increases the dissolution rate and saturation solubility. Similarly, loading of glabridin in MSNs improves the saturation solubility and dissolution velocity [496]. The biological activity, including anticancer activity, of polyphenols and flavonoids obtained from black chokeberry fruits is efficient compared to the free forms when loaded in MCM-41 and ZnO-MCM-41 [497] Co-delivery of topotecan and quercetin by MSNs results in pH-responsive release, subsequently increasing the intracellular release in cancer cells. Ultimately, it induces notable molecular activation (structural changes in tumor cell: endoplasmic reticulum, nucleus, and mitochondria) leading to cancer cell death [264]. Similar evidence has been obtained with targeted delivery of epigallocatechin-3-gallate-loaded MSNs for breast cancer treatment in vivo [266].

6. Conclusions and Future Perspective

Engineered MSNs with a variety of nanostructures are important inorganic nanocarriers for drug delivery in nanomedicine applications. MSNs have various unique physiochemical properties, including high pore volume, high specific surface area and porosity. In addition, various organic functional groups can be used for their surface modification by facile processes. MSNs are generally accepted to have good biocompatibility, being safe and showing no-significant side effects. The toxicity of MSNs as in the case of any drug or nanomaterial depends on dose/concentration, material properties, application routes. The degree of toxicity is low as indicated by several studies if the synthesis is performed in optimized conditions or overdose is avoided. Additionally, according to many animal studies, the toxicity of MSNs can diminish by optimizing the synthesis parameters and surface modification. Most in vivo studies generate data stipulating that the suggested average dose of 50 mg/kg is well tolerated in animals and safe without any toxicity or apparent abnormalities. This is considered as an adequate dose to be used, e.g., in cancer therapy. This dose can be increased for oral route administration compared to intraperitoneal or intravenous injection. Importantly, the use of MSN-drug-loaded nanoformulations can allow the use of an even higher dose (three or more times) [174]. As with other nanomaterials, for future translation to clinical applications, the safety aspects of MSNs should be considered carefully for each type because many nanostructures are reported. Recently, the first clinical trial in humans was conducted with oral delivery of fenofibrate formulation based on the ordered mesoporous silica [33].

MSNs can be used as multifunctional targeted anticancer delivery systems, delivering a variety of drugs, therapeutic proteins, and antibodies. Furthermore, due to their nanoporous structure, MSNs have a high loading capacity for therapeutic agents and are excellent nanocarriers for internal- and external-responsive release of drugs (e.g., pH, GSH, redox, light, magnetic direction, and ultrasound). The available data indicate that the use of MSNs as prodrug nanocarriers can overcome the present barriers in their application: poor water solubility, low bioavailability, and insufficient targeting. Therefore, the available literature suggests a high potential of MSNs as natural prodrug delivery vehicles. The present pre-clinical and clinical tests show that MSNs are promising drug delivery carriers from a biocompatibility/safety perspective, opening the door towards the clinical nanomedicine application for cancer therapy.

For future research directions, we suggest the importance of co-delivery systems in which two or more anticancer natural prodrugs are combined, as well as exploring thousands of natural prodrugs that have not been thoroughly investigated yet. Furthermore, scientists can investigate loading MSNs with crude extract from plant materials. This can also be explored in synergistic therapy with crude extract containing many prodrug components together. Particularly promising prodrug substances are essential oils applied using MSN-based delivery systems. Their traditional use is only limited to cosmetics and some pharmaceutical applications. The essential oil nanoformulations will add value to cancer therapy.

The core–shell nanoformulations containing a core of MSNs loaded with prodrugs and a shell of organic substances, such as chitosan, Arabic gum, or others, are highly recommended to establish prodrug delivery systems. As an important parameter, the stability and dispersibility of nanoformulations should be taken into consideration because they affect the biological performance and therapeutic actions. Additionally, we think that the large-scale production for each type of MSNs will lead to obtaining safe material by optimizing and stabilizing the material parameters. In our opinion, animal and reported clinical studies open the doors to develop MSNs-based nanoformulations to be translated into clinical evaluations for cancers soon.

Author Contributions: Conceptualization, K.A. and W.L.; literature review, K.A.; writing—original draft preparation, K.A.; writing-review and editing, K.A. and W.L.; visualization, K.A. and W.L.; supervision, W.L. Both authors have read and agreed to the published version of the manuscript.

Funding: This work was funded by the Institute of High Pressure Physics (IHPP), Polish Academy of Sciences (PAS), Poland and The APC was also funded by IHPP.

Institutional Review Board Statement: Not applicable.

Informed Consent Statement: Not applicable.

Acknowledgments: We would like to thank the Institute of High Pressure Physics (IHPP), Polish Academy of Sciences (PAS), Poland, for the financial support.

Conflicts of Interest: The authors declare no conflict of interest regarding the publication of this paper.

References

1. Vallet-Regi, M.; Rámila, A.; del Real, R.P.; Pérez-Pariente, J. A New Property of MCM-41: Drug Delivery System. *Chem. Mater.* **2001**, *13*, 308–311. [CrossRef]
2. Kresge, C.T.; Leonowicz, M.E.; Roth, W.J.; Vartuli, J.C.; Beck, J.S. Ordered mesoporous molecular sieves synthesized by a liquid-crystal template mechanism. *Nature* **1992**, *359*, 710–712. [CrossRef]
3. Gonçalves, M.C. Sol-Gel Silica Nanoparticles in Medicine: A Natural Choice. Design, Synthesis and Products. *Molecules* **2018**, *23*, 2021. [CrossRef]
4. Pednekar, P.P.; Godiyal, S.C.; Jadhav, K.R.; Kadam, V.J. Chapter 23—Mesoporous silica nanoparticles: A promising multifunctional drug delivery system. In *Nanostructures for Cancer Therapy*; Ficai, A., Grumezescu, A.M., Eds.; Elsevier: Amsterdam, The Netherlands, 2017; pp. 593–621.
5. Le Hoang Doan, T.; Mai, N.X.D.; Matsumoto, K.; Tamanoi, F. Chapter 4—Tumor Targeting and Tumor Growth Inhibition Capability of Mesoporous Silica Nanoparticles in Mouse Models. In *The Enzymes*; Tamanoi, F., Ed.; Academic Press: Cambridge, MA, USA, 2018; Volume 44, pp. 61–82.
6. Mitran, R.-A.; Deaconu, M.; Matei, C.; Berger, D. Chapter 11—Mesoporous Silica as Carrier for Drug-Delivery Systems. In *Nanocarriers for Drug Delivery*; Mohapatra, S.S., Ranjan, S., Dasgupta, N., Mishra, R.K., Thomas, S., Eds.; Elsevier: Amsterdam, The Netherlands, 2019; pp. 351–374.
7. Mekaru, H.; Lu, J.; Tamanoi, F. Development of mesoporous silica-based nanoparticles with controlled release capability for cancer therapy. *Adv. Drug Deliv. Rev.* **2015**, *95*, 40–49. [CrossRef]
8. Slowing, I.I.; Vivero-Escoto, J.L.; Wu, C.-W.; Lin, V.S.Y. Mesoporous silica nanoparticles as controlled release drug delivery and gene transfection carriers. *Adv. Drug Deliv. Rev.* **2008**, *60*, 1278–1288. [CrossRef]
9. Mamaeva, V.; Sahlgren, C.; Lindén, M. Mesoporous silica nanoparticles in medicine—Recent advances. *Adv. Drug Deliv. Rev.* **2013**, *65*, 689–702. [CrossRef]
10. Narayan, R.; Nayak, U.Y.; Raichur, A.M.; Garg, S. Mesoporous Silica Nanoparticles: A Comprehensive Review on Synthesis and Recent Advances. *Pharmaceutics* **2018**, *10*, 118. [CrossRef]
11. Kwon, S.; Singh, R.K.; Perez, R.A.; Abou Neel, E.A.; Kim, H.W.; Chrzanowski, W. Silica-based mesoporous nanoparticles for controlled drug delivery. *J. Tissue Eng.* **2013**, *4*, 2041731413503357. [CrossRef]
12. Liong, M.; Lu, J.; Kovochich, M.; Xia, T.; Ruehm, S.G.; Nel, A.E.; Tamanoi, F.; Zink, J.I. Multifunctional inorganic nanoparticles for imaging, targeting, and drug delivery. *ACS Nano* **2008**, *2*, 889–896. [CrossRef]
13. Pérez-Esteve, É.; Ruiz-Rico, M.; de la Torre, C.; Llorca, E.; Sancenón, F.; Marcos, M.D.; Amorós, P.; Guillem, C.; Martínez-Máñez, R.; Barat, J.M. Stability of different mesoporous silica particles during an in vitro digestion. *Microporous Mesoporous Mater.* **2016**, *230*, 196–207. [CrossRef]
14. Riikonen, J.; Xu, W.; Lehto, V.-P. Mesoporous systems for poorly soluble drugs—Recent trends. *Int. J. Pharm.* **2018**, *536*, 178–186. [CrossRef] [PubMed]
15. Maleki, A.; Kettiger, H.; Schoubben, A.; Rosenholm, J.M.; Ambrogi, V.; Hamidi, M. Mesoporous silica materials: From physicochemical properties to enhanced dissolution of poorly water-soluble drugs. *J. Control. Release* **2017**, *262*, 329–347. [CrossRef]
16. Ambrogi, V.; Perioli, L.; Pagano, C.; Latterini, L.; Marmottini, F.; Ricci, M.; Rossi, C. MCM-41 for furosemide dissolution improvement. *Microporous Mesoporous Mater.* **2012**, *147*, 343–349. [CrossRef]
17. Yang, G.; Li, Z.; Wu, F.; Chen, M.; Wang, R.; Zhu, H.; Li, Q.; Yuan, Y. Improving Solubility and Bioavailability of Breviscapine with Mesoporous Silica Nanoparticles Prepared Using Ultrasound-Assisted Solution-Enhanced Dispersion by Supercritical Fluids Method. *Int. J. Nanomed.* **2020**, *15*, 1661–1675. [CrossRef] [PubMed]
18. McCarthy, C.A.; Ahern, R.J.; Dontireddy, R.; Ryan, K.B.; Crean, A.M. Mesoporous silica formulation strategies for drug dissolution enhancement: A review. *Expert Opin. Drug Deliv.* **2016**, *13*, 93–108. [CrossRef] [PubMed]
19. Kumar, D.; Sailaja Chirravuri, S.V.; Shastri, N.R. Impact of surface area of silica particles on dissolution rate and oral bioavailability of poorly water soluble drugs: A case study with aceclofenac. *Int. J. Pharm.* **2014**, *461*, 459–468. [CrossRef]
20. Huang, Y.; Zhao, X.; Zu, Y.; Wang, L.; Deng, Y.; Wu, M.; Wang, H. Enhanced Solubility and Bioavailability of Apigenin via Preparation of Solid Dispersions of Mesoporous Silica Nanoparticles. *Iran. J. Pharm. Res.* **2019**, *18*, 168–182.
21. Zhang, Q.; Wang, X.; Li, P.-Z.; Nguyen, K.T.; Wang, X.-J.; Luo, Z.; Zhang, H.; Tan, N.S.; Zhao, Y. Biocompatible, Uniform, and Redispersible Mesoporous Silica Nanoparticles for Cancer-Targeted Drug Delivery In Vivo. *Adv. Funct. Mater.* **2014**, *24*, 2450–2461. [CrossRef]

22. Argyo, C.; Weiss, V.; Bräuchle, C.; Bein, T. Multifunctional Mesoporous Silica Nanoparticles as a Universal Platform for Drug Delivery. *Chem. Mater.* **2014**, *26*, 435–451. [CrossRef]
23. Lu, J.; Liong, M.; Li, Z.; Zink, J.I.; Tamanoi, F. Biocompatibility, Biodistribution, and Drug-Delivery Efficiency of Mesoporous Silica Nanoparticles for Cancer Therapy in Animals. *Small* **2010**, *6*, 1794–1805. [CrossRef] [PubMed]
24. Kwon, D.; Cha, B.G.; Cho, Y.; Min, J.; Park, E.B.; Kang, S.J.; Kim, J. Extra-Large Pore Mesoporous Silica Nanoparticles for Directing in Vivo M2 Macrophage Polarization by Delivering IL-4. *Nano Lett.* **2017**, *17*, 2747–2756. [CrossRef] [PubMed]
25. Malvindi, M.A.; Brunetti, V.; Vecchio, G.; Galeone, A.; Cingolani, R.; Pompa, P.P. SiO2 nanoparticles biocompatibility and their potential for gene delivery and silencing. *Nanoscale* **2012**, *4*, 486–495. [CrossRef]
26. Abeer, M.M.; Rewatkar, P.; Qu, Z.; Talekar, M.; Kleitz, F.; Schmid, R.; Lindén, M.; Kumeria, T.; Popat, A. Silica nanoparticles: A promising platform for enhanced oral delivery of macromolecules. *J. Control. Release* **2020**, *326*, 544–555. [CrossRef] [PubMed]
27. Diab, R.; Canilho, N.; Pavel, I.A.; Haffner, F.B.; Girardon, M.; Pasc, A. Silica-based systems for oral delivery of drugs, macromolecules and cells. *Adv. Colloid Interface Sci.* **2017**, *249*, 346–362. [CrossRef] [PubMed]
28. Mohammadpour, R.; Cheney, D.L.; Grunberger, J.W.; Yazdimamaghani, M.; Jedrzkiewicz, J.; Isaacson, K.J.; Dobrovolskaia, M.A.; Ghandehari, H. One-year chronic toxicity evaluation of single dose intravenously administered silica nanoparticles in mice and their Ex vivo human hemocompatibility. *J. Control. Release* **2020**, *324*, 471–481. [CrossRef]
29. Fu, C.; Liu, T.; Li, L.; Liu, H.; Chen, D.; Tang, F. The absorption, distribution, excretion and toxicity of mesoporous silica nanoparticles in mice following different exposure routes. *Biomaterials* **2013**, *34*, 2565–2575. [CrossRef]
30. Huang, X.; Li, L.; Liu, T.; Hao, N.; Liu, H.; Chen, D.; Tang, F. The shape effect of mesoporous silica nanoparticles on biodistribution, clearance, and biocompatibility in vivo. *ACS Nano* **2011**, *5*, 5390–5399. [CrossRef]
31. Watermann, A.; Brieger, J. Mesoporous Silica Nanoparticles as Drug Delivery Vehicles in Cancer. *Nanomaterials* **2017**, *7*, 189. [CrossRef]
32. Vallet-Regí, M.; Colilla, M.; Izquierdo-Barba, I.; Manzano, M. Mesoporous Silica Nanoparticles for Drug Delivery: Current Insights. *Molecules* **2018**, *23*, 47. [CrossRef]
33. Bukara, K.; Schueller, L.; Rosier, J.; Martens, M.A.; Daems, T.; Verheyden, L.; Eelen, S.; Van Speybroeck, M.; Libanati, C.; Martens, J.A.; et al. Ordered mesoporous silica to enhance the bioavailability of poorly water-soluble drugs: Proof of concept in man. *Eur. J. Pharm. Biopharm.* **2016**, *108*, 220–225. [CrossRef]
34. Cragg, G.M.; Newman, D.J. Plants as a source of anti-cancer agents. *J. Ethnopharmacol.* **2005**, *100*, 72–79. [CrossRef] [PubMed]
35. Harvey, A.L. Natural products in drug discovery. *Drug Discov. Today* **2008**, *13*, 894–901. [CrossRef] [PubMed]
36. Hostettmann, K.; Marston, A. The Search for New Drugs from Higher Plants. *Chim. Int. J. Chem.* **2007**, *61*, 322–326. [CrossRef]
37. Atanasov, A.G.; Waltenberger, B.; Pferschy-Wenzig, E.M.; Linder, T.; Wawrosch, C.; Uhrin, P.; Temml, V.; Wang, L.; Schwaiger, S.; Heiss, E.H.; et al. Discovery and resupply of pharmacologically active plant-derived natural products: A review. *Biotechnol. Adv.* **2015**, *33*, 1582–1614. [CrossRef]
38. Ji, H.-F.; Li, X.-J.; Zhang, H.-Y. Natural products and drug discovery. *EMBO Rep.* **2009**, *10*, 194–200. [CrossRef]
39. Watkins, R.; Wu, L.; Zhang, C.; Davis, R.M.; Xu, B. Natural product-based nanomedicine: Recent advances and issues. *Int. J. Nanomed.* **2015**, *10*, 6055–6074. [CrossRef]
40. Aljuffali, I.A.; Fang, C.L.; Chen, C.H.; Fang, J.Y. Nanomedicine as a Strategy for Natural Compound Delivery to Prevent and Treat Cancers. *Curr. Pharm. Des.* **2016**, *22*, 4219–4231. [CrossRef]
41. Fonseca-Santos, B.; Chorilli, M. The uses of resveratrol for neurological diseases treatment and insights for nanotechnology based drug delivery systems. *Int. J. Pharm.* **2020**, 119832. [CrossRef]
42. AbouAitah, K.; Swiderska-Sroda, A.; Farghali, A.A.; Wojnarowicz, J.; Stefanek, A.; Gierlotka, S.; Opalinska, A.; Allayeh, A.K.; Ciach, T.; Lojkowski, W. Folic acid-conjugated mesoporous silica particles as nanocarriers of natural prodrugs for cancer targeting and antioxidant action. *Oncotarget* **2018**, *9*, 26466–26490. [CrossRef]
43. AbouAitah, K.; Hassan, H.A.; Swiderska-Sroda, A.; Gohar, L.; Shaker, O.G.; Wojnarowicz, J.; Opalinska, A.; Smalc-Koziorowska, J.; Gierlotka, S.; Lojkowski, W. Targeted Nano-Drug Delivery of Colchicine against Colon Cancer Cells by Means of Mesoporous Silica Nanoparticles. *Cancers* **2020**, *12*, 144. [CrossRef]
44. Shahein, S.A.; Aboul-Enein, A.M.; Higazy, I.M.; Abou-Elella, F.; Lojkowski, W.; Ahmed, E.R.; Mousa, S.A.; AbouAitah, K. Targeted anticancer potential against glioma cells of thymoquinone delivered by mesoporous silica core-shell nanoformulations with pH-dependent release. *Int. J. Nanomed.* **2019**, *14*, 5503–5526. [CrossRef]
45. Bisht, S.; Feldmann, G.; Soni, S.; Ravi, R.; Karikar, C.; Maitra, A.; Maitra, A. Polymeric nanoparticle-encapsulated curcumin ("nanocurcumin"): A novel strategy for human cancer therapy. *J. Nanobiotechnol.* **2007**, *5*, 3. [CrossRef] [PubMed]
46. Pool, H.; Quintanar, D.; Figueroa, J.D.D.; Marinho Mano, C.; Bechara, J.E.H.; Godínez, L.A.; Mendoza, S. Antioxidant Effects of Quercetin and Catechin Encapsulated into PLGA Nanoparticles. *J. Nanomater.* **2012**, *2012*, 145380. [CrossRef]
47. Fang, Q.; Sculley, J.; Zhou, H.C.J.; Zhu, G. 5.01—Porous Metal–Organic Frameworks. In *Comprehensive Nanoscience and Technology*; Andrews, D.L., Scholes, G.D., Wiederrecht, G.P., Eds.; Academic Press: Amsterdam, The Netherlands, 2011; pp. 1–20.
48. Sing, K.S.W. Reporting physisorption data for gas/solid systems. *Pure Appl. Chem.* **1982**, *54*, 2201–2218. [CrossRef]
49. Sing, K.S.W. Reporting physisorption data for gas/solid systems with special reference to the determination of surface area and porosity (Recommendations 1984). *Pure Appl. Chem.* **1985**, *57*, 603–619. [CrossRef]

50. Beck, J.S.; Vartuli, J.C.; Roth, W.J.; Leonowicz, M.E.; Kresge, C.T.; Schmitt, K.D.; Chu, C.T.W.; Olson, D.H.; Sheppard, E.W.; McCullen, S.B.; et al. A new family of mesoporous molecular sieves prepared with liquid crystal templates. *J. Am. Chem. Soc.* **1992**, *114*, 10834–10843. [CrossRef]
51. Inagaki, S.; Fukushima, Y.; Kuroda, K. Synthesis of highly ordered mesoporous materials from a layered polysilicate. *J. Chem. Soc. Chem. Commun.* **1993**, 680–682. [CrossRef]
52. Hoffmann, F.; Cornelius, M.; Morell, J.; Fröba, M. Silica-Based Mesoporous Organic–Inorganic Hybrid Materials. *Angew. Chem. Int. Ed.* **2006**, *45*, 3216–3251. [CrossRef]
53. Ryoo, R.; Kim, J.M.; Ko, C.H.; Shin, C.H. Disordered Molecular Sieve with Branched Mesoporous Channel Network. *J. Phys. Chem.* **1996**, *100*, 17718–17721. [CrossRef]
54. Zhou, B.; Li, C.Y.; Qi, N.; Jiang, M.; Wang, B.; Chen, Z.Q. Pore structure of mesoporous silica (KIT-6) synthesized at different temperatures using positron as a nondestructive probe. *Appl. Surf. Sci.* **2018**, *450*, 31–37. [CrossRef]
55. Deka, J.R.; Lin, Y.-H.; Kao, H.-M. Ordered cubic mesoporous silica KIT-5 functionalized with carboxylic acid groups for dye removal. *RSC Adv.* **2014**, *4*, 49061–49069. [CrossRef]
56. Zhao, D.; Feng, J.; Huo, Q.; Melosh, N.; Fredrickson, G.H.; Chmelka, B.F.; Stucky, G.D. Triblock Copolymer Syntheses of Mesoporous Silica with Periodic 50 to 300 Angstrom Pores. *Science* **1998**, *279*, 548. [CrossRef] [PubMed]
57. Widenmeyer, M.; Anwander, R. Pore Size Control of Highly Ordered Mesoporous Silica MCM-48. *Chem. Mater.* **2002**, *14*, 1827–1831. [CrossRef]
58. Lin, L.-C.; Thirumavalavan, M.; Wang, Y.-T.; Lee, J.-F. Surface area and pore size tailoring of mesoporous silica materials by different hydrothermal treatments and adsorption of heavy metal ions. *Colloids Surf. A Physicochem. Eng. Asp.* **2010**, *369*, 223–231. [CrossRef]
59. Polshettiwar, V.; Cha, D.; Zhang, X.; Basset, J.M. High-Surface-Area Silica Nanospheres (KCC-1) with a Fibrous Morphology. *Angew. Chem. Int. Ed.* **2010**, *49*, 9652–9656. [CrossRef] [PubMed]
60. Bayal, N.; Singh, B.; Singh, R.; Polshettiwar, V. Size and Fiber Density Controlled Synthesis of Fibrous Nanosilica Spheres (KCC-1). *Sci. Rep.* **2016**, *6*, 24888. [CrossRef] [PubMed]
61. Zhang, S.; Qian, Y.; Ahn, W.-S. Catalytic dehydrogenation of formic acid over palladium nanoparticles immobilized on fibrous mesoporous silica KCC-1. *Chin. J. Catal.* **2019**, *40*, 1704–1712. [CrossRef]
62. Zarei, F.; Marjani, A.; Soltani, R. Novel and green nanocomposite-based adsorbents from functionalised mesoporous KCC-1 and chitosan-oleic acid for adsorption of Pb(II). *Eur. Polym. J.* **2019**, *119*, 400–409. [CrossRef]
63. Soleymani, J.; Hasanzadeh, M.; Somi, M.H.; Shadjou, N.; Jouyban, A. Highly sensitive and specific cytosensing of HT 29 colorectal cancer cells using folic acid functionalized-KCC-1 nanoparticles. *Biosens. Bioelectron.* **2019**, *132*, 122–131. [CrossRef]
64. Abbasy, L.; Mohammadzadeh, A.; Hasanzadeh, M.; Ehsani, M.; Mokhtarzadeh, A. Biosensing of prostate specific antigen (PSA) in human plasma samples using biomacromolecule encapsulation into KCC-1-npr-NH2: A new platform for prostate cancer detection. *Int. J. Biol. Macromol.* **2020**, *154*, 584–595. [CrossRef]
65. Ali, Z.; Tian, L.; Zhao, P.; Zhang, B.; Ali, N.; Khan, M.; Zhang, Q. Immobilization of lipase on mesoporous silica nanoparticles with hierarchical fibrous pore. *J. Mol. Catal. B Enzym.* **2016**, *134*, 129–135. [CrossRef]
66. Follmann, H.D.M.; Oliveira, O.N.; Martins, A.C.; Lazarin-Bidóia, D.; Nakamura, C.V.; Rubira, A.F.; Silva, R.; Asefa, T. Nanofibrous silica microparticles/polymer hybrid aerogels for sustained delivery of poorly water-soluble camptothecin. *J. Colloid Interface Sci.* **2020**, *567*, 92–102. [CrossRef] [PubMed]
67. Peng, H.; Wang, D.; Xu, L.; Wu, P. One-pot synthesis of primary amides on bifunctional Rh(OH)x/TS-1@KCC-1 catalysts. *Chin. J. Catal.* **2013**, *34*, 2057–2065. [CrossRef]
68. AbouAitah, K.E.A.; Farghali, A.A.; Swiderska-Sroda, A.; Lojkowski, W.; Razin, A.M. Mesoporous silica materials in drug delivery system: pH/glutathione-responsive release of poorly water-soluble pro-drug quercetin from two and three-dimensional pore-structure nanoparticles. *J. Nanomed. Nanotechnol.* **2016**, 7. [CrossRef]
69. AbouAitah, K.E.A.; Farghali, A.A.; Swiderska-Sroda, A.; Lojkowski, W.; Razin, A.M. pH-controlled release system for curcumin based on functionalized dendritic mesoporous silica nanoparticles. *J. Nanomed. Nanotechnol.* **2016**, *7*, 1–11.
70. Lin, J.; Peng, C.; Ravi, S.; Siddiki, A.K.M.N.A.; Zheng, J.; Balkus, K.J. Biphenyl Wrinkled Mesoporous Silica Nanoparticles for pH-Responsive Doxorubicin Drug Delivery. *Materials* **2020**, *13*, 1998. [CrossRef]
71. Moon, D.-S.; Lee, J.-K. Tunable Synthesis of Hierarchical Mesoporous Silica Nanoparticles with Radial Wrinkle Structure. *Langmuir* **2012**, *28*, 12341–12347. [CrossRef]
72. Wang, R.; Habib, E.; Zhu, X.X. Synthesis of wrinkled mesoporous silica and its reinforcing effect for dental resin composites. *Dent. Mater.* **2017**, *33*, 1139–1148. [CrossRef]
73. Maity, A.; Polshettiwar, V. Dendritic Fibrous Nanosilica for Catalysis, Energy Harvesting, Carbon Dioxide Mitigation, Drug Delivery, and Sensing. *ChemSusChem* **2017**, *10*, 3866–3913. [CrossRef]
74. Szczęśniak, B.; Choma, J.; Jaroniec, M. Major advances in the development of ordered mesoporous materials. *Chem. Commun.* **2020**, *56*, 7836–7848. [CrossRef]
75. Xu, C.; Lei, C.; Yu, C. Mesoporous Silica Nanoparticles for Protein Protection and Delivery. *Front. Chem.* **2019**, *7*, 290. [CrossRef]
76. Douroumis, D.; Onyesom, I.; Maniruzzaman, M.; Mitchell, J. Mesoporous silica nanoparticles in nanotechnology. *Crit. Rev. Biotechnol.* **2013**, *33*, 229–245. [CrossRef]

77. Wu, S.-H.; Mou, C.-Y.; Lin, H.-P. Synthesis of mesoporous silica nanoparticles. *Chem. Soc. Rev.* **2013**, *42*, 3862–3875. [CrossRef] [PubMed]
78. Farjadian, F.; Roointan, A.; Mohammadi-Samani, S.; Hosseini, M. Mesoporous silica nanoparticles: Synthesis, pharmaceutical applications, biodistribution, and biosafety assessment. *Chem. Eng. J.* **2019**, *359*, 684–705. [CrossRef]
79. Castillo, R.R.; Lozano, D.; González, B.; Manzano, M.; Izquierdo-Barba, I.; Vallet-Regí, M. Advances in mesoporous silica nanoparticles for targeted stimuli-responsive drug delivery: An update. *Expert Opin. Drug Deliv.* **2019**, *16*, 415–439. [CrossRef] [PubMed]
80. Paris, J.L.; Vallet-Regí, M. Mesoporous Silica Nanoparticles for Co-Delivery of Drugs and Nucleic Acids in Oncology: A Review. *Pharmaceutics* **2020**, *12*, 526. [CrossRef]
81. Aquib, M.; Farooq, M.A.; Banerjee, P.; Akhtar, F.; Filli, M.S.; Boakye-Yiadom, K.O.; Kesse, S.; Raza, F.; Maviah, M.B.J.; Mavlyanova, R.; et al. Targeted and stimuli-responsive mesoporous silica nanoparticles for drug delivery and theranostic use. *J. Biomed. Mater. Res. Part A* **2019**, *107*, 2643–2666. [CrossRef]
82. Hadipour Moghaddam, S.P.; Mohammadpour, R.; Ghandehari, H. In vitro and in vivo evaluation of degradation, toxicity, biodistribution, and clearance of silica nanoparticles as a function of size, porosity, density, and composition. *J. Control. Release* **2019**, *311–312*, 1–15. [CrossRef]
83. Li, Z.; Zhang, Y.; Feng, N. Mesoporous silica nanoparticles: Synthesis, classification, drug loading, pharmacokinetics, biocompatibility, and application in drug delivery. *Expert Opin. Drug Deliv.* **2019**, *16*, 219–237. [CrossRef]
84. Nieto, A.; Colilla, M.; Balas, F.; Vallet-Regí, M. Surface Electrochemistry of Mesoporous Silicas as a Key Factor in the Design of Tailored Delivery Devices. *Langmuir* **2010**, *26*, 5038–5049. [CrossRef]
85. Vallet-Regí, M.; Balas, F.; Arcos, D. Mesoporous Materials for Drug Delivery. *Angew. Chem. Int. Ed.* **2007**, *46*, 7548–7558. [CrossRef] [PubMed]
86. Rahikkala, A.; Rosenholm, J.M.; Santos, H.A. Chapter 16—Biofunctionalized Mesoporous Silica Nanomaterials for Targeted Drug Delivery. In *Biomedical Applications of Functionalized Nanomaterials*; Sarmento, B., das Neves, J., Eds.; Elsevier: Amsterdam, The Netherlands, 2018; pp. 489–520.
87. Stein, A.; Melde, B.J.; Schroden, R.C. Hybrid Inorganic–Organic Mesoporous Silicates—Nanoscopic Reactors Coming of Age. *Adv. Mater.* **2000**, *12*, 1403–1419. [CrossRef]
88. Tarn, D.; Ashley, C.E.; Xue, M.; Carnes, E.C.; Zink, J.I.; Brinker, C.J. Mesoporous Silica Nanoparticle Nanocarriers: Biofunctionality and Biocompatibility. *Acc. Chem. Res.* **2013**, *46*, 792–801. [CrossRef] [PubMed]
89. Huh, S.; Wiench, J.W.; Yoo, J.-C.; Pruski, M.; Lin, V.S.Y. Organic Functionalization and Morphology Control of Mesoporous Silicas via a Co-Condensation Synthesis Method. *Chem. Mater.* **2003**, *15*, 4247–4256. [CrossRef]
90. Lu, J.; Liong, M.; Zink, J.I.; Tamanoi, F. Mesoporous Silica Nanoparticles as a Delivery System for Hydrophobic Anticancer Drugs. *Small* **2007**, *3*, 1341–1346. [CrossRef] [PubMed]
91. Sayari, A.; Hamoudi, S. Periodic Mesoporous Silica-Based Organic–Inorganic Nanocomposite Materials. *Chem. Mater.* **2001**, *13*, 3151–3168. [CrossRef]
92. Wu, S.-H.; Hung, Y.; Mou, C.-Y. Mesoporous silica nanoparticles as nanocarriers. *Chem. Commun.* **2011**, *47*, 9972–9985. [CrossRef] [PubMed]
93. Manzanares, D.; Ceña, V. Endocytosis: The Nanoparticle and Submicron Nanocompounds Gateway into the Cell. *Pharmaceutics* **2020**, *12*, 371. [CrossRef]
94. Kou, L.; Sun, J.; Zhai, Y.; He, Z. The endocytosis and intracellular fate of nanomedicines: Implication for rational design. *Asian J. Pharm. Sci.* **2013**, *8*, 1–10. [CrossRef]
95. Borbás, E.; Sinkó, B.; Tsinman, O.; Tsinman, K.; Kiserdei, É.; Démuth, B.; Balogh, A.; Bodák, B.; Domokos, A.; Dargó, G.; et al. Investigation and Mathematical Description of the Real Driving Force of Passive Transport of Drug Molecules from Supersaturated Solutions. *Mol. Pharm.* **2016**, *13*, 3816–3826. [CrossRef]
96. Doherty, G.J.; McMahon, H.T. Mechanisms of Endocytosis. *Annu. Rev. Biochem.* **2009**, *78*, 857–902. [CrossRef] [PubMed]
97. Rewatkar, P.; Kumeria, T.; Popat, A. Chapter 5—Size, shape and surface charge considerations of orally delivered nanomedicines. In *Nanotechnology for Oral Drug Delivery*; Martins, J.P., Santos, H.A., Eds.; Academic Press: Cambridge, MA, USA, 2020; pp. 143–176.
98. He, C.; Hu, Y.; Yin, L.; Tang, C.; Yin, C. Effects of particle size and surface charge on cellular uptake and biodistribution of polymeric nanoparticles. *Biomaterials* **2010**, *31*, 3657–3666. [CrossRef] [PubMed]
99. McMahon, H.T.; Boucrot, E. Molecular mechanism and physiological functions of clathrin-mediated endocytosis. *Nat. Rev. Mol. Cell Biol.* **2011**, *12*, 517–533. [CrossRef] [PubMed]
100. Sahay, G.; Alakhova, D.Y.; Kabanov, A.V. Endocytosis of nanomedicines. *J. Control. Release* **2010**, *145*, 182–195. [CrossRef]
101. Foroozandeh, P.; Aziz, A.A. Insight into Cellular Uptake and Intracellular Trafficking of Nanoparticles. *Nanoscale Res. Lett.* **2018**, *13*, 339. [CrossRef]
102. Gustafson, H.H.; Holt-Casper, D.; Grainger, D.W.; Ghandehari, H. Nanoparticle Uptake: The Phagocyte Problem. *Nano Today* **2015**, *10*, 487–510. [CrossRef]
103. Lu, F.; Wu, S.-H.; Hung, Y.; Mou, C.-Y. Size Effect on Cell Uptake in Well-Suspended, Uniform Mesoporous Silica Nanoparticles. *Small* **2009**, *5*, 1408–1413. [CrossRef]

104. Gratton, S.E.A.; Ropp, P.A.; Pohlhaus, P.D.; Luft, J.C.; Madden, V.J.; Napier, M.E.; DeSimone, J.M. The effect of particle design on cellular internalization pathways. *Proc. Natl. Acad. Sci. USA* **2008**, *105*, 11613–11618. [CrossRef]
105. Min, Y.; Akbulut, M.; Kristiansen, K.; Golan, Y.; Israelachvili, J. The role of interparticle and external forces in nanoparticle assembly. In *Nanoscience and Technology: A Collection of Reviews from Nature Journals*; World Scientific: Singapore, 2010; pp. 38–49.
106. Wei, P.; Zhang, L.; Lu, Y.; Man, N.; Wen, L. C60 (Nd) nanoparticles enhance chemotherapeutic susceptibility of cancer cells by modulation of autophagy. *Nanotechnology* **2010**, *21*, 495101. [CrossRef]
107. Song, L.; Wengang, L.; Niveen, M.K. Stimuli responsive nanomaterials for controlled release applications. *Nanotechnol. Rev.* **2012**, *1*, 493–513. [CrossRef]
108. Behzadi, S.; Serpooshan, V.; Tao, W.; Hamaly, M.A.; Alkawareek, M.Y.; Dreaden, E.C.; Brown, D.; Alkilany, A.M.; Farokhzad, O.C.; Mahmoudi, M. Cellular uptake of nanoparticles: Journey inside the cell. *Chem. Soc. Rev.* **2017**, *46*, 4218–4244. [CrossRef] [PubMed]
109. Biswas, A.K.; Islam, M.R.; Choudhury, Z.S.; Mostafa, A.; Kadir, M.F. Nanotechnology based approaches in cancer therapeutics. *Adv. Nat. Sci. Nanosci. Nanotechnol.* **2014**, *5*, 043001. [CrossRef]
110. Neuberger, T.; Schöpf, B.; Hofmann, H.; Hofmann, M.; von Rechenberg, B. Superparamagnetic nanoparticles for biomedical applications: Possibilities and limitations of a new drug delivery system. *J. Magn. Magn. Mater.* **2005**, *293*, 483–496. [CrossRef]
111. Maruyama, K. Intracellular targeting delivery of liposomal drugs to solid tumors based on EPR effects. *Adv. Drug Deliv. Rev.* **2011**, *63*, 161–169. [CrossRef]
112. Maeda, H.; Wu, J.; Sawa, T.; Matsumura, Y.; Hori, K. Tumor vascular permeability and the EPR effect in macromolecular therapeutics: A review. *J. Control. Release* **2000**, *65*, 271–284. [CrossRef]
113. Haddick, L.; Zhang, W.; Reinhard, S.; Möller, K.; Engelke, H.; Wagner, E.; Bein, T. Particle-Size-Dependent Delivery of Antitumoral miRNA Using Targeted Mesoporous Silica Nanoparticles. *Pharmaceutics* **2020**, *12*, 505. [CrossRef]
114. Yang, Y.; Karmakar, S.; Zhang, J.; Yu, M.; Mitter, N.; Yu, C. Synthesis of SBA-15 rods with small sizes for enhanced cellular uptake. *J. Mater. Chem. B* **2014**, *2*, 4929–4934. [CrossRef]
115. Zhu, M.; Nie, G.; Meng, H.; Xia, T.; Nel, A.; Zhao, Y. Physicochemical Properties Determine Nanomaterial Cellular Uptake, Transport, and Fate. *Acc. Chem. Res.* **2013**, *46*, 622–631. [CrossRef]
116. Panariti, A.; Miserocchi, G.; Rivolta, I. The effect of nanoparticle uptake on cellular behavior: Disrupting or enabling functions? *Nanotechnol. Sci. Appl.* **2012**, *5*, 87–100. [CrossRef]
117. Adjei, I.M.; Sharma, B.; Labhasetwar, V. Nanoparticles: Cellular uptake and cytotoxicity. *Adv. Exp. Med. Biol* **2014**, *811*, 73–91. [CrossRef]
118. Marano, F.; Hussain, S.; Rodrigues-Lima, F.; Baeza-Squiban, A.; Boland, S. Nanoparticles: Molecular targets and cell signalling. *Arch. Toxicol.* **2011**, *85*, 733–741. [CrossRef] [PubMed]
119. Fröhlich, E. The role of surface charge in cellular uptake and cytotoxicity of medical nanoparticles. *Int. J. Nanomed.* **2012**, *7*, 5577–5591. [CrossRef] [PubMed]
120. Allen, T.M.; Austin, G.A.; Chonn, A.; Lin, L.; Lee, K.C. Uptake of liposomes by cultured mouse bone marrow macrophages: Influence of liposome composition and size. *Biochim. Biophys. Acta (BBA) Biomembr.* **1991**, *1061*, 56–64. [CrossRef]
121. Arvizo, R.R.; Miranda, O.R.; Thompson, M.A.; Pabelick, C.M.; Bhattacharya, R.; Robertson, J.D.; Rotello, V.M.; Prakash, Y.S.; Mukherjee, P. Effect of Nanoparticle Surface Charge at the Plasma Membrane and Beyond. *Nano Lett.* **2010**, *10*, 2543–2548. [CrossRef]
122. Wang, B.; Zhang, L.; Bae, S.C.; Granick, S. Nanoparticle-induced surface reconstruction of phospholipid membranes. *Proc. Natl. Acad. Sci. USA* **2008**, *105*, 18171–18175. [CrossRef]
123. Dausend, J.; Musyanovych, A.; Dass, M.; Walther, P.; Schrezenmeier, H.; Landfester, K.; Mailänder, V. Uptake Mechanism of Oppositely Charged Fluorescent Nanoparticles in HeLa Cells. *Macromol. Biosci.* **2008**, *8*, 1135–1143. [CrossRef]
124. Jambhrunkar, S.; Qu, Z.; Popat, A.; Yang, J.; Noonan, O.; Acauan, L.; Ahmad Nor, Y.; Yu, C.; Karmakar, S. Effect of Surface Functionality of Silica Nanoparticles on Cellular Uptake and Cytotoxicity. *Mol. Pharm.* **2014**, *11*, 3642–3655. [CrossRef]
125. Baghirov, H.; Karaman, D.; Viitala, T.; Duchanoy, A.; Lou, Y.-R.; Mamaeva, V.; Pryazhnikov, E.; Khiroug, L.; de Lange Davies, C.; Sahlgren, C.; et al. Feasibility Study of the Permeability and Uptake of Mesoporous Silica Nanoparticles across the Blood-Brain Barrier. *PLoS ONE* **2016**, *11*, e0160705. [CrossRef]
126. Trewyn, B.G.; Nieweg, J.A.; Zhao, Y.; Lin, V.S.Y. Biocompatible mesoporous silica nanoparticles with different morphologies for animal cell membrane penetration. *Chem. Eng. J.* **2008**, *137*, 23–29. [CrossRef]
127. Huang, X.; Teng, X.; Chen, D.; Tang, F.; He, J. The effect of the shape of mesoporous silica nanoparticles on cellular uptake and cell function. *Biomaterials* **2010**, *31*, 438–448. [CrossRef]
128. Dias, D.R.; Moreira, A.F.; Correia, I.J. The effect of the shape of gold core–mesoporous silica shell nanoparticles on the cellular behavior and tumor spheroid penetration. *J. Mater. Chem. B* **2016**, *4*, 7630–7640. [CrossRef] [PubMed]
129. Pada, A.-K.; Desai, D.; Sun, K.; Prakirth Govardhanam, N.; Törnquist, K.; Zhang, J.; Rosenholm, J.M. Comparison of Polydopamine-Coated Mesoporous Silica Nanorods and Spheres for the Delivery of Hydrophilic and Hydrophobic Anticancer Drugs. *Int. J. Mol. Sci.* **2019**, *20*, 3408. [CrossRef] [PubMed]
130. Hao, N.; Li, L.; Tang, F. Shape matters when engineering mesoporous silica-based nanomedicines. *Biomater. Sci.* **2016**, *4*, 575–591. [CrossRef] [PubMed]

131. Tang, F.; Li, L.; Chen, D. Mesoporous Silica Nanoparticles: Synthesis, Biocompatibility and Drug Delivery. *Adv. Mater.* **2012**, *24*, 1504–1534. [CrossRef]
132. Niculescu, V.-C. Mesoporous Silica Nanoparticles for Bio-Applications. *Front. Mater.* **2020**, *7*. [CrossRef]
133. Hosseinpour, S.; Walsh, L.J.; Xu, C. Biomedical application of mesoporous silica nanoparticles as delivery systems: A biological safety perspective. *J. Mater. Chem. B* **2020**, *8*, 9863–9876. [CrossRef]
134. Trewyn, B.G.; Giri, S.; Slowing, I.I.; Lin, V.S.Y. Mesoporous silica nanoparticle based controlled release, drug delivery, and biosensor systems. *Chem. Commun.* **2007**, 3236–3245. [CrossRef]
135. Manzano, M.; Colilla, M.; Vallet-Regí, M. Drug delivery from ordered mesoporous matrices. *Expert Opin Drug Deliv* **2009**, *6*, 1383–1400. [CrossRef]
136. Vivero-Escoto, J.L.; Slowing, I.I.; Trewyn, B.G.; Lin, V.S.Y. Mesoporous Silica Nanoparticles for Intracellular Controlled Drug Delivery. *Small* **2010**, *6*, 1952–1967. [CrossRef]
137. Asefa, T.; Tao, Z. Biocompatibility of Mesoporous Silica Nanoparticles. *Chem. Res. Toxicol.* **2012**, *25*, 2265–2284. [CrossRef]
138. Park, J.-H.; Gu, L.; von Maltzahn, G.; Ruoslahti, E.; Bhatia, S.N.; Sailor, M.J. Biodegradable luminescent porous silicon nanoparticles for in vivo applications. *Nat. Mater.* **2009**, *8*, 331–336. [CrossRef] [PubMed]
139. Hudson, S.P.; Padera, R.F.; Langer, R.; Kohane, D.S. The biocompatibility of mesoporous silicates. *Biomaterials* **2008**, *29*, 4045–4055. [CrossRef] [PubMed]
140. Yildirim, A.; Ozgur, E.; Bayindir, M. Impact of mesoporous silica nanoparticle surface functionality on hemolytic activity, thrombogenicity and non-specific protein adsorption. *J. Mater. Chem. B* **2013**, *1*, 1909–1920. [CrossRef] [PubMed]
141. Garrido-Cano, I.; Candela-Noguera, V.; Herrera, G.; Cejalvo, J.M.; Lluch, A.; Marcos, M.D.; Sancenon, F.; Eroles, P.; Martínez-Máñez, R. Biocompatibility and internalization assessment of bare and functionalised mesoporous silica nanoparticles. *Microporous Mesoporous Mater.* **2021**, 310. [CrossRef]
142. He, Q.; Zhang, Z.; Gao, F.; Li, Y.; Shi, J. In vivo Biodistribution and Urinary Excretion of Mesoporous Silica Nanoparticles: Effects of Particle Size and PEGylation. *Small* **2011**, *7*, 271–280. [CrossRef]
143. Yu, T.; Hubbard, D.; Ray, A.; Ghandehari, H. In vivo biodistribution and pharmacokinetics of silica nanoparticles as a function of geometry, porosity and surface characteristics. *J. Control. Release* **2012**, *163*, 46–54. [CrossRef]
144. Li, L.; Liu, T.; Fu, C.; Tan, L.; Meng, X.; Liu, H. Biodistribution, excretion, and toxicity of mesoporous silica nanoparticles after oral administration depend on their shape. *Nanomed. Nanotechnol. Biol. Med.* **2015**, *11*, 1915–1924. [CrossRef]
145. Zhao, Y.; Wang, Y.; Ran, F.; Cui, Y.; Liu, C.; Zhao, Q.; Gao, Y.; Wang, D.; Wang, S. A comparison between sphere and rod nanoparticles regarding their in vivo biological behavior and pharmacokinetics. *Sci. Rep.* **2017**, *7*, 4131. [CrossRef]
146. Janßen, H.C.; Warwas, D.P.; Dahlhaus, D.; Meißner, J.; Taptimthong, P.; Kietzmann, M.; Behrens, P.; Reifenrath, J.; Angrisani, N. In vitro and in vivo accumulation of magnetic nanoporous silica nanoparticles on implant materials with different magnetic properties. *J. Nanobiotechnol.* **2018**, *16*, 96. [CrossRef]
147. Li, H.; Wu, X.; Yang, B.; Li, J.; Xu, L.; Liu, H.; Li, S.; Xu, J.; Yang, M.; Wei, M. Evaluation of biomimetically synthesized mesoporous silica nanoparticles as drug carriers: Structure, wettability, degradation, biocompatibility and brain distribution. *Mater. Sci. Eng. C* **2019**, *94*, 453–464. [CrossRef]
148. Cho, M.; Cho, W.-S.; Choi, M.; Kim, S.J.; Han, B.S.; Kim, S.H.; Kim, H.O.; Sheen, Y.Y.; Jeong, J. The impact of size on tissue distribution and elimination by single intravenous injection of silica nanoparticles. *Toxicol. Lett.* **2009**, *189*, 177–183. [CrossRef] [PubMed]
149. Hornung, V.; Bauernfeind, F.; Halle, A.; Samstad, E.O.; Kono, H.; Rock, K.L.; Fitzgerald, K.A.; Latz, E. Silica crystals and aluminum salts activate the NALP3 inflammasome through phagosomal destabilization. *Nat. Immunol.* **2008**, *9*, 847–856. [CrossRef] [PubMed]
150. Jones, L.H.P.; Handreck, K.A. Silica In Soils, Plants, and Animals. In *Advances in Agronomy*; Norman, A.G., Ed.; Academic Press: Cambridge, MA, USA, 1967; Volume 19, pp. 107–149.
151. Rosenholm, J.M.; Mamaeva, V.; Sahlgren, C.; Lindén, M. Nanoparticles in targeted cancer therapy: Mesoporous silica nanoparticles entering preclinical development stage. *Nanomedicine* **2012**, *7*, 111–120. [CrossRef] [PubMed]
152. Martin, K.R. Silicon: The Health Benefits of a Metalloid. In *Interrelations between Essential Metal Ions and Human Diseases*; Sigel, A., Sigel, H., Sigel, R.K.O., Eds.; Springer: Dordrecht, The Netherlands, 2013; pp. 451–473.
153. Ehrlich, H.; Demadis, K.D.; Pokrovsky, O.S.; Koutsoukos, P.G. Modern Views on Desilicification: Biosilica and Abiotic Silica Dissolution in Natural and Artificial Environments. *Chem. Rev.* **2010**, *110*, 4656–4689. [CrossRef] [PubMed]
154. Martin, K.R. The chemistry of silica and its potential health benefits. *J. Nutr. Health Aging* **2007**, *11*, 94–97. [PubMed]
155. Croissant, J.G.; Fatieiev, Y.; Khashab, N.M. Degradability and Clearance of Silicon, Organosilica, Silsesquioxane, Silica Mixed Oxide, and Mesoporous Silica Nanoparticles. *Adv. Mater.* **2017**, *29*, 1604634. [CrossRef]
156. Carlisle, E.M. Silicon: A Possible Factor in Bone Calcification. *Science* **1970**, *167*, 279. [CrossRef]
157. Jugdaohsingh, R. Silicon and bone health. *J. Nutr Health Aging* **2007**, *11*, 99–110.
158. Benezra, M.; Penate-Medina, O.; Zanzonico, P.B.; Schaer, D.; Ow, H.; Burns, A.; DeStanchina, E.; Longo, V.; Herz, E.; Iyer, S.; et al. Multimodal silica nanoparticles are effective cancer-targeted probes in a model of human melanoma. *J. Clin. Investig.* **2011**, *121*, 2768–2780. [CrossRef]
159. Quan, G.; Pan, X.; Wang, Z.; Wu, Q.; Li, G.; Dian, L.; Chen, B.; Wu, C. Lactosaminated mesoporous silica nanoparticles for asialoglycoprotein receptor targeted anticancer drug delivery. *J. Nanobiotechnol.* **2015**, *13*, 7. [CrossRef]

160. Napierska, D.; Thomassen, L.C.J.; Lison, D.; Martens, J.A.; Hoet, P.H. The nanosilica hazard: Another variable entity. *Part. Fibre Toxicol.* **2010**, *7*, 39. [CrossRef] [PubMed]
161. Di Pasqua, A.J.; Sharma, K.K.; Shi, Y.-L.; Toms, B.B.; Ouellette, W.; Dabrowiak, J.C.; Asefa, T. Cytotoxicity of mesoporous silica nanomaterials. *J. Inorg. Biochem.* **2008**, *102*, 1416–1423. [CrossRef] [PubMed]
162. Lee, S.; Yun, H.-S.; Kim, S.-H. The comparative effects of mesoporous silica nanoparticles and colloidal silica on inflammation and apoptosis. *Biomaterials* **2011**, *32*, 9434–9443. [CrossRef] [PubMed]
163. Li, Y.; Sun, L.; Jin, M.; Du, Z.; Liu, X.; Guo, C.; Li, Y.; Huang, P.; Sun, Z. Size-dependent cytotoxicity of amorphous silica nanoparticles in human hepatoma HepG2 cells. *Toxicol. In Vitro* **2011**, *25*, 1343–1352. [CrossRef]
164. Liu, T.; Li, L.; Teng, X.; Huang, X.; Liu, H.; Chen, D.; Ren, J.; He, J.; Tang, F. Single and repeated dose toxicity of mesoporous hollow silica nanoparticles in intravenously exposed mice. *Biomaterials* **2011**, *32*, 1657–1668. [CrossRef]
165. Carvalho, G.C.; Sábio, R.M.; de Cássia Ribeiro, T.; Monteiro, A.S.; Pereira, D.V.; Ribeiro, S.J.L.; Chorilli, M. Highlights in Mesoporous Silica Nanoparticles as a Multifunctional Controlled Drug Delivery Nanoplatform for Infectious Diseases Treatment. *Pharm. Res.* **2020**, *37*, 191. [CrossRef]
166. Petushkov, A.; Ndiege, N.; Salem, A.K.; Larsen, S.C. Chapter 7—Toxicity of Silica Nanomaterials: Zeolites, Mesoporous Silica, and Amorphous Silica Nanoparticles. In *Advances in Molecular Toxicology*; Fishbein, J.C., Ed.; Elsevier: Amsterdam, The Netherlands, 2010; Volume 4, pp. 223–266.
167. Murugadoss, S.; Lison, D.; Godderis, L.; Van Den Brule, S.; Mast, J.; Brassinne, F.; Sebaihi, N.; Hoet, P.H. Toxicology of silica nanoparticles: An update. *Arch. Toxicol.* **2017**, *91*, 2967–3010. [CrossRef]
168. Croissant, J.G.; Fatieiev, Y.; Almalik, A.; Khashab, N.M. Mesoporous Silica and Organosilica Nanoparticles: Physical Chemistry, Biosafety, Delivery Strategies, and Biomedical Applications. *Adv. Healthc. Mater.* **2018**, *7*, 1700831. [CrossRef]
169. Nash, T.; Allison, A.C.; Harington, J.S. Physico-Chemical Properties of Silica in Relation to its Toxicity. *Nature* **1966**, *210*, 259–261. [CrossRef]
170. Zhang, H.; Dunphy, D.R.; Jiang, X.; Meng, H.; Sun, B.; Tarn, D.; Xue, M.; Wang, X.; Lin, S.; Ji, Z.; et al. Processing Pathway Dependence of Amorphous Silica Nanoparticle Toxicity: Colloidal vs Pyrolytic. *J. Am. Chem. Soc.* **2012**, *134*, 15790–15804. [CrossRef]
171. Bhavsar, D.; Patel, V.; Sawant, K. Systematic investigation of in vitro and in vivo safety, toxicity and degradation of mesoporous silica nanoparticles synthesized using commercial sodium silicate. *Microporous Mesoporous Mater.* **2019**, *284*, 343–352. [CrossRef]
172. Rascol, E.; Daurat, M.; Da Silva, A.; Maynadier, M.; Dorandeu, C.; Charnay, C.; Garcia, M.; Lai-Kee-Him, J.; Bron, P.; Auffan, M.; et al. Biological Fate of Fe3O4 Core-Shell Mesoporous Silica Nanoparticles Depending on Particle Surface Chemistry. *Nanomaterials* **2017**, *7*, 162. [CrossRef]
173. Rascol, E.; Pisani, C.; Dorandeu, C.; Nyalosaso, J.L.; Charnay, C.; Daurat, M.; Da Silva, A.; Devoisselle, J.-M.; Gaillard, J.-C.; Armengaud, J.; et al. Biosafety of Mesoporous Silica Nanoparticles. *Biomimetics* **2018**, *3*, 22. [CrossRef]
174. Nasr, S.S.; Nasra, M.M.A.; Hazzah, H.A.; Abdallah, O.Y. Mesoporous silica nanoparticles, a safe option for silymarin delivery: Preparation, characterization, and in vivo evaluation. *Drug Deliv. Transl. Res.* **2019**, *9*, 968–979. [CrossRef] [PubMed]
175. Rawat, N.; Sandhya; Subaharan, K.; Eswaramoorthy, M.; Kaul, G. Comparative in vivo toxicity assessment places multiwalled carbon nanotubes at a higher level than mesoporous silica nanoparticles. *Toxicol. Ind. Health* **2016**, *33*, 182–192. [CrossRef] [PubMed]
176. Lee, S.; Kim, M.S.; Lee, D.; Kwon, T.K.; Khang, D.; Yun, H.S.; Kim, S.H. The comparative immunotoxicity of mesoporous silica nanoparticles and colloidal silica nanoparticles in mice. *Int. J. Nanomed.* **2013**, *8*, 147–158. [CrossRef]
177. Limnell, T.; Santos, H.A.; Mäkilä, E.; Heikkilä, T.; Salonen, J.; Murzin, D.Y.; Kumar, N.; Laaksonen, T.; Peltonen, L.; Hirvonen, J. Drug delivery formulations of ordered and nonordered mesoporous silica: Comparison of three drug loading methods. *J. Pharm. Sci.* **2011**, *100*, 3294–3306. [CrossRef] [PubMed]
178. Rosenholm, J.M.; Lindén, M. Towards establishing structure-activity relationships for mesoporous silica in drug delivery applications. *J. Control. Release* **2008**, *128*, 157–164. [CrossRef] [PubMed]
179. Zhang, Z.; Wang, L.; Wang, J.; Jiang, X.; Li, X.; Hu, Z.; Ji, Y.; Wu, X.; Chen, C. Mesoporous Silica-Coated Gold Nanorods as a Light-Mediated Multifunctional Theranostic Platform for Cancer Treatment. *Adv. Mater.* **2012**, *24*, 1418–1423. [CrossRef] [PubMed]
180. She, X.; Chen, L.; Li, C.; He, C.; He, L.; Kong, L. Functionalization of Hollow Mesoporous Silica Nanoparticles for Improved 5-FU Loading. *J. Nanomater.* **2015**, *2015*, 872035. [CrossRef]
181. Doadrio, J.C.; Sousa, E.M.B.; Izquierdo-Barba, I.; Doadrio, A.L.; Perez-Pariente, J.; Vallet-Regí, M. Functionalization of mesoporous materials with long alkyl chains as a strategy for controlling drug delivery pattern. *J. Mater. Chem.* **2006**, *16*, 462–466. [CrossRef]
182. Balas, F.; Manzano, M.; Horcajada, P.; Vallet-Regí, M. Confinement and Controlled Release of Bisphosphonates on Ordered Mesoporous Silica-Based Materials. *J. Am. Chem. Soc.* **2006**, *128*, 8116–8117. [CrossRef] [PubMed]
183. Ibrahim, A.H.; Smått, J.-H.; Govardhanam, N.P.; Ibrahim, H.M.; Ismael, H.R.; Afouna, M.I.; Samy, A.M.; Rosenholm, J.M. Formulation and optimization of drug-loaded mesoporous silica nanoparticle-based tablets to improve the dissolution rate of the poorly water-soluble drug silymarin. *Eur. J. Pharm. Sci.* **2020**, *142*, 105103. [CrossRef] [PubMed]
184. He, Y.; Liang, S.; Long, M.; Xu, H. Mesoporous silica nanoparticles as potential carriers for enhanced drug solubility of paclitaxel. *Mater. Sci. Eng. C* **2017**, *78*, 12–17. [CrossRef] [PubMed]

185. Zhou, Y.; Quan, G.; Wu, Q.; Zhang, X.; Niu, B.; Wu, B.; Huang, Y.; Pan, X.; Wu, C. Mesoporous silica nanoparticles for drug and gene delivery. *Acta Pharm. Sin. B* **2018**, *8*, 165–177. [CrossRef]
186. Cheng, C.-A.; Deng, T.; Lin, F.-C.; Cai, Y.; Zink, J.I. Supramolecular Nanomachines as Stimuli-Responsive Gatekeepers on Mesoporous Silica Nanoparticles for Antibiotic and Cancer Drug Delivery. *Theranostics* **2019**, *9*, 3341–3364. [CrossRef]
187. Torney, F.; Trewyn, B.G.; Lin, V.S.Y.; Wang, K. Mesoporous silica nanoparticles deliver DNA and chemicals into plants. *Nat. Nanotechnol.* **2007**, *2*, 295–300. [CrossRef]
188. Giri, S.; Trewyn, B.G.; Stellmaker, M.P.; Lin, V.S.Y. Stimuli-Responsive Controlled-Release Delivery System Based on Mesoporous Silica Nanorods Capped with Magnetic Nanoparticles. *Angew. Chem. Int. Ed.* **2005**, *44*, 5038–5044. [CrossRef]
189. Slowing, I.I.; Vivero-Escoto, J.L.; Trewyn, B.G.; Lin, V.S.Y. Mesoporous silica nanoparticles: Structural design and applications. *J. Mater. Chem.* **2010**, *20*, 7924–7937. [CrossRef]
190. Lai, C.-Y.; Trewyn, B.G.; Jeffinija, D.M.; Jeftinija, K.; Xu, S.; Jeftinija, S.; Lin, V.S.Y. A Mesoporous Silica Nanosphere-Based Carrier System with Chemically Removable CdS Nanoparticle Caps for Stimuli-Responsive Controlled Release of Neurotransmitters and Drug Molecules. *J. Am. Chem. Soc.* **2003**, *125*, 4451–4459. [CrossRef]
191. Chang, B.; Sha, X.; Guo, J.; Jiao, Y.; Wang, C.; Yang, W. Thermo and pH dual responsive, polymer shell coated, magnetic mesoporous silica nanoparticles for controlled drug release. *J. Mater. Chem.* **2011**, *21*, 9239–9247. [CrossRef]
192. Chang, B.; Chen, D.; Wang, Y.; Chen, Y.; Jiao, Y.; Sha, X.; Yang, W. Bioresponsive Controlled Drug Release Based on Mesoporous Silica Nanoparticles Coated with Reductively Sheddable Polymer Shell. *Chem. Mater.* **2013**, *25*, 574–585. [CrossRef]
193. Croissant, J.G.; Zhang, D.; Alsaiari, S.; Lu, J.; Deng, L.; Tamanoi, F.; AlMalik, A.M.; Zink, J.I.; Khashab, N.M. Protein-gold clusters-capped mesoporous silica nanoparticles for high drug loading, autonomous gemcitabine/doxorubicin co-delivery, and in-vivo tumor imaging. *J. Control. Release* **2016**, *229*, 183–191. [CrossRef] [PubMed]
194. Saleh, T.; Soudi, T.; Shojaosadati, S.A. Aptamer functionalized curcumin-loaded human serum albumin (HSA) nanoparticles for targeted delivery to HER-2 positive breast cancer cells. *Int. J. Biol. Macromol.* **2019**, *130*, 109–116. [CrossRef]
195. Iraji, S.; Ganji, F.; Rashidi, L. Surface modified mesoporous silica nanoparticles as sustained-release gallic acid nano-carriers. *J. Drug Deliv. Sci. Technol.* **2018**, *47*, 468–476. [CrossRef]
196. Ma'mani, L.; Nikzad, S.; Kheiri-Manjili, H.; Al-Musawi, S.; Saeedi, M.; Askarlou, S.; Foroumadi, A.; Shafiee, A. Curcumin-loaded guanidine functionalized PEGylated I3ad mesoporous silica nanoparticles KIT-6: Practical strategy for the breast cancer therapy. *Eur. J. Med. Chem.* **2014**, *83*, 646–654. [CrossRef]
197. Szegedi, Á.; Shestakova, P.; Trendafilova, I.; Mihayi, J.; Tsacheva, I.; Mitova, V.; Kyulavska, M.; Koseva, N.; Momekova, D.; Konstantinov, S.; et al. Modified mesoporous silica nanoparticles coated by polymer complex as novel curcumin delivery carriers. *J. Drug Deliv. Sci. Technol.* **2019**, *49*, 700–712. [CrossRef]
198. Sattary, M.; Amini, J.; Hallaj, R. Antifungal activity of the lemongrass and clove oil encapsulated in mesoporous silica nanoparticles against wheat's take-all disease. *Pestic. Biochem. Physiol.* **2020**, *170*, 104696. [CrossRef]
199. Song, Y.; Zhou, B.; Du, X.; Wang, Y.; Zhang, J.; Ai, Y.; Xia, Z.; Zhao, G. Folic acid (FA)-conjugated mesoporous silica nanoparticles combined with MRP-1 siRNA improves the suppressive effects of myricetin on non-small cell lung cancer (NSCLC). *Biomed. Pharmacother.* **2020**, *125*, 109561. [CrossRef]
200. Li, T.; Chen, X.; Liu, Y.; Fan, L.; Lin, L.; Xu, Y.; Chen, S.; Shao, J. pH-Sensitive mesoporous silica nanoparticles anticancer prodrugs for sustained release of ursolic acid and the enhanced anti-cancer efficacy for hepatocellular carcinoma cancer. *Eur. J. Pharm. Sci.* **2017**, *96*, 456–463. [CrossRef]
201. Lungare, S.; Hallam, K.; Badhan, R.K.S. Phytochemical-loaded mesoporous silica nanoparticles for nose-to-brain olfactory drug delivery. *Int. J. Pharm.* **2016**, *513*, 280–293. [CrossRef] [PubMed]
202. Sapino, S.; Ugazio, E.; Gastaldi, L.; Miletto, I.; Berlier, G.; Zonari, D.; Oliaro-Bosso, S. Mesoporous silica as topical nanocarriers for quercetin: Characterization and in vitro studies. *Eur. J. Pharm. Biopharm.* **2015**, *89*, 116–125. [CrossRef]
203. Kundu, M.; Chatterjee, S.; Ghosh, N.; Manna, P.; Das, J.; Sil, P.C. Tumor targeted delivery of umbelliferone via a smart mesoporous silica nanoparticles controlled-release drug delivery system for increased anticancer efficiency. *Mater. Sci. Eng. C* **2020**, *116*, 111239. [CrossRef]
204. Zhao, Q.; Wu, B.; Shang, Y.; Huang, X.; Dong, H.; Liu, H.; Chen, W.; Gui, R.; Li, J. Development of a nano-drug delivery system based on mesoporous silica and its anti-lymphoma activity. *Appl. Nanosci.* **2020**, *10*, 3431–3442. [CrossRef]
205. Angelos, S.; Khashab, N.M.; Yang, Y.-W.; Trabolsi, A.; Khatib, H.A.; Stoddart, J.F.; Zink, J.I. pH Clock-Operated Mechanized Nanoparticles. *J. Am. Chem. Soc.* **2009**, *131*, 12912–12914. [CrossRef] [PubMed]
206. Patel, K.; Angelos, S.; Dichtel, W.R.; Coskun, A.; Yang, Y.-W.; Zink, J.I.; Stoddart, J.F. Enzyme-Responsive Snap-Top Covered Silica Nanocontainers. *J. Am. Chem. Soc.* **2008**, *130*, 2382–2383. [CrossRef] [PubMed]
207. Hernandez, R.; Tseng, H.-R.; Wong, J.W.; Stoddart, J.F.; Zink, J.I. An Operational Supramolecular Nanovalve. *J. Am. Chem. Soc.* **2004**, *126*, 3370–3371. [CrossRef]
208. Angelos, S.; Johansson, E.; Stoddart, J.F.; Zink, J.I. Mesostructured Silica Supports for Functional Materials and Molecular Machines. *Adv. Funct. Mater.* **2007**, *17*, 2261–2271. [CrossRef]
209. Khashab, N.M.; Belowich, M.E.; Trabolsi, A.; Friedman, D.C.; Valente, C.; Lau, Y.; Khatib, H.A.; Zink, J.I.; Stoddart, J.F. pH-Responsive mechanised nanoparticles gated by semirotaxanes. *Chem. Commun.* **2009**, 5371–5373. [CrossRef]
210. Croissant, J.; Zink, J.I. Nanovalve-Controlled Cargo Release Activated by Plasmonic Heating. *J. Am. Chem. Soc.* **2012**, *134*, 7628–7631. [CrossRef]

211. Croissant, J.; Chaix, A.; Mongin, O.; Wang, M.; Clément, S.; Raehm, L.; Durand, J.-O.; Hugues, V.; Blanchard-Desce, M.; Maynadier, M.; et al. Two-Photon-Triggered Drug Delivery via Fluorescent Nanovalves. *Small* **2014**, *10*, 1752–1755. [CrossRef] [PubMed]
212. Ambrogio, M.W.; Thomas, C.R.; Zhao, Y.-L.; Zink, J.I.; Stoddart, J.F. Mechanized Silica Nanoparticles: A New Frontier in Theranostic Nanomedicine. *Acc. Chem. Res.* **2011**, *44*, 903–913. [CrossRef] [PubMed]
213. Gan, Q.; Lu, X.; Yuan, Y.; Qian, J.; Zhou, H.; Shi, J.; Liu, C. A magnetic, reversible pH-responsive nanogated ensemble based on Fe3O4 nanoparticles-capped mesoporous silica. *Biomaterials* **2011**, *32*, 1932–1942. [CrossRef] [PubMed]
214. Liu, R.; Zhang, Y.; Zhao, X.; Agarwal, A.; Mueller, L.J.; Feng, P. pH-responsive nanogated ensemble based on gold-capped mesoporous silica through an acid-labile acetal linker. *J. Am. Chem. Soc.* **2010**, *132*, 1500–1501. [CrossRef]
215. Liu, M.; Sun, X.; Liao, Z.; Li, Y.; Qi, X.; Qian, Y.; Fenniri, H.; Zhao, P.; Shen, J. Zinc oxide end-capped Fe(3)O(4)@mSiO(2) core-shell nanocarriers as targeted and responsive drug delivery system for chemo-/ions synergistic therapeutics. *Drug Deliv.* **2019**, *26*, 732–743. [CrossRef]
216. Liu, M.C.; Liu, B.; Chen, X.L.; Lin, H.C.; Sun, X.Y.; Lu, J.Z.; Li, Y.Y.; Yan, S.Q.; Zhang, L.Y.; Zhao, P. Calcium carbonate end-capped, folate-mediated Fe(3)O(4)@mSiO(2) core-shell nanocarriers as targeted controlled-release drug delivery system. *J. Biomater. Appl.* **2018**, *32*, 1090–1104. [CrossRef]
217. Butler, K.S.; Durfee, P.N.; Theron, C.; Ashley, C.E.; Carnes, E.C.; Brinker, C.J. Protocells: Modular Mesoporous Silica Nanoparticle-Supported Lipid Bilayers for Drug Delivery. *Small* **2016**, *12*, 2173–2185. [CrossRef]
218. Kumar, P.; Tambe, P.; Paknikar, K.M.; Gajbhiye, V. Mesoporous silica nanoparticles as cutting-edge theranostics: Advancement from merely a carrier to tailor-made smart delivery platform. *J. Control. Release* **2018**, *287*, 35–57. [CrossRef]
219. Bakhshian Nik, A.; Zare, H.; Razavi, S.; Mohammadi, H.; Torab Ahmadi, P.; Yazdani, N.; Bayandori, M.; Rabiee, N.; Izadi Mobarakeh, J. Smart drug delivery: Capping strategies for mesoporous silica nanoparticles. *Microporous Mesoporous Mater.* **2020**, *299*, 110115. [CrossRef]
220. Baeza, A.; Colilla, M.; Vallet-Regí, M. Advances in mesoporous silica nanoparticles for targeted stimuli-responsive drug delivery. *Expert Opin. Drug Deliv.* **2015**, *12*, 319–337. [CrossRef]
221. Manzano, M.; Vallet-Regí, M. Mesoporous silica nanoparticles in nanomedicine applications. *J. Mater. Sci. Mater. Med.* **2018**, *29*, 65. [CrossRef] [PubMed]
222. Ahmadi Nasab, N.; Hassani Kumleh, H.; Beygzadeh, M.; Teimourian, S.; Kazemzad, M. Delivery of curcumin by a pH-responsive chitosan mesoporous silica nanoparticles for cancer treatment. *Artif. Cellsnanomed. Biotechnol.* **2018**, *46*, 75–81. [CrossRef] [PubMed]
223. Mishra, S.; Manna, K.; Kayal, U.; Saha, M.; Chatterjee, S.; Chandra, D.; Hara, M.; Datta, S.; Bhaumik, A.; Das Saha, K. Folic acid-conjugated magnetic mesoporous silica nanoparticles loaded with quercetin: A theranostic approach for cancer management. *RSC Adv.* **2020**, *10*, 23148–23164. [CrossRef]
224. Rashidi, L.; Vasheghani-Farahani, E.; Rostami, K.; Ganji, F.; Fallahpour, M. Mesoporous silica nanoparticles with different pore sizes for delivery of pH-sensitive gallic acid. *Asia-Pac. J. Chem. Eng.* **2014**, *9*, 845–853. [CrossRef]
225. Feng, Y.; Li, N.-X.; Yin, H.-L.; Chen, T.-Y.; Yang, Q.; Wu, M. Thermo- and pH-responsive, Lipid-coated, Mesoporous Silica Nanoparticle-based Dual Drug Delivery System To Improve the Antitumor Effect of Hydrophobic Drugs. *Mol. Pharm.* **2019**, *16*, 422–436. [CrossRef]
226. Fu, J.; Zhu, Y. Lysosomes activating chain reactions against cancer cells with a pH-switched prodrug/procatalyst co-delivery nanosystem. *J. Mater. Chem. B* **2017**, *5*, 996–1004. [CrossRef]
227. Russo, A.; DeGraff, W.; Friedman, N.; Mitchell, J.B. Selective modulation of glutathione levels in human normal versus tumor cells and subsequent differential response to chemotherapy drugs. *Cancer Res.* **1986**, *46*, 2845–2848.
228. Lin, J.-T.; Ye, Q.-B.; Yang, Q.-J.; Wang, G.-H. Hierarchical bioresponsive nanocarriers for codelivery of curcumin and doxorubicin. *Colloids Surf. B Biointerfaces* **2019**, *180*, 93–101. [CrossRef]
229. Xu, X.; Lü, S.; Gao, C.; Feng, C.; Wu, C.; Bai, X.; Gao, N.; Wang, Z.; Liu, M. Self-fluorescent and stimuli-responsive mesoporous silica nanoparticles using a double-role curcumin gatekeeper for drug delivery. *Chem. Eng. J.* **2016**, *300*, 185–192. [CrossRef]
230. Vaghasiya, K.; Ray, E.; Sharma, A.; Katare, O.P.; Verma, R.K. Matrix Metalloproteinase-Responsive Mesoporous Silica Nanoparticles Cloaked with Cleavable Protein for "Self-Actuating" On-Demand Controlled Drug Delivery for Cancer Therapy. *ACS Appl. Bio Mater.* **2020**, *3*, 4987–4999. [CrossRef]
231. Baeza, A.; Guisasola, E.; Ruiz-Hernández, E.; Vallet-Regí, M. Magnetically Triggered Multidrug Release by Hybrid Mesoporous Silica Nanoparticles. *Chem. Mater.* **2012**, *24*, 517–524. [CrossRef]
232. Wang, Z.; Wang, Y.S.; Chang, Z.M.; Li, L.; Zhang, Y.; Lu, M.M.; Zheng, X.; Li, M.; Shao, D.; Li, J.; et al. Berberine-loaded Janus nanocarriers for magnetic field-enhanced therapy against hepatocellular carcinoma. *Chem. Biol. Drug Des.* **2017**, *89*, 464–469. [CrossRef] [PubMed]
233. Asgari, M.; Miri, T.; Soleymani, M.; Barati, A. A novel method for in situ encapsulation of curcumin in magnetite-silica core-shell nanocomposites: A multifunctional platform for drug delivery and magnetic hyperthermia therapy. *J. Mol. Liq.* **2020**, 114731. [CrossRef]
234. Zhu, Y.; Tao, C. DNA-capped Fe3O4/SiO2 magnetic mesoporous silica nanoparticles for potential controlled drug release and hyperthermia. *RSC Adv.* **2015**, *5*, 22365–22372. [CrossRef]
235. Mal, N.K.; Fujiwara, M.; Tanaka, Y. Photocontrolled reversible release of guest molecules from coumarin-modified mesoporous silica. *Nature* **2003**, *421*, 350–353. [CrossRef] [PubMed]

236. Ferris, D.P.; Zhao, Y.-L.; Khashab, N.M.; Khatib, H.A.; Stoddart, J.F.; Zink, J.I. Light-Operated Mechanized Nanoparticles. *J. Am. Chem. Soc.* **2009**, *131*, 1686–1688. [CrossRef]
237. Martínez-Carmona, M.; Baeza, A.; Rodriguez-Milla, M.A.; García-Castro, J.; Vallet-Regí, M. Mesoporous silica nanoparticles grafted with a light-responsive protein shell for highly cytotoxic antitumoral therapy. *J. Mater. Chem. B* **2015**, *3*, 5746–5752. [CrossRef]
238. Kuang, G.; Zhang, Q.; He, S.; Liu, Y. Curcumin-loaded PEGylated mesoporous silica nanoparticles for effective photodynamic therapy. *RSC Adv.* **2020**, *10*, 24624–24630. [CrossRef]
239. Li, X.D.; Wang, Z.; Wang, X.R.; Shao, D.; Zhang, X.; Li, L.; Ge, M.F.; Chang, Z.M.; Dong, W.F. Berberine-loaded Janus gold mesoporous silica nanocarriers for chemo/radio/photothermal therapy of liver cancer and radiation-induced injury inhibition. *Int. J. Nanomed.* **2019**, *14*, 3967–3982. [CrossRef]
240. Yu, T.; Tong, L.; Ao, Y.; Zhang, G.; Liu, Y.; Zhang, H. Novel design of NIR-triggered plasmonic nanodots capped mesoporous silica nanoparticles loaded with natural capsaicin to inhibition of metastasis of human papillary thyroid carcinoma B-CPAP cells in thyroid cancer chemo-photothermal therapy. *J. Photochem. Photobiol. B* **2019**, *197*, 111534. [CrossRef]
241. Sirsi, S.R.; Borden, M.A. State-of-the-art materials for ultrasound-triggered drug delivery. *Adv. Drug Deliv. Rev.* **2014**, *72*, 3–14. [CrossRef] [PubMed]
242. Wang, J.; Pelletier, M.; Zhang, H.; Xia, H.; Zhao, Y. High-Frequency Ultrasound-Responsive Block Copolymer Micelle. *Langmuir* **2009**, *25*, 13201–13205. [CrossRef] [PubMed]
243. Paris, J.L.; Cabañas, M.V.; Manzano, M.; Vallet-Regí, M. Polymer-Grafted Mesoporous Silica Nanoparticles as Ultrasound-Responsive Drug Carriers. *ACS Nano* **2015**, *9*, 11023–11033. [CrossRef] [PubMed]
244. Paris, J.L.; de la Torre, P.; Victoria Cabañas, M.; Manzano, M.; Grau, M.; Flores, A.I.; Vallet-Regí, M. Vectorization of ultrasound-responsive nanoparticles in placental mesenchymal stem cells for cancer therapy. *Nanoscale* **2017**, *9*, 5528–5537. [CrossRef] [PubMed]
245. Li, X.; Wang, Z.; Xia, H. Ultrasound Reversible Response Nanocarrier Based on Sodium Alginate Modified Mesoporous Silica Nanoparticles. *Front. Chem.* **2019**, *7*, 59. [CrossRef] [PubMed]
246. Luo, Z.; Ding, X.; Hu, Y.; Wu, S.; Xiang, Y.; Zeng, Y.; Zhang, B.; Yan, H.; Zhang, H.; Zhu, L.; et al. Engineering a Hollow Nanocontainer Platform with Multifunctional Molecular Machines for Tumor-Targeted Therapy in Vitro and in Vivo. *ACS Nano* **2013**, *7*, 10271–10284. [CrossRef] [PubMed]
247. Matsumura, Y.; Maeda, H. A new concept for macromolecular therapeutics in cancer chemotherapy: Mechanism of tumoritropic accumulation of proteins and the antitumor agent smancs. *Cancer Res.* **1986**, *46*, 6387–6392. [PubMed]
248. Nakamura, H.; Fang, J.; Maeda, H. Development of next-generation macromolecular drugs based on the EPR effect: Challenges and pitfalls. *Expert Opin. Drug Deliv.* **2015**, *12*, 53–64. [CrossRef] [PubMed]
249. Danhier, F.; Feron, O.; Préat, V. To exploit the tumor microenvironment: Passive and active tumor targeting of nanocarriers for anti-cancer drug delivery. *J. Control. Release* **2010**, *148*, 135–146. [CrossRef]
250. Peer, D.; Karp, J.M.; Hong, S.; Farokhzad, O.C.; Margalit, R.; Langer, R. Nanocarriers as an emerging platform for cancer therapy. *Nat. Nanotechnol* **2007**, *2*, 751–760. [CrossRef]
251. Philipp, A.; Meyer, M.; Wagner, E. Extracellular targeting of synthetic therapeutic nucleic acid formulations. *Curr. Gene* **2008**, *8*, 324–334. [CrossRef] [PubMed]
252. Ang, C.Y.; Tan, S.Y.; Zhao, Y. Recent advances in biocompatible nanocarriers for delivery of chemotherapeutic cargoes towards cancer therapy. *Org. Biomol. Chem.* **2014**, *12*, 4776–4806. [CrossRef] [PubMed]
253. Mickler, F.M.; Möckl, L.; Ruthardt, N.; Ogris, M.; Wagner, E.; Bräuchle, C. Tuning nanoparticle uptake: Live-cell imaging reveals two distinct endocytosis mechanisms mediated by natural and artificial EGFR targeting ligand. *Nano Lett.* **2012**, *12*, 3417–3423. [CrossRef] [PubMed]
254. Rosenholm, J.M.; Peuhu, E.; Bate-Eya, L.T.; Eriksson, J.E.; Sahlgren, C.; Lindén, M. Cancer-Cell-Specific Induction of Apoptosis Using Mesoporous Silica Nanoparticles as Drug-Delivery Vectors. *Small* **2010**, *6*, 1234–1241. [CrossRef] [PubMed]
255. Zhang, J.; Yuan, Z.F.; Wang, Y.; Chen, W.H.; Luo, G.F.; Cheng, S.X.; Zhuo, R.X.; Zhang, X.Z. Multifunctional envelope-type mesoporous silica nanoparticles for tumor-triggered targeting drug delivery. *J. Am. Chem. Soc.* **2013**, *135*, 5068–5073. [CrossRef]
256. Shen, Y.; Li, M.; Liu, T.; Liu, J.; Xie, Y.; Zhang, J.; Xu, S.; Liu, H. A dual-functional HER2 aptamer-conjugated, pH-activated mesoporous silica nanocarrier-based drug delivery system provides in vitro synergistic cytotoxicity in HER2-positive breast cancer cells. *Int. J. Nanomed.* **2019**, *14*, 4029–4044. [CrossRef]
257. Zhao, Q.; Liu, J.; Zhu, W.; Sun, C.; Di, D.; Zhang, Y.; Wang, P.; Wang, Z.; Wang, S. Dual-stimuli responsive hyaluronic acid-conjugated mesoporous silica for targeted delivery to CD44-overexpressing cancer cells. *Acta Biomater.* **2015**, *23*, 147–156. [CrossRef]
258. Brevet, D.; Gary-Bobo, M.; Raehm, L.; Richeter, S.; Hocine, O.; Amro, K.; Loock, B.; Couleaud, P.; Frochot, C.; Morère, A.; et al. Mannose-targeted mesoporous silica nanoparticles for photodynamic therapy. *Chem. Commun.* **2009**, 1475–1477. [CrossRef]
259. Gisbert-Garzarán, M.; Vallet-Regí, M. Influence of the Surface Functionalization on the Fate and Performance of Mesoporous Silica Nanoparticles. *Nanomaterials* **2020**, *10*, 916. [CrossRef]
260. Li, N.; Wang, Z.; Zhang, Y.; Zhang, K.; Xie, J.; Liu, Y.; Li, W.; Feng, N. Curcumin-loaded redox-responsive mesoporous silica nanoparticles for targeted breast cancer therapy. *Artif. Cells Nanomed. Biotechnol.* **2018**, *46*, 921–935. [CrossRef]

261. Malekmohammadi, S.; Hadadzadeh, H.; Farrokhpour, H.; Amirghofran, Z. Immobilization of gold nanoparticles on folate-conjugated dendritic mesoporous silica-coated reduced graphene oxide nanosheets: A new nanoplatform for curcumin pH-controlled and targeted delivery. *Soft Matter* **2018**, *14*, 2400–2410. [CrossRef]
262. Fang, J.; Zhang, S.; Xue, X.; Zhu, X.; Song, S.; Wang, B.; Jiang, L.; Qin, M.; Liang, H.; Gao, L. Quercetin and doxorubicin co-delivery using mesoporous silica nanoparticles enhance the efficacy of gastric carcinoma chemotherapy. *Int. J. Nanomed.* **2018**, *13*, 5113–5126. [CrossRef] [PubMed]
263. Kumar, B.N.P.; Puvvada, N.; Rajput, S.; Sarkar, S.; Mahto, M.K.; Yallapu, M.M.; Pathak, A.; Emdad, L.; Das, S.K.; Reis, R.L.; et al. Targeting of EGFR, VEGFR2, and Akt by Engineered Dual Drug Encapsulated Mesoporous Silica-Gold Nanoclusters Sensitizes Tamoxifen-Resistant Breast Cancer. *Mol. Pharm.* **2018**, *15*, 2698–2713. [CrossRef] [PubMed]
264. Murugan, C.; Rayappan, K.; Thangam, R.; Bhanumathi, R.; Shanthi, K.; Vivek, R.; Thirumurugan, R.; Bhattacharyya, A.; Sivasubramanian, S.; Gunasekaran, P.; et al. Combinatorial nanocarrier based drug delivery approach for amalgamation of anti-tumor agents in breast cancer cells: An improved nanomedicine strategy. *Sci. Rep.* **2016**, *6*, 34053. [CrossRef] [PubMed]
265. Sarkar, A.; Ghosh, S.; Chowdhury, S.; Pandey, B.; Sil, P.C. Targeted delivery of quercetin loaded mesoporous silica nanoparticles to the breast cancer cells. *Biochim. Biophys. Acta* **2016**, *1860*, 2065–2075. [CrossRef]
266. Ding, J.; Yao, J.; Xue, J.; Li, R.; Bao, B.; Jiang, L.; Zhu, J.J.; He, Z. Tumor-Homing Cell-Penetrating Peptide Linked to Colloidal Mesoporous Silica Encapsulated (-)-Epigallocatechin-3-gallate as Drug Delivery System for Breast Cancer Therapy in Vivo. *ACS Appl. Mater. Interfaces* **2015**, *7*, 18145–18155. [CrossRef]
267. Hu, Y.; Wang, Z.; Qiu, Y.; Liu, Y.; Ding, M.; Zhang, Y. Anti-miRNA21 and resveratrol-loaded polysaccharide-based mesoporous silica nanoparticle for synergistic activity in gastric carcinoma. *J. Drug Target.* **2019**, *27*, 1135–1143. [CrossRef]
268. Del Favero, G.; Bialas, F.; Grabher, S.; Wittig, A.; Bräuer, B.; Gerthsen, D.; Echalier, C.; Kamalov, M.; Marko, D.; Becker, C.F.W. Silica particles with a quercetin–R5 peptide conjugate are taken up into HT-29 cells and translocate into the nucleus. *Chem. Commun.* **2019**, *55*, 9649–9652. [CrossRef]
269. Havel, H.A. Where Are the Nanodrugs? An Industry Perspective on Development of Drug Products Containing Nanomaterials. *AAPS J.* **2016**, *18*, 1351–1353. [CrossRef]
270. Havel, H.; Finch, G.; Strode, P.; Wolfgang, M.; Zale, S.; Bobe, I.; Youssoufian, H.; Peterson, M.; Liu, M. Nanomedicines: From Bench to Bedside and Beyond. *AAPS J.* **2016**, *18*, 1373–1378. [CrossRef]
271. Tran, S.; DeGiovanni, P.J.; Piel, B.; Rai, P. Cancer nanomedicine: A review of recent success in drug delivery. *Clin. Transl. Med.* **2017**, *6*, 44. [CrossRef] [PubMed]
272. Cragg, G.M.; Pezzuto, J.M. Natural Products as a Vital Source for the Discovery of Cancer Chemotherapeutic and Chemopreventive Agents. *Med. Princ. Pract. Int. J. Kuwait Univ. Health Sci. Cent.* **2016**, *25* (Suppl. S2), 41–59. [CrossRef] [PubMed]
273. Nwodo, J.N.; Ibezim, A.; Simoben, C.V.; Ntie-Kang, F. Exploring Cancer Therapeutics with Natural Products from African Medicinal Plants, Part II: Alkaloids, Terpenoids and Flavonoids. *Anticancer Agents Med. Chem.* **2016**, *16*, 108–127. [CrossRef] [PubMed]
274. Tapiero, H.; Tew, K.D.; Ba, G.N.; Mathé, G. Polyphenols: Do they play a role in the prevention of human pathologies? *Biomed. Pharm.* **2002**, *56*, 200–207. [CrossRef]
275. Sak, K. Cytotoxicity of dietary flavonoids on different human cancer types. *Pharmacogn. Rev.* **2014**, *8*, 122–146. [CrossRef] [PubMed]
276. Huang, M.; Lu, J.J.; Huang, M.Q.; Bao, J.L.; Chen, X.P.; Wang, Y.T. Terpenoids: Natural products for cancer therapy. *Expert Opin. Investig. Drugs* **2012**, *21*, 1801–1818. [CrossRef]
277. Amawi, H.; Ashby, C.R., Jr.; Tiwari, A.K. Cancer chemoprevention through dietary flavonoids: What's limiting? *Chin. J. Cancer* **2017**, *36*, 50. [CrossRef]
278. Kumar, V.; Bhatt, P.C.; Rahman, M.; Kaithwas, G.; Choudhry, H.; Al-Abbasi, F.A.; Anwar, F.; Verma, A. Fabrication, optimization, and characterization of umbelliferone β-D-galactopyranoside-loaded PLGA nanoparticles in treatment of hepatocellular carcinoma: In vitro and in vivo studies. *Int. J. Nanomed.* **2017**, *12*, 6747–6758. [CrossRef]
279. Seca, A.M.L.; Pinto, D. Plant Secondary Metabolites as Anticancer Agents: Successes in Clinical Trials and Therapeutic Application. *Int. J. Mol. Sci.* **2018**, *19*, 263. [CrossRef]
280. Rajesh, E.; Sankari, L.S.; Malathi, L.; Krupaa, J.R. Naturally occurring products in cancer therapy. *J. Pharm. Bioallied. Sci.* **2015**, *7*, S181–S183. [CrossRef]
281. Demain, A.L.; Vaishnav, P. Natural products for cancer chemotherapy. *Microb. Biotechnol.* **2011**, *4*, 687–699. [CrossRef]
282. Reddy, L.; Odhav, B.; Bhoola, K.D. Natural products for cancer prevention: A global perspective. *Pharmacol. Ther.* **2003**, *99*, 1–13. [CrossRef]
283. Zubair, H.; Azim, S.; Ahmad, A.; Khan, M.A.; Patel, G.K.; Singh, S.; Singh, A.P. Cancer Chemoprevention by Phytochemicals: Nature's Healing Touch. *Molecules* **2017**, *22*, 395. [CrossRef] [PubMed]
284. Burnett, J.; Newman, B.; Sun, D. Targeting cancer stem cells with natural products. *Curr. Drug Targets* **2012**, *13*, 1054–1064. [CrossRef] [PubMed]
285. Kashyap, D.; Tuli, H.S.; Yerer, M.B.; Sharma, A.; Sak, K.; Srivastava, S.; Pandey, A.; Garg, V.K.; Sethi, G.; Bishayee, A. Natural product-based nanoformulations for cancer therapy: Opportunities and challenges. *Semin. Cancer Biol.* **2019**. [CrossRef] [PubMed]
286. Kashyap, D.; Sharma, A.; Tuli, H.S.; Sak, K.; Punia, S.; Mukherjee, T.K. Kaempferol—A dietary anticancer molecule with multiple mechanisms of action: Recent trends and advancements. *J. Funct. Foods* **2017**, *30*, 203–219. [CrossRef]

287. Harborne, J.B. Classes and functions of secondary products from plants. In *Chemicals from Plants*; World Scientific/Imperial College Press: Singapore, 1999; pp. 1–25.
288. Rahman, M.; Ahmad, M.Z.; Kazmi, I.; Akhter, S.; Afzal, M.; Gupta, G.; Sinha, V.R. Emergence of nanomedicine as cancer targeted magic bullets: Recent development and need to address the toxicity apprehension. *Curr. Drug Discov. Technol.* **2012**, *9*, 319–329. [CrossRef]
289. Rahman, M.; Ahmad, M.Z.; Kazmi, I.; Akhter, S.; Afzal, M.; Gupta, G.; Jalees Ahmed, F.; Anwar, F. Advancement in multifunctional nanoparticles for the effective treatment of cancer. *Expert Opin. Drug Deliv.* **2012**, *9*, 367–381. [CrossRef]
290. Bobo, D.; Robinson, K.J.; Islam, J.; Thurecht, K.J.; Corrie, S.R. Nanoparticle-Based Medicines: A Review of FDA-Approved Materials and Clinical Trials to Date. *Pharm. Res.* **2016**, *33*, 2373–2387. [CrossRef]
291. Leonarduzzi, G.; Testa, G.; Sottero, B.; Gamba, P.; Poli, G. Design and development of nanovehicle-based delivery systems for preventive or therapeutic supplementation with flavonoids. *Curr. Med. Chem.* **2010**, *17*, 74–95. [CrossRef]
292. Jeetah, R.; Bhaw-Luximon, A.; Jhurry, D. Nanopharmaceutics: Phytochemical-based controlled or sustained drug-delivery systems for cancer treatment. *J. Biomed. Nanotechnol.* **2014**, *10*, 1810–1840. [CrossRef]
293. Gohulkumar, M.; Gurushankar, K.; Rajendra Prasad, N.; Krishnakumar, N. Enhanced cytotoxicity and apoptosis-induced anticancer effect of silibinin-loaded nanoparticles in oral carcinoma (KB) cells. *Mater. Sci. Eng. C Mater. Biol. Appl.* **2014**, *41*, 274–282. [CrossRef] [PubMed]
294. Khan, N.; Bharali, D.J.; Adhami, V.M.; Siddiqui, I.A.; Cui, H.; Shabana, S.M.; Mousa, S.A.; Mukhtar, H. Oral administration of naturally occurring chitosan-based nanoformulated green tea polyphenol EGCG effectively inhibits prostate cancer cell growth in a xenograft model. *Carcinogenesis* **2014**, *35*, 415–423. [CrossRef] [PubMed]
295. Majumdar, D.; Jung, K.-H.; Zhang, H.; Nannapaneni, S.; Wang, X.; Amin, A.R.M.R.; Chen, Z.; Chen, Z.G.; Shin, D.M. Luteolin nanoparticle in chemoprevention: In vitro and in vivo anticancer activity. *Cancer Prev. Res.* **2014**, *7*, 65–73. [CrossRef] [PubMed]
296. El-Far, A.H.; Al Jaouni, S.K.; Li, W.; Mousa, S.A. Protective Roles of Thymoquinone Nanoformulations: Potential Nanonutraceuticals in Human Diseases. *Nutrients* **2018**, *10*, 1369. [CrossRef] [PubMed]
297. Ballout, F.; Habli, Z.; Rahal, O.N.; Fatfat, M.; Gali-Muhtasib, H. Thymoquinone-based nanotechnology for cancer therapy: Promises and challenges. *Drug Discov. Today* **2018**, *23*, 1089–1098. [CrossRef]
298. Hazra, B.; Kumar, B.; Biswas, S.; Pandey, B.N.; Mishra, K.P. Enhancement of the tumour inhibitory activity, in vivo, of diospyrin, a plant-derived quinonoid, through liposomal encapsulation. *Toxicol. Lett.* **2005**, *157*, 109–117. [CrossRef] [PubMed]
299. Anand, P.; Sundaram, C.; Jhurani, S.; Kunnumakkara, A.B.; Aggarwal, B.B. Curcumin and cancer: An "old-age" disease with an "age-old" solution. *Cancer Lett.* **2008**, *267*, 133–164. [CrossRef]
300. Nirmala, C.; Puvanakrishnan, R. Protective role of curcumin against isoproterenol induced myocardial infarction in rats. *Mol. Cell. Biochem.* **1996**, *159*, 85–93. [CrossRef]
301. Jordan, W.C.; Drew, C.R. Curcumin—A natural herb with anti-HIV activity. *J. Natl. Med. Assoc.* **1996**, *88*, 333.
302. Phan, T.T.; See, P.; Lee, S.T.; Chan, S.Y. Protective effects of curcumin against oxidative damage on skin cells in vitro: Its implication for wound healing. *J. Trauma* **2001**, *51*, 927–931. [CrossRef] [PubMed]
303. Lim, G.P.; Chu, T.; Yang, F.; Beech, W.; Frautschy, S.A.; Cole, G.M. The Curry Spice Curcumin Reduces Oxidative Damage and Amyloid Pathology in an Alzheimer Transgenic Mouse. *J. Neurosci.* **2001**, *21*, 8370. [CrossRef] [PubMed]
304. Gupta, S.C.; Patchva, S.; Koh, W.; Aggarwal, B.B. Discovery of curcumin, a component of golden spice, and its miraculous biological activities. *Clin. Exp. Pharmacol. Physiol.* **2012**, *39*, 283–299. [CrossRef] [PubMed]
305. Arablou, T.; Kolahdouz-Mohammadi, R. Curcumin and endometriosis: Review on potential roles and molecular mechanisms. *Biomed. Pharm.* **2018**, *97*, 91–97. [CrossRef]
306. Ak, T.; Gülçin, İ. Antioxidant and radical scavenging properties of curcumin. *Chem. Biol. Interact.* **2008**, *174*, 27–37. [CrossRef]
307. Sharma, O.P. Antioxidant activity of curcumin and related compounds. *Biochem. Pharm.* **1976**, *25*, 1811–1812. [CrossRef]
308. Bhattacharyya, S.; Mandal, D.; Sen, G.S.; Pal, S.; Banerjee, S.; Lahiry, L.; Finke, J.H.; Tannenbaum, C.S.; Das, T.; Sa, G. Tumor-induced oxidative stress perturbs nuclear factor-kappaB activity-augmenting tumor necrosis factor-alpha-mediated T-cell death: Protection by curcumin. *Cancer Res.* **2007**, *67*, 362–370. [CrossRef]
309. Sandur, S.K.; Pandey, M.K.; Sung, B.; Ahn, K.S.; Murakami, A.; Sethi, G.; Limtrakul, P.; Badmaev, V.; Aggarwal, B.B. Curcumin, demethoxycurcumin, bisdemethoxycurcumin, tetrahydrocurcumin and turmerones differentially regulate anti-inflammatory and anti-proliferative responses through a ROS-independent mechanism. *Carcinogenesis* **2007**, *28*, 1765–1773. [CrossRef]
310. De, R.; Kundu, P.; Swarnakar, S.; Ramamurthy, T.; Chowdhury, A.; Nair, G.B.; Mukhopadhyay, A.K. Antimicrobial activity of curcumin against Helicobacter pylori isolates from India and during infections in mice. *Antimicrob. Agents Chemother.* **2009**, *53*, 1592–1597. [CrossRef]
311. Mun, S.H.; Joung, D.K.; Kim, Y.S.; Kang, O.H.; Kim, S.B.; Seo, Y.S.; Kim, Y.C.; Lee, D.S.; Shin, D.W.; Kweon, K.T.; et al. Synergistic antibacterial effect of curcumin against methicillin-resistant Staphylococcus aureus. *Phytomedicine* **2013**, *20*, 714–718. [CrossRef]
312. Neelofar, K.; Shreaz, S.; Rimple, B.; Muralidhar, S.; Nikhat, M.; Khan, L.A. Curcumin as a promising anticandidal of clinical interest. *Can. J. Microbiol.* **2011**, *57*, 204–210. [CrossRef] [PubMed]
313. Khalil, O.A.K.; de Faria Oliveira, O.M.M.; Vellosa, J.C.R.; de Quadros, A.U.; Dalposso, L.M.; Karam, T.K.; Mainardes, R.M.; Khalil, N.M. Curcumin antifungal and antioxidant activities are increased in the presence of ascorbic acid. *Food Chem.* **2012**, *133*, 1001–1005. [CrossRef]

314. Tomeh, M.A.; Hadianamrei, R.; Zhao, X. A Review of Curcumin and Its Derivatives as Anticancer Agents. *Int. J. Mol. Sci.* **2019**, *20*, 1033. [CrossRef] [PubMed]
315. Chen, J.; He, Z.M.; Wang, F.L.; Zhang, Z.S.; Liu, X.Z.; Zhai, D.D.; Chen, W.D. Curcumin and its promise as an anticancer drug: An analysis of its anticancer and antifungal effects in cancer and associated complications from invasive fungal infections. *Eur. J. Pharm.* **2016**, *772*, 33–42. [CrossRef]
316. Ravindranath, V.; Chandrasekhara, N. Absorption and tissue distribution of curcumin in rats. *Toxicology* **1980**, *16*, 259–265. [CrossRef]
317. Ravindranath, V.; Chandrasekhara, N. In vitro studies on the intestinal absorption of curcumin in rats. *Toxicology* **1981**, *20*, 251–257. [CrossRef]
318. Ravindranath, V.; Chandrasekhara, N. Metabolism of curcumn-studies with [3H]curcumin. *Toxicology* **1981**, *22*, 337–344. [CrossRef]
319. Gupta, N.K.; Dixit, V.K. Bioavailability Enhancement of Curcumin by Complexation with Phosphatidyl Choline. *J. Pharm. Sci.* **2011**, *100*, 1987–1995. [CrossRef] [PubMed]
320. Bollu, V.S.; Barui, A.K.; Mondal, S.K.; Prashar, S.; Fajardo, M.; Briones, D.; Rodríguez-Diéguez, A.; Patra, C.R.; Gómez-Ruiz, S. Curcumin-loaded silica-based mesoporous materials: Synthesis, characterization and cytotoxic properties against cancer cells. *Mater. Sci. Eng. C* **2016**, *63*, 393–410. [CrossRef]
321. Datz, S.; Engelke, H.; Schirnding, C.V.; Nguyen, L.; Bein, T. Lipid bilayer-coated curcumin-based mesoporous organosilica nanoparticles for cellular delivery. *Microporous Mesoporous Mater.* **2016**, *225*, 371–377. [CrossRef]
322. Rahmatolahzadeh, R.; Hamadanian, M.; Ma'mani, L.; Shafiee, A. Aspartic acid functionalized PEGylated MSN@GO hybrid as an effective and sustainable nano-system for in-vitro drug delivery. *Adv. Med. Sci.* **2018**, *63*, 257–264. [CrossRef] [PubMed]
323. Song, Y.; Cai, L.; Tian, Z.; Wu, Y.; Chen, J. Phytochemical Curcumin-Coformulated, Silver-Decorated Melanin-like Polydopamine/Mesoporous Silica Composites with Improved Antibacterial and Chemotherapeutic Effects against Drug-Resistant Cancer Cells. *ACS Omega* **2020**, *5*, 15083–15094. [CrossRef] [PubMed]
324. Gao, J.; Fan, K.; Jin, Y.; Zhao, L.; Wang, Q.; Tang, Y.; Xu, H.; Liu, Z.; Wang, S.; Lin, J.; et al. PEGylated lipid bilayer coated mesoporous silica nanoparticles co-delivery of paclitaxel and curcumin leads to increased tumor site drug accumulation and reduced tumor burden. *Eur. J. Pharm. Sci.* **2019**, *140*, 105070. [CrossRef] [PubMed]
325. Sun, X.; Wang, N.; Yang, L.-Y.; Ouyang, X.-K.; Huang, F. Folic Acid and PEI Modified Mesoporous Silica for Targeted Delivery of Curcumin. *Pharmaceutics* **2019**, *11*, 430. [CrossRef]
326. Mashayekhi, S.; Rasoulpoor, S.; Shabani, S.; Esmaeilizadeh, N.; Serati-Nouri, H.; Sheervalilou, R.; Pilehvar-Soltanahmadi, Y. Curcumin-loaded mesoporous silica nanoparticles/nanofiber composites for supporting long-term proliferation and stemness preservation of adipose-derived stem cells. *Int. J. Pharm.* **2020**, *587*, 119656. [CrossRef] [PubMed]
327. He, Y.; Shao, L.; Usman, I.; Hu, Y.; Pan, A.; Liang, S.; Xu, H. A pH-responsive dissociable mesoporous silica-based nanoplatform enabling efficient dual-drug co-delivery and rapid clearance for cancer therapy. *Biomater. Sci.* **2020**, *8*, 3418–3429. [CrossRef]
328. Wibowo, F.R.; Saputra, O.A.; Lestari, W.W.; Koketsu, M.; Mukti, R.R.; Martien, R. pH-Triggered Drug Release Controlled by Poly(Styrene Sulfonate) Growth Hollow Mesoporous Silica Nanoparticles. *ACS Omega* **2020**, *5*, 4261–4269. [CrossRef]
329. Kong, Z.L.; Kuo, H.P.; Johnson, A.; Wu, L.C.; Chang, K.L.B. Curcumin-Loaded Mesoporous Silica Nanoparticles Markedly Enhanced Cytotoxicity in Hepatocellular Carcinoma Cells. *Int. J. Mol. Sci.* **2019**, *20*, 2918. [CrossRef]
330. Harini, L.; Srivastava, S.; Gnanakumar, G.P.; Karthikeyan, B.; Ross, C.; Krishnakumar, V.; Kannan, V.R.; Sundar, K.; Kathiresan, T. An ingenious non-spherical mesoporous silica nanoparticle cargo with curcumin induces mitochondria-mediated apoptosis in breast cancer (MCF-7) cells. *Oncotarget* **2019**, *10*, 1193–1208. [CrossRef]
331. Chen, C.; Sun, W.; Wang, X.; Wang, Y.; Wang, P. Rational design of curcumin loaded multifunctional mesoporous silica nanoparticles to enhance the cytotoxicity for targeted and controlled drug release. *Mater. Sci. Eng. C* **2018**, *85*, 88–96. [CrossRef]
332. Lv, Y.; Li, J.; Chen, H.; Bai, Y.; Zhang, L. Glycyrrhetinic acid-functionalized mesoporous silica nanoparticles as hepatocellular carcinoma-targeted drug carrier. *Int. J. Nanomed.* **2017**, *12*, 4361–4370. [CrossRef] [PubMed]
333. Harini, L.; Karthikeyan, B.; Srivastava, S.; Suresh, S.B.; Ross, C.; Gnanakumar, G.; Rajagopal, S.; Sundar, K.; Kathiresan, T. Polyethylenimine-modified curcumin-loaded mesoporus silica nanoparticle (MCM-41) induces cell death in MCF-7 cell line. *IET Nanobiotechnol.* **2017**, *11*, 57–61. [CrossRef] [PubMed]
334. Tiwari, N.; Nawale, L.; Sarkar, D.; Badiger, M.V. Carboxymethyl Cellulose-Grafted Mesoporous Silica Hybrid Nanogels for Enhanced Cellular Uptake and Release of Curcumin. *Gels* **2017**, *3*, 8. [CrossRef] [PubMed]
335. Wang, J.; Wang, Y.; Liu, Q.; Yang, L.; Zhu, R.; Yu, C.; Wang, S. Rational Design of Multifunctional Dendritic Mesoporous Silica Nanoparticles to Load Curcumin and Enhance Efficacy for Breast Cancer Therapy. *ACS Appl. Mater. Interfaces* **2016**, *8*, 26511–26523. [CrossRef]
336. Kotcherlakota, R.; Barui, A.K.; Prashar, S.; Fajardo, M.; Briones, D.; Rodríguez-Diéguez, A.; Patra, C.R.; Gómez-Ruiz, S. Curcumin loaded mesoporous silica: An effective drug delivery system for cancer treatment. *Biomater. Sci.* **2016**, *4*, 448–459. [CrossRef]
337. Li, Y.; Yao, J.; Han, C.; Yang, J.; Chaudhry, M.T.; Wang, S.; Liu, H.; Yin, Y. Quercetin, Inflammation and Immunity. *Nutrients* **2016**, *8*, 167. [CrossRef]
338. Davis, J.M.; Murphy, E.A.; Carmichael, M.D. Effects of the dietary flavonoid quercetin upon performance and health. *Curr. Sports Med. Rep.* **2009**, *8*, 206–213. [CrossRef]
339. Lamson, D.W.; Brignall, M.S. Antioxidants and cancer, part 3: Quercetin. *Altern. Med. Rev.* **2000**, *5*, 196–208.

340. Boots, A.W.; Haenen, G.R.; Bast, A. Health effects of quercetin: From antioxidant to nutraceutical. *Eur. J. Pharm.* **2008**, *585*, 325–337. [CrossRef]
341. Choi, H.J.; Song, J.H.; Park, K.S.; Kwon, D.H. Inhibitory effects of quercetin 3-rhamnoside on influenza A virus replication. *Eur. J. Pharm. Sci.* **2009**, *37*, 329–333. [CrossRef]
342. Rotelli, A.E.; Guardia, T.; Juárez, A.O.; de la Rocha, N.E.; Pelzer, L.E. Comparative study of flavonoids in experimental models of inflammation. *Pharm. Res.* **2003**, *48*, 601–606. [CrossRef]
343. Kumar, B.; Gupta, S.K.; Nag, T.C.; Srivastava, S.; Saxena, R.; Jha, K.A.; Srinivasan, B.P. Retinal neuroprotective effects of quercetin in streptozotocin-induced diabetic rats. *Exp. Eye Res.* **2014**, *125*, 193–202. [CrossRef] [PubMed]
344. Hu, X.T.; Ding, C.; Zhou, N.; Xu, C. Quercetin protects gastric epithelial cell from oxidative damage in vitro and in vivo. *Eur. J. Pharm.* **2015**, *754*, 115–124. [CrossRef] [PubMed]
345. Aguirre, L.; Arias, N.; Teresa Macarulla, M.; Gracia, A.; Portillo, M.P. Beneficial effects of quercetin on obesity and diabetes. *Open Nutraceuticals J.* **2011**, *4*, 189–198.
346. Yang, L.; Hu, Z.; Zhu, J.; Liang, Q.; Zhou, H.; Li, J.; Fan, X.; Zhao, Z.; Pan, H.; Fei, B. Systematic Elucidation of the Mechanism of Quercetin against Gastric Cancer via Network Pharmacology Approach. *BioMed Res. Int.* **2020**, *2020*, 3860213. [CrossRef] [PubMed]
347. Xu, D.; Hu, M.J.; Wang, Y.Q.; Cui, Y.L. Antioxidant Activities of Quercetin and Its Complexes for Medicinal Application. *Molecules* **2019**, *24*, 1123. [CrossRef]
348. Rauf, A.; Imran, M.; Khan, I.A.; Ur-Rehman, M.; Gilani, S.A.; Mehmood, Z.; Mubarak, M.S. Anticancer potential of quercetin: A comprehensive review. *Phytother. Res.* **2018**, *32*, 2109–2130. [CrossRef]
349. Chun, O.K.; Chung, S.J.; Song, W.O. Estimated dietary flavonoid intake and major food sources of U.S. adults. *J. Nutr.* **2007**, *137*, 1244–1252. [CrossRef]
350. Gugler, R.; Leschik, M.; Dengler, H.J. Disposition of quercetin in man after single oral and intravenous doses. *Eur. J. Clin. Pharm.* **1975**, *9*, 229–234. [CrossRef]
351. Egert, S.; Wolffram, S.; Bosy-Westphal, A.; Boesch-Saadatmandi, C.; Wagner, A.E.; Frank, J.; Rimbach, G.; Mueller, M.J. Daily quercetin supplementation dose-dependently increases plasma quercetin concentrations in healthy humans. *J. Nutr.* **2008**, *138*, 1615–1621. [CrossRef]
352. Thangasamy, T.; Sittadjody, S.; Burd, R. Quercetin: A potential complementary and alternative cancer therapy. In *Complementary and Alternative Therapies and the Aging Population*; Elsevier: Amsterdam, The Netherlands, 2009; pp. 563–584.
353. Novo, M.C.; Osugui, L.; dos Reis, V.O.; Longo-Maugéri, I.M.; Mariano, M.; Popi, A.F. Blockage of Wnt/β-catenin signaling by quercetin reduces survival and proliferation of B-1 cells in vitro. *Immunobiology* **2015**, *220*, 60–67. [CrossRef] [PubMed]
354. Sharmila, G.; Bhat, F.A.; Arunkumar, R.; Elumalai, P.; Raja Singh, P.; Senthilkumar, K.; Arunakaran, J. Chemopreventive effect of quercetin, a natural dietary flavonoid on prostate cancer in in vivo model. *Clin. Nutr.* **2014**, *33*, 718–726. [CrossRef] [PubMed]
355. Vafadar, A.; Shabaninejad, Z.; Movahedpour, A.; Fallahi, F.; Taghavipour, M.; Ghasemi, Y.; Akbari, M.; Shafiee, A.; Hajighadimi, S.; Moradizarmehri, S.; et al. Quercetin and cancer: New insights into its therapeutic effects on ovarian cancer cells. *Cell. Biosci.* **2020**, *10*, 32. [CrossRef]
356. Fernández-Palanca, P.; Fondevila, F.; Méndez-Blanco, C.; Tuñón, M.J.; González-Gallego, J.; Mauriz, J.L. Antitumor Effects of Quercetin in Hepatocarcinoma In Vitro and In Vivo Models: A Systematic Review. *Nutrients* **2019**, *11*, 2875. [CrossRef] [PubMed]
357. Jana, N.; Břetislav, G.; Pavel, S.; Pavla, U. Potential of the Flavonoid Quercetin to Prevent and Treat Cancer—Current Status of Research. *Klin. Onkol.* **2018**, *31*, 184–190. [CrossRef] [PubMed]
358. Ward, A.B.; Mir, H.; Kapur, N.; Gales, D.N.; Carriere, P.P.; Singh, S. Quercetin inhibits prostate cancer by attenuating cell survival and inhibiting anti-apoptotic pathways. *World J. Surg. Oncol.* **2018**, *16*, 108. [CrossRef] [PubMed]
359. Tang, S.M.; Deng, X.T.; Zhou, J.; Li, Q.P.; Ge, X.X.; Miao, L. Pharmacological basis and new insights of quercetin action in respect to its anti-cancer effects. *Biomed. Pharm.* **2020**, *121*, 109604. [CrossRef]
360. Murakami, A.; Ashida, H.; Terao, J. Multitargeted cancer prevention by quercetin. *Cancer Lett.* **2008**, *269*, 315–325. [CrossRef]
361. Cai, X.; Fang, Z.; Dou, J.; Yu, A.; Zhai, G. Bioavailability of quercetin: Problems and promises. *Curr. Med. Chem.* **2013**, *20*, 2572–2582. [CrossRef]
362. Niazvand, F.; Orazizadeh, M.; Khorsandi, L.; Abbaspour, M.; Mansouri, E.; Khodadadi, A. Effects of Quercetin-Loaded Nanoparticles on MCF-7 Human Breast Cancer Cells. *Medicina* **2019**, *55*, 114. [CrossRef]
363. Nam, J.-S.; Sharma, A.R.; Nguyen, L.T.; Chakraborty, C.; Sharma, G.; Lee, S.-S. Application of Bioactive Quercetin in Oncotherapy: From Nutrition to Nanomedicine. *Molecules* **2016**, *21*, 108. [CrossRef] [PubMed]
364. Baksi, R.; Singh, D.P.; Borse, S.P.; Rana, R.; Sharma, V.; Nivsarkar, M. In vitro and in vivo anticancer efficacy potential of Quercetin loaded polymeric nanoparticles. *Biomed. Pharmacother.* **2018**, *106*, 1513–1526. [CrossRef] [PubMed]
365. Lou, M.; Zhang, L.-N.; Ji, P.-G.; Feng, F.-Q.; Liu, J.-H.; Yang, C.; Li, B.-F.; Wang, L. Quercetin nanoparticles induced autophagy and apoptosis through AKT/ERK/Caspase-3 signaling pathway in human neuroglioma cells: In vitro and in vivo. *Biomed. Pharmacother.* **2016**, *84*, 1–9. [CrossRef]
366. Rajesh Kumar, S.; Priyatharshni, S.; Babu, V.N.; Mangalaraj, D.; Viswanathan, C.; Kannan, S.; Ponpandian, N. Quercetin conjugated superparamagnetic magnetite nanoparticles for in-vitro analysis of breast cancer cell lines for chemotherapy applications. *J. Colloid Interface Sci.* **2014**, *436*, 234–242. [CrossRef]

367. Ren, K.-W.; Li, Y.-H.; Wu, G.; Ren, J.-Z.; Lu, H.-B.; Li, Z.-M.; Han, X.-W. Quercetin nanoparticles display antitumor activity via proliferation inhibition and apoptosis induction in liver cancer cells. *Int. J. Oncol.* **2017**, *50*, 1299–1311. [CrossRef] [PubMed]
368. Xu, G.; Li, B.; Wang, T.; Wan, J.; Zhang, Y.; Huang, J.; Shen, Y. Enhancing the anti-ovarian cancer activity of quercetin using a self-assembling micelle and thermosensitive hydrogel drug delivery system. *RSC Adv.* **2018**, *8*, 21229–21242. [CrossRef]
369. Liu, M.; Fu, M.; Yang, X.; Jia, G.; Shi, X.; Ji, J.; Liu, X.; Zhai, G. Paclitaxel and quercetin co-loaded functional mesoporous silica nanoparticles overcoming multidrug resistance in breast cancer. *Colloids Surf. B Biointerfaces* **2020**, *196*, 111284. [CrossRef] [PubMed]
370. Huang, C.; Chen, T.; Zhu, D.; Huang, Q. Enhanced Tumor Targeting and Radiotherapy by Quercetin Loaded Biomimetic Nanoparticles. *Front. Chem.* **2020**, *8*, 225. [CrossRef]
371. Shao, M.; Chang, C.; Liu, Z.; Chen, K.; Zhou, Y.; Zheng, G.; Huang, Z.; Xu, H.; Xu, P.; Lu, B. Polydopamine coated hollow mesoporous silica nanoparticles as pH-sensitive nanocarriers for overcoming multidrug resistance. *Colloids Surf. B Biointerfaces* **2019**, *183*, 110427. [CrossRef]
372. Ko, J.-H.; Sethi, G.; Um, J.-Y.; Shanmugam, M.K.; Arfuso, F.; Kumar, A.P.; Bishayee, A.; Ahn, K.S. The Role of Resveratrol in Cancer Therapy. *Int. J. Mol. Sci.* **2017**, *18*, 2589. [CrossRef]
373. Shukla, Y.; Singh, R. Resveratrol and cellular mechanisms of cancer prevention. *Ann. N. Y. Acad. Sci.* **2011**, *1215*, 1–8. [CrossRef] [PubMed]
374. Patel, K.R.; Brown, V.A.; Jones, D.J.; Britton, R.G.; Hemingway, D.; Miller, A.S.; West, K.P.; Booth, T.D.; Perloff, M.; Crowell, J.A.; et al. Clinical pharmacology of resveratrol and its metabolites in colorectal cancer patients. *Cancer Res.* **2010**, *70*, 7392–7399. [CrossRef] [PubMed]
375. Kjaer, T.N.; Ornstrup, M.J.; Poulsen, M.M.; Jørgensen, J.O.; Hougaard, D.M.; Cohen, A.S.; Neghabat, S.; Richelsen, B.; Pedersen, S.B. Resveratrol reduces the levels of circulating androgen precursors but has no effect on, testosterone, dihydrotestosterone, PSA levels or prostate volume. A 4-month randomised trial in middle-aged men. *Prostate* **2015**, *75*, 1255–1263. [CrossRef] [PubMed]
376. Ma, D.S.L.; Tan, L.T.-H.; Chan, K.-G.; Yap, W.H.; Pusparajah, P.; Chuah, L.-H.; Ming, L.C.; Khan, T.M.; Lee, L.-H.; Goh, B.-H. Resveratrol-Potential Antibacterial Agent against Foodborne Pathogens. *Front. Pharmacol.* **2018**, *9*, 102. [CrossRef]
377. Perrone, D.; Fuggetta, M.P.; Ardito, F.; Cottarelli, A.; De Filippis, A.; Ravagnan, G.; De Maria, S.; Lo Muzio, L. Resveratrol (3,5,4′-trihydroxystilbene) and its properties in oral diseases. *Exp. Med.* **2017**, *14*, 3–9. [CrossRef]
378. Jang, M.; Cai, L.; Udeani, G.O.; Slowing, K.V.; Thomas, C.F.; Beecher, C.W.; Fong, H.H.; Farnsworth, N.R.; Kinghorn, A.D.; Mehta, R.G.; et al. Cancer chemopreventive activity of resveratrol, a natural product derived from grapes. *Science* **1997**, *275*, 218–220. [CrossRef]
379. Jung, C.M.; Heinze, T.M.; Schnackenberg, L.K.; Mullis, L.B.; Elkins, S.A.; Elkins, C.A.; Steele, R.S.; Sutherland, J.B. Interaction of dietary resveratrol with animal-associated bacteria. *FEMS Microbiol. Lett.* **2009**, *297*, 266–273. [CrossRef]
380. Fernández-Mar, M.I.; Mateos, R.; García-Parrilla, M.C.; Puertas, B.; Cantos-Villar, E. Bioactive compounds in wine: Resveratrol, hydroxytyrosol and melatonin: A review. *Food Chem.* **2012**, *130*, 797–813. [CrossRef]
381. Athar, M.; Back, J.H.; Tang, X.; Kim, K.H.; Kopelovich, L.; Bickers, D.R.; Kim, A.L. Resveratrol: A review of preclinical studies for human cancer prevention. *Toxicol. Appl. Pharm.* **2007**, *224*, 274–283. [CrossRef]
382. Sawda, C.; Moussa, C.; Turner, R.S. Resveratrol for Alzheimer's disease. *Ann. N. Y. Acad. Sci.* **2017**, *1403*, 142–149. [CrossRef]
383. Gülçin, İ. Antioxidant properties of resveratrol: A structure–activity insight. *Innov. Food Sci. Emerg. Technol.* **2010**, *11*, 210–218. [CrossRef]
384. De Sá Coutinho, D.; Pacheco, M.T.; Frozza, R.L.; Bernardi, A. Anti-Inflammatory Effects of Resveratrol: Mechanistic Insights. *Int. J. Mol. Sci.* **2018**, *19*, 1812. [CrossRef] [PubMed]
385. Gao, X.; Xu, Y.X.; Janakiraman, N.; Chapman, R.A.; Gautam, S.C. Immunomodulatory activity of resveratrol: Suppression of lymphocyte proliferation, development of cell-mediated cytotoxicity, and cytokine production. *Biochem. Pharm.* **2001**, *62*, 1299–1308. [CrossRef]
386. Trung, L.Q.; An, D.T.T. Is Resveratrol a Cancer Immunomodulatory Molecule? *Front. Pharmacol.* **2018**, *9*, 1255. [CrossRef] [PubMed]
387. Berge, G.; Øvrebø, S.; Eilertsen, E.; Haugen, A.; Mollerup, S. Analysis of resveratrol as a lung cancer chemopreventive agent in A/J mice exposed to benzo[a]pyrene. *Br. J. Cancer* **2004**, *91*, 1380–1383. [CrossRef] [PubMed]
388. Yu, Y.H.; Chen, H.A.; Chen, P.S.; Cheng, Y.J.; Hsu, W.H.; Chang, Y.W.; Chen, Y.H.; Jan, Y.; Hsiao, M.; Chang, T.Y.; et al. MiR-520h-mediated FOXC2 regulation is critical for inhibition of lung cancer progression by resveratrol. *Oncogene* **2013**, *32*, 431–443. [CrossRef] [PubMed]
389. Yin, H.T.; Tian, Q.Z.; Guan, L.; Zhou, Y.; Huang, X.E.; Zhang, H. In vitro and in vivo evaluation of the antitumor efficiency of resveratrol against lung cancer. *Asian Pac. J. Cancer Prev.* **2013**, *14*, 1703–1706. [CrossRef] [PubMed]
390. Roy, S.K.; Chen, Q.; Fu, J.; Shankar, S.; Srivastava, R.K. Resveratrol inhibits growth of orthotopic pancreatic tumors through activation of FOXO transcription factors. *PLoS ONE* **2011**, *6*, e25166. [CrossRef] [PubMed]
391. Lin, H.C.; Chen, Y.F.; Hsu, W.H.; Yang, C.W.; Kao, C.H.; Tsai, T.F. Resveratrol helps recovery from fatty liver and protects against hepatocellular carcinoma induced by hepatitis B virus X protein in a mouse model. *Cancer Prev. Res.* **2012**, *5*, 952–962. [CrossRef]
392. Carbó, N.; Costelli, P.; Baccino, F.M.; López-Soriano, F.J.; Argilés, J.M. Resveratrol, a natural product present in wine, decreases tumour growth in a rat tumour model. *Biochem. Biophys. Res. Commun.* **1999**, *254*, 739–743. [CrossRef]

393. Chatterjee, K.; Mukherjee, S.; Vanmanen, J.; Banerjee, P.; Fata, J.E. Dietary Polyphenols, Resveratrol and Pterostilbene Exhibit Antitumor Activity on an HPV E6-Positive Cervical Cancer Model: An in vitro and in vivo Analysis. *Front. Oncol.* **2019**, *9*, 352. [CrossRef] [PubMed]
394. Huderson, A.C.; Myers, J.N.; Niaz, M.S.; Washington, M.K.; Ramesh, A. Chemoprevention of benzo(a)pyrene-induced colon polyps in ApcMin mice by resveratrol. *J. Nutr. Biochem.* **2013**, *24*, 713–724. [CrossRef] [PubMed]
395. Wang, T.T.; Hudson, T.S.; Wang, T.C.; Remsberg, C.M.; Davies, N.M.; Takahashi, Y.; Kim, Y.S.; Seifried, H.; Vinyard, B.T.; Perkins, S.N.; et al. Differential effects of resveratrol on androgen-responsive LNCaP human prostate cancer cells in vitro and in vivo. *Carcinogenesis* **2008**, *29*, 2001–2010. [CrossRef] [PubMed]
396. Bove, K.; Lincoln, D.W.; Tsan, M.F. Effect of resveratrol on growth of 4T1 breast cancer cells in vitro and in vivo. *Biochem. Biophys. Res. Commun.* **2002**, *291*, 1001–1005. [CrossRef] [PubMed]
397. Garvin, S.; Ollinger, K.; Dabrosin, C. Resveratrol induces apoptosis and inhibits angiogenesis in human breast cancer xenografts in vivo. *Cancer Lett.* **2006**, *231*, 113–122. [CrossRef]
398. Bhat, K.P.; Lantvit, D.; Christov, K.; Mehta, R.G.; Moon, R.C.; Pezzuto, J.M. Estrogenic and antiestrogenic properties of resveratrol in mammary tumor models. *Cancer Res.* **2001**, *61*, 7456–7463.
399. Nguyen, A.V.; Martinez, M.; Stamos, M.J.; Moyer, M.P.; Planutis, K.; Hope, C.; Holcombe, R.F. Results of a phase I pilot clinical trial examining the effect of plant-derived resveratrol and grape powder on Wnt pathway target gene expression in colonic mucosa and colon cancer. *Cancer Manag. Res.* **2009**, *1*, 25–37.
400. Howells, L.M.; Berry, D.P.; Elliott, P.J.; Jacobson, E.W.; Hoffmann, E.; Hegarty, B.; Brown, K.; Steward, W.P.; Gescher, A.J. Phase I randomized, double-blind pilot study of micronized resveratrol (SRT501) in patients with hepatic metastases–safety, pharmacokinetics, and pharmacodynamics. *Cancer Prev. Res.* **2011**, *4*, 1419–1425. [CrossRef]
401. Cottart, C.H.; Nivet-Antoine, V.; Laguillier-Morizot, C.; Beaudeux, J.L. Resveratrol bioavailability and toxicity in humans. *Mol. Nutr. Food Res.* **2010**, *54*, 7–16. [CrossRef]
402. Patel, K.R.; Scott, E.; Brown, V.A.; Gescher, A.J.; Steward, W.P.; Brown, K. Clinical trials of resveratrol. *Ann. N. Y. Acad. Sci.* **2011**, *1215*, 161–169. [CrossRef]
403. Johnson, J.J.; Nihal, M.; Siddiqui, I.A.; Scarlett, C.O.; Bailey, H.H.; Mukhtar, H.; Ahmad, N. Enhancing the bioavailability of resveratrol by combining it with piperine. *Mol. Nutr. Food Res.* **2011**, *55*, 1169–1176. [CrossRef] [PubMed]
404. Pangeni, R.; Sahni, J.K.; Ali, J.; Sharma, S.; Baboota, S. Resveratrol: Review on therapeutic potential and recent advances in drug delivery. *Expert Opin. Drug Deliv.* **2014**, *11*, 1285–1298. [CrossRef]
405. Ansari, K.A.; Vavia, P.R.; Trotta, F.; Cavalli, R. Cyclodextrin-based nanosponges for delivery of resveratrol: In vitro characterisation, stability, cytotoxicity and permeation study. *AAPS Pharmscitech.* **2011**, *12*, 279–286. [CrossRef] [PubMed]
406. Nastiti, C.; Ponto, T.; Mohammed, Y.; Roberts, M.S.; Benson, H.A.E. Novel Nanocarriers for Targeted Topical Skin Delivery of the Antioxidant Resveratrol. *Pharmaceutics* **2020**, *12*, 108. [CrossRef] [PubMed]
407. Lee, C.W.; Yen, F.L.; Huang, H.W.; Wu, T.H.; Ko, H.H.; Tzeng, W.S.; Lin, C.C. Resveratrol nanoparticle system improves dissolution properties and enhances the hepatoprotective effect of resveratrol through antioxidant and anti-inflammatory pathways. *J. Agric. Food Chem* **2012**, *60*, 4662–4671. [CrossRef]
408. Chaudhary, Z.; Subramaniam, S.; Khan, G.M.; Abeer, M.M.; Qu, Z.; Janjua, T.; Kumeria, T.; Batra, J.; Popat, A. Encapsulation and Controlled Release of Resveratrol Within Functionalized Mesoporous Silica Nanoparticles for Prostate Cancer Therapy. *Front. Bioeng. Biotechnol.* **2019**, *7*, 225. [CrossRef] [PubMed]
409. Summerlin, N.; Qu, Z.; Pujara, N.; Sheng, Y.; Jambhrunkar, S.; McGuckin, M.; Popat, A. Colloidal mesoporous silica nanoparticles enhance the biological activity of resveratrol. *Colloids Surf. B Biointerfaces* **2016**, *144*, 1–7. [CrossRef]
410. Song, D.; Hao, J.; Fan, D. Biological properties and clinical applications of berberine. *Front. Med.* **2020**. [CrossRef]
411. Cicero, A.F.; Baggioni, A. Berberine and Its Role in Chronic Disease. *Adv. Exp. Med. Biol* **2016**, *928*, 27–45. [CrossRef]
412. Schor, J.; Fabno, N. Clinical Applications for Berberine: Potential therapeutic applications in metabolic syndrome, type 2 diabetes, and dyslipidemia. *Nat. Med. J.* **2012**, *4*. Available online: https://www.naturalmedicinejournal.com/print/587 (accessed on 1 January 2021).
413. Zych, M.; Wojnar, W.; Kielanowska, M.; Folwarczna, J.; Kaczmarczyk-Sedlak, I. Effect of Berberine on Glycation, Aldose Reductase Activity, and Oxidative Stress in the Lenses of Streptozotocin-Induced Diabetic Rats In Vivo-A Preliminary Study. *Int. J. Mol. Sci.* **2020**, *21*, 4278. [CrossRef] [PubMed]
414. Liu, W.; Liu, P.; Tao, S.; Deng, Y.; Li, X.; Lan, T.; Zhang, X.; Guo, F.; Huang, W.; Chen, F.; et al. Berberine inhibits aldose reductase and oxidative stress in rat mesangial cells cultured under high glucose. *Arch. Biochem. Biophys.* **2008**, *475*, 128–134. [CrossRef]
415. Zhu, N.; Li, J.; Li, Y.; Zhang, Y.; Du, Q.; Hao, P.; Cao, X.; Li, L. Berberine Protects Against Simulated Ischemia/Reperfusion Injury-Induced H9C2 Cardiomyocytes Apoptosis In Vitro and Myocardial Ischemia/Reperfusion-Induced Apoptosis In Vivo by Regulating the Mitophagy-Mediated HIF-1α/BNIP3 Pathway. *Front. Pharm.* **2020**, *11*, 367. [CrossRef]
416. Zhao, G.L.; Yu, L.M.; Gao, W.L.; Duan, W.X.; Jiang, B.; Liu, X.D.; Zhang, B.; Liu, Z.H.; Zhai, M.E.; Jin, Z.X.; et al. Berberine protects rat heart from ischemia/reperfusion injury via activating JAK2/STAT3 signaling and attenuating endoplasmic reticulum stress. *Acta Pharm. Sin.* **2016**, *37*, 354–367. [CrossRef]
417. Kuo, C.-L.; Chi, C.-W.; Liu, T.-Y. The anti-inflammatory potential of berberine in vitro and in vivo. *Cancer Lett.* **2004**, *203*, 127–137. [CrossRef] [PubMed]

418. Wang, Y.; Yi, X.; Ghanam, K.; Zhang, S.; Zhao, T.; Zhu, X. Berberine decreases cholesterol levels in rats through multiple mechanisms, including inhibition of cholesterol absorption. *Metabolism* **2014**, *63*, 1167–1177. [CrossRef] [PubMed]
419. Xu, J.; Long, Y.; Ni, L.; Yuan, X.; Yu, N.; Wu, R.; Tao, J.; Zhang, Y. Anticancer effect of berberine based on experimental animal models of various cancers: A systematic review and meta-analysis. *BMC Cancer* **2019**, *19*, 589. [CrossRef]
420. Yin, J.; Xing, H.; Ye, J. Efficacy of berberine in patients with type 2 diabetes mellitus. *Metab. Clin. Exp.* **2008**, *57*, 712–717. [CrossRef]
421. Cicero, A.; Ertek, S. Metabolic and cardiovascular effects of berberine: From preclinical evidences to clinical trial results. *Clin. Lipidol.* **2009**, *4*, 553–563. [CrossRef]
422. Cicero, A.F.G.; Colletti, A. Role of phytochemicals in the management of metabolic syndrome. *Phytomedicine* **2016**, *23*, 1134–1144. [CrossRef]
423. Cristiana, C.; Placido, F.; Silvia, S.; Aldo Roda and Arrigo, F.G.C. Berberine: New Insights from Pharmacological Aspects to Clinical Evidences in the Management of Metabolic Disorders. *Curr. Med. Chem.* **2016**, *23*, 1460–1476. [CrossRef]
424. Wang, Y.; Liu, Y.; Du, X.; Ma, H.; Yao, J. The Anti-Cancer Mechanisms of Berberine: A Review. *Cancer Manag. Res.* **2020**, *12*, 695–702. [CrossRef] [PubMed]
425. Sahibzada, M.U.K.; Sadiq, A.; Faidah, H.S.; Khurram, M.; Amin, M.U.; Haseeb, A.; Kakar, M. Berberine nanoparticles with enhanced in vitro bioavailability: Characterization and antimicrobial activity. *Drug Des. Dev. Ther.* **2018**, *12*, 303–312. [CrossRef] [PubMed]
426. Mirhadi, E.; Rezaee, M.; Malaekeh-Nikouei, B. Nano strategies for berberine delivery, a natural alkaloid of Berberis. *Biomed. Pharm.* **2018**, *104*, 465–473. [CrossRef] [PubMed]
427. Deng, J.; Wu, Z.; Zhao, Z.; Wu, C.; Yuan, M.; Su, Z.; Wang, Y.; Wang, Z. Berberine-Loaded Nanostructured Lipid Carriers Enhance the Treatment of Ulcerative Colitis. *Int. J. Nanomed.* **2020**, *15*, 3937–3951. [CrossRef]
428. Yue, J.; Wang, Z.; Shao, D.; Chang, Z.; Hu, R.; Li, L.; Luo, S.-Z.; Dong, W.-F. Cancer cell membrane-modified biodegradable mesoporous silica nanocarriers for berberine therapy of liver cancer. *RSC Adv.* **2018**, *8*, 40288–40297. [CrossRef]
429. Schneider-Stock, R.; Fakhoury, I.H.; Zaki, A.M.; El-Baba, C.O.; Gali-Muhtasib, H.U. Thymoquinone: Fifty years of success in the battle against cancer models. *Drug Discov. Today* **2014**, *19*, 18–30. [CrossRef]
430. Gurung, R.L.; Lim, S.N.; Khaw, A.K.; Soon, J.F.; Shenoy, K.; Mohamed Ali, S.; Jayapal, M.; Sethu, S.; Baskar, R.; Hande, M.P. Thymoquinone induces telomere shortening, DNA damage and apoptosis in human glioblastoma cells. *PLoS ONE* **2010**, *5*, e12124. [CrossRef]
431. Gali-Muhtasib, H.; Ocker, M.; Kuester, D.; Krueger, S.; El-Hajj, Z.; Diestel, A.; Evert, M.; El-Najjar, N.; Peters, B.; Jurjus, A.; et al. Thymoquinone reduces mouse colon tumor cell invasion and inhibits tumor growth in murine colon cancer models. *J. Cell Mol. Med.* **2008**, *12*, 330–342. [CrossRef]
432. Jakaria, M.; Cho, D.Y.; Ezazul Haque, M.; Karthivashan, G.; Kim, I.S.; Ganesan, P.; Choi, D.K. Neuropharmacological Potential and Delivery Prospects of Thymoquinone for Neurological Disorders. *Oxid. Med. Cell. Longev.* **2018**, *2018*, 1209801. [CrossRef]
433. Ahmad, A.; Mishra, R.K.; Vyawahare, A.; Kumar, A.; Rehman, M.U.; Qamar, W.; Khan, A.Q.; Khan, R. Thymoquinone (2-Isoprpyl-5-methyl-1, 4-benzoquinone) as a chemopreventive/anticancer agent: Chemistry and biological effects. *Saudi Pharm. J.* **2019**, *27*, 1113–1126. [CrossRef] [PubMed]
434. Al-Majed, A.A.; Al-Omar, F.A.; Nagi, M.N. Neuroprotective effects of thymoquinone against transient forebrain ischemia in the rat hippocampus. *Eur. J. Pharmacol.* **2006**, *543*, 40–47. [CrossRef] [PubMed]
435. Umar, S.; Zargan, J.; Umar, K.; Ahmad, S.; Katiyar, C.K.; Khan, H.A. Modulation of the oxidative stress and inflammatory cytokine response by thymoquinone in the collagen induced arthritis in Wistar rats. *Chem. Biol. Interact.* **2012**, *197*, 40–46. [CrossRef] [PubMed]
436. Woo, C.C.; Kumar, A.P.; Sethi, G.; Tan, K.H.B. Thymoquinone: Potential cure for inflammatory disorders and cancer. *Biochem. Pharmacol.* **2012**, *83*, 443–451. [CrossRef]
437. Asaduzzaman Khan, M.; Tania, M.; Fu, S.; Fu, J. Thymoquinone, as an anticancer molecule: From basic research to clinical investigation. *Oncotarget* **2017**, *8*, 51907–51919. [CrossRef]
438. Chaieb, K.; Kouidhi, B.; Jrah, H.; Mahdouani, K.; Bakhrouf, A. Antibacterial activity of Thymoquinone, an active principle of Nigella sativa and its potency to prevent bacterial biofilm formation. *BMC Complement. Altern. Med.* **2011**, *11*, 29. [CrossRef]
439. Kassab, R.B.; El-Hennamy, R.E. The role of thymoquinone as a potent antioxidant in ameliorating the neurotoxic effect of sodium arsenate in female rat. *Egypt. J. Basic Appl. Sci.* **2017**, *4*, 160–167. [CrossRef]
440. Bule, M.; Nikfar, S.; Amini, M.; Abdollahi, M. The antidiabetic effect of thymoquinone: A systematic review and meta-analysis of animal studies. *Food Res. Int.* **2020**, *127*, 108736. [CrossRef]
441. El-Najjar, N.; Ketola, R.A.; Nissilä, T.; Mauriala, T.; Antopolsky, M.; Jänis, J.; Gali-Muhtasib, H.; Urtti, A.; Vuorela, H. Impact of protein binding on the analytical detectability and anticancer activity of thymoquinone. *J. Chem. Biol.* **2011**, *4*, 97–107. [CrossRef]
442. Pathan, S.A.; Jain, G.K.; Zaidi, S.M.; Akhter, S.; Vohora, D.; Chander, P.; Kole, P.L.; Ahmad, F.J.; Khar, R.K. Stability-indicating ultra-performance liquid chromatography method for the estimation of thymoquinone and its application in biopharmaceutical studies. *Biomed. Chromatogr.* **2011**, *25*, 613–620. [CrossRef]
443. Salmani, J.M.; Asghar, S.; Lv, H.; Zhou, J. Aqueous solubility and degradation kinetics of the phytochemical anticancer thymoquinone; probing the effects of solvents, pH and light. *Molecules* **2014**, *19*, 5925–5939. [CrossRef] [PubMed]
444. Darakhshan, S.; Bidmeshki Pour, A.; Hosseinzadeh Colagar, A.; Sisakhtnezhad, S. Thymoquinone and its therapeutic potentials. *Pharm. Res.* **2015**, *95–96*, 138–158. [CrossRef] [PubMed]

445. Rathore, C.; Upadhyay, N.; Kaundal, R.; Dwivedi, R.P.; Rahatekar, S.; John, A.; Dua, K.; Tambuwala, M.M.; Jain, S.; Chaudari, D.; et al. Enhanced oral bioavailability and hepatoprotective activity of thymoquinone in the form of phospholipidic nano-constructs. *Expert Opin. Drug Deliv.* **2020**, *17*, 237–253. [CrossRef] [PubMed]
446. Abukhader, M.M.; Khan, S.A. Thymoquinone and Nanoparticles: A Promising Approach for the Clinical Trials. *J. Bionanosci.* **2017**, *11*, 258–265. [CrossRef]
447. Goel, S.; Mishra, P. Thymoquinone loaded mesoporous silica nanoparticles retard cell invasion and enhance in vitro cytotoxicity due to ROS mediated apoptosis in HeLa and MCF-7 cell lines. *Mater. Sci. Eng. C Mater. Biol. Appl.* **2019**, *104*, 109881. [CrossRef]
448. Fahmy, H.M.; Fathy, M.M.; Abd-elbadia, R.A.; Elshemey, W.M. Targeting of Thymoquinone-loaded mesoporous silica nanoparticles to different brain areas: In vivo study. *Life Sci.* **2019**, *222*, 94–102. [CrossRef]
449. Kahkeshani, N.; Farzaei, F.; Fotouhi, M.; Alavi, S.S.; Bahramsoltani, R.; Naseri, R.; Momtaz, S.; Abbasabadi, Z.; Rahimi, R.; Farzaei, M.H.; et al. Pharmacological effects of gallic acid in health and diseases: A mechanistic review. *Iran. J. Basic Med. Sci.* **2019**, *22*, 225–237. [CrossRef]
450. Li, Z.-J.; Liu, M.; Dawuti, G.; Dou, Q.; Ma, Y.; Liu, H.-G.; Aibai, S. Antifungal Activity of Gallic Acid In Vitro and In Vivo. *Phytother. Res.* **2017**, *31*, 1039–1045. [CrossRef]
451. Subramanian, A.P.; John, A.A.; Vellayappan, M.V.; Balaji, A.; Jaganathan, S.K.; Supriyanto, E.; Yusof, M. Gallic acid: Prospects and molecular mechanisms of its anticancer activity. *RSC Adv.* **2015**, *5*, 35608–35621. [CrossRef]
452. Akbari, G. Molecular mechanisms underlying gallic acid effects against cardiovascular diseases: An update review. *Avicenna J. Phytomed.* **2020**, *10*, 11–23.
453. Gao, J.; Hu, J.; Hu, D.; Yang, X. A Role of Gallic Acid in Oxidative Damage Diseases: A Comprehensive Review. *Nat. Prod. Commun.* **2019**, *14*, 1934578X19874174. [CrossRef]
454. Shabani, S.; Rabiei, Z.; Amini-Khoei, H. Exploring the multifaceted neuroprotective actions of gallic acid: A review. *Int. J. Food Prop.* **2020**, *23*, 736–752. [CrossRef]
455. Badhani, B.; Sharma, N.; Kakkar, R. Gallic acid: A versatile antioxidant with promising therapeutic and industrial applications. *RSC Adv.* **2015**, *5*, 27540–27557. [CrossRef]
456. de Cristo Soares Alves, A.; Mainardes, R.M.; Khalil, N.M. Nanoencapsulation of gallic acid and evaluation of its cytotoxicity and antioxidant activity. *Mater. Sci. Eng. C Mater. Biol. Appl.* **2016**, *60*, 126–134. [CrossRef] [PubMed]
457. Khan, B.A.; Mahmood, T.; Menaa, F.; Shahzad, Y.; Yousaf, A.M.; Hussain, T.; Ray, S.D. New Perspectives on the Efficacy of Gallic Acid in Cosmetics & Nanocosmeceuticals. *Curr. Pharm. Des.* **2018**, *24*, 5181–5187. [CrossRef] [PubMed]
458. Zhao, Y.; Li, D.; Zhu, Z.; Sun, Y. Improved Neuroprotective Effects of Gallic Acid-Loaded Chitosan Nanoparticles Against Ischemic Stroke. *Rejuvenation Res.* **2019**, *23*, 284–292. [CrossRef]
459. Shah, S.T.; Yehya, W.A.; Saad, O.; Simarani, K.; Chowdhury, Z.; Alhadi, A.A.; Al-Ani, L.A. Surface Functionalization of Iron Oxide Nanoparticles with Gallic Acid as Potential Antioxidant and Antimicrobial Agents. *Nanomaterials* **2017**, *7*, 306. [CrossRef]
460. Nagpal, K.; Singh, S.K.; Mishra, D.N. Nanoparticle mediated brain targeted delivery of gallic acid: In vivo behavioral and biochemical studies for improved antioxidant and antidepressant-like activity. *Drug Deliv.* **2012**, *19*, 378–391. [CrossRef]
461. Lewandowski, D.; Ruszkowski, P.; Pińska, A.; Schroeder, G.; Kurczewska, J. SBA-15 Mesoporous Silica Modified with Gallic Acid and Evaluation of Its Cytotoxic Activity. *PLoS ONE* **2015**, *10*, e0132541. [CrossRef]
462. Rashidi, L.; Vasheghani-Farahani, E.; Soleimani, M.; Atashi, A.; Rostami, K.; Gangi, F.; Fallahpour, M.; Tahouri, M.T. A cellular uptake and cytotoxicity properties study of gallic acid-loaded mesoporous silica nanoparticles on Caco-2 cells. *J. Nanopart. Res.* **2014**, *16*, 2285. [CrossRef]
463. Lammari, N.; Louaer, O.; Meniai, A.H.; Elaissari, A. Encapsulation of Essential Oils via Nanoprecipitation Process: Overview, Progress, Challenges and Prospects. *Pharmaceutics* **2020**, *12*, 431. [CrossRef] [PubMed]
464. Sharifi-Rad, J.; Sureda, A.; Tenore, G.C.; Daglia, M.; Sharifi-Rad, M.; Valussi, M.; Tundis, R.; Loizzo, M.R.; Ademiluyi, A.O.; Sharifi-Rad, R.; et al. Biological Activities of Essential Oils: From Plant Chemoecology to Traditional Healing Systems. *Molecules* **2017**, *22*, 70. [CrossRef] [PubMed]
465. Elshafie, H.S.; Camele, I. An Overview of the Biological Effects of Some Mediterranean Essential Oils on Human Health. *BioMed Res. Int.* **2017**, *2017*, 9268468. [CrossRef] [PubMed]
466. Baser, K.H.C.; Buchbauer, G. *Handbook of Essential Oils: Science, Technology, and Applications*; CRC Press: Boca Raton, FL, USA, 2015.
467. Ali, B.; Al-Wabel, N.A.; Shams, S.; Ahamad, A.; Khan, S.A.; Anwar, F. Essential oils used in aromatherapy: A systemic review. *Asian Pac. J. Trop. Biomed.* **2015**, *5*, 601–611. [CrossRef]
468. Dhifi, W.; Bellili, S.; Jazi, S.; Bahloul, N.; Mnif, W. Essential Oils' Chemical Characterization and Investigation of Some Biological Activities: A Critical Review. *Medicines* **2016**, *3*, 25. [CrossRef]
469. Andrade, M.A.; Braga, M.A.; Cesar, P.H.S.; Trento, M.V.C.; Espósito, M.A.; Silva, L.F.; Marcussi, S. Anticancer Properties of Essential Oils: An Overview. *Curr. Cancer Drug Targets* **2018**, *18*, 957–966. [CrossRef]
470. Edris, A.E. Pharmaceutical and therapeutic Potentials of essential oils and their individual volatile constituents: A review. *Phytother. Res.* **2007**, *21*, 308–323. [CrossRef]
471. Blowman, K.; Magalhães, M.; Lemos, M.F.L.; Cabral, C.; Pires, I.M. Anticancer Properties of Essential Oils and Other Natural Products. *Evid.-Based Complement. Altern. Med.* **2018**, *2018*, 3149362. [CrossRef]
472. Gautam, N.; Mantha, A.K.; Mittal, S. Essential Oils and Their Constituents as Anticancer Agents: A Mechanistic View. *BioMed Res. Int.* **2014**, *2014*, 154106. [CrossRef]

473. Fitsiou, E.; Pappa, A. Anticancer Activity of Essential Oils and Other Extracts from Aromatic Plants Grown in Greece. *Antioxidants* **2019**, *8*, 290. [CrossRef]
474. Bhalla, Y.; Gupta, V.K.; Jaitak, V. Anticancer activity of essential oils: A review. *J. Sci. Food Agric.* **2013**, *93*, 3643–3653. [CrossRef] [PubMed]
475. Bayala, B.; Bassole, I.H.; Scifo, R.; Gnoula, C.; Morel, L.; Lobaccaro, J.-M.A.; Simpore, J. Anticancer activity of essential oils and their chemical components—A review. *Am. J. Cancer Res.* **2014**, *4*, 591–607. [PubMed]
476. Manjamalai, A.; Kumar, M.J.; Grace, V.M. Essential oil of Tridax procumbens L induces apoptosis and suppresses angiogenesis and lung metastasis of the B16F-10 cell line in C57BL/6 mice. *Asian Pac. J. Cancer Prev.* **2012**, *13*, 5887–5895. [CrossRef]
477. Manjamalai, A.; Grace, V.M. The chemotherapeutic effect of essential oil of Plectranthus amboinicus (Lour) on lung metastasis developed by B16F-10 cell line in C57BL/6 mice. *Cancer Investig.* **2013**, *31*, 74–82. [CrossRef] [PubMed]
478. Turek, C.; Stintzing, F.C. Stability of Essential Oils: A Review. *Compr. Rev. Food Sci. Food Saf.* **2013**, *12*, 40–53. [CrossRef]
479. Froiio, F.; Ginot, L.; Paolino, D.; Lebaz, N.; Bentaher, A.; Fessi, H.; Elaissari, A. Essential Oils-Loaded Polymer Particles: Preparation, Characterization and Antimicrobial Property. *Polymers* **2019**, *11*, 17. [CrossRef] [PubMed]
480. Ali, H.; Al-Khalifa, A.R.; Aouf, A.; Boukhebti, H.; Farouk, A. Effect of nanoencapsulation on volatile constituents, and antioxidant and anticancer activities of Algerian Origanum glandulosum Desf. essential oil. *Sci. Rep.* **2020**, *10*, 2812. [CrossRef]
481. Attallah, O.A.; Shetta, A.; Elshishiny, F.; Mamdouh, W. Essential oil loaded pectin/chitosan nanoparticles preparation and optimization via Box–Behnken design against MCF-7 breast cancer cell lines. *RSC Adv.* **2020**, *10*, 8703–8708. [CrossRef]
482. De Matos, S.P.; Teixeira, H.F.; de Lima, Á.A.N.; Veiga-Junior, V.F.; Koester, L.S. Essential Oils and Isolated Terpenes in Nanosystems Designed for Topical Administration: A Review. *Biomolecules* **2019**, *9*, 138. [CrossRef]
483. Melendez-Rodriguez, B.; Figueroa-Lopez, K.J.; Bernardos, A.; Martínez-Máñez, R.; Cabedo, L.; Torres-Giner, S.; Lagaron, J.M. Electrospun Antimicrobial Films of Poly(3-hydroxybutyrate-co-3-hydroxyvalerate) Containing Eugenol Essential Oil Encapsulated in Mesoporous Silica Nanoparticles. *Nanomaterials* **2019**, *9*, 227. [CrossRef]
484. Ebadollahi, A.; Sendi, J.J.; Aliakbar, A. Efficacy of Nanoencapsulated Thymus eriocalyx and Thymus kotschyanus Essential Oils by a Mesoporous Material MCM-41 Against Tetranychus urticae (Acari: Tetranychidae). *J. Econ. Entomol.* **2017**, *110*, 2413–2420. [CrossRef] [PubMed]
485. Janatova, A.; Bernardos, A.; Smid, J.; Frankova, A.; Lhotka, M.; Kourimská, L.; Pulkrabek, J.; Kloucek, P. Long-term antifungal activity of volatile essential oil components released from mesoporous silica materials. *Ind. Crop. Prod.* **2015**, *67*, 216–220. [CrossRef]
486. Jobdeedamrong, A.; Jenjob, R.; Crespy, D. Encapsulation and Release of Essential Oils in Functional Silica Nanocontainers. *Langmuir* **2018**, *34*, 13235–13243. [CrossRef] [PubMed]
487. Kim, M.; Yeom, Y.E.; Kim, D.; Kim, J.; Lee, C. Delayed Volatilization of Lavender Essential Oil Using Mesoporous Silica Nanoparticles. *Polymer* **2019**, *43*, 327–330. [CrossRef]
488. Jin, L.; Teng, J.; Hu, L.; Lan, X.; Xu, Y.; Sheng, J.; Song, Y.; Wang, M. Pepper fragrant essential oil (PFEO) and functionalized MCM-41 nanoparticles: Formation, characterization, and bactericidal activity. *J. Sci. Food Agric.* **2019**, *99*, 5168–5175. [CrossRef]
489. Bravo Cadena, M.; Preston, G.M.; Van der Hoorn, R.A.L.; Townley, H.E.; Thompson, I.P. Species-specific antimicrobial activity of essential oils and enhancement by encapsulation in mesoporous silica nanoparticles. *Ind. Crop. Prod.* **2018**, *122*, 582–590. [CrossRef]
490. Bernardos, A.; Marina, T.; Žáček, P.; Pérez-Esteve, É.; Martínez-Mañez, R.; Lhotka, M.; Kouřimská, L.; Pulkrábek, J.; Kloucek, P. Antifungal effect of essential oil components against Aspergillus niger when loaded into silica mesoporous supports. *J. Sci. Food Agric.* **2015**, *95*, 2824–2831. [CrossRef] [PubMed]
491. Chan, A.C.; Bravo Cadena, M.; Townley, H.E.; Fricker, M.D.; Thompson, I.P. Effective delivery of volatile biocides employing mesoporous silicates for treating biofilms. *J. R. Soc. Interface* **2017**, *14*, 20160650. [CrossRef]
492. Crespo-Ortiz, M.P.; Wei, M.Q. Antitumor activity of artemisinin and its derivatives: From a well-known antimalarial agent to a potential anticancer drug. *J. Biomed. Biotechnol.* **2012**, *2012*, 247597. [CrossRef]
493. Chen, J.; Guo, Z.; Wang, H.B.; Zhou, J.J.; Zhang, W.J.; Chen, Q.W. Multifunctional mesoporous nanoparticles as pH-responsive Fe(2+) reservoirs and artemisinin vehicles for synergistic inhibition of tumor growth. *Biomaterials* **2014**, *35*, 6498–6507. [CrossRef]
494. Kumar, A.; Sharma, P.R.; Mondhe, D.M. Potential anticancer role of colchicine-based derivatives: An overview. *Anticancer Drugs* **2017**, *28*, 250–262. [CrossRef]
495. Cauda, V.; Engelke, H.; Sauer, A.; Arcizet, D.; Bräuchle, C.; Rädler, J.; Bein, T. Colchicine-Loaded Lipid Bilayer-Coated 50 nm Mesoporous Nanoparticles Efficiently Induce Microtubule Depolymerization upon Cell Uptake. *Nano Lett.* **2010**, *10*, 2484–2492. [CrossRef]
496. Hespeler, D.; Kaltenbach, J.; Pyo, S.M. Glabridin smartPearls—Silica selection, production, amorphous stability and enhanced solubility. *Int. J. Pharm.* **2019**, *561*, 228–235. [CrossRef]
497. Buda, V.; Brezoiu, A.M.; Berger, D.; Pavel, I.Z.; Muntean, D.; Minda, D.; Dehelean, C.A.; Soica, C.; Diaconeasa, Z.; Folescu, R.; et al. Biological Evaluation of Black Chokeberry Extract Free and Embedded in Two Mesoporous Silica-Type Matrices. *Pharmaceutics* **2020**, *12*, 838. [CrossRef] [PubMed]

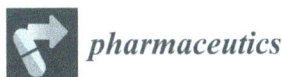

Review

The Therapeutic Efficacy of Dendrimer and Micelle Formulations for Breast Cancer Treatment

Sibusiso Alven and Blessing Atim Aderibigbe *

Department of Chemistry, University of Fort Hare, Alice Campus, Eastern Cape 5700, South Africa; 201214199@ufh.ac.za
* Correspondence: baderibigbe@ufh.ac.za or blessingaderibigbe@gmail.com; Tel.: +27-4060-222-66

Received: 16 August 2020; Accepted: 16 October 2020; Published: 15 December 2020

Abstract: Breast cancer is among the most common types of cancer in women and it is the cause of a high rate of mortality globally. The use of anticancer drugs is the standard treatment approach used for this type of cancer. However, most of these drugs are limited by multi-drug resistance, drug toxicity, poor drug bioavailability, low water solubility, poor pharmacokinetics, etc. To overcome multi-drug resistance, combinations of two or more anticancer drugs are used. However, the combination of two or more anticancer drugs produce toxic side effects. Micelles and dendrimers are promising drug delivery systems that can overcome the limitations associated with the currently used anticancer drugs. They have the capability to overcome drug resistance, reduce drug toxicity, improve the drug solubility and bioavailability. Different classes of anticancer drugs have been loaded into micelles and dendrimers, resulting in targeted drug delivery, sustained drug release mechanism, increased cellular uptake, reduced toxic side effects of the loaded drugs with enhanced anticancer activity in vitro and in vivo. This review article reports the biological outcomes of dendrimers and micelles loaded with different known anticancer agents on breast cancer in vitro and in vivo.

Keywords: breast cancer; micelles; dendrimers; anticancer drugs; drug delivery; doxorubicin; platinum drug; methotrexate

1. Introduction

Cancer is a life-threatening disease characterized by abnormal and uncontrolled cell proliferation, which can invade other organs of the body [1]. Approximately 90–95% of cancer cases are attributed to genetic mutation and 5–10% cases are caused by inherited genetic mutations [2]. The World Health Organisation (WHO) reported 9 million cancer-related deaths in 2018, which occurred mostly in Asia and Africa. Types of cancer are classified based on the body organ affected, and some examples of cancer types include breast, lung, liver, colorectal, skin, brain, stomach, and pancreatic cancer, etc. [3,4].

Among the cancer types, breast cancer is common in women, and it has been reported to be the cause of approximately 627,000 deaths in the world annually [5]. There were 230,000 breast cancer cases diagnosed in the United States alone with over 40,000 deaths, and it is identified as the second common cause of cancer-related death in women [6]. The mortality rate relating to breast cancer has decreased over the past 20 years by 30% due to consistent progress in drug development, which has resulted in an improved survival rate of 90% [7]. Despite the improvements in the survival rate in some developed countries, metastatic breast tumor is still challenging to treat with a predictable overall survival rate of only 23% [8]. The main pathways that are involved in breast cancer metastases and development are not well understood.

Breast cancer is classified into three subtypes based on the occurrence and absence of three receptors present in the tumor cells: (i). hormone receptor (HR) positive breast cancer (express progesterone and estrogen receptors), (ii). Oncogene human epidermal growth factor 2 (HER-2/neu), and (iii). Triple-negative breast cancer (TNBC) (negative for expression of progesterone, estrogen, and HER-2/neu) [9,10]. The TNBC is the worst chronic breast tumor subtype. Several methods used to treat cancer include chemotherapy, hormonal therapy, radiotherapy, immunotherapy, and surgery [11]. Chemotherapy is one of the best treatment methods used to combat breast cancer subtypes, although it suffers from several shortcomings [12].

Chemotherapy is the most utilized approach, and recently it involves the combination of two or more anticancer agents to overcome the development of drug resistance. The shortcomings of chemotherapy include multi-drug resistance, drug toxicity, poor drug bioavailability, low water solubility, and poor pharmacokinetic parameters [13]. Polymeric nanocarriers are effective potential systems that can be utilized for targeted drug delivery. Their capability to overcome the shortcomings of anticancer drugs that are associated with chemotherapy is promising. They are drug delivery systems formulated from polymer-based materials and are used to deliver different types of bioactive agents (e.g., hydrophilic and hydrophobic drugs) to the targeted biological environment. There are various types of polymeric nanocarriers utilized for the delivery of bioactive agents resulting in improved therapeutic outcomes such as polymeric nanoparticles [14–18], nanoliposomes [19–22], nanocapsules [23], polymer prodrugs [24–29], nanogels [30], hydrogels [31], dendrimers [32,33], and micelles [34–37]. Polymeric nanocarriers offer several unique and potent advantages: improved drug solubility, enhanced drug biodegradability, bioavailability, and biocompatibility, improved patient compliance, controlled and sustained drug release kinetics, preservation of the drug efficacy during plasma circulation, reduced drug toxicity, and overcome drug resistance [34,38]. Due to the unique features of polymeric nanocarriers, this review will report the in vitro and in vivo biological efficacy of micelles and dendrimers designed for the treatment of breast cancer.

2. Breast Cancer and Its Chemotherapy

Among the subtypes of breast cancer, 60% of breast cancer cases are HR-positive breast tumors, and HER-2/neu constitute around 20% of all breast cancer cases. Approximately 20% of breast cancer cases are TNBC [39]. Breast cancer-related symptoms include a change in the shape and size of breast, skin dimpling, swollen lymph nodes, red patch of the skin, a lump in the breast, discharge of fluid from the nipple, bone pain, and shortness of breath [40]. Several factors that contribute to breast cancer include obesity, early age menstruation, smoking, inherited genes mutations, ionizing radiation, lack of exercise, etc. [41]. Breast cancer therapies presently used are chemotherapy, radiation therapy, immunotherapy, surgery, hormone therapy, and antibody therapy [42,43]. These therapies have short and long-term consequences that affect patients' quality of life [43].

Anticancer drugs (Figure 1, Table 1) act by interfering with the abnormal, uncontrolled cell division and are cell cycle phase non-specific or specific [43,44]. Cell cycle phase-specific bioactive agents include the plant alkaloids (e.g., vinca alkaloids and taxanes) and the antimetabolites (e.g., fluorouracil (**1**), methotrexate (**2**)) [45]. Antimetabolites are very effective in the S-phase of cell division, and they act specifically on cells involved in the formation of new cells from the synthesis of new DNA. Plant alkaloids are effective in the S- and M-phases. Fluorouracil acts as a thymidylate synthase inhibitor by interfering with DNA replication. Vinca alkaloids (e.g., vincristine (**3**)) bind with microtubule assembly, destroying chromosome segregation during mitosis. The taxanes (e.g., paclitaxel (**4**), docetaxel (**5**)) prevent the normal functioning of microtubule during mitosis and hinders cell division [45].

Alkylating agents are cell cycle phase non-specific bioactive agents, and their examples include cyclophosphamide (cytoxan (**6**)), they target the replicating cells' DNA. Other examples of alkylating agents are platinum drugs (e.g., carboplatin (**7**), cisplatin (**8**) and oxaliplatin (**9**))) which are responsible for the inhibition of DNA synthesis in cancer cells. Anti-tumor antibiotics are also cell cycle phase non-specific bioactive agents (e.g., epirubicin (**10**), doxorubicin (**11**) and camptothecin (**12**)). They prevent RNA (ribonucleic acid) synthesis by binding with the DNA, thereby distorting the DNA structure [46]. Other chemotherapeutic agents employed for breast tumor chemotherapy include tamoxifen (**13**) a selective estrogen-receptor modulator) administered to the patient with ER-positive breast tumor, and it acts as an estrogen antagonist. Another drug used to treat breast cancer is arimidex (**14**) which hinders aromatase action. It is administered to postmenopausal women diagnosed with hormone-receptor-positive, metastatic hormone-receptor-positive breast cancer, and advanced-stage breast cancer. Trastuzumab ((**15**), a biological response modifier) acts as a HER2 protein inhibitor on breast cancer cells, terminate cell division, and causes apoptosis and cell stasis [46].

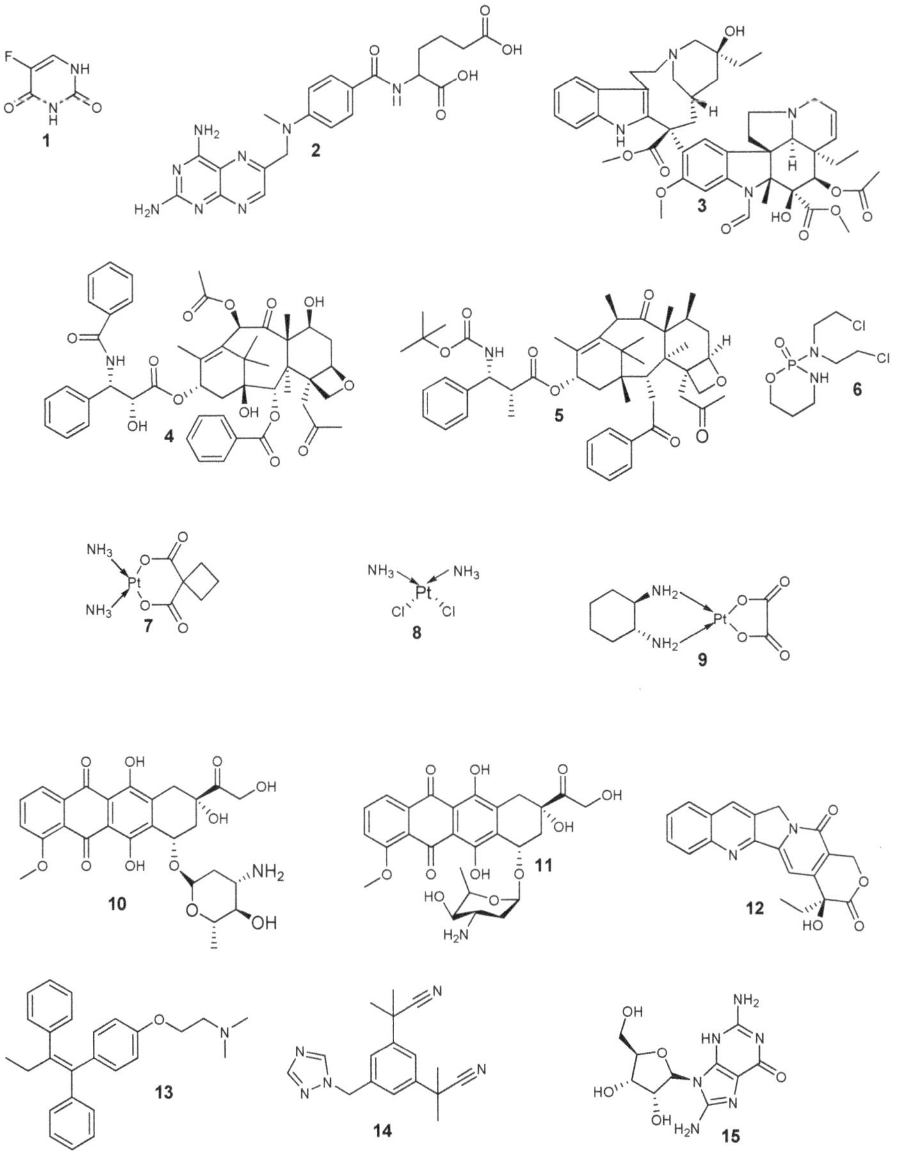

Figure 1. Anticancer drugs used for the treatment of breast cancer: fluorouracil (**1**), methotrexate (**2**), vincristine (**3**), paclitaxel (**4**), docetaxel (**5**), cytoxan (**6**), carboplatin (**7**), cisplatin (**8**), oxaliplatin (**9**), epirubicin (**10**), doxorubicin (**11**), camptothecin (**12**), tamoxifen (**13**), arimidex (**14**) and trastuzumab (**15**).

Table 1. Classification of anticancer drugs and their side effects.

Anticancer Drugs	Drug Class	Mode of Action	Side Effects
Doxorubicin Epirubicin Camptothecin	Antitumor antibiotics	Binds to DNA and prevent DNA synthesis. They cause changes in the chromatin structure via inhibition of topoisomerase II.	Vomiting/nausea, weight loss, alopecia, thrombocytopenia, neutropenia, anorexia, and impaired immunity.
Cyclophosphamide (Cytoxan)	Alkylating agent Anti-neoplastic drug	Result in cross-linkage in DNA strands. Inhibit DNA biosynthesis and cell division.	Severe vomiting/nausea, neurotoxicity, pulmonary fibrosis, immune suppression, and alopecia.
Paclitaxel (taxol) Docetaxel (Taxotere)	Plant alkaloids Taxane class	Hinders microtubule disassembly and increase microtubule assembly. Terminate cell division in metaphase.	Leutropenia, hypersensitivity, anaphylaxis, thrombocytopenia, myalgias, fatigue, neutropenia, arthralgias, stomatitis, and Peripheral neuropathy
Vincristine	Vinca alkaloids Mitotic inhibitor	Binds to mitotic tubules and prevent the formation of microtubule in the mitotic spindle, inhibits mitosis I metaphase.	Mucositis, leukopenis, weight change, neurotoxicity, constipation, fatigue, secondary neoplasm, and thrombocytopenia
5-Fluorouracil	Pyrimidine antimetabolite	Inhibits enzyme formation needed for the synthesis of DNA.	Thrombocytopenia, peripheral neuropathy, mucositis, anaemia, neutropenia, neurotoxicity, cerebellar ataxia, and skin changes
Cisplatin Carboplatin	Platinum drugs	Inhibits the synthesis of DNA and prevents cell replication.	Ototoxicity, neurotoxicity, cardiotoxicity, nephrotoxicity, myelosuppression, neutropenia, and delayed hypersensitivity
Arimidex	aromatase inhibitor	Hinders aromatase, which intermediates transformation of androstenedione to estrone, which is then converted to estradiol.	Pain, mild nausea, vaginal dryness, osteoporosis, chest pain, increased risk for fractures, oedema, weakness, mild diarrhea, headache, and arthralgias
Tamoxifen	Selective estrogen receptor modulator	Strives with estrogen for receptor binding	Vaginal discharge, altered menses, amenorrhea, cough oedema, bone pain, musculoskeletal pain, dizziness, and endometrial hyperplasia.
Bevacizumab	Monoclonal antibody biological modifier	Binds to HER2 positive cancer cells and bring them up to be destroyed by the immune system. Cell proliferation inhibition.	Weakness, pain, flu-like symptoms, chills, diarrhea, abdominal pain, back pain, anorexia, congestive heart failure, and left ventricular cardiac dysfunction

All the aforementioned anticancer drugs can affect healthy cells (e.g., bone marrow, and hair follicle, etc.), resulting in significant and frequent adverse effects that include alopecia, loss of appetite, vomiting, and nausea, thrombocytopenia, neuropathy, mucositis, myelosuppression-induced anemia, etc. [47]. The chemotherapeutic drugs are employed to target the rapid division of cancer cells; various cells in the human body rapidly divide in a normal manner, such as the digestive tract cells and hair follicle cells, which are also affected by the chemotherapeutics. Also, the widespread distribution and short half-life of anticancer drugs require more dosing, resulting in increased side effects [47]. The anticancer drugs' side effects are due to their non-targeted and non-specific nature that result in the healthy cells/tissue exposure to their toxic side effects. Polymeric nanocarriers are promising candidates that can be employed to overcome the shortcomings of currently used anticancer drugs. Hence this review article is focused on polymeric micelles and dendrimers nanocarriers loaded with anticancer drugs for breast tumor targeting.

3. Micelles and Dendrimers Nanoformulations That Are Currently in the Clinical Trials

Micelles display excellent features such as good tumor-targeted delivery, making them suitable as a drug delivery system with high translational potential. Some micelle-based systems are presently under various phases of clinical assessment (Table 2), but most of them are still under preclinical evaluation [48]. Genexol®-PM and NK105 were developed to improve the water solubility and therapeutic efficacy of paclitaxel and irinotecan (topoisomerase-I inhibitor). Genexol®-PM is known as the copolymer micelle made up of mPEG-PDLLA solubilizer. Its enhanced water solubilizing efficiency of 25% is higher than the formulation, Taxol®. In addition, this micelle formulation has a greater maximum tolerated dose when compared to Taxol® [48]. Furthermore, Genexol®-PM exhibits higher cellular internalization and good inhibition of P-glycoprotein, and decreased myelo-suppression when compared to Taxol®. Presently, Genexol®-PM has been approved for clinical application in South Korea, Hungary, and Bulgaria, and it is being assessed in Phase II clinical trials in the USA. It is sold under the trade name Cynviloq™ [48,49].

NK105 is a micelle formulation developed from PEG-poly(aspartic acid) copolymer and 4-phenyl-1-butanol to improve its hydrophilicity. It delivers loaded paclitaxel to solid tumors [50]. Tumor maximum concentration of these micelles was higher than paclitaxel when screened on HT-29 colon tumor model. Nippon Kayaku Co. Ltd. (Tokyo, Japan), a certified company in Japan, began phase II clinical trial of NK105 [50]. NK012 micelle formulation is composed of conjugated drug SN38 (irinotecan hydrochloride) with poly(L-glutamic acid) fragment of PEG–P(Glu) block copolymer. Despite its significant cytotoxicity against several cancer cell lines screened, NK012 micelle is an effective micellar system with an average particle size of 20 nm and the drug loading capacity of approximately 20% [51]. Two clinical trial phases were completed independently in the USA and Japan, with no serious dose-dependent side effects. Based on these findings, NK012 micelles are currently under phase II clinical trial [51].

The micelle products NC-6300, NK911, and NC-6004 are formulated for the delivery of epirubicin, doxorubicin, and cisplatin, respectively [52]. The antitumor activity of NC-6300 with a significant decrease in cardiac toxicity in the phase I clinical evaluation in 2013 revealed that the formulation is safe and tolerable [53]. NK911 formulation in a clinical trial at the National Cancer Centre Hospital in Japan, Tokyo, showed the recommended dose and minimum toxicity dose of 50 and 67 mg/m^2, respectively [53]. The NC-4016 micelles formulation containing DACH-platinum was reported to be stable in physiological environments with prolonged blood plasma circulation after bolus administration resulting in more than 1000-fold increase in blood plasma concentration between 0 to 3 days when compared to free oxaliplatin during preclinical evaluations. Phase I clinical study commenced in 2013 at the University of Texas MD Anderson Cancer Centre in the USA in patients with advanced lymphoma or solid tumor [54]. NC-6004 (Nanoplatin™) was evaluated at phase I/II clinical trial in patients with advanced solid tumour to evaluate its safe dose, safety, efficacy, and tolerability [55]. Seventeen patients with advanced solid tumour types were administered the formulation intravenously with a starting dose of 10 mg m^{-2} which was increased to 120 mg/m^2. The maximum tolerated dose of 120 mg/m^2 and a recommended dose of 90 mg/m^2 was reported. The sustained release of cisplatin after administration contributed to the low toxicity of the formulation.

SP1049C micellar formulation has been reported to overcome multidrug resistance in a clinical trial [56]. It is composed of Pluronic L61 and Pluronic F127. It is loaded with doxorubicin. Pluronic L61 inhibits the efflux mechanism of P-glycoprotein, while pluronic F127 enhances the stability of the formulation. The biodistribution of the formulation was similar to the free doxorubicin in the liver, blood plasma, kidney, lungs, and heart. The cytotoxicity of the formulation was significant against a brain tumor. Its effective therapeutic outcomes were reported in preclinical studies, phase I and II clinical trials in patients with advanced adenocarcinoma of gastroesophageal and oesophagus junctions. It is a registered chemotherapeutic agent for the treatment of metastatic adenocarcinoma [56].

On the other hand, the use of dendrimer-based nanocarriers for cancer therapy is beneficial. A lot is left to be discovered and addressed to confirm their efficacy in cancer treatment [57]. One of the antitumor dendrimer formulations that have succeeded from preclinical evaluation to Phase I clinical study is DEP® docetaxel. DEP® docetaxel formulated from PEGylated PLL dendrimer has shown promising results in clinical trials revealing the efficacy of dendrimer systems [58]. Other dendrimers currently under clinical studies are DEP®cabazitaxel, ImDendrim, and MAG-Tn3 [59].

Table 2. Clinical status of polymeric micelles and dendrimers nanoformulations.

Nanocarriers	Product/Trade Name	Copolymer Composition	Entrapped Drug	Cancer Therapy	Clinical Trial Phase	Ref
Micelles	Genexol®-PM/Cynviloq™	mPEG-PDLLA	Paclitaxel	Lung and Breast Cancer	Phase IV	[48,49]
Micelles	NK105	PEG-poly(aspartic acid) copolymer	Paclitaxel	Breast, colon, and gastric cancer	Phase III	[50]
Micelles	NK012	poly(L-glutamic acid)	Irinotecan	TNBC and small lung cancer	Phase II	[51]
Micelles	NC-6300	PEG-b-poly(aspartate-hydrazone)	Epirubicin	Breast and liver cancer	Phase I	[53]
Micelles	NK911	PEG-P (Asp)-DOX	Doxorubicin	Solid tumors	Phase II	[53]
Micelles	NC-4016	PEG-b-poly(β-glutamic acid)	Oxaliplatin	Solid Tumor	Phase I	[54]
Micelles	NC-6004	PEG-b-poly(L-glutamic acid)	Cisplatin	Pancreatic cancer	Phase III	[55]
Micelles	siRNA micelles	siRNA	siRNA	Lung Cancer	Phase I	[55]
Micelles	SP1049C	Pluronic L61 and F127	Doxorubicin	Adenocarcinoma	Phase III	[56]
Dendrimers	DEP® docetaxel	PEGylated PLL	Docetaxel	breast, Lung, Prostate, and ovarian cancer	Phase I	[58]
Dendrimers	DEP® cabazitaxel	Polylysine	Cabazitaxel	Testicular, ovarian, breast, bladder, and head and neck	Phase I/11	[59]
Dendrimers	ImDendrim	Polylysine	188Rerhenium complex	Liver cancer	Phase I	[59]
Dendrimers	MAG-Tn3	Carbohydrate peptide lysine	Vaccine composed of tri Tn glycotope	Breast cancer	Phase I	[59]

4. Dendrimers for Breast Cancer Therapy

Dendrimers are nanocarriers with hyperbranched, spherical, and three-dimensional (Figure 2a). Different anticancer drugs have been loaded into dendrimers for the treatment of breast cancer (Figure 2b) (Table 3) [60,61]. They are utilized in biomedical applications for drug delivery of bioactive agents such as antimalarial, anticancer, antiviral, antiprotozoal, antitubercular drugs, etc. Their well-defined surface functional groups and globular nanosize in the range of 1–10 nm makes them useful for drug delivery [62]. Polymeric dendrimer is of great interest in biomedical applications such as polyamidoamine (PAMAM) dendrimers due to their low toxicity [62,63]. These nanocarriers have successfully delivered chemotherapeutic agents and in theranostic applications in chemotherapy [64]. Other types of dendrimers used in biomedical applications, especially in oncology include poly-lysine, PPI, phosphorus, and carbosilane dendrimers. Polylysine (PLL) is one of the amphiphilic dendrimers with branched structure based on penta-functional core molecules obtained by functionalization of positively charged basic amino acids like lysine or β-amino-alanine [65]. PLL demonstrates a remarkable new group of molecules since they have a small size and are made of natural components that are more easily internalized than those based on synthetic molecules. Cationic PLL dendrimers are useful in numerous biomedical applications, such as carriers for antitumor drugs (5-fluorouracil etc.) [65]. Poly (propyleneimine) (PPI) dendrimers are highly branched macromolecules with symmetric architecture, and they have been widely studied for DNA delivery. These dendrimers can enhance transfection efficiency by endocytosis and direct transport into the cell nucleus [66]. Phosphorous and carbosilane dendrimers are inorganic dendrimers with interesting biomedical applications. These dendrimers demonstrate therapeutic effects against many cancer types and can be loaded with different anticancer drugs for drug delivery [67,68].

The other advantages of dendrimers in chemotherapy include enhanced drug efficacy, improved drug biocompatibility, reduced drug toxicity, and controlled and sustained drug release kinetics [69–72].

4.1. Dendrimers Loaded with Doxorubicin

Dendrimers can overcome the toxic side effects of doxorubicin by promoting sustained release profile (Table 3). Guo and co-workers formulated hyaluronic acid (HA)-modified amine-terminated fourth-generation PAMAM dendrimers for co-delivery of doxorubicin and cisplatin [73]. The TEM images of the drug-loaded dendrimers displayed spherical shaped morphology. The dual drug-loaded dendrimers displayed a mean particle size of 91 ± 2.18 nm, a negative surface charge of −24 ± 7.6 mV, and a polydispersity index (PDI) of 0.35 ± 0.06. The dendrimers' drug loading efficiency was 13.6% and 18.3% for cisplatin and doxorubicin, respectively [73]. The drug release studies of PAMAM dendrimers in an acidic tumor condition and physiological environment (pH 7.4) in vitro showed no release of both drugs within 2 and 24 h, respectively, demonstrating that co-loaded dendrimers were sufficiently stable to avoid drug clearance from the blood plasma before reaching the target tissue. The cellular uptake studies of the formulation in MDA-MB-231 and MCF-7 breast cancer cell models using confocal scanning microscopy showed that the cellular uptake was time-dependent. The antitumor analysis in vitro of HA modified co-loaded PAMAM dendrimers and plain co-loaded PAMAM dendrimers were evaluated on both cancer cell lines using MTT assay. The modified co-loaded drug dendrimers showed good anticancer efficacy of 58% cell death while the plain co-loaded dendrimers showed 49% cell death on MDA-MB-231 cells [73]. PAMAM dendrimers uptake into cancer cells is via a clathrin-mediated uptake passageway followed by rapid transport to the cellular compartments such as (endosomes and lysosomes) [74]. The modified dual drug-loaded dendrimers were stable, and their uptake was via the lysosome-mediated pathway. It also enhanced drug accumulation in the tumor tissue when compared to the free drug solutions. After 24 h of distribution studies, no drugs were observed in the kidneys and the heart, revealing the reduced side effects of the formulation. The in vivo antitumor studies in tumor-bearing BALB/c mice showed that the modified dual drug-loaded dendrimer formulation exhibited significant antitumor effect. The study revealed the synergistic efficacy of co-delivery of anticancer drugs using dendrimers [73].

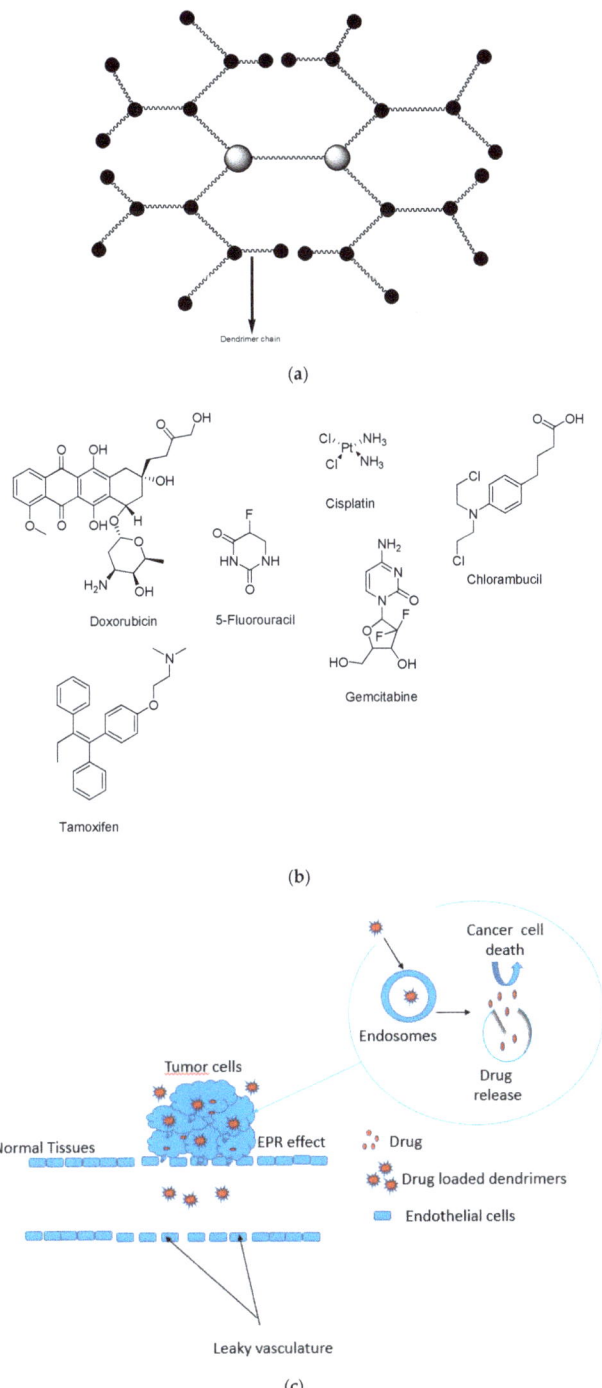

Figure 2. (**a**): A schematic diagram of a dendrimer. (**b**): Structures of some anticancer drugs which have been loaded into dendrimers. (**c**): Drug uptake from dendrimer into tumor cells via EPR effect.

Incorporating doxorubicin into dendrimers can also result in targeted drug delivery to the cancer cells, and the nature of the targeting moiety plays an important role. Chittasupho et al. prepared CXCR4 targeted dendrimers encapsulated with an antitumor antibiotic, doxorubicin, using PAMAM dendrimers [75]. The encapsulation and drug loading capacity of doxorubicin in the PAMAM dendrimers were 97.25 ± 0.04 and 3.40 ± 0.04%, respectively. The in vitro drug release kinetics of the doxorubicin from the dendrimers was quick at pH 5.0 compared to pH 7.4. After 2 h of treatment, the uptake of the formulation into BT-549-Luc cells was 10.7 (for 0.25 mg/mL), 11.5 (for 0.5 mg/mL), and 13.2 (for 1 mg/mL) fold higher when compared to the dendrimer without a targeting moiety. The uptake of the formulation into T47D cells were 3.0 (0.25 mg/mL), 4.6 (0.5 mg/mL), and 4.3 (1 mg/mL)-fold higher when compared to the dendrimer without a targeting moiety. The IC_{50} values of the drug-loaded dendrimer on BT-549 after 12 h were 25.2 µg/mL compared to the free drug, which was 72.6 µg/mL. The free drug did not display any cytotoxic effect on the T47D cells, but the IC_{50} values of the drug-loaded dendrimer on the cell lines after 120 h was 124.4 µg/mL [75]. The cellular uptake of the dendrimers into T47D and BT-549-Luc breast tumor cell was time and concentration-dependent. The cytotoxicity of the doxorubicin-loaded polymeric dendrimer was potent compared to the free doxorubicin and unloaded dendrimers. The cyclic pentapeptide, FC131 [(cyclo)(D-Tyr-Arg-Arg-L-3-(2-naphthyl)alanine-Gly)] incorporated into the formulation is a potent antagonist of CXCR4, an important chemokine receptor that is involved in the metastasis of cancers. The presence of FC131 in the formulation inhibited BT-549-Luc cells migration resulting from reduced interactions between SDF-1α and CXCR4 receptors [75].

Dendrimers are also potent systems to combat multi-drug resistant breast cancer. Wang et al. formulated pluronic F68-incorporated PAMAM dendrimer conjugates loaded with doxorubicin. The in vivo and in vitro anticancer studies revealed doxorubicin pluronic F68-PAMAM dendrimers increased antitumor efficacy against MCF-7/ADR cancer cells by caveolae-mediated endocytosis. They significantly increased apoptosis by regulating gene expression and mitochondrial function [76]. The use of pH-sensitive linkers for the incorporation of drugs to dendrimers is a promising approach. Kojima et al. prepared collagen peptide-modified dendrimers encapsulated with doxorubicin for breast cancer treatment. The drug was incorporated via a pH degradable linker. The diffusion of the drug from the dendrimers was reduced. The reduced release of the drug is effective in overcoming drug resistance. The dendrimers exhibited significant anticancer efficacy against MCF-7 and MDA-MB-231 breast cancer cells with in vivo attenuated metastatic activity. MDA-MB-231 cells were more sensitive to the formulation when compared to MCF-7 cells. The dendrimer inhibited tumor growth significantly [77].

Similar findings on the effect of the linkers on the release profile of DOX was also reported by Kaminskas et al. [78]. Generation 5 PEGylated polylysine dendrimers composed of an outer generation of L-lysine or succinimyldipropyldiamine (SPN) loaded with doxorubicin via 4-(hydrazinosulfonyl) benzoic acid (HSBA) linker. The release of DOX from the formulation was slow with a release of less than 10% of DOX in pH 7.4 buffer for 3 days. However, a 100% release of DOX was significant in pH 5. The formulation retained the cytotoxic properties of the loaded DOX in vitro. The clearance patterns of both the DOX conjugated dendrimers were similar to the free DOX. However, the SPN dendrimers showed reduced metabolic lability and increased uptake into RES organs compared to the equivalent all-lysine dendrimers. In vivo studies of the formulations in rats bearing Walker 256 tumours revealed a high uptake into the tumour tissue. The labile HSBA linker influenced the targeted drug delivery mechanism of DOX to tumours [78]. The size of the dendrimers is also crucial in their therapeutic outcomes. Mehta et al. investigated the influence of dendrimer generation (G4 and G5) and PEG lengths (of 570 and 1100 Da) on selected factors such as the pharmacokinetics, drug release kinetics, tumor biodistribution, and anticancer activity. The PEGylated polylysine dendrimers were conjugated with doxorubicin using a cathepsin-B cleavable valine-citrulline linker. The largest G5 PEG1100 dendrimer good tumor and retention was good but the drug release was slow, thereby limiting its anticancer activity. The smallest G4 PEG570 dendrimer was significantly efficient in cathepsin-mediated doxorubicin release, but its systemic exposure and tumor uptake were limited.

The intermediate-sized dendrimer displayed better drug release kinetics, tumor uptake, systemic exposure, and good retention. These findings revealed the influence of the PEG molecular weight and dendrimer size on the therapeutic efficacy of the dendrimer formulations [79].

Dox is passively transported via the cellular membrane, which makes it prone to efflux pumps [80]. It is not specifically targeted to the tumour but affects the growth of other cell types in the body, thereby resulting in a compromised immune system. The use of dendrimers for the delivery of DOX offers several advantages, such as prevent drug clearance from the blood plasma before reaching the target tissue [73,75]. It also enhances drug accumulation in the tumor tissues and inhibits drug distribution to healthy tissues/organs [73,78]. The linkers used to incorporate DOX influenced its rate of release from the formulation and its uptake into cancer tissues [75,77–79]. The dendrimer formulations loaded with DOX were specific and effective against some breast cancer cell lines [77]. Generally, the release of DOX from the dendrimer formulations was enhanced at acidic pH [73]. The dendrimer size also plays a crucial role in the therapeutic efficacy of dendrimer formulations [79].

4.2. Dendrimers Loaded with Oligodeoxynucleotides

Gene delivery using dendrimers have been reported to be an effective approach resulting in enhanced biological outcomes (Table 3). Wang and co-workers synthesized G4 PAMAM dendrimers loaded with antisense oligodeoxynucleotides for gene delivery in the treatment of breast cancer. Incorporating antisense oligodeoxynucleotides to the dendrimers reduced its toxicity, enhanced its stability binding and inhibits its capability to bind to the erythrocytes and BSA. The cellular uptake of the antisense oligodeoxynucleotides from the dendrimers was high in MDA-MB-231 breast tumor cells. In vivo anticancer experiment using human breast tumor xenograft mice model showed that these dendrimers possess a high capacity of accumulating antisense oligodeoxynucleotides, thereby hindering the tumor vascularization [81]. Similar high cellular uptake of dendrimer-based formulations was also reported by Chen and co-workers. Breast cancer cellular uptake of oligodeoxynucleotide nanoparticles formed in the presence of polypropyleneimine dendrimers was studied. The confocal microscopy results demonstrated higher cellular uptake of oligodeoxynucleotide loaded dendrimers by MDA-MB-231 breast cancer cells compared to free oligodeoxynucleotide. The cellular uptake of G-4 and G-5 dendrimers by the breast cancer cell (MDA-MB-231) was facile. G-1 to G-3 dendrimers exhibited lower zeta potential (5.2–6.5 mV) compared to G-4 and G-5 dendrimers which were in the range of (12–18 mV). The cellular uptake of dendrimers was facile, suggesting that the structure and charge density are essential in cellular transport [82].

Furthermore, the coating of dendrimers promotes targeted drug delivery, thereby inhibiting rapid drug clearance. Pourianazar and Gunduz formulated PAMAM dendrimer-coated magnetic nanoparticles entrapped with CpG oligodeoxynucleotide for breast cancer treatment. The particle size analysis displayed an average particle size of approximately 40 ± 10 nm. The cytotoxicity experiment of the dendrimer nanoparticles using MTT assay demonstrated induced cell death in SKBR3 and MDA-MB231 breast tumor cells, indicating that the dendrimers are suitable as targeted nanocarriers for the delivery of CpG oligodeoxynucleotide. The magnetic core of the dendrimer is ideal for targeted delivery. The formulation displayed high apoptotic capability. The loading of CpG- oligodeoxynucleotide into the magnetic nanoparticles is crucial for targeted delivery to the tumor, where the nanoparticles undergo endocytosis leading to their uptake in the endosomal sites. The mechanism mentioned earlier inhibits their rapid clearance by nucleases [83]. Xin and co-workers formulated G4 PAMAM dendrimers loaded with antisense oligodeoxynucleotide for breast cancer targeting. The G4 PAMAM dendrimers loaded with antisense oligodeoxynucleotide displayed a reduced copy number of Cyclooxygenase-2 mRNA and protein expression in the tumor tissue and the microvessel density in the tumor cells was also reduced with a significant tumor growth inhibition. The formulation displayed a high transfection rate, induced apoptosis with a G0/G1 cell cycle arrest [84].

Antisense and siRNA oligonucleotides are developed for the inhibition of target gene expression. Some dendrimers designed for Antisense and siRNA oligonucleotides incorporation display some toxicity in vitro on human erythrocytes [81]. However, the covalent linkage between G4PAMAM and antisense oligodeoxynucleotides enhanced the stability of dendrimer formulation with reduced toxicity. The dendrimers are useful in protecting therapeutic genes from destruction by enzymes, revealing the potency of dendrimers for transfection in gene manipulation [81]. The cellular uptake of dendrimers is attributed to their sizes and zeta potential. Dendrimers with significantly lower potential in the range of (5.2–6.5 mV) were not taken up by the breast cancer cells [82]. Loading CpG oligodeoxynucleotide in the magnetic core of the dendrimer resulted in targeted drug delivery with the capability to hinder rapid clearance [83]. G4 PAMAM dendrimers loaded with antisense oligodeoxynucleotide reduced the copy number of Cyclooxygenase-2 mRNA and protein expression in the tumor tissue and the microvessel density in the tumor cells resulting in a significant tumor growth inhibition [84].

4.3. Dendrimers Loaded with Trastuzumab

Dendrimers have also been designed for targeted delivery of trastuzumad (Table 3). Kulhari et al. formulated PAMAM dendrimers grafted with trastuzumab for targeted delivery to HER2-positive breast cancer. Dendrimers can cause hemolysis via binding to the erythrocytes via electrostatic interaction resulting in toxicity and reduced bioavailability. The in vitro drug release profile of the drug loaded dendrimers was sustained when compared to the control (Taxotere) over a period of 2 days. Hemolytic toxicity analysis revealed that trastuzumab-encapsulated dendrimers lowered hemolysis than the free dendrimers, showing concentration-dependent hemolysis. The cytotoxicity analysis in vitro of trastuzumab-encapsulated dendrimers showed low cell viability (approximately 36.2%) on MDA-MB-231 and MDA-MB-453 cancer cells when compared to those treated with docetaxel-loaded dendrimers (cell viability of approximately 57.6%) after 2 days [85]. Drug-loaded dendrimers display cell specificity, making them promising systems that can overcome drug toxicity. Miyano et al. prepared the G6 lysine dendrimers entrapped with trastuzumab for specific cellular internalization in HER2-positive breast cancer cells. The DLS analysis of the dendrimers displayed an average particle size of approximately 5–6 nm with negative zeta potentials and low PDI. The targeting efficiency showed that trastuzumab-loaded dendrimers bind specifically to SKBR3 breast cancer cells (HER2-positive) in a dose-dependent mode with a low binding affinity to MCF-7 cells (HER2-negative). The cellular internalization analysis demonstrated that these dendrimers were significantly internalized in SKBR3 breast tumor cells and then transferred to lysosomes [86]. Dendrimers are also designed for combination therapy with a combination of two anticancer drugs. Marcinkowska et al. developed PAMAM dendrimers for targeted binding to membrane receptors, HER-2 that are overexpressed in cancer cells. Over 20% of breast cancer displays an overexpression of HER-2 human epidermal growth factor receptor. The dendrimers were loaded with trastuzumab together with either docetaxel or paclitaxel via succinic acid linker. The formulation was highly toxic toward the HER-2-positive SKBR-3 cells but displayed low toxicity towards HER-2-negative MCF-7 cells. The accumulation of trastuzumab was rapid in HER-2-positive SKBR-3 cell line when compared to the HER-2-negative MCF-7 cells which is influenced by the nature of incorporation via PEG linker into the dendrimer. However, a high amount of PAMAM- paclitaxel-trastuzumab dendrimer was significant in the HER-2-negative MCF-7 cells. The formulation selective binding of the PAMAM- docetaxel -trastuzumab conjugate on HER-2-positive SKBR-3 cells only was significant [87]. The pH-sensitive linker used made the formulation less stable in an acidic environment of the cancer cells. The dendrimer displayed high specific targeting to the HER-2-positive SKBR-3 cells. Trastuzumab, a recombinant, humanised IG1 monoclonal antibody, binds selectively to the human epidermal growth factor receptor 2 (EGFR2) and blocks the receptor hindering the uncontrolled proliferation of HER-2-positive cancer cells. The inhibition of the proliferation results in cell cycle arrest in the G1 phase making the combination of trastuzumab with other classes an attractive approach to develop potent anticancer drugs. The conjugation of dendrimer influences its biodistribution and specific targeting capability, thereby reducing toxicity. The combination of trastuzumad with neratinib using dendrimers is also effective against drug resistance and useful for targeted drug delivery. Aleanizy et al. formulated trastuzumab-grafted dendrimers loaded with neratinib for dual treatment of breast cancer to reduce drug resistance and promote targeted therapy [88]. Trastuzumab was conjugated to the surface of the dendrimer via maleimide-poly(ethylene) glycol-*N*-hydroxysuccinimide linker. In vitro analysis of the SKBR-3 cell viability after 48 h was 40%, 36%, and 33% for neratinib, neratinib-conjugated-dendrimers, and neratinib-loaded-dendrimers-trastuzumab, respectively. The affinity of trastuzumab to the HER2 receptors expressed in SKBR-3 cells promoted the internalization of the formulation via receptor-mediated endocytosis [88]. Chan and co-workers formulated diethylenetriaminepentaacetic acid-modified G4 PAMAM dendrimers conjugated with trastuzumab and nuclear translocation sequence (NTS) for breast cancer therapy. These dendrimers demonstrated retained HER2 immunoreactivity and were internalized in the nucleus of the breast cancer cells. The in vitro cytotoxicity analysis of G4 PAMAM dendrimers conjugated with trastuzumab and NTS exhibited potential anticancer activity against MDA-MB-231 and SK-Br-3 breast cancer cell lines [89]. Oddone and co-workers prepared and evaluated cellular uptake of PAMAM G4. 5 dendrimers loaded with florescein isothiocyanated in BALB/c mice breast tumors and murine breast cancer cells. The dynamic light scattering (DLS) analysis demonstrated the hydrodynamic particle size of 96.3 ± 1.4 nm with a PDI value of approximately 0.0296 ± 0.0171, and TEM results showed the particle size distribution of 44.2 ± 9.2 nm. The cellular uptake studies of PAMAM G4. 5 demonstrated significant uptake by the 4T1 cancer breast cells in vitro, and BALB/c mice breast tumors in vivo [90]. The type of drug conjugated to a dendrimer can influence its specific targeting capability. The conjugation of trastuzumab into dendrimers with selected classes of anticancer drugs can enhance its superior application for the treatment of some breast cancers due to the specific targeting mechanism into the tumor cells.

4.4. Dendrimers Loaded with Other Anticancer Drugs

Other anticancer drugs have been successfully loaded into dendrimers with good therapeutic outcomes on breast cancer (Table 3). Bielawski and co-workers formulated G3 PAMAM dendrimers loaded with chlorambucil [91]. Chlorambucil use is limited by its toxic side effects. The in vitro anticancer assessment revealed that the chlorambucil-entrapped dendrimers decreased the cell viability in both the estrogen receptor-negative (MDA-MB-231) and estrogen receptor-positive (MCF-7) breast tumor cell lines. The cytotoxic effect was concentration-dependent in both breast cancer cells. The dendrimers loaded with chlorambucil was more effective when compared to the free chlorambucil in both breast tumor models. The drug-loaded dendrimers IC_{50} values after 1 day of incubation in MDA-MB-231 and MCF-7 cells were 15 ± 2 nM and 25 ± 2 nM respectively, when compared to the free drug, which was 86 ± 2 nM and 88 ± 2 nM, respectively on both cancer cell lines. The formulation displayed stronger inhibition of collagen biosynthesis when compared to the free drug, chlorambucil. One characteristic feature of breast cancer cells is their interaction with extracellular matrix proteins is deregulated. Collagen is useful for the integrity of the connective tissue. A decreased amount of collagen in extracellular matrix can promote the movement and invasion of neoplastic cells, thereby contributing to the inhibition of cell growth and also the induction of apoptosis [92]. Studies using annexin V-FITC detected apoptosis by a fluorescent microscopy assay. It showed that the formulation hindered cancer cell proliferation by increasing the number of necrotic and apoptotic cells [91].

The number of terminal branches, hydrophilicity, and the dendrimers size positively influence their therapeutic outcomes. Abdel-Rahman and Al-Abd synthesized thermo-responsive dendrimers composed of tetrabromohydroquinone as the core and anticancer drug with branched oligoethylene glycol [93]. The thermoresponsive behavior studies at room temperature showed that all the polymeric dendrimers were aqueous-soluble. The lower critical solution temperature (LCST) of the dendrimers was in the range of 28–36 °C. The anticancer efficacy of the dendrimers was evaluated in vitro on the MCF-7 cancer cell model employing SRB-U assay and all the dendrimers exhibited significant cytotoxic effect with IC_{50} values ranging between 1.1 and 25.4 μg/mL. The resistant fractions of MCF-7 breast cancer cells to the formulation was in the range of 1.97–11.22%. The most potent dendrimers displayed an IC_{50} value of 1.1 μg/mL. The cellular uptake mechanism of the formulation and its cytotoxic effect was induced by an increase in the number of terminal branches and the interaction of the dendrimer lipid bilayer [93]. Factors to be considered when designing dendrimers include hydrophilicity in which increasing the hydrophilicity of the formulation reduce their penetration via the cell membrane; increasing the number of terminal branches, increases the cytotoxic effect of the formulation against cancer cells; increasing the dendrimer size will decrease the penetration of the formulation via the cell membrane.

Dendrimers loaded with metal-based nanoparticles have also been reported to be suitable for MR/CT molecular imaging of breast cancer cells. The currently used clinically contrast agents suffer from limitations such as renal toxicity at high concentrations, short imaging time, and non-specificity. Li and co-workers designed multifunctional dendrimer-based gold nanoparticles modified with PEG monomethyl ether and gadolinium chelate for breast cancer therapy [94]. Dendrimer-based metal nanoparticles were effective as a dual-modality contrast agent for MR/CT molecular imaging of breast cancer cells in vitro and in vivo. They were also found to be non-cytotoxic when used at a concentration of 0–50 µM. Their cellular uptake was efficient in vitro after incubation and in vivo in xenograft tumor model after intravenous injection of the formulation. The low uptake of gold nanoparticles in the liver and kidney indicates the capability of the NPs to escape the reticuloendothelial system in the liver and pass via the renal filter, thereby promoting an efficient uptake of the particles into the tumor by a passive EPR effect. The high uptake of the gold particle in the tumor region up to 0.276 g/kg ± 0.006 g/kg after 1 h of intravenous administration promoted effective MR/CT imaging of the tumors. Furthermore, the biodistribution of the formulation in the blood revealed their long blood circulation time with 0.0080 g/kg of the formulation in the blood 24 h after administration. The prolonged blood circulation time is attributed to the modification of PEG moieties on the dendrimer surface, which enhanced specific uptake by the reticuloendothelial system [94]. Despite the findings obtained, there is still a pressing need to evaluate the biodistribution behavior of the nanoparticles over an extended period of time.

Finlay et al. formulated PAMAM-RNA dendrimer complex to treat breast cancer by targeting TWIST1 transcription factor, which regularly is overexpressed in severe breast cancer. The cellular uptake of the siRNA loaded PAMAM dendrimers by the TNBC cells was effective, thereby causing significant inhibition of TWIST1 related target genes. Furthermore, the dendrimers' capability to deliver siRNA to xenograft orthotopic tumor model was significant. siRNA was present in the tumor for over a period of four hours after treatment [95]. TWIST1 is a potentially clinically therapeutic target for the treatment of metastatic breast cancer [96]. However, the use of TWIST1 knockdown via PAMAM dendrimer-delivered siRNA is not suitable as a sole treatment for metastatic breast cancer. It can be used as an adjuvant therapy to reduce migration/invasion, chemoresistance, and antiapoptotic capability common with aggressive cancers.

Winnicka et al. formulated and evaluated the effect of G2 and G3 PAMAM dendrimers on human breast cancer cell lines. The in vitro anticancer study demonstrated that the G2 PMAMAM dendrimers possessed significant cytotoxic efficacy with an IC$_{50}$ value of 140 ± 2 µM and 153 ± 3 µM against MDA-MB-231 and MCF-7 after 1 day of incubation and 99 ± 2µM and 120 ± 3 µM for G3 PAMAM, respectively. The inhibition in cell viability of the dendrimers was influenced by their apoptosis induction capability [97]. Dendrimers are useful in improving the water solubility of the incorporated drugs. Debnath et al. prepared dendrimers loaded with curcumin for the treatment of breast cancer. These dendrimers enhanced the water insolubility of curcumin. In vitro cytotoxicity analysis using MTT assay showed good anticancer activity of curcumin-loaded dendrimers against BT549 and SKBr3 breast cancer cell lines by inducing cellular apoptosis via caspase-3 activation [98]. The use of curcumin is limited by its poor water solubility and bioavailability. Incorporating it into dendrimers enhanced its water solubility with significant anticancer activity. Yao and co-workers designed polylysine dendrimer encapsulated with PHSCN peptide for breast cancer therapy. The in vitro anticancer analysis of peptide-loaded dendrimers exhibited a higher cytotoxic effect. In vivo, the formulation inhibited the extravasation of MDA-MB-231 and SUM-149 PT in the lungs of mice. PHSCN dendrimer was

700- to 1100-fold more effective than the PHSCN peptide, and they were effective in preventing the formation of metastatic colonies. The dendrimer capability to target the activated α5β1 integrins of the tumor cells without affecting the unactivated α5β1 receptors of healthy tissues indicate its potential to prolong the life span of patients with metastatic breast cancer [99]. The dendrimer displayed specific targeting capability. Lozano-Cruz et al. also reported loaded curcumin in the core of a "bow-tie" cationic carbosilane dendrimer. The dendrimers were highly soluble in water, retained the antioxidant activity of curcumin, and induced significant cytotoxic effect against MCF-7 cancer cells compared to the free curcumin [100]. The dendritic wedges played an important role in the anticancer and antioxidant activity of the dendrimers.

Winnicka et al. synthesized G3 PAMAM dendrimers incorporated with modified glycosides (proscillaridin A and digoxin) for the treatment of breast cancer. The in vitro cytotoxicity analysis of the dendrimers displayed improved anticancer efficacy against MDA-MB-231 and MCF-7 by the induction of significant cellular apoptosis compared to the apoptosis caused by the modified glycosides [101]. Mei et al. prepared PAMAM dendrimers co-loaded with 5-fluorouracil and antisense micro-RNA 21 gene for in vitro breast cancer cell suppression. micro-RNA 21 (miR-21) is overexpressed in breast cancer. The antisense inhibition of miRNA function is used to knockdown miRNA causing a significant inhibition of cell growth. The in vitro cytotoxicity results showed that the incorporation of micro-RNA 21 greatly enhanced the anticancer sensitivity of 5-fluorouracil in the MCF-7 cancer cells by effectively stimulating apoptosis and inhibiting the migration ability of MCF-7 breast cancer cells [102].

Zhang et al. synthesized PAMAM-NH_2 dendrimers to reverse multidrug-resistant breast cancer cells (MCF-7/ADR cells). The in vitro cytotoxicity analysis of PAMAM-NH_2 dendrimers demonstrated significant concentration-dependent toxicity with the cell viability being more than 85% at low concentration of (10–50 μg/mL) after 3 days, revealing the low anticancer effect of the dendrimer against MCF-7/ADR breast cancer cells at low concentration. The cell viability was decreased at a high PAMAM-NH_2 concentration of 100–1000 μg/mL, confirming concentration-dependent toxicity [103]. P-gp and MDR-associated protein influenced higher PAMAM-NH_2 exocytosis with lower PAMAM-NH_2 endocytosis in the MCF-7/ADR cells than MCF-7 cells. The dendrimer degraded in the lysosomal vesicles of the MCF-7/ADR cells than in the MCF-7 cells. Dendrimers are promising systems that display high-efficiency transportation in sensitive and resistant cells.

Zhang and co-workers designed enzyme-responsive PEGylated lysine peptide dendrimers loaded with gemcitabine. The in vitro drug release profile of the dendrimers was significantly faster, with a release of approximately 80% gemcitabine in the tumor environment within 24 h. The drug release profile was influenced by the enzyme-cleavable linker, glycyl phenylalanyl leucyl glycine tetra-peptide used to conjugate the drug. The in vivo cytotoxicity experiment of gemcitabine loaded dendrimers using 4T1 murine breast cancer model indicated significant suppressed relative tumor volume of approximately 86.17 ± 38.27% and 2-fold higher tumor growth inhibition value of about 90% when compared to gemcitabine [104]. The nature of the linker used in the dendrimer influences their drug release profile.

Matai and Gopinath formulated hydrophobic myristic acid modified G5 PAMAM dendrimers for the delivery of tamoxifen in vitro to breast cancer cells [105]. The in vitro drug release profile at acidic condition (pH 5.5) of the tumor microenvironment showed sustained release of tamoxifen from the PAMAM dendrimer. Cellular uptake experiments showed that these dendrimers target the lysosome of the cancer cells. Furthermore, the anticancer analysis of dendrimers loaded with tamoxifen using MTT assay showed high inhibitory effects in MCF-7 human breast cancer cell lines [105]. The random grafting of lipid-like myristic acid chains to the surface of the dendrimers improved the stability and solubility of the loaded drug significantly. The myristoyl groups increased the cellular uptake and reduced the cytotoxicity of formulation.

Table 3. A summary of polymeric dendrimers nanocarriers loaded with anticancer drugs for breast targeting.

Polymers	Anticancer Drugs	Breast Cancer Models	Therapeutic Outcomes	References
PAMAM	Doxorubicin and cisplatin	MDA-MB-231 and MCF-7	The HA modified polymeric dendrimers showed good anticancer efficacy of when compared to the unmodified dendrimers	[73]
PAMAM	Doxorubicin	T47D and BT-549-Luc	High cellular uptake and binding.	[75]
pluronic F68- PAMAM	Doxorubicin	MCF-7/ADR	Improved antitumor activity	[76]
Collagen	Doxorubicin	MCF-7 and MDA-MB-231	Potential anticancer efficacy	[77]
PAMAM	Antisense oligodeoxynucleotides	MDA-MB-231	High cellular accumulation of the loaded drug.	[81]
polypropyleneimine	Oligodeoxynucleotide nanoparticles	MDA-MB-231	High cellular uptake	[82]
PAMAM	CpG oligodeoxynucleotide	SKBR3 and MDA-MB231	Decreased cell viability.	[83]
PAMAM	Antisense oligodeoxynucleotide	-	Growth tumor inhibition	[84]
PAMAM	Trastuzumab	MDA-MB-231 and MDA-MB-453	Sustained drug release profile and reduced breast cancer cell viability.	[85]
polylysine	Trastuzumab	SKBR3 and MCF-7	High cellular internalization	[86]
PAMAM	Trastuzumab	MDA-MB-231 and SK-Br-3	Increased anticancer efficacy	[89]
PAMAM	Florescein isothiocyanated	4T1	Good cellular uptake	[90]
oligoethylene glycol	Tetrabromohydroquinone	MCF-7	Potent cytotoxicity efficacy against breast tumor.	[93]
PEG	Au nanoparticles	MCF-7	Excellent antitumor efficacy.	[94]
PAMAM	siRNA	SUM1315	High cellular uptake.	[95]
PAMAM	-	MDA-MB-231 and MCF-7	Good cytotoxicity	[97]
-	Curcumin	BT549 and SKBr3	Good anticancer activity	[98]
polylysine	PHSCN peptide	MDA-MB-231 and SUM-149	High cytotoxicity	[99]
PAMAM	Proscillaridin A and digoxin	MDA-MB-231 and MCF-7	High cell apoptosis	[101]
PAMAM	5-fluorouracil	MCF-7	Improved anticancer efficacy	[102]
PAMAM-NH2	-	MCF-7/ADR	Concentration-dependent cytotoxicity	[103]
PEG	Gemcitabine	4T1	Suppressed tumor volume	[104]
PAMAM	Tamoxifen	MCF-7	High cancer cell inhibitory effect	[105]

Zhou et al. developed hyperbranched polyglycerol derivative (HPG-C18) and dendritic poly(L-lysine) for the codelivery of docetaxel and MMP-9 siRNA plasmid into tumor cells. The dendrimers were prepared by click reaction between azido-modified hyperbranched polyglycerol derivative and propargyl. The formulation displayed good gene delivery capability in vitro, which occurred via the induction of a decrease in MMP-9 protein expression in MCF-7 cells. The dendrimer displayed a significant apoptosis to breast cancer cells when compared to docetaxel or MMP-9. In vivo studies indicated that the codelivery of docetaxel or MMP-9 resulted in enhanced tumor inhibition [106].

4.5. Limitations of Dendrimers

The clinical translation of dendrimers is not rapid due to several limitations. Drugs are loaded into dendrimers via physical encapsulation or conjugation to the surface of the dendrimers [107]. Chemical conjugation can enhance drug loading, and the use of selective linkers results in targeted drug delivery. However, this drug loading approach can limit the availability of the drug that can be modified and can also significantly reduce the potency of the incorporated drug [108]. Furthermore, conjugating too many drugs on a dendrimer can increase the polydispersity index [73]. It also results in a slow drug release profile, which can reduce the efficacy of the conjugated drug. Guo et al. reported drug release studies of drug-loaded dendrimers in an acidic tumor condition and physiological environment in vitro and no release of both drugs within 2 and 24 h [73]. Although the finding demonstrates the high stability of the co-loaded dendrimers in blood plasma, the delayed drug release revealed that the linkers used did not promote rapid drug release in the tumor environment and could limit the anticancer activity of the formulation. Similar findings have been reported on the slow release of DOX and tamoxifen from the PAMAM dendrimer [77,78,105]. In another research report, a slow release of DOX from G5 PEG1100 dendrimer was reported to limit the anticancer activity of the formulation [79]. However, it is important to mention that the slow release of the drug from the dendrimers can overcome drug resistance and drug toxicity.

The physical encapsulation of drugs into dendrimer offers several advantages, such as ease of loading [109]. However, it often results in a large initial burst and inconsistent drug release, low stability upon storage, low-drug loading, premature drug release, etc. [108,109]. This is often reported as a rapid drug release in the first few hours [75]. PAMAMs are toxic, and their toxicity is overcome via modification of their structure. Dendrimers with cationic groups display significant toxicity when administered at high doses [108,110]. The surface charge of cationic dendrimers influences their strong interaction with anionic lipid bilayers by electrostatic interactions resulting in the formation of holes known as nanopores in the cell membranes with high cellular toxicity [111]. Furthermore, positively charged dendrimers have also been reported to be toxic which limits their use [112]. However, the surface modification of dendrimers has made them suitable for biological applications. Dendrimers such as poly(propylene imine) and poly(amido amine) containing terminal primary amines are characterized by generation and concentration-dependent toxicity [108]. Several surface modifications have been performed on dendrimers to enhance their specific targeting capability.

Polyethylene glycol modification increases the biocompatibility of dendrimers by prolonging the blood circulation time of dendrimers in vivo and also tumor accumulation through the enhanced permeability and retention (EPR) effect [41]. Kaminskas et al. modified the surface of dendrimers using PEG, which resulted in the reduced metabolic lability and increased uptake into the tumors [78]. Mehta et al. reported PEGylated polylysine dendrimers. The largest G5 PEG1100 dendrimers displayed good tumor uptake and retention. However, the drug release was slow, thereby limiting the anticancer activity of the formulation. The smallest G4 PEG570 dendrimer tumor uptake was limited, and the intermediate-sized dendrimer displayed significant tumor uptake and good retention. The PEG molecular weight and the dendrimer size had a significant effect on the therapeutic efficacy of the dendrimer formulations [79]. PEG is also used as a drug spacer. Aleanizy et al. reported trastuzumab-grafted dendrimers. The drug was conjugated to the surface of dendrimer via maleimide-poly(ethylene) glycol-N-hydroxysuccinimide linker to promote internalization of the formulation via receptor-mediated endocytosis [88]. Zhang et al. reported PEGylated lysine peptide dendrimers loaded with gemcitabine via the enzyme-cleavable linker, glycyl phenylalanyl leucyl glycine tetra-peptide. The uptake of the drug into the tumor was high, with a tumor growth inhibition value of over 90% compared to gemcitabine [104]. Dendrimer was modified with PEG and loaded with gold nanoparticles for MR/CT molecular imaging of breast cancer cells. The uptake of the gold nanoparticles into the liver and kidney was low indicating the nanoparticles escaped the reticuloendothelial system in the liver. The uptake of the gold particle into the tumor was high promoting effective MR/CT imaging of the tumors. The formulation displayed prolonged blood circulation time attributed to the modification of PEG moieties on the dendrimer surface [94].

Dendrimers also suffer from other limitations, such as inadequate tumor accumulation and rapid systemic clearance [79,82,108]. PAMAM dendrimers (G2–G4) were reported to display rapid renal clearance, and some of them were taken up by the kidney [113]. The rapid elimination of some dendrimers from plasma circulation insufficient tumor accumulation [108]. The use of targeting moieties has been reported to be a unique approach to promote targeting drug delivery to the tumor [75,84,105]. A variability of therapeutics outcomes from animal studies results from the diversity of animal models used, different duration of treatment, etc. Some strains of animal models react differently to the tested formulations, and some of the animals may have the capability to display adaptation that can withstand the toxic side effects of the tested formulations. The use of different strains of animals influences the data interpretation, toxicity profiles, etc. [110].

5. Polymeric Micelles

Micelles are self-assembled or colloidal nanoparticles/nanocarriers with a mean particle size ranging from 5 to 100 nm [114,115]. They consist of surfactants or amphiphiles and are composed of two different parts: hydrophobic tails and a hydrophilic head (Figure 3a) [116,117]. The concentration whereby the micelles are produced is called critical micelle concentration [118]. Several factors affect the production of the micelles, such as temperature, the solvent used, size of the hydrophobic domain in the amphiphilic molecule, and the concentration of amphiphiles [116]. The advantages of micelles in drug delivery include high drug loading capacity, high drug encapsulation efficiency, high drug cellular uptake due to the micellar nanosize (Figure 3b), improved drug stability, and they are easily eliminated from the biological environment after biodegradation, protect normal body cells from drug toxicity, useful for combination therapy, and they improve pharmacokinetic parameters of encapsulated drugs [119–121]. Different anticancer drugs have been loaded into micelles resulting inan improved anticancer activity of the loaded drugs in vitro and in vivo (Figure 3c,d) (Table 4).

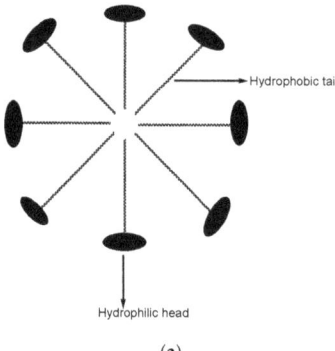

(a)

Figure 3. *Cont.*

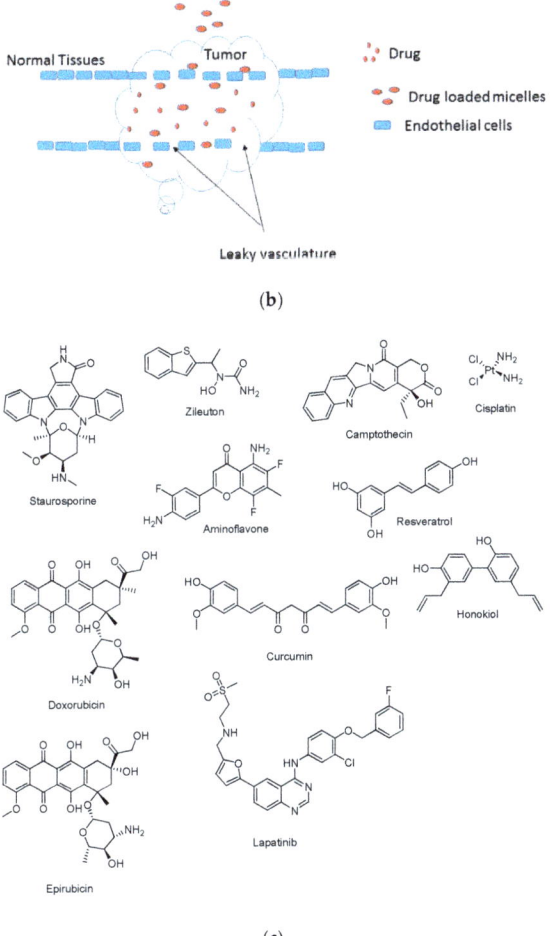

Figure 3. *Cont.*

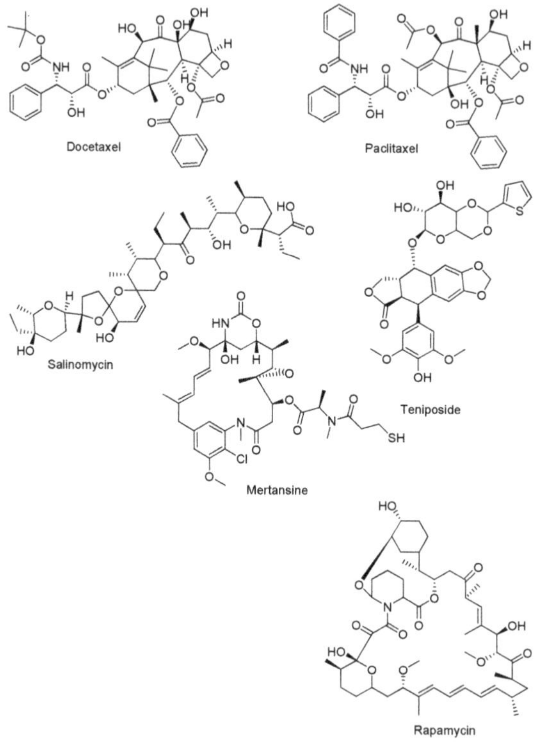

[Chemical structures shown: Docetaxel, Paclitaxel, Salinomycin, Mertansine, Teniposide, Rapamycin]

(d)

Figure 3. (**a**): Schematic diagram of polymeric micelles. (**b**): A schematic diagram illustrating the uptake of micelles formulation into tumor cells. (**c**): Structures of some anticancer drugs loaded into micelles. (**d**): Structures of some anticancer drugs loaded into micelles.

5.1. Polymeric Micelles Loaded with Docetaxel

Loading docetaxel into micelles has been reported by several researchers to result in good therapeutic outcomes in vitro and in vivo when compared to the free drug, docetaxel (Table 4). It has been designed for combination therapy and sustained release profile of both loaded drugs. Guo et al. prepared methoxylpoly(ethylene glycol)-poly(D,L-lactide) copolymer (mPEG-PDLA)-based micelles co-loaded with docetaxel and resveratrol at a 1:1 fixed ratio for drug-resistant breast tumor therapy [122]. The average particle size and PDI of the mPEG-PDLA micelles were 17.1 ± 3.2 nm and 0.27 ± 0.01, respectively. The % drug loading of docetaxel and resveratrol in the polymeric micelles was 16.87 and 16.89%, respectively. The TEM results showed spherical morphology, which was uniform, and the particle size was in the range of 20–50 nm. The in vitro drug release profiles were fast for both drugs in the first 12 h at physiological pH of 7.4. After 12 h, the drug release mechanism was slow, and the cumulative release of both drugs was almost 80% in 3 days. Combining both drugs at a ratio of 1:1 (w/w) resulted in a significant synergistic effect against the MCF-7 cells. The loading of both drugs in the micelles resulted in prolonged drug release profiles and improved cytotoxicity in vitro [122]. The cytotoxicity assessment in vitro of the blank mPEG-PDLA-based micelles in MCF-7 breast tumor cells using MTT assay showed a non-cytotoxic effect indicating their safety and biocompatibility of the micelles. The co-loaded polymeric micelles demonstrated the highest cytotoxic efficacy that resulted in 70% of the MCF-7 cell death, which was greater than the activity of micelles loaded with the same concentration of either docetaxel or resveratrol. Furthermore, the pharmacokinetic study in vivo of co-loaded polymeric micelles demonstrated that these polymeric micelles mostly prolonged the exposure period of docetaxel and resveratrol in the blood plasma circulation. The $AUC_{(0 \to t)}$ value of the micelles loaded with docetaxel was 3.0-fold higher than the free drug in vivo after intravenous administration [122]. Lang et al. formulated tumor-environment-responsive micelles entrapped with docetaxel for metastatic breast tumor treatment [123]. These micelles were prepared from amphiphilic copolymer, poly((1,4-butanediol)-diacrylate-b-N,N-diisopropylethylenediamine)-peptide-polyethylene glycol (PEG) (BD-peptide-PEG), matrix metallo-proteinase (MMP)-responsive polymer, and poly((1,4-butanediol)-diacrylate-b-N,N-diisopropyl-ethylenediamine)-polyethyleneimine (BD-PEI). The drug encapsulation efficiency and drug loading of the micelles were 80.54% and 9.81%, respectively. The average particle size was 24.36 nm, with a surface charge of 1.44 mV. The cellular uptake assessment of micelles displayed higher cellular uptake in the 4T1 breast cancer model in vivo than the cell culture medium in vitro. The polymeric micelles were cytotoxic in 4T1 breast cancer cells, indicating that polymeric micelles are specific and important as a drug delivery system. The drug release from the micelles formulation in acidic endo/lysosomes is via the dissociation of the micelle resulting from the protonation of the hydrophobic block. The drug-loaded micelle inhibited primary tumor growth and pulmonary metastasis effectively with a prolonged circulation time. Its efficient uptake into tumor cells is a promising approach for treating metastatic breast cancer [123].

Drug-loaded micelles can be designed to be dose-dependent. Logie et al. evaluated taxane-binding peptide-modified micelles encapsulated with docetaxel employing poly(D,L-lactide-co-2-methyl-2-carboxytrimethylene carbonate) [124]. The average particle size of the micelle was 121 ± 25 nm, with a distribution of 0.15 ± 0.03. The pharmacokinetic profiles of the free drug and the polymeric micelles showed a significant reduction in the concentration of plasma immediately after administration, and displayed modest enhancement of the parameters of pharmacokinetic for 7 h. The in vivo cytotoxicity studies of docetaxel loaded micelles against MDA-MB-231/H2N breast tumor model in mice showed a 72% tumor growth inhibition at a higher dose (8 mg/kg), while at a lower dose (5 mg/kg), a 50% tumor growth inhibition was visible which is the same as the free drug in a lower dose [124]. The concentration of the formulation used in vivo influenced their cytotoxic effects. Hu et al. formulated micelles from methacrylated block copolymer holding monomethoxy PEG encapsulated with docetaxel [125]. The in vitro drug release kinetics showed a sustained docetaxel release from these polymeric micelles at physiological environments (pH 7.4), due to the covalent conjugation via a hydrolyzable linker. Furthermore, the in vivo antitumor study in mice bearing MDA-MB-231 breast cancer xenografts showed potent chemotherapeutic activity compared to free docetaxel (Taxotere) [125]. The nature of the linker used for the conjugation influenced the drug release profile of the formulation. A sustained release profile is suitable for drug delivery systems to overcome drug toxicity.

Li and co-workers formulated Lyp-1 modified PEI derivative-PCL-g-PEI-based micelles co-loaded with docetaxel and near infrared (NIR) dye (IR820) for breast cancer chemotherapy [126]. The average particle size was 38 nm with a surface charge of +5 mV. The in vitro drug release profile indicated that docetaxel and IR820 were released slowly from the micelles, when compared to the free drugs, docetaxel and IR820, respectively. The Lyp-1 modified dual drug-loaded micelles demonstrated high growth inhibition of 4T1 breast tumor cells when compared to the free drug and unmodified micelles [126]. Kutty and Feng prepared D-α-cetuximab-conjugated tocopheryl polyethylene glycol succinate (TPGS)-based micelles loaded with docetaxel for the treatment of triple-negative breast cancer (TNBC) therapy. The cytotoxicity analysis demonstrated that the anticancer effects of docetaxel could be greatly improved by incorporating it into the cetuximab-conjugated TPGS micelles. The cytotoxic effect of the formulation was 223.8 and 205.6-fold higher than the control (Taxotere®) on the MDA-MB-231 and MDA-MB-468 breast cancer cell lines, respectively revealing the efficacy of the micelles [127].

Drug-loaded micelles display enhanced oral drug availability. Wang et al. formulated PEG–PCL-based micelle hydrogels for oral drug delivery of docetaxel for breast cancer treatment. The particle size was 20 nm with approximately 7.76% drug loading capacity, which enhanced docetaxel absorption in the intestine tract. The pharmacokinetic analysis showed that docetaxel-loaded micelle-hydrogel significantly enhanced the oral drug bioavailability by 10-fold when compared to docetaxel-loaded micelles. The cytotoxicity analysis demonstrated that the docetaxel-micelle hydrogels were effective in inhibiting the tumor growth in 4T1 breast cancer model, and decreased systemic toxicity [128]. Micelles have been reported to exhibit significant tumor growth. Tan et al. formulated and evaluated mPEG-polyester micelles loaded with docetaxel for breast cancer treatment. The concentration of docetaxel-loaded mPEG-polyester micelles uptake in the tumor tissue and plasma was high when compared to the free docetaxel. In addition, the docetaxel entrapped micelles demonstrated higher tumor growth inhibition when compared to the free docetaxel in vitro and in vivo [129].

Drug-loaded micelles are effective in suppressing breast cancer metastasis. Li et al. formulated small-sized mPEG$_{2000}$-b-PDLLA$_{1300}$ micelles incorporated with docetaxel for breast cancer metastasis suppression. The cytotoxicity analysis demonstrated that the drug loaded micelles revealed similar activity as the free drug, docetaxel in cellular growth suppression of the primary tumors with a significant anticancer activity in 4T1 mouse breast tumor metastasis model [130]. Raza et al. synthesized Dextran-PLGA-incorporated docetaxel micelles for the treatment of breast cancer. The micelles average particle size was 96.5 nm, with a drug encapsulation of 54.85%. The in vitro cytotoxicity experiment showed that the anticancer activity of docetaxel incorporated in the micelles against MDA-MB-231 and MCF-7 cell lines was improved by 100%. The pharmacokinetic profile of the formulation revealed 16-fold enhanced bioavailability with a AUC$_{(0-\infty)}$ of 16367.39 µg·mL^{-1}·h when compared to the free drug, which was 1206.75 µg·mL^{-1}·h. The drug clearance of the formulation was reduced, revealing the extended residence of the drug in the biological system with the half-life of the drug increased by 5-fold, when compared to the free drug [131]. Kutty et al. formulated cetuximab conjugated TPGS micelles encapsulated with docetaxel for TNBC therapy. The ex vivo and in vivo cytotoxicity analysis of micelles showed the effective targeted and hindered EGFR-overexpressing on MDA-MB-231 TNBC breast tumor cell lines. The micelles accumulated in the tumours after administration via intravenous injection, and it was retained for 24 h. The uptake of the micelles was via receptor-mediated endocytosis. The tumours treated with the micelles exhibited improved cell cycle arrest and attenuated proliferation [132]. Koo et al. formulated docetaxel-loaded EG-PLys-PPhe micelles for breast cancer treatment. It was composed of a core-shell containing redox-responsive shell-specific cross-links and loaded with docetaxel [133]. The drug release was influenced by the concentration of glutathione, which resulted in a reductive cleavage of the disulfide cross-links in the shell domains. The in vivo tissue distribution and tumor accumulation of the formulation labeled with a near-infrared fluorescence (NIRF) dye, showed enhanced tumor-targeted ability of the formulation with prolonged stable circulation in the blood and enhanced permeation and retention (EPR) effect. The therapeutic efficacy of the formulation was enhanced in tumor-bearing mice when compared to the free drug [133]. Muthu et al. formulated TPGS micelles of transferrin co-loaded with docetaxel and ultra-bright gold nanoclusters. The in vitro anticancer studies demonstrated that these micelles were 71.73 times more effective when compared to the control (Taxotere®) after 24 h of incubation with the MDA-MB-231-luc breast cancer cells [134]. Tan et al. reported novel MPEG-PDLLA-PLL copolymer micelles for drug delivery of docetaxel to breast cancer cells. The in vitro and in vivo anticancer studies using MTT assay and mice model, respectively, demonstrated that these micelles were efficient in tumor cell growth inhibition against subcutaneous 4T1 and MCF-7 breast cancer cell lines [135].

Zhang and co-workers formulated PEG-b-PLGA copolymer micelles co-loaded with docetaxel and chloroquine for breast cancer targeting. The in vitro cytotoxicity analysis of docetaxel loaded PEG-b-PLGA micelles and dual drug-loaded PEG-b-PLGA micelles after 24 h of incubation with MCF-7 cancer cells showed an IC$_{50}$ value of 22.30 ± 1.32 and 1.75 ± 0.43 mg/mL, respectively, which demonstrated a 12-fold more efficient treatment of the dual drug loaded micelles when compared to loading a single drug in the micelles formulation. Combining docetaxel with chloroquine in the micelle formulation significantly improved the cytotoxic effect [136]. Jun and co-workers prepared docetaxel loaded micelles utilizing tripodal cyclotriphosphazene amphiphilile [NP(PEG750)(GlyPheLeu)$_2$Et]$_3$ as a carrier. The in vivo studies on xenograft model demonstrated complete tumor suppression of the MDA-MB-231 breast cancer cells at a lower dose of 5 mg/kg compared to Taxotere® [137]. Enteshari et al. prepared poly(styrenemaleic acid)-poly(amide-ether-ester-imide) co-polymeric nanomicelles encapsulated with docetaxel for breast cancer treatment. The results from these micelles showed considerably inhibited tumor growth of MC4-L2 breast tumors induced in BALB/c mice and increased animal survival when compared to the free docetaxel [138]. Varshosaz and co-workers formulated magnetic polyvinyl caprolactam–polyvinyl acetate–PEG micelles entrapped with docetaxel and Fe_3O_4 nanoparticles for breast cancer treatment [139]. The average particle size was 144.3 nm, with a negative zeta potential of −2.58 mV and 70% drug-loading efficiency. The in vitro cytotoxicity analysis of docetaxel loaded polymeric using MTT assay displayed significantly more anticancer activity when compared to the free drug on MDA-MB-231 and MCF-7 breast cancer cells, but the blank magnetic polymeric micelles displayed no cytotoxic effect on the normal fibroblast cells [139].

Zheng and co-workers formulated polypeptide cationic micelles of PEG-PLL-PLLeu for co-delivery of docetaxel and siRNA-Bcl-2 for breast tumor therapy. The anticancer analysis demonstrated that the dual drug-loaded micelles revealed down-regulation of the anti-apoptotic Bcl-2 gene and improved antitumor efficacy with a smaller dose of docetaxel, resulting in the inhibition of tumor growth of MCF-7 breast cancer xenograft murine model when compared to the docetaxel and siRNA [140]. Tong et al. formulated phospholipid-based micelles loaded with docetaxel $mPEG_{2000}$-distearoylphosphatidylethanolamine (DSPE) for the treatment of breast cancer. The micelles showed drug loading capacity of 3.14 ± 0.13% and encapsulation efficiency of 97.31 ± 2.95%. The cytotoxicity analysis demonstrated that docetaxel loaded micelles displayed similar antiproliferative efficacy as the control, (Taxotere®) in vitro. The formulation displayed good antitumor activity when compared to Taxotere® in vivo against MCF-7 breast tumor induced nude mice, which can be attributed to the passive targeting of the cancer cells by the polymeric micelles [141].

Docetaxel is used either alone or in combination with other anticancer drugs for the treatment of cancers such as breast, ovarian, etc. [142]. It has side effects such as neutropenia, fluid retention, gastrointestinal complications etc. [143]. The incorporation of docetaxel into formulations of micelles improved its therapeutic efficacy. The micelles loaded with docetaxel displayed particle sizes in the range of 17.1–121 nm. The formulation displayed sustained drug release profile [122], improved bioavailability after intravenous administration [122,131], prolonged circulation time [123], inhibited tumor growth at high dose [121], enhanced oral drug bioavailability [127], tumor targeted capability [133,138], displayed similar effect with a clinically approved drug [141]. Docetaxel has been combined with some anticancer drugs in micelles formulation such as resveratrol [122], and chloroquine [136] for breast cancer treatment.

5.2. Polymeric Micelles Loaded with Doxorubicin

Doxorubicin is used either alone or in combination with other anticancer drugs for the treatment of cancers such as bladder, breast, ovarian, etc. [144]. It exhibits low oral bioavailability, permeability, and acute toxicity to normal tissue. It has side effects such as cardiotoxicity that is not reversible and nephrotoxicity [145]. The incorporation of doxorubicin into formulations of micelles improved its therapeutic efficacy (Table 4).

Micelles loaded with DOX that displayed a pH-dependent drug release profile. Gao and co-workers formulated zwitterionic pH-responsive polymeric micelles for drug delivery of doxorubicin using hyaluronic acid (HA) as a nanocarrier [146]. The drug loading capacity and encapsulation efficiency of the HA micelles were 84.3% and 68.9%, respectively. The drug release mechanisms in vitro of the micelle loaded with doxorubicin were evaluated at pH 7.4 (physiological environment) and pH 5.0 (lysosome of cancer cells). The doxorubicin release from the micelle was slow, and it was less than 30% after 24 h at pH 7.4 while it was quick at pH 5.0 before 12 h and was 70% after 24 h. The in vitro anticancer studies of the drug-loaded polymeric micelles and individual drug against MCF-7 breast tumor cells utilizing a CCK-8 assay demonstrated that doxorubicin-loaded micelles exhibited higher growth inhibition (IC_{50} value in the range of 1.85–1.97 µg/mL) when compared to the free doxorubicin

(IC$_{50}$ value of 2.33 µg/mL). The cellular uptake assessment showed a successful uptake of the micelle formulation in the MCF-7 cells. Furthermore, in vivo anticancer studies showed that the drug-loaded micelles displayed significant tumor growth inhibition of approximately 80% when compared to the NaCl group (used as control) [146]. The formulation quick release in acidic pH inhibited the growth of the tumor and improved the cytotoxic effect.

Gao et al. formulated polymeric micelles using two polymers: poly(L-histidine) (PHis) (Mn 4700)-*b*-PEG (Mn 2000) and poly(L-lactide) (PLLA)(Mn 3000)-*b*-PEG(Mn 2000)-folate for the delivery of doxorubicin [147]. In vivo studies showed the absence of tumor metastasis in the lung and heart after treatment with the micelle formulation. The micelles suppressed the proliferation of cancer cells and inhibited tumor growth and cancer cell metastasis. Using folic acid as a targeting moiety combined with the pH-sensitive core phase carrier promoted targeted drug delivery and triggered drug release at the tumor sites. The pH-sensitive folate conjugated micelle loaded with DOX is a promising approach for the treatment of cancer metastasis. The encapsulation of DOX in the core of the micelle also protected the normal tissues from being exposed to the side effects of DOX [147]. The cytotoxicity of free DOX was higher than that of DOX carried by PLLA-*b*-PEG and PHis-*b*-PEG micelles. The cytotoxicity of DOX-loaded PHis-*b*-PEG was higher than DOX-loaded PLLA-*b*-PEG micelle because pH-dependent drug release from pH-sensitive PHis-*b*-PEG micelle at pH 6.8 when compared to the pH-insensitive PLLA-*b*-PEG micelle. The blank micelles did not display any cytotoxic effect on 4T1 cells revealing the biocompatible nature of the micelles.

Zhao et al. formulated micelles entrapped with an antitumor antibiotic, doxorubicin, for the eradication of cancer stem cells in TNBC utilizing pluronic block copolymers [141]. The antitumor effects of the free drug and polymeric micelles were evaluated against cancer stem cells in TNBC in vitro. The cytotoxicity efficacy of the drug-loaded micelles against MDA-MB-231 and MDA-MB-468 and potency in reducing the development of a colony of cancer stem cells when compared to free doxorubicin was studied. Furthermore, polymeric micelles were potent in tumor growth inhibition in vivo in the orthotopic tumor models formed from cancer stem cells, confirming polymeric micelles as potential therapeutics against TNBC [148]. Bae et al. prepared micelles for co-delivery of doxorubicin and phosphatidylinositol-3 kinase inhibitor wortmannin using PEG-*b*-poly(aspartate hydrazide) copolymers as a polymeric nanocarriers [149]. The particle size of the polymeric micelles employing DLS was less than 100 nm, which is preferable for tumor-specific drug delivery in vivo. The cytotoxicity evaluation in vitro against MCF-7 cells demonstrated that the anticancer efficacy was time- and dose-dependent and the cell viability was effectively suppressed after 3 days of incubation by dual drug-loaded polymeric micelles when compared to individual drug-loaded polymeric micelles and the free drugs [149]. Zhang and co-workers formulated crosslinked glutathione-sensitive carboxymethyl chitosan micelles co-loaded with doxorubicin and cisplatin for breast tumor therapy. The in vitro drug release profile demonstrated that these micelles were highly glutathione-sensitive. The cytotoxicity experiments showed that the dual drug-loaded micelles displayed high synergistic chemotherapeutic efficacy against HeLa cancer cells when compared to doxorubicin-loaded micelles, free doxorubicn, and plain polymeric micelles [150]. Varshosaz et al. formulated magnetic folate-dextran-retinoic acid micelles encapsulated with doxorubicin. The in vitro cytotoxicity analysis of doxorubicin-loaded polymeric micelles employing MTT assay showed good anticancer activity against MDA-MB-468 and MCF-7 breast tumor cells [151].

Lv et al. prepared amphiphilic PEG$_{2k}$-PLA$_{5k}$ micelles loaded with a combination of doxorubicin and curcumin to treat MDR breast cancer. The dual drug-loaded micelles displayed low efflux rate of doxorubicin, high cellular uptake, and high down-regulation of P-glycoprotein and inhibition of ATP activity. The co-loaded micelles also displayed high tumor accumulation and inhibitory effect on the tumor growth in xenograft model of drug-resistant MCF-7/ADR cells when compared to the free drugs revealing the efficacy of micelles loaded with two drugs [152]. Cuong and co-workers synthesized doxorubicin-loaded PEG-PCL-PEG micelles loaded with doxorubicin for breast cancer therapy. The circulation time of doxorubicin-loaded polymeric micelles in the plasma was prolonged when compared to the free doxorubicin in vivo. The tumor growth of MCF-7 breast cancer cells in nude mice was suppressed by multiple doses of the drug-loaded micelles when compared to multiple doses of free doxorubicin [153]. Yu and co-worker formulated amphiphilic diblock polymeric micelles loaded with doxorubicin to reverse doxorubicin resistance in breast cancer. The in vivo cytotoxicity analysis of the polymeric micelles demonstrated significant growth inhibition of doxorubicin-resistant MCF-7/ADR breast cancer in an orthotopic tumor-bearing mouse model [154].

Lee and co-workers reported folate modified PLLA/PEG polymeric micelles loaded with doxorubicin for resistant breast cancer therapy. The micelles displayed more than 90% anticancer efficacy in doxorubicin resistant MCF-7/DOX^R breast cancer cells. Furthermore, the in vivo antitumor experiments in the MCF-7/DOX^R xenograft model showed that the accumulated doxorubicin level of modified micelles in solid tumors was 20 times higher than free drug and 3 times higher than the unmodified polymeric micelles group [155]. Varshosaz and co-workers synthesized Pluronic® F127-poly (methyl vinyl ether-alt-maleic acid) copolymer-based micelles entrapped with doxorubicin for breast cancer targeting [156]. The in vitro drug release profile at pH 5.5 and pH 7.4 after 4 h was sustained. However, doxorubicin release mechanism from the micelles was faster in pH 5.5 when compared to pH 7.4 demonstrating that after the cellular internalization of drug-loaded micelles into the cytosol of cancer cells, the pH of lysosomes can stimulate the fast doxorubicin release from the micelles. The in vitro cytotoxicity analysis demonstrated that the micelles loaded with doxorubicin destroyed approximately 48.9 ± 1.7% of MCF-7 breast tumor cells when compared to the free doxorubicin which destroyed 36.4 ± 1.1% of these breast tumor cells [156].

Sun et al. synthesized doxorubicin loaded PAA-g-PEG graft micelles for the treatment of breast carcinoma [157]. The in vivo cytotoxicity analysis of the drug-loaded micelles in 4T1 tumor induced nude mice breast carcinoma subcutaneous model demonstrated high accumulation of the formulation in the tumor than the free doxorubicin with a reduced distribution to important tissues. The anticancer effect of the polymeric micelles was importantly better when compared to the free doxorubicin, as confirmed by the tumor volume and body weight changes of the tumor-bearing mice [157]. Shuai et al. formulated micelles based on block copolymers of poly (ε-caprolactone) and PEG for the delivery of doxorubicin. Hemolytic experiments displayed that the free doxorubicin caused approximately 11% hemolysis at 200 μm/mL while no hemolysis was observed with the doxorubicin-loaded micelles at the same doxorubicin concentration of 200 μm/mL. The in vitro cytotoxicity study demonstrated that the micelles displayed a time-delayed anticancer activity in MCF-7 breast cancer cells because cancer cell viability was approximately 80% on 4th day and it drastically decreased on the 5th day at a concentration range between 0.01–10 μM [158]. Cuong and co-workers formulated folate-modified star-shaped PEG–PCL micelles loaded with doxorubicin for human breast cancer targeting. The cellular uptake analysis showed that the uptake of decorated micelle incorporated with doxorubicin was higher than the free drug in human MCF-7 breast tumor cells in a time-dependent manner. Furthermore, the experiment revealed that these folate-decorated star-shaped PEG–PCL micelles were non-toxic and are potential nanocarriers for cancer therapy [159]. Another study by Cuong and co-workers demonstrated that doxorubicin-incorporated micelles of a star-shaped poly(ε-caprolactone)-polyphosphoester block co-polymer significantly improved antitumor efficacy in MCF-7/drug-resistant breast cancer cells and MCF-7/drug-sensitive breast cancer cells after incubation in vitro [160].

Zhou et al. formulated micelles entrapped with doxorubicin from dextran and indomethacin for breast cancer treatment. These micelles demonstrated uniform size distribution with a mean diameter of 50 nm. The in vivo studies on male BALB/c nude mice bearing resistant MCF-7 breast xenograft tumor cells showed that the micelles significantly inhibited the tumor growth when compared to the control (saline) and doxorubicin [161]. Liao et al. prepared PEG–PCL cetuximab-immunomicelles encapsulated with doxorubicin and superparamagnetic iron oxide for EGFR-overexpressing breast tumor cell targeting. The in vitro anticancer analysis utilizing a MTT assay showed that the A431 breast cancer cells are highly sensitive to drug-loaded micelles when compared to MDA-MB-453 breast tumor cells. Furthermore, EGFR-overexpressing A431 cells, immunomicelles exhibited significant inhibitory effects on cell growth when the doxorubicin concentration was more than 2 μg/mL [162]. Chen et al. formulated micellar doxorubicin nanoparticles of mPEG-PCL-graft-cellulose to overcome MDR breast cancer cells. The flow cytometry and confocal laser scanning microscopy (CLSM) analysis in MCF7/ADR cells demonstrated more efficient endocytosis of the micellar doxorubicin nanoparticles in these cancer cells when compared to the diffusion of the free doxorubicin into the cytoplasm of the cancer cells. These results revealed that the doxorubicin loaded mPEG-PCL-g-cellulose micelles were effective in overcoming P-glycoprotein efflux in MDR breast tumor cells [163].

Zeng and co-workers prepared hyperbranched block poly-2,2-bis(methylol) propionic acid (bis-MPA)-PEG micelles for the delivery of doxorubicin in breast tumor cells. The particle size analysis of micelles using DLS and TEM showed an average hydrodynamic diameter in the range of 90–130 nm. The in vitro drug release profile from the drug-loaded polymeric micelles at physiological conditions was a biphasic release mechanism, with an initial slight burst drug release followed by a sustained release. The cytotoxicity analysis using MTT assay demonstrated that the anticancer efficacy of micelles was concentration dependent because the cell viability of MCF-7 and MDA-MB-468 breast cancer cells was decreased as the concentration of doxorubicin-loaded micelles increased [164]. Cheng et al. formulated amphiphilic poly(Îμ-caprolactone) micellar nanoparticles loaded with doxorubicin for breast cancer therapy. The in vitro cytotoxicity of the drug loaded micelles was higher against MCF-7 human breast cancer cells when compared to the plain micelles when incubated at a temperature increased above the LCST [165].

Danhier et al. formulated vitamin E-based tocopherol succinate (TOS)-TPGS micelles encapsulated with doxorubicin for breast tumor treatment [166]. The mean particle size of 78 nm with a negative surface charge of −7 mV. The in vitro cytotoxicity evaluation of doxorubicin-loaded micelles showed that they exhibited higher anticancer activity when compared to the free doxorubicin against MCF-7 breast tumor cells after 24 h. Furthermore, the in vivo anticancer analysis revealed a 100% long-time survival of MCF-7 and CT26 induced mice treated with the micelles loaded with doxorubicin when compared to the free drug [166]. Liu and co-workers synthesized mPEG-PLA micellar nanoparticles co-loaded with doxorubicin and gemcitabine for synergistic anticancer efficacy on breast cancer cells. The in vitro cytotoxicity analysis of the co-loaded micelles using MTT assay exhibited significant synergistic anticancer effect against MCF-7 breast cancer cells [167]. Cagel et al. formulated micelles from Tetronic T1107, Pluronic F127, TPGS, and incorporated doxorubicin resulting in improved cytotoxicity on breast cancer cell lines. The in vitro drug release was significantly high at an acidic tumor microenvironment of pH 5.5 when compared to the physiological environment of pH 7.4. The in vitro cytotoxicity analysis of the micelles revealed higher anticancer efficacy against TNBC cells (MDA-MB- 231) when compared to the control (Doxil®) [168].

Chen and co-workers formulated Pluronic-based functional micelles co-loaded with doxorubicin and paclitaxel for MDR breast cancer treatment [169]. The in vitro drug release profile was sustained for both drugs. The co-loaded micelles significantly reduced the cell viability of MCF-7 cancer cells when compared to a single drug-loaded micelles. Furthermore, the in vivo antitumor analysis revealed high anticancer activity in MCF-7/ADR tumor-bearing mice for the dual drug-loaded micelles when compared to the combined administration of doxorubicin and paclitaxel [169]. Wang et al. designed MPEG-PCL-4-formylbenzoic acid (FBA) micellar nanoparticles for combination therapy of paclitaxel and doxorubicin. The combination resulted in synergistic antitumor efficacy against MCF-7 breast cancer cells when compared to the single drug-loaded micelles and the free drugs [170].

5.3. Polymeric Micelles Loaded with Paclitaxel

Paclitaxel is used for the treatment of various types of cancers, including breast cancer. The resistance of breast cancer to paclitaxel is due to certain genes, ABC transporters, etc. [171,172]. Some of the side effects of paclitaxel include peripheral neuropathy, poor solubility, etc. which are responsible for more research on its use in several preclinical and clinical studies [171]. The incorporation of paclitaxel into micelles have been reported to improve its therapeutic outcomes in vitro and in vivo (Table 4).

Wang et al. designed and evaluated carboxymethyl chitosan-rhein polymeric micelles for oral delivery of paclitaxel [173]. The entrapment efficiency and drug loading of paclitaxel in chitosan-based micelles were 86.99 ± 12.26% and 35.24 ± 1.58%, respectively. The drug-loaded polymeric micelles improved the paclitaxel bioavailability. The drug release profile of polymeric micelles was sustained with a slowed drug release of 66.14% in 2 days at physiological conditions in vitro. The in vitro synergistic anticancer studies against the cancer cells between paclitaxel and chitosan-rhein conjugates was assessed utilizing MCF-7 cancer cells. Cell viability outcomes demonstrated a dose-dependent toxicity of paclitaxel. In addition, the low cytotoxic effect of the polymeric micelles was observed at experimental doses. The IC_{50} value of paclitaxel-loaded polymeric micelles and free paclitaxel in MCF-7 cells was 17.62 nM and 30.70 nM for 3 days, respectively [173]. The sustained release profile of the formulation has the potential to overcome drug resistance. Zajdel et al. prepared polylactide-*co*-poly(ethylene glycol) micelles loaded with a combination of paclitaxel and lapatinib. The micelles diameter was 20 nm in diameter and spherical morphology. The biodistribution, cellular uptake, circulation time and the efficacy of the micelles was influenced by the morphology. Over 8.0% and 8.7% of paclitaxel and lapatinib was released from the micelles after 1 h. After 24 h, the release of paclitaxel was 61.2% while the release of lapatinib was 27.6%. The high release of paclitaxel is attributed to factors such as diffusion, higher molar mass and higher loading content compared to lapatinib. The micellar system passively targeted the cancer cells by enhanced permeability and retention effect. The drug-loaded micelles displayed enhanced cytotoxic effects compared to the free drugs after 48 h and 72 h on MCF-7 cell lines. The drug combination using the micelles showed synergistic effects by reducing the viability of HER-2 negative breast cancer cell lines [174]. Wu and co-workers prepared and evaluated folate targeted biodegradable polymeric MPEG-*b*-P(LA-*co*-DHC/FA) micelles loaded with paclitaxel for breast cancer cell targeting [175]. The in vivo antitumor results in EMT-6 breast cancer cell line showed that the mean tumor masses were 0.18, 0.33, and 0.49 g for the drug-loaded polymeric micelles, free paclitaxel, and saline (control), respectively, indicating the potent anticancer efficacy of micelles when compared to free drug and control. Furthermore, the tumor growth inhibition of the three formulation groups was 66.1, 36.6, and 1.0%, respectively [168].

Wang et al. formulated pH-sensitive micelles using poly(2-ethyl-2-oxazoline)-poly(D,L-lactide) for the combination of paclitaxel and honokiol. The mean particle size was in the range of 41–44 nm with PDI that is less than 0.3, indicating the good stability of the micelles and their potential capability to deliver drugs to the tumor. TEM image of polymeric micelles was sphere-shaped with uniform particle size. The drug release profile from the formulation was fast followed by a slow and sustained drug release of both loaded drugs for 2 days at pH 5.4 and 7.4. The in vitro antitumor studies of the polymeric micelles were studied in the MCF-7/ADR breast cancer line employing SRB assay. The anticancer results showed that the cell viability was in the range of 99.5 ± 11.5%–100.0 ± 7.92% at a polymeric micelle concentration of 14.31 µg/mL, followed by a rapid decrease [176].

Oda et al. designed lyophilized diethylenetriaminepentaacetic acid-functionalized micelles encapsulated with paclitaxel utilizing 1,2-distearoyl-sn-glycero-3-phosphoethanolamine-N [methoxy(polyethyleneglycol)-2000] as a polymer. The lyophilization route did not alter the biological and physicochemical properties of polymeric micelles. Furthermore, the biodistribution profile of polymeric micelles displayed high uptake in the spleen, liver, and kidney in mice-bearing 4T1 tumor, indicating that polymeric micelles can be easily eliminated via these routes [177]. Zhang et al. formulated and evaluated polymeric micelles entrapped with paclitaxel that is based on poly(ε-caprolactone)-poly(ethylene glycol)-poly(ε-caprolactone) triblock copolymers [178]. The anticancer outcomes of drug-loaded polymeric micelles in the EMT6 breast tumor model showed that the cell viability was lower at 3 days by 2–10 times when compared to day 1, indicating the drug capability to kill tumor cells effectively and it also revealed that there no need for a prolonged exposure period [178].

Zhang and co-workers formulated octreotide modified PEG-*b*-PCL-based micelles encapsulated with paclitaxel or salinomycin for breast tumor therapy. The average particle size of the polymeric micelles ranged between 25 and 30 nm with an encapsulation efficiency of more than 90%. The in vitro cytotoxicity analysis of dual drug-loaded micelles demonstrated stronger growth inhibition against MCF-7 breast cancer cells when compared to the free drugs and the single drug-loaded micelles [179]. Yin and co-workers formulated hyaluronic acid-based amphiphilic micelles co-loaded with hydrophobic paclitaxel and hydrophilic AURKA specific siRNA for breast cancer treatment. The in vivo anticancer analysis using BalB/c nude mice bearing MDA-MB- 231 tumors demonstrated that the volume of the tumors in mice that received polymeric micelles encapsulated with paclitaxel or si-AURKA specific siRNA were notably smaller than the mice treated with the controls (saline and Taxol®). Furthermore, the mice treated with co-loaded micelles showed the synergistic antitumor effect of the loaded drugs [180]. Wang et al. formulated PEG-PDLLA micelles loaded with paclitaxel for breast cancer therapy. The in vivo imaging demonstrated that the polymeric micelles had outstanding specific cancer cells targeting effect and improved drug accumulation. The in vivo and in vitro antitumor experiments demonstrated that the paclitaxel-loaded micelles possessed high inhibition of the cancer cells and cell apoptosis on MDA-MB-231 breast cancer cells [181].

Kelishady and co-workers formulated Pluronic F127 polymeric micelles co-loaded with paclitaxel and lapatinib for the treatment of metastatic breast cancer [182]. The in vitro drug release profile of the micelles showed a burst release of 43% of PTX and 24% of lapatinib in the first 2 h, followed by a sustained drug release mechanism for 25 h. The in vitro anticancer analysis showed that the dual drug-loaded micelles significantly suppressed the proliferation of resistant T-47D breast cancer cell lines with IC_{50} value of 0.6 ± 0.1 µg/mL when compared to the free drug combination mixture of paclitaxel and lapatinib that showed an IC_{50} value of 6.7 ± 1.2 µg/mL [182]. Hou et al. formulated novel Soluplus®-Solutol® HS15 binary mixed micelles loaded with paclitaxel. The in vivo anticancer experiments using male nude mice bearing MDA-MB-231 breast cancer cells demonstrated that these micelles achieved higher antitumor efficacy of 57.66% when compared to 41.13% of the free paclitaxel [183]. The hyaluronic acid-shelled acid-activatable paclitaxel micelles designed by Zhong and co-workers were effective in vivo against mice induced with MCF-7 human breast tumor with little adverse effects. The formulation completely inhibited the growth of the tumor with 100% survival rate over 55 days [184].

Hasenstein et al. formulated a PEG-PLA multidrug-loaded micelle called Triolimus containing paclitaxel, 17-AAG, and rapamycin. The drug-loaded micelle significantly inhibited MDA-MB-231 and 549 breast cancer tumor growth in vivo when compared to the micelles loaded with paclitaxel alone [185]. Lee et al. performed a phase II clinical trial of monomethoxy poly(ethylene glycol)-block-poly(D,L-lactide) micelle called Genexol-PM encapsulated with paclitaxel for metastatic breast cancer therapy in 41 patients. The results from this clinical studies demonstrated that 37 patients who were administered the formulation via intravenous infusion at a dosage of 300 mg/m^2 for a period of three weeks as a first-line chemotherapy therapy for their metastatic breast cancer showed a response rate of 59.5% and two responses were observed in four breast cancer patients treated in the second-line setting for their metastatic cancer. Febrile neutropenia was not reported in any of the patients [186]. Mei and co-workers formulated α-conotoxin ImI modified PEG-DSPE micelles loaded with paclitaxel. The micelles displayed higher anticancer efficacy by inducing significant cell apoptosis and significant antitumor activity in MCF-7 tumor-bearing mice [187]. Liu et al. prepared PLGA-*g*-dextran micelles encapsulated with paclitaxel for breast cancer therapy. These micelles demonstrated higher anticancer efficacy against MCF-7 breast cancer cells than the control, (Taxol®) in vitro showing that paclitaxel loaded PLGA-*g*-dextran micelles can overcome the multidrug resistance in human breast carcinoma cells [188]. Yang et al. formulated micellar drug delivery systems that are based on poly(ethylene glycol)-benzoic imine-poly(g-benzyl-L-aspartate)-*b*-poly(1-vinylimidazole) block copolymer (PPBV) layer detachment for co-delivery of paclitaxel and curcumin. The in vivo cytotoxicity using the mice bearing subcutaneous MCF-7 breast tumors demonstrated that the average tumor volume after treatment with the dual drug-loaded PPBV micelles was 6.6, 5.4, 5.2, and 4.7-fold smaller when compared to those treated with 0.9% NaCl, a combination of paclitaxel and curcumin, PPBV micelles loaded with paclitaxel alone, and PPBV micelles loaded with curcumin alone, respectively [189]. Han et al. formulated and evaluated HA-based micelle conjugates loaded with paclitaxel for breast tumor therapy. The cellular uptake analysis revealed that the HA micelles loaded with paclitaxel could be specifically and efficiently internalized into 4T1 breast cancer cells via endocytosis. In vitro cytotoxicity analysis showed that the paclitaxel loaded micelles enhanced the selectivity of paclitaxel for destroying the 4T1 cancer cells when compared to the free paclitaxel [190].

Wang and co-workers formulated MCF-7 cell-specific phage protein modified PEG-phosphatidylethanolamine micelles loaded with paclitaxel for breast cancer targeting. The fluorescence microscopy demonstrated that MCF-7 targeted phage micelles were bound to the target cells, MCF-7 when compared to the non-target cells. The in vitro cytotoxicity analysis of the micelles loaded with paclitaxel exhibited a significant higher antitumor efficacy on MCF-7 breast cancer cells than the free paclitaxel [191]. Bernabeu et al. formulated mixed micelles that are based on two copolymers of polyvinyl caprolactam–polyvinyl acetate–PEG (Soluplus®) and TPGS for the incorporation of paclitaxel with improved anticancer activity on breast cancer cell lines. The in vitro cytotoxicity experiments showed that the mixed micelles loaded with paclitaxel demonstrated superior anticancer efficacy when compared to the free paclitaxel solution against MCF-7 and TNBC cells (MDA-MB-231) [192]. Chen et al. formulated poly (β-amino ester) copolymer micelles loaded with paclitaxel for breast cancer metastasis treatment. The in vivo and in vitro cytotoxicity studies of micelles showed that the micelles induced drug cellular uptake and significant MDA-MB-231 breast cancer cell disruption and suppressed breast tumor metastasis [193].

Wang and co-workers prepared PEG-PE–based micellar nanoparticles loaded with paclitaxel. The micellar nanoparticles demonstrated improved antitumor activity by promoting enhanced cell apoptosis against MCF-7 and reduced breast cancer cell proliferation [194]. Wang et al. also synthesized biodegradable mPEG-poly(caprolactone) micelles for co-delivery of paclitaxel and honokiol. The in vitro drug release profile was a sustained release of both drugs from the micelles. The in vitro cytotoxicity analysis and the cellular uptake studies of the co-loaded micelles showed an increased antitumor activity on the 4T1 breast cancer cells by promoting cell apoptosis and higher cellular uptake by the breast cancer cells [195]. Lang et al. formulated polymeric micelles loaded with paclitaxel for improved metastatic breast cancer therapy. The in vivo cytotoxicity studies of the micelles demonstrated 15-fold higher intratumor paclitaxel accumulation when compared to the commercially available paclitaxel, and achieved a growth tumor inhibition rate of 96.8% on the 4T1 metastatic breast cancer mice model [196]. Wang and workers reported folate modified pluronic copolymer micelles encapsulated with paclitaxel. Their anticancer activity on MDR MCF-7 ADR breast cancer cells was high when compared to paclitaxel solution [197]. The finding revealed the efficacy of using targeting moiety.

Lu et al. synthesized PEG-derivatized embelin as a nanomicellar drug delivery system loaded with paclitaxel for breast cancer therapy. The in vitro cell uptake of the micelles by the cancer cells were significantly high. The in vitro antitumor analysis demonstrated that paclitaxel loaded micelles revealed higher levels of antitumor effect on 4T1.2 breast cancer cells when compared to Taxol formulation [198]. Zhu et al. synthesized low-density lipoprotein–N-succinyl chitosan–cystamine–urocanic acid micelles for the co-delivery of paclitaxel and siRNA. The in vitro cellular uptake analysis demonstrated an initial significant accumulation of the co-loaded micelles in lyso/endosomes and a gradual diffusion into the entire cytoplasm of MCF-7 breast tumor cells. The in vivo cytotoxicity studies of micelles co-loaded with paclitaxel and siRNA using MCF-7 breast tumor-bearing nude mice showed the superior anticancer efficacy revealing a synergistic anticancer effect of combining paclitaxel and siRNA, when compared to the paclitaxel loaded micelles and siRNA loaded micelles [199].

5.4. Polymeric Micelles Loaded with Curcumin

The clinical use of curcumin remains a challenge resulting from its poor solubility, bioavailability, and stability. To improve its bioavailability and solubility, it is loaded into nanoparticles such as Chen et al. formulated phosphorylated calixarene-based micelles loaded with curcumin for TNBC treatment [200]. The DLS analysis of curcumin loaded micelles demonstrated a mean particle size of 3.86 ± 0.32 nm with a negative zeta potential of −25.18 ± 5.74 mV and PDI value of 0.125 ± 0.078, revealing a narrow size distribution. The encapsulation efficiency and drug loading capacity were 95.40 ± 4.50 and 17.10 ± 1.25%, respectively. The in vitro drug release profile was slow at pH 7.4 and fast at pH 5.5, indicating continuous sustained drug release pattern and prolonged release at neutral pH. The in vitro cytotoxicity studies using the MTT assay demonstrated concentration-dependent pattern against BT-549 breast cancer cells with IC_{50} value of 2.67 ± 0.40 µg/mL for curcumin loaded micelles, 9.78 ± 0.51 µg/mL for curcumin, and 194.35 ± 23.87 µg/mL for plain micelles. The similar anticancer trends were reported in MCF-7 breast tumor cells. Furthermore, the in vivo drug release studies using mice bearing BT-549 tumors demonstrated improved sustained curcumin release around the tumor mass at 24 h after intratumoral injection, revealing curcumin loaded micelles can potentially accumulate at the tumor environment. Loading curcumin into the micelles facilitated curcumin capability to hinder the nuclear activity of androgen receptor, induce cell cycle arrest and apoptosis. These mechanisms mentioned above contributed to the formulation ability to inhibit the growth of BT-549 tumor xenografts in mice, without causing any significant side effects during the 14 days of treatment [200].

Huang and co-workers formulated PEGylated micelles co-encapsulated with curcumin and doxorubicin, exerting a synergistic effect in MDR breast tumor cells. The micelles showed a mean particle size of 90.64 ± 0.15 nm and a negative surface charge of −15.3 ± 0.8 mV. The in vitro cytotoxicity of polymeric micelles was high with a IC_{50} value of 3.10 µg/mL when compared to free doxorubicin (IC_{50} of 31.99 µg/mL). Moreover, the micelles exhibited high cellular uptake and reduced cellular efflux. The combination index of the dual drug-loaded micelles was 0.17, which shows a strong synergistic anticancer activity against MCF-7/ADR breast cancer cells [201]. Jung and co-workers formulated epidermal growth factor-modified DSPE-PEG phospholipid micelle nanoparticles loaded with curcumin for breast cancer treatment. The micelle was conjugated with epidermal growth factor for specific targeting of epidermal growth factor receptors overexpressed on TNBC. The in vitro cytotoxicity study on MDA-MB-468 breast cancer cells revealed that the highest dose tested of 10 µM of free curcumin and curcumin loaded micelles significantly reduced cell viability to 41.5 ± 2.8 and 63.1 ± 8.3%, respectively [202]. Medel et al. prepared curcumin-bortezomib loaded mPEG-b-PLA-based miceller nanoparticles for synergistic anticancer efficacy. The in vitro cellular uptake analysis of the nanoparticles with an average particle of 100–150 nm size showed a maximum cellular uptake by the MDA-MB 231 and MCF-7 breast cancer cells after 3 h, which can result in potential anticancer effects [203].

Liu et al. formulated MPEG-PCL copolymer micelles loaded with curcumin for breast tumor therapy. The DLS analysis of curcumin loaded micelles demonstrated an average particle size of 28.2 ± 1.8 nm with PDI of 0.136 ± 0.050 and surface charge of −0.41 ± 0.25 mV. The TEM results exhibited spherical-shaped morphology in aqueous solution, and the results were consistent with that of particle size analysis. The drug loading capacity and encapsulation efficiency of curcumin loaded micelles were 14.84 ± 0.11% and 98.91 ± 0.70%, respectively. The drug-loaded micelles exhibited higher anticancer activity against 4T1 breast tumor cells in vitro when compared to free curcumin in a dose-dependent manner [204]. The formulation was effective in the inhibition of tumor growth, spontaneous pulmonary metastasis and extended the life span of the 4T1 breast tumor model.

5.5. Polymeric Micelles Loaded with Platinum Drugs

Platinum-based drugs cause apoptosis by penetrating into the nucleus of cancer cells resulting in the formation of adducts with DNA. However, their use is limited pharmacologically by toxicity and poor water solubility. Wan and co-workers formulated poly (2-oxazoline)-based micelles co-loaded with cisplatin and paclitaxel for breast tumor treatment [205]. The pharmacokinetic analysis showed that the dual drug-loaded polymeric micelles increased the plasma half-life of each drug when compared to the single drug loaded micelles. The in vivo cytotoxicity experiments of the dual drug-loaded micelles demonstrated the superior anticancer efficacy of the dual drug-loaded micelles when compared to single drug-loaded micelles or drug solutions against multidrug resistant breast cancer LCC-6-MDR orthotopic tumor models [205]. Ahmad et al. designed MPEG-block-Poly (L-glutamic acid-*co*-L-phenylalanine) micelle nanoparticles loaded with cisplatin for human breast cancer treatment. The in vitro drug release profile showed that 30% of cisplatin was released at physiological pH and 39% of the drug was released at acidic pH of the lysosome. The in vitro anticancer studies employing MTT viability assay displayed that the cell proliferation inhibition of polymeric micelle nanoparticle against ZR-75-30 human breast cancer cells was time- and dose-dependent. The micelle nanoparticles indicated more inhibition with low IC_{50} values on ZR-75-30 cell line when compared to the plain micelles and free drug. The formulation displayed high stability and extended blood circulation time [206].

Wang and co-workers formulated folate-modified mPEG-*b*-poly(L-lactide-*co*-2-methyl-2-carboxylpropylene carbonate-platinum (II) complex micelles. The particle size analysis of the micelles exhibited the average particle size that ranged between 100–200 nm. The drug molecules were loaded in the core part of the micelles, and the folic acid moiety was designed on the corona of the micelles for targeted drug delivery. Folic acid receptors are overexpressed on breast cancers making it a good targeting moiety. The cytotoxicity was evaluated using MTT assay which demonstrated very little antitumor effect for the plain polymeric micelles against MCF-7 breast cancer cells. The drug content from the micelle was significant at the tumor site. The micelles exhibited prolonged blood circulation when compared to the free drug [207].

5.6. Polymeric Micelles Loaded with Other Anticancer Drugs

Other types of anticancer drugs have been loaded into prepared micelles which revealed the efficacy of micelles for the treatment of breast cancer (Table 4). Teniposide, a semisynthetic derivative of podophyllotoxin damages the DNA in the replication process with the induction of cellular apoptosis. However, it exhibits low water solubility and is administered as an injection. Some side effects are hypersensitivity reactions, tachycardia, etc. Its elimination is rapid, with a widespread distribution to normal organs and tumor tissue, thereby decreasing its therapeutic efficacy with increased side effects [208,209].

Chu and co-worker prepared and evaluated polymeric micelles encapsulated with teniposide that are based on monomethoxy-poly(ethylene glycol)-poly(e-caprolactone-*co*-D,L-lactide) (MPEG-PCLA) copolymers for breast cancer therapy [210]. The mean particle size was 29.6 ± 0.3 nm, with a negative surface charge of −0.980 mV. The encapsulation efficiency and drug loading were 92.63 ± 2.05% and 18.53 ± 0.41%, respectively. The in vitro drug release profile of the micelles at physiological condition (pH 7.4) was slowed and sustained with about 33% and 78% release of teniposide from the polymeric micelles in the first 8 h and 72 h, respectively. The in vitro anticancer assessment of the drug-loaded micelles using MCF-7 cancer cell lines and MTT assay for 2 days showed that the drug-loaded micelles significantly inhibited cell growth with (IC_{50} value = 3.248 µg/mL) when compared to the free drug (IC_{50} value = 5.342 µg/mL) in a dose-dependent manner. Furthermore, the in vivo evaluation using the MCF-7-bearing nude mice model showed smaller relative tumor volumes for those groups treated with teniposide-loaded polymeric micelles than those treated with individual teniposide [210]. The teniposide-loaded MPEG-PCLA micelles improved the water solubility, reduced the toxicity, and enhanced the antitumor activity of teniposide. However, there is a need for further studies.

Epirubicin administration have been reported to present high relapse rate resulting from the presence of a subpopulation of cancer cells, known as cancer stem-like cells. These cells are resistant to the currently used conventional therapies. Zhang et al. formulated polymeric micelles co-loaded with epirubicin and staurosporine that are based on poly(ethylene glycol)-*b*-poly(aspartate-hydrazide-epirubicin) copolymer for the treatment of breast cancer. The cytotoxicity studies of polymeric micelles indicated potent chemotherapeutic activity against premature orthotopic 4T1-luc breast cancer cells in vitro with prolonged survival [211]. The formulation reduced cancer stem-like cells fraction in these tumors, thereby extending the survival of mice. These findings indicate the potential of micelles in eradicating breast cancer cells and cancer stem-like cells, which will result in the prevention and recurrence of the cancer thereby improving patient survival.

Min et al. formulated and assessed MPEG-poly(β-amino ester)-based micelles encapsulated with camptothecin for breast tumor therapy. The pH of the tumor environment was the targeted site for the delivery of the loaded drug. The drug release was quick from the polymeric micelles in the acidic conditions simulating a tumor environment. The cytotoxicity results in vitro demonstrated that the plain polymeric micelles demonstrated significantly 100% cell viability of MDA-MB231 breast cancer cells even in higher concentrations confirming non-toxicity of micelles in the normal body. On the other hand, drug-loaded micelles showed low cell viability on MDA-MB231 breast cancer cells [212].

The extracellular pH at the solid tumor site is reported to be 6.8 when compared to the normal tissue with a pH of 7.4. Designing a pH-sensitive drug delivery is a good approach that can result in pH-responsiveness at the target tumor tissues. Most prepared pH-responsive delivery systems promote rapid drug release into the inner part of tumor cells [213,214]. However, endosomal pH-responsive micelles are not specific to the target cancer cells because the pH is the same as that of the normal cells endosomal acid which is below 6.5. There is still a need to improve the pH-responsiveness of micelles in weak acidic tumor microenvironment, and tumor accumulation in vivo.

Chida et al. formulated pH-responsive PEG-*b*-poly(β-benzyl L-aspartate) (PEG-*b*-PBLA)-based micelles encapsulated with anthracycline drug, epirubicin for breast cancer metastasis treatment. The in vitro drug release studies demonstrated that epirubicin was released from the polymeric micelles in a pH-dependent pattern with a low drug release mechanism at pH 7.4 (physiological condition). The epirubicin release kinetics was gradually fast with decreasing pH values until pH 6.7 (tumor microenvironment condition), and further increased at pH 5.5 (endosomal environment). The antitumor studies of polymeric micelles loaded with epirubicin against axillary lymph node metastasis (ALNM) of MDA-MB-231 TNBC demonstrated their potential to inhibit the growth of the spreading primary tumor and the growth of ALNM, through efficient drug activation promoted by the intratumoral acidic environment [215]. The release mechanism of the micelles inhibited the spread of cancer.

Gener and co-workers designed and evaluated micelles that are based on amphiphilic polymer Pluronic® F127 loaded with Zileuton™ for breast cancer treatment. The in vivo and in vitro antitumor studies showed the drug-loaded polymeric micelles significant tumor growth inhibition in MDA-MB-231 and MCF-7 and breast cancer cell models when compared to the free Zileuton™. Furthermore, the polymeric micelles inhibited the circulation of breast tumor cells in the blood plasma effectively, and by doing so, significantly blocked metastatic spread [216]. The formulation eliminated cancer stem cells in the blood stream and reduced the number of cancer stem cells in the tumor in vivo. Eliminated cancer stem cells are usually replaced by new cells for tumor survival and propagation [217]. The capability of the micelles to eliminate cancer stem cell stream and metastatic spread is promising. These findings suggest that the formulation will show synergistic efficacy if combined with potent cytotoxic agents and is potentially a good approach to overcome cancer reoccurrence.

Lamch and co-workers formulated and evaluated in vitro the copolymers Pluronic-based micelles loaded with photofrin II® for breast and ovarian cancer therapy. The research involved the evaluation of suitable conditions for photodynamic reaction and apoptosis in human cancer cells. The effect of Photofrin II®-loaded micelle formulation on the integrity of the cancer and human erythrocytes and cancer cells was also studied to determine the bioavailability of these nanocarriers in intravenous administration. The in vitro cytotoxicity studies of polymeric micelles exhibited superior pro-apoptotic and cytotoxic efficacy against MCF-7 tumor cells when compared to photofrin II® [218].

Polymeric micelles are useful for efficient delivery of the loaded drug to the tumor cells and is also useful in reducing the effective drug concentration, which is suitable to diminish the side effects of the loaded anticancer drugs. The size of the micelles play a huge role in their uptake and formulation containing Photofrin II® with the size below 20 nm were delivered inside the breast MCF-7/WT (caspase-3 deficient) cells efficiently. The results indicate that the administration of the formulation is potentially useful for the treatment of resistant cancers after irradiation.

Marcos and co-workers formulated and evaluated polymeric micelles that are based on poly(ethylene oxide)-poly(propylene oxide)-poly(ethylene oxide) triblock copolymers encapsulated with N-(2-hydroxyphenyl)-2-propylpentanamide for breast cancer targeting. The in vitro drug release kinetics of drug-entrapped micelles followed Weibull's drug release model, demonstrating sustained drug release mechanism. The cytotoxicity effect of the polymeric micelles was significant in MDA-MB-231 [219]. N-(2-hydroxyphenyl)-2-propylpentanamide, has good anticancer activity against MDA-MB-231 cells but its low water solubility limit its therapeutic effectiveness. The incorporation of the drug into the micelles enhanced the water solubility by 23- and 31-fold. The hydrodynamic diameter of the formulation was 30 nm. The micelles improved the solubility of the drug forming stable aggregates and enhanced the drug release with a good maintenance. The sustained release system induced cell death and increased the drug administration time. Lu and co-workers prepared and evaluated micelles that are based on polylactide-b-(poly(2-hydroxyethyl acrylate-co-2-chloroethylmethacrylate-co-fluorescein-O-methacrylate)) (PLA-P(HEA-CEMA-F)) loaded with ruthenium complexes. The in vitro antitumor studies of the drug-loaded polymeric micelles in MDA-MB-231 and MCF-7 cancer cell models displayed enhanced anti-metastatic effect when compared to the free drugs and the tumor growth inhibition of drug-loaded micelles was 10 times higher when compared to the free drug [220]. Ruthenium complexes such as [Ru(η^6-p-cymene)Cl$_2$(PTA)] are not active against primary tumors but are effective in reducing metastasis. Their clearance rate from vital organs, their capability to reduce the progression of cancer in vivo, and their low toxicity make them useful for further studies [221]. The selectively targeted behavior of the micelle formulations on metastatic tumor cells limited the metastases of cancer.

Table 4. A summary of micelles loaded with anticancer drugs.

Polymers	Drugs	Cancer Cell Lines	Therapeutic Outcomes	References
mPEG-PDLA	Docetaxel and resveratrol	MCF-7	Improved pharmacokinetic parameters, good biocompatibility, and safety.	[122]
BD-Peptide-PEG and BD-PEI	Docetaxel	4T1	High cellular uptake	[123]
Poly(D,L-lactide-co-2-methyl-2-carboxy-trimethylene carbonate)	Docetaxel	MDA-MB-231/H2N	High tumor growth inhibition and improvement in pharmacokinetic parameters	[124]
Monomethoxy PEG	Docetaxel	MDA-MB-231	Sustained in vitro drug release profile and potent in vivo antitumor efficacy.	[125]
PCL-g-PEI	Docetaxel and NIR dye	4T1	High tumor growth inhibition	[126]
TPGS	Docetaxel	MDA-MB-231 and MDA-MB-468	Greatly enhanced anticancer activity	[127]
PEG-PCL	Docetaxel	4T1	High tumor growth inhibition and decreased systemic toxicity	[128]
mPEG-polyester	Docetaxel	-	High tumor growth inhibition	[129]
mPEG$_{2000}$-b-PDLLA$_{1300}$	Docetaxel	4T1	greater anticancer activity	[130]
PLGA	Docetaxel	MDA-MB-231 and MCF-7	Improved antitumor activity	[131]
TPGS	Docetaxel	MDA-MB-231	Hindering of EGFR-overexpressing tumor cell lines	[132]
PLys-PPhe	Docetaxel	-	Improved tumor specificity	[133]
TPGS	Docetaxel	MDA-MB-231	High antitumor efficacy	[134]
MPEG-PDLLA-PLL	Docetaxel	4T1 and MCF-7	High tumor growth inhibition	[135]
PEG-b-PLGA	Docetaxel and chloroquine	MCF-7	Good anticancer activity	[136]

Table 4. Cont.

Polymers	Drugs	Cancer Cell Lines	Therapeutic Outcomes	References
[NP(PEG750)(GlyPheLeu)$_2$Et]$_3$	Docetaxel	MDA-MB-231	Excellent anticancer efficacy	[137]
Poly(styrene maleic acid)-poly (amide-ether-ester-imide)	Docetaxel	MC4-L2	High tumor inhibition and increased survival in vivo	[138]
Polyvinyl caprolactam–polyvinyl acetate–PEG	Docetaxel and Fe$_3$O$_4$	MDA-MB-231 and MCF-7	Good anticancer activity	[139]
PEG-PLL-PLLeu	Docetaxel and siRNA-Bcl-2	MCF-7	Improved antitumor efficacy	[140]
mPEG2000-DSPE	Docetaxel	MCF-7	Better antitumor activity	[141]
HA	Doxorubicin	MCF-7	High tumor growth inhibition	[146]
Phis-PEG and PLLA-PEG	Doxorubicin	4T1	Moderate anticancer activity	[147]
Pluronic block copolymers	Doxorubicin	MDA-MB-231 and MDA-MB-468	Potent tumor growth inhibition	[148]
PEG-poly(aspartate hydrazide) block copolymers	Doxorubicin and wortmannin	MCF-7	Small particle size which is suitable for tumor-specific drug delivery	[149]
Carboxymethyl chitosan	Doxorubicin and cisplatin	HeLa	Synergistic anticancer effect	[150]
Dextran-retinoic acid	Doxorubicin	MDA-MB-468 and MCF-7	Good antitumor activity	[151]
PEG$_{2k}$-PLA$_{5k}$	Doxorubicin and curcumin	MCF-7/ADR	Higher tumor accumulation and tumor growth inhibitory effect	[152]
PEG-PCL-PEG	Doxorubicin	MCF-7	Suppressed tumor cells	[153]
-	Doxorubicin	MCF-7/ADR	Potential tumor growth inhibition	[154]
PLLA/PEG	Doxorubicin	MCF-7/DOX^R	High cytotoxicity	[155]
Pluronic® F127-poly (methyl-vinyl ether-alt-maleic acid) copolymer	Doxorubicin	MCF-7	Sustained drug release kinetics with good anticancer activity	[156]
PAA-g-PEG	Doxorubicin	4T1	High tumor accumulation	[157]
Poly (ε-caprolactone)-PEG	Doxorubicin	MCF-7	Time-delayed anticancer activity	[158]
PEG–PCL	Doxorubicin	MCF-7	High drug cellular uptake	[159]
Poly(ε-caprolactone)-polyphospho-ester	Doxorubicin	MCF-7	Improved antitumor activity	[160]
Dextran and indomethacin	Doxorubicin	MCF-7	Potential tumor growth inhibition	[161]
PEG-PCL	Doxorubicin and iron oxide	A431 and MDA-MB-453	Significant tumor inhibitory effect	[162]
mPEG-PCL-g-cellulose	Doxorubicin	MCF7/ADR	Good cellular internalization	[163]
Poly 2,2-bis (methylol) propionic acid (bis-MPA)-PEG	Doxorubicin	MCF-7 and MDA-MB-468	Concentration-dependent anticancer activity	[164]
Poly (Іμ-caprolactone)	Doxorubicin	MCF-7	Higher antitumor activity	[165]
TPGS	Doxorubicin	MCF-7	100% long-term survival of the treated mice	[166]
mPEG-PLA	Doxorubicin and gemcitabine	MCF-7	Synergistic anticancer efficacy	[167]
Tetronic T1107, Pluronic F127, and TPGS	Doxorubicin	MDA-MB-231	High anticancer efficacy	[168]
Pluronic	Doxorubicin and paclitaxel	MCF-7	Decreased cancer cell viability	[169]
MPEG-PCL-4-FBA	Doxorubicin and paclitaxel	MCF-7	Synergistic antitumor efficacy	[170]
Carboxymethyl chitosan	Paclitaxel	MCF-7	Improved oral drug bioavailability and synergistic anticancer activity.	[173]
Poly(2-oxazoline)-	Paclitaxel and cisplatin	LCC-6-MDR	Extended of the average lifespan of animals models in vivo	[174]
MPEG-b-P(LA-co-DHC/FA)	Paclitaxel	EMT-6	Reduced tumor mass and high tumor growth inhibition	[175]
Poly(2-ethyl-2-oxazoline)-poly(D,L-lactide)-	Paclitaxel and honokiol	MCF-7/ADR	Decreased cancer cell viability and small particle size which is beneficial for tumor-targeted drug delivery	[176]
1,2-distearoyl-sn-glycero-3-phosphoethanol-amine-N-[methoxy(PEGl)-2000]	Paclitaxel	4T1	Great potential for theranostic application in the breast cancer therapy	[177]
Poly(ε-caprolactone)-PEG-poly(ε-caprolactone) triblock copolymers	Paclitaxel	EMT6	Low cell viability	[178]
PEG-b-PCL	Paclitaxel and salinomycin	MCF-7	High tumor growth inhibition	[179]
HA	paclitaxel and hydrophilic AURKA	MDA-MB-231	Decreased tumor volume	[180]
PEG-PDLLA	Paclitaxel	MDA-MB-231	Significant tumor growth inhibition and cell apoptosis	[181]
Pluronic F127	Paclitaxel and lapatinib	T-47D	Suppressed proliferation of breast cancer cell	[182]

Table 4. Cont.

Polymers	Drugs	Cancer Cell Lines	Therapeutic Outcomes	References
Soluplus®—Solutol® HS15	Paclitaxel	MDA-MB-231	Good anticancer efficacy	[183]
HA	Paclitaxel	MCF-7	Good anticancer activity with reduced drug toxicity	[184]
PEG-PLA	Paclitaxel, 17-AAG, and Rapamycin	MDA-MB-231 and 549	High tumor growth inhibition	[185]
mPEG-b-poly(D,L-lactide)	Paclitaxel	-	Good clinical response rate	[186]
PEG-DSPE	Paclitaxel	MCF-7	Greater anticancer activity	[187]
PLGA-g-dextran	Paclitaxel	MCF-7	High anticancer efficacy	[188]
PPBV	Paclitaxel and curcumin	MCF-7	Small tumor volume	[189]
HA	Paclitaxel	4T1	Good cellular uptake	[190]
PEG-phosphatidyl-ethanolamine	Paclitaxel	MCF-7	High antitumor efficacy	[191]
Caprolactam–polyvinyl acetate–PEG and TPGS	Paclitaxel	MCF-7 and MDA-MB-231	Superior anticancer efficacy	[192]
Poly(β-amino ester)	Paclitaxel	MDA-MB-231	Good cellular uptake and suppression of the tumor metastasis	[193]
PEG-PE	Paclitaxel	MCF-7	Enhanced anticancer activity	[194]
mPEG-poly(capro-lactone)	Paclitaxel and honokiol	4T1	High cellular uptake and increased anticancer efficacy	[195]
-	Paclitaxel	4T1	High growth inhibition on tumor metastasis	[196]
Pluronic	Paclitaxel	MCF-7	High anticancer activity	[197]
PEG	Paclitaxel	4T1.2	High anticancer activity	[198]
lipoprotein-N-succinyl chitosan–cystamine–urocanic acid	Paclitaxel and siRNA	MCF-7	Superior anticancer activity	[199]
phosphorylated calixarene	Curcumin	BT-549	Concentration-dependent cytotoxicity	[200]
PEG	Curcumin and doxorubicin	MCF-7/ADR	High synergistic anticancer activity	[201]
DSPE-PEG	Curcumin	MDA-MB-468	Decreased cancer cell viability	[202]
mPEG-b-PLA-	Curcumin and bortezomib	MDA-MB-231 and MCF-7	Maximum cellular uptake	[203]
MPEG-PCL	Curcumin	4T1	High anticancer activity	[204]
poly (2-oxazoline)	Cisplatin and paclitaxel	LCC-6-MDR	Prolonged plasma half-life and superior antitumor activity.	[205]
MPEG-block-poly (L-glutamic acid-co-L-phenylalanine)	Cisplatin	ZR-75-30	Inhibition of cancer cell proliferation	[206]
mPEG-b-poly(L-lactide-co-2-methyl-2-carboxyl-propylene carbonate	Platinum (II) drug	MCF-7	Dose-dependent cytotoxicity	[207]
MPEG-PCLA copolymer	Teniposide	MCF-7	Significant cell growth inhibition and reduced tumor volumes in vivo	[210]
PEG-b-poly(aspartate-hydrazide-epirubicin) copolymer	Epirubicin and staurosporine	orthotopic 4T1-luc	Potent anticancer efficacy and prolonged animal survival.	[211]
MPEG-poly(β-amino ester) copolymer	Camptothecin	MDA-MB231	Non-toxicity of the plain micelles and low cell viability for drug-loaded micelles	[212]
PEG-b-PBLA	Epirubicin	MDA-MB-231	Good tumor growth inhibition and suppression of ALNM	[215]
Pluronic® F127	Zileuton™	MDA-MB-231 and MCF-7	Significant tumor growth inhibition and inhibition of metastatic spread and cancer cell blood circulation.	[216]
Pluronic	Photofrin II®	MCF-7	Improved in vitro pro-apoptotic and cytotoxic activity	[218]
Poly(ethylene oxide)-poly(propylene oxide)-poly(ethylene oxide) triblock copolymers	N-(2-Hydroxy-phenyl)-2-propyl-pentanamide	MDA-MB-231	Sustained drug release mechanism and anti-proliferative properties	[219]
PLA-P(HEA-CEMA-F)	Ruthenium complexes	MDA-MB-231 and MCF-7	Improved anti-metastatic effect and tumor growth inhibition	[220]
PAMAM-PLA	Aminoflavone	MDA-MB-468 and BT474	Decreased cancer cell viability	[222]
Dendron	Endoxifen	-	Sustained drug release and improved permeation through skin	[223]
PEG	Mertansine	MDA-MB-231	Suppressed tumor growth	[224]

Brinkman et al. formulated 12 amino acid peptide targeting epidermal growth factor receptor (EGFR) modified unimolecular PAMAM-PLA micelle nanoparticles loaded with aminoflavone for TNBC treatment. The in vitro cellular uptake studies showed that the modified polymeric micelles accumulated to a greater amount in the cytoplasm of MDA-MB-468 TNBC cells than the non-modified micelles. The in vitro cytotoxicity analysis demonstrated a significant decrease in cell viability of MDA-MB-468 and BT474 breast cancer cells that are incubated with modified micelle nanoparticles when compared to the unmodified micelles and free aminoflavone [222]. The micelles excellent stability and preferentially drug uptake at endosomal pH levels when compared to the blood pH suggest that they are potential therapeutics for EGFR-overexpressing triple negative breast cancer. Yang and co-workers formulated dendron-based micelles for topical delivery of endoxifen for estrogen-positive breast cancer treatment. Endoxifen is effective for the treatment and the prevention of estrogen-positive breast cancer; but its oral formulation induced severe side effects. The in vitro drug release profile demonstrated sustained release of endoxifen from the dendron-based micelles for 6 days. Micelles significantly improved the permeation of endoxifen through the mouse skin (up to 20-fold) and human skin (up to 4-fold). These results revealed that dendron-based micelles are useful for the topical delivery of endoxifen, providing a potential alternative administration method for chemoprevention of breast cancer [223]. Zhong and co-workers formulated cRGD-decorated, redox-activatable micellar mertansine prodrug to deliver mertansine to $\alpha v \beta 3$ integrin overexpressed triple negative breast cancer. The cytotoxicity analysis showed that these micelles effectively suppressed MDA-MB-231 breast tumor growth without causing obvious side effects, as revealed by the body weight loss and histological analysis [224]. The formulation was effective in targeting and delivering of mertansine to $\alpha_v \beta_3$ integrin overexpressing triple negative breast cancer with a potent tumor growth inhibition. These findings reveal the high affinity of the formulation to MDA-MB-231 cells and high intracellular drug release effective for potent antitumor effect; high stability and good targeting ability of the formulation resulting in high accumulation in the cancer cells; high effective inhibition of the tumor growth and reduced systemic toxicity when compared to the free mertansine showing its promising use for the treatment of triple negative breast cancer.

5.7. Limitations of Micelles

Micelles offer two distinct features when compared to other drug delivery systems, such as their small size (hydrodynamic sizes less than 50 nm) [225]. Its small particle sizes are suitable for good cellular uptake, blood circulation, tumor tissue penetration, and efficient internalization in cancer cells [225,226]. Their small size has improved the performance of the encapsulated drug in vivo due to the enhanced permeability and retention (EPR) effect [225,227]. They are also feasible for large-scale prooduction. It has well-defined molecular structures and good assembly behaviors. Micelle formulations are simple to produce at a large scale [228]. Polymeric micelles are useful for the delivery of hydrophobic and hydrophilic drugs to the target site. Their good stability, slow dissociation extend their circulation times, and their specific accumulation in the tumor tissues [229]. Small hydrophobic drugs are solubilized in the inner hydrophobic core of micelles, and their outer hydrophilic shell protects the drug from scavengers by the mononuclear phagocytic system [230,231]. Despite the distinct properties of micelles reported by several researchers, they are also limited due to their capability to undergo dilution resulting in dissociation when administered intravenously into the blood environment. The factor mentioned above is attributed to a shift from equilibrium to a unimer state and binding of the proteins to the unimeric components [231]. The protein binding can result in a burst release effect of the encapsulated drugs into the bloodstream, thereby nullifying the unique properties of micelles such as high drug loading, targeting capability, and prolonged blood circulation [225,229]. It can result in drug biodistribution that is favourable and toxicity with therapeutic outcomes similar to the free drugs [232]. Taxotere®, a micellar formulation displayed reduced therapeutic outcomes after intravenous administration resulting from its quick removal from the blood circulation [225].

The structural stability of micelles is affected by the physiological environment. Injection of micelles into the bloodstream results in them undergoing changes, including the disruption of the micellar structure via hydrolysis of the linkers etc. The disruption of the micellar causes a premature release of the encapsulated drug and the uptake of the drug in healthy tissues/organs, thereby inducing severe side effects and reducing the therapeutic efficacy of the loaded drug [233]. One strategic approach to improve the stability of micelles by cross-linking the micelles to afford a rigid micellar structure and prolonged blood circulation. Guo et al. reported mPEG-PDLA micelles with hydrophilic surface composed of PEG chain, which enhanced the micelles capability of escaping from the reticuloendothelial system, resulting in a slower clearance. A preferential accumulation of the formulation was significant in the tumors due to the enhanced permeability and prolonged circulation time [122]. Lang et al. coated the surface of the micelles with PEG, resulting in targeted drug delivery to the tumor and enhanced drug uptake [123]. Hu et al. reported Core-crosslinked polymeric micelles that promoted a 100% tumour-free survival [125]. Crosslinking of the micelles have resulted in them having distinct features such as prolonged circulation [122,123], efficient uptake into the tumor tissues with good retention [122,123,132], sustained drug release [125], and increased drug bioavailability [128,131,141].

6. Conclusions

This review reports the therapeutic biological outcomes (in vivo and in vitro) of dendrimers and micelles, as nanocarriers loaded with anticancer drugs on breast cancer. The nanocarriers exhibited distinct properties that revealed their capability to overcome the shortcomings of chemotherapeutic agents such as drug toxicity, multi-drug resistance, low drug cellular uptake, poor drug solubility, and drug bioavailability. The drug release profiles from the micelles and dendrimers were generally sustained at physiological conditions resulting in their low toxicity to the healthy cells and fast drug release at tumor conditions resulting in high cytotoxicity and uptake in the breast cancer cells. Furthermore, the polymeric nanocarriers exhibited high cellular uptake, important growth inhibition, inhibited metastases, and improved pharmacokinetic parameters (such as prolonged drug blood circulation). Although these systems show promising chemotherapeutic outcomes in breast tumor in vitro and in vivo in the reported preclinical studies, there is a serious need for further studies in order for these systems to reach clinical trial phases.

Author Contributions: Conceptualization, S.A. and B.A.A.; methodology, S.A. and B.A.A.; investigation, S.A. and B.A.A.; writing—original draft preparation, S.A. and B.A.A.; writing—review and editing, S.A. and B.A.A.; supervision, B.A.A.; funding acquisition, B.A.A. All authors have read and agreed to the published version of the manuscript.

Funding: The financial assistance of the Medical Research Council and National Research Foundation, South Africa towards this research are hereby acknowledged. The views and opinions expressed in this manuscript are those of the authors and not of MRC or NRF.

Conflicts of Interest: The authors declare no conflict of interest.

References

1. Singh, S.; Sharma, B.; Kanwar, S.S.; Kumar, A. Lead Phytochemicals for Anticancer Drug Development. *Front. Plant Sci.* **2016**, *7*, 1667. [CrossRef] [PubMed]
2. Anand, P.; Kunnumakara, A.B.; Sundaram, C.; Harikumar, K.B.; Tharakan, S.T.; Lai, O.S.; Sung, B.; Aggarwal, B.B. Cancer is a preventable disease that requires major lifestyle changes. *Pharm. Res.* **2008**, *25*, 2097–2116. [CrossRef] [PubMed]
3. Okuhara, T.; Ishikawa, H.; Urakubo, A.; Hayakama, M.; Yamaki, T.; Tarayama, T.; Kuchi, T. Cancer information needs according to cancer type: A content analysis of data from Japan's largest cancer information website. *Prev. Med. Rep.* **2018**, *12*, 245–252. [CrossRef] [PubMed]
4. Peter, S.; Aderibigbe, B.A. Ferrocene-Based Compounds with Antimalaria/Anticancer Activity. *Molecules* **2019**, *24*, 3604. [CrossRef]
5. Feng, S.; Chien, S. Chemotherapeutic engineering: Application and further development of chemical engineering principles for chemotherapy of cancer and other diseases. *Chem. Eng. Sci.* **2003**, *58*, 4087–4114. [CrossRef]
6. International Agency for Research. *Latest Global Cancer Data: Cancer Burden Rises to 18.1 Million New Cases and 9.6 Million Cancer Deaths in 2018*; International Agency for Research on Cancer: Lyon, France, 2018.

7. Siegel, R.; Ward, E.; Brawley, O.; Jemal, A. Cancer statistics, 2011: The impact of eliminating socioeconomic and racial disparities on premature cancer deaths. *CA Cancer J. Clin.* **2011**, *61*, 212–236. [CrossRef]
8. Tinoco, G.; Warsch, S.; Glück, S.; Avancha, K.; Montero, A.J. Treating Breast Cancer in the 21st Century: Emerging Biological Therapies. *J. Cancer* **2013**, *4*, 117–132. [CrossRef]
9. American Cancer Society. *Cancer Facts and Figures*; American Cancer Society: Atlanta, GA, USA, 2011.
10. Carlson, R.W.; Allred, D.C.; Anderson, B.O.; Burstein, H.J.; Carter, W.B.; Edge, S.B.; Erban, J.K.; Farrar, W.B.; Goldstein, L.J.; Gradishar, W.J.; et al. Breast cancer. Clinical practice guidelines in oncology. *J. Natl. Compr. Cancer Netw.* **2009**, *7*, 122–192. [CrossRef]
11. Peng, J.; Chen, J.; Xie, F.; Bao, W.; Xu, H.; Wang, H.; Xu, Y.; Du, Z. Herceptin-conjugated paclitaxel loaded PCL-PEG worm-like nanocrystal micelles for the combinatorial treatment of HER2-positive breast cancer. *Biomaterials* **2019**, *222*, 119420. [CrossRef]
12. Chang, L.; Weiner, L.S.; Hartman, S.J.; Horvath, S.; Jeste, D.; Mischel, P.S.; Kado, D.M. Breast cancer treatment and its effects on aging. *J. Geriatr. Oncol.* **2019**, *10*, 346–355. [CrossRef]
13. Alven, S.; Nqoro, X.; Buyana, B.; Aderibigbe, B.A. Polymer-Drug Conjugate, a Potential Therapeutic to Combat Breast and Lung Cancer. *Pharmaceutics* **2020**, *12*, 406. [CrossRef] [PubMed]
14. Rania, M.H.; Abdelkader, A.M.; Sherweit, H.E.; Eman, S.M.; Noha, A.G.; Salma, A.; Tarek, E.; Rosaline, A.; Maha, F.; Abdullah, I.E.; et al. Dual stimuli-responsive polypyrrole nanoparticles for anticancer therapy. *J. Drug Deliv. Sci. Technol.* **2018**, *47*, 176–180.
15. Ma, W.; Xu, A.; Ying, J.; Li, B.; Jin, Y. Biodegradable core-shell copolymer-phospholipid nanoparticles for combination chemotherapy: An in vitro study. *J. Biomed. Nanotechnol.* **2015**, *11*, 1193–1200. [CrossRef] [PubMed]
16. Li, Z.; Zhu, J.; Wang, Y.; Zhou, M.; Li, D.; Zheng, S.; Luo, C.; Zhang, H.; Zhong, L.; Li, W.; et al. In situ apolipoprotein E-enriched corona guides dihydroartemisinin-decorating nanoparticles towards LDLr-mediated tumor-homing chemotherapy. *Asian J. Pharm. Sci.* **2019**, 2. [CrossRef]
17. Liu, L.; Wei, Y.; Zhai, S.; Chen, Q.; Xing, D. Dihydroartemisinin and transferrin dual-dressed nano-graphene oxide for a pH-triggered chemotherapy. *Biomaterials* **2015**, *62*, 35–46. [CrossRef]
18. Nguyen, H.T.; Tran, T.H.; Kim, J.O.; Yong, C.S.; Nguyen, C.N. Enhancing the in vitro anti-cancer efficacy of artesunate by loading into poly-D,L-lactide-*co*-glycolide (PLGA) nanoparticles. *Arch. Pharm. Res.* **2015**, *38*, 716–724. [CrossRef]
19. Jieqing, M.; Rongfa, G.; Haitao, S.; Fei, L.; Chaogeng, X.; Mingqi, L.; Tianshu, K. Comparison of anticancer activity between lactoferrin nanoliposome and lactoferrin in Caco-2 cells in vitro. *Food Chem. Toxicol.* **2013**, *59*, 72–77.
20. Zucker, D.; Andriyanov, A.V.; Steiner, A.; Raviv, U.; Barenholz, Y. Characterization of PEGylated nanoliposomes co-remotely loaded with topotecan and vincristine: Relating structure and pharmacokinetics to therapeutic efficacy. *J. Control. Release* **2012**, *160*, 281–289. [CrossRef]
21. Nancy, D.; Samantha, M.; Jason, T.; Cynthia, L.; Vasilios, P.; Elena, G.; Christopher, W.E.; Lia, L.; Walid, S.K.; Omid, G.; et al. Nanoliposome targeting in breast cancer is influenced by the tumor microenvironment. *Nanomed. Nanotechnol. Biol. Med.* **2019**, *17*, 71–81.
22. Perillo, E.; Allard-vannier, E.; Falanga, A.; Stiuso, P.; Teresa, M.; Galdiero, M.; Galdiero, S.; Chourpa, I. Quantitative and qualitative effect of gH625 on the nanoliposome-mediated delivery of mitoxantrone anticancer drug to HeLa cells. *Int. J. Pharm.* **2015**, *488*, 59–66. [CrossRef]
23. Liang, X.-J.; Chen, C.; Zhao, Y.; Wang, P.C. Circumventing Tumor Resistance to Chemotherapy by Nanotechnology. *Methods Mol. Biol.* **2010**, *596*, 467–488.
24. Larson, L.; Ghandehari, H. Polymeric Conjugates Drug Delivery. *Chem. Mater.* **2012**, *24*, 840–953. [CrossRef] [PubMed]
25. Alven, S.; Aderibigbe, B.A.; Balogun, M.O.; Matshe, W.M.R.; Ray, S.S. Polymer-drug conjugates containing antimalarial drugs and antibiotics. *J. Drug Deliv. Sci. Technol.* **2019**, *53*, 101171. [CrossRef]
26. Cai, H.; Wang, X.; Zhang, H.; Sun, L.; Pan, D.; Gong, Q.; Gu, Z.; Luo, K. Enzyme-sensitive biodegradable and multifunctional polymeric conjugate as theranostic nanomedicine. *Appl. Mater. Today* **2018**, *11*, 207–218. [CrossRef]

27. Vogus, D.R.; Evans, M.E.; Pusuluri, A.; Barajas, A.; Zhang, M.; Krishnan, V.; Nowak, M.; Menegatti, S.; Helgeson, M.E.; Squires, T.M.; et al. A hyaluronic acid conjugate engineered to synergistically and sequentially deliver gemcitabine and doxorubicin to treat triple negative breast cancer. *J. Control. Release* **2017**, *267*, 191–202. [CrossRef] [PubMed]
28. Armiñán, A.; Palomino-Schätzlein, M.; Deladriere, C.; Arroyo-Crespo, J.J.; Vicente-Ruiz, S.; Vicent, M.J.; Pineda-Lucena, A. Metabolomics facilitates the discrimination of the specific anti-cancer effects of free- and polymer-conjugated doxorubicin in breast cancer models. *Biomaterials* **2018**, *162*, 144–153. [CrossRef] [PubMed]
29. Zhou, H.; Lv, S.; Zhang, D.; Deng, M.; Zhang, X.; Tang, Z. A polypeptide based podophyllotoxin conjugate for the treatment of multi drug resistant breast cancer with enhanced efficiency and minimal toxicity. *Acta Biomater.* **2018**, *73*, 388–399. [CrossRef] [PubMed]
30. Sultana, F.; Imran-Ul-Haque, M.M.; Arafat, M.; Sharmin, S. An overview of nanogel drug delivery system. *J. Appl. Pharm. Sci.* **2013**, *3*, S95–S105.
31. Martin, L.; Wilson, C.G.; Koosha, F.; Tetley, L.; Gray, A.; Senel, S.; Uchegbu, I.F. The release of model macromolecules may be controlled by the hydrophobicity of palmitoyl glycol chitosan hydrogels. *J. Control. Release* **2002**, *80*, 87–100. [CrossRef]
32. Namazi, H.; Adeli, M. Dendrimers of citric acid and poly (ethylene glycol) as the new drug-delivery agents. *Biomaterials* **2005**, *26*, 1175–1183. [CrossRef]
33. Saluja, V.; Mankoo, A.; Saraogi, G.K.; Tambuwala, M.M.; Mishra, V. Smart dendrimers: Synergizing the targeting of anticancer bioactives. *J. Drug Deliv. Sci. Technol.* **2019**, *52*, 15–26. [CrossRef]
34. Manjili, H.K.; Malvandi, H.; Mousavi, M.S.; Attari, E.; Danafar, H. In vitro and in vivo delivery of artemisinin loaded PCL–PEG–PCL micelles and its pharmacokinetic study. *Artif. Cells Nanomed. Biotechnol.* **2018**, *46*, 926–936. [CrossRef] [PubMed]
35. Ramazani, A.; Keramati, M.; Malvandi, H.; Danafar, H.; Kheiri Manjili, H. Preparation and in vivo evaluation of anti-plasmodial properties of artemisinin-loaded PCL-PEG-PCL nanoparticles. *Pharm. Dev. Technol.* **2017**. [CrossRef] [PubMed]
36. Yao, Q.; Liu, Y.; Kou, L.; Tu, Y.; Tang, X.; Zhu, L. Tumor-targeted drug delivery and sensitization by MMP2-responsive polymeric micelles. *Nanomed. Nanotechnol. Biol. Med.* **2019**, *19*, 71–80. [CrossRef]
37. Movellan, J.; Urban, P.; Moles, E.; Fuente, J.M.; Sierra, T.; Serrano, J.L.; Fernandez-busquetts, X. Amphiphilic dendritic derivatives as nanocarriers for the targeted delivery of antimalarial drugs. *Biomaterials* **2014**, *13*, 7940–7950. [CrossRef]
38. Bhadra, D.; Bhadra, S.; Jain, N.K. Pegylated Lysine Based Copolymeric Dendritic Micelles For Solubilization And Delivery Of Artemether. *J. Pharm. Pharm. Sci.* **2005**, *8*, 467–482.
39. Anders, C.; Carey, L. Biology, metastatic patterns, and treatment of patients with triple-negative breast cancer. *Clin. Breast Cancer* **2009**, *9*, S73–S81. [CrossRef]
40. Ikhuoria, E.B.; Bach, C. Introduction to Breast Carcinogenesis Symptoms, Risks Factors, Treatment and Management. *Eur. J. Eng. Res. Sci.* **2018**, *3*, 58–66. [CrossRef]
41. Humberto, P.J.; Marilie, D.G.; Hope, L.E.; Jia, C.; Antonia, M.C.; Alfred, I.N.; Regina, M.S.; Mary, S.W.; Susan, L.T. Urinary concentrations of environmental phenols and their associations with breast cancer incidence and mortality following breast cancer. *Environ. Int.* **2019**, *130*, 104890.
42. Lee, S. Human serum albumin: A nanomedicine platform targeting breast cancer cells. *J. Drug Deliv. Sci. Technol.* **2019**, *52*, 652–659. [CrossRef]
43. Smoot, B.; Wampler, M.; Topp, K.S. Breast Cancer Treatments and Complications: Implications for Rehabilitation. *Rehabil. Oncol.* **2009**, *27*. [CrossRef]
44. Nurgali, K.; Jagoe, R.T.; Abalo, R. Editorial: Adverse Effects of Cancer Chemotherapy: Anything New to Improve Tolerance and Reduce Sequelae? *Front. Pharmacol.* **2018**, *9*, 245. [CrossRef] [PubMed]
45. Bedell, C. A changing paradigm for cancer treatment: The advent of new oral chemotherapy agents. *Clin. J. Oncol. Nurs.* **2003**, *7*, 5–9. [CrossRef] [PubMed]
46. Birner, A. Pharmacology of oral chemotherapy agents. *Clin. J. Oncol. Nurs.* **2003**, *7*, 11–19. [CrossRef]
47. Shapiro, D.E.; Boggs, S.R.; Rodrigue, J.R.; Urry, H.L.; Algina, J.J.; Hellman, R.; Ewen, F. Stage II breast cancer: Differences between four coping patterns in side effects during adjuvant chemotherapy. *J. Psychosom. Res.* **1997**, *43*, 143–157. [CrossRef]

48. Cabral, H.; Kataoka, K. Progress of drug-loaded polymeric micelles into clinical studies. *J. Control. Release* **2014**, *19*, 465–476. [CrossRef]
49. Lua, Y.; Park, K. Polymeric micelles and alternative nanonized delivery vehicles for poorly soluble drugs. *Int. J. Pharm.* **2013**, *453*, 198–214. [CrossRef]
50. Kato, K.; Chin, K.; Yoshikawa, T.; Yamaguchi, K.; Tsuji, Y.; Esaki, T. Phase II study of NK105, a paclitaxel incorporating micellar nanoparticle, for previously treated advanced or recurrent gastric cancer. *Investig. New Drugs* **2012**, *30*, 1621–1627. [CrossRef]
51. Fields, J.S.; Burris, H.A.; Infante, J.R.; Greco, F.A.; Spigel, D.R.; Kawamura, S.; Ishioka, T.; Yamazaki, H.; Bendell, J.C. A phase I study of NK012 in combination with 5 fluorouracil with or without leucovorin in patients (pts) with advanced solid tumors. *J. Clin. Oncol.* **2012**, *30*. [CrossRef]
52. Deshmukh, A.S.; Chauhan, P.N.; Noolvi, M.N.; Chaturvedi, K.; Ganguly, K.; Shukla, S.S.; Nadagouda, M.N.; Aminabhavi, T.M. Polymeric micelles: Basic research to clinical practice. *Int. J. Pharm.* **2017**, *532*, 249–268. [CrossRef]
53. Takahashi, A.; Yamamoto, Y.; Yasunaga, M.; Koga, Y.; Kuroda, J.; Takigahira, M.; Harada, M.; Saito, H.; Hayashi, T.; Kato, Y.; et al. NC-6300, an epirubicin-incorporating micelle, extends the antitumor effect and reduces the cardiotoxicity of epirubicin. *Cancer Sci.* **2013**, *104*, 920–925. [CrossRef]
54. Gong, J.; Chen, M.; Zheng, Y.; Wang, S.; Wang, Y. Polymeric micelles drug delivery system in oncology. *J. Control. Release* **2012**, *159*, 312–323. [CrossRef] [PubMed]
55. Plummer, R.; Wilson, R.H.; Calvert, H.; Boddy, A.V.; Griffin, M.; Sludden, J.; Tilby, M.J.; Eatock, M.; Pearson, D.G.; Ottley, C.J.; et al. A Phase I clinical study of cisplatin-incorporated polymeric micelles (NC-6004) in patients with solid tumours. *Br. J. Cancer* **2011**, *104*, 593–598. [CrossRef] [PubMed]
56. Valle, J.W.; Armstrong, A.; Newman, C.; Alakhov, V.; Pietrzynski, G.; Brewer, J. A phase 2 study of SP1049C, doxorubicin in P-glycoprotein- targeting pluronics in patients with advanced adeno-carcinoma of the esophagus and gastro esophageal junction. *Investig. New Drugs* **2011**, *29*, 1029–1037. [CrossRef]
57. Mendes, L.P.; Pan, J.; Torchilin, V.P. Dendrimers as Nanocarriers for Nucleic Acid and Drug Delivery in Cancer Therapy. *Molecules* **2017**, *22*, 1401. [CrossRef] [PubMed]
58. StarPharma DEP™ Docetaxel. Available online: https://starpharma.com/drug_delivery/dep_docetaxel (accessed on 5 May 2020).
59. Dias, A.P.; Santos, S.S.; da Silva, J.V.; Parise-Filhoa, R.; Ferreira, E.I.; Seoud, O.E.; Giaroll, J. Dendrimers in the context of nanomedicine. *Int. J. Pharm.* **2020**, *573*, 118814. [CrossRef]
60. Alven, S.; Aderibigbe, B.A. Combination Therapy Strategies for the Treatment. *Molecules* **2019**, *24*, 3601. [CrossRef]
61. Narmani, A.; Mohammadnejad, J.; Yavari, K. Synthesis and evaluation of polyethylene glycol- and folic acid-conjugated polyamidoamine G4 dendrimer as nanocarrier. *J. Drug Deliv. Sci. Technol.* **2019**, *50*, 278–286. [CrossRef]
62. Uram, Ł.; Filipowicz, A.; Misiorek, M.; Pienkowska, N.; Markowicz, J.; Walajtys-Rode, E.; Wolowiec, S. Biotinylated PAMAM G3 dendrimer conjugated with celecoxib and/or Fmoc-L-Leucine and its cytotoxicity for normal and cancer human cell lines. *Eur. J. Pharm. Sci.* **2018**, *124*, 1–9. [CrossRef]
63. Qiu, L.Y.; Bae, Y.H. Polymer architecture and drug delivery. *Pharm. Res.* **2006**, *23*. [CrossRef]
64. Li, J.; Liang, H.; Liu, J.; Wang, Z. Poly (amidoamine)(PAMAM) dendrimer mediated delivery of drug and pDNA/siRNA for cancer therapy. *Int. J. Pharm.* **2018**, *546*, 215–225. [CrossRef] [PubMed]
65. Janiszewska1, J.; Posadas, I.; Játiva, P.; Bugaj-Zarebska, M.; Urbanczyk-Lipkowska, Z.; Ceña, V. Second Generation Amphiphilic Poly-Lysine Dendrons Inhibit Glioblastoma Cell Proliferation without Toxicity for Neurons or Astrocytes. *PLoS ONE* **2016**, *11*, e0165704. [CrossRef] [PubMed]
66. Gorzkiewicz, M.; Konopka, M.; Janaszewska, A.; Tarasenko, I.I.; Nadezhda, N.; Sheveleva, N.N.; Gajeke, A.; Neelov, I.M.; Klajnert-Maculewicz, B. Application of new lysine-based peptide dendrimers D3K2 and D3G2 for gene delivery: Specifi cytotoxicity to cancer cells and transfection in vitro. *Bioinorg. Chem.* **2020**, *95*, 103504. [CrossRef]
67. Caminade, A.-M. Phosphorus Dendrimers as Nanotools against Cancers. *Molecules* **2020**, *25*, 3333. [CrossRef]
68. Liu, M.; Frechet, J. Designing dendrimers for drug delivery. *Pharm. Sci. Technol. Today* **1999**, *2*, 393–401. [CrossRef]
69. Shrivastava, P.K.; Singh, R.; Shrivastava, S.K. Polyamidoamine dendrimer and dextran conjugates: Preparation, characterization, and in vitro and in vivo evaluation. *Chem. Pap.* **2010**, *64*, 592–601. [CrossRef]

70. Aqil, F.; Munagala, R.; Jeyabalan, J.; Vadhanam, M.V. Bioavailability of phytochemicals and its enhancement by drug delivery systems. *Cancer Lett.* **2013**, *334*, 133–141. [CrossRef]
71. Ghalandarlaki, N.; Alizadeh, A.M.; Ashkani-esfahani, S. Nanotechnology-Applied Curcumin for Different Diseases Therapy. *BioMed Res. Int.* **2014**, *2014*, 394264. [CrossRef]
72. Gha, M.; Dehghan, G.; Baradaran, B.; Zarebkohan, A.; Mansoori, B.; Soleymani, J.; Dolatabadi, J.; Ezzati, N.; Hamblin, M.R. Co-delivery of curcumin and Bcl-2 siRNA by PAMAM dendrimers for enhancement of the therapeutic efficacy in HeLa cancer cells. *Colloids Surf. B Biointerfaces* **2020**, *188*, 110762.
73. Guo, X.; Kang, X.; Wang, Y.; Zhang, X.; Li, C.; Liu, Y.; Du, L. Co-delivery of cisplatin and doxorubicin by covalently conjugating with polyamidoamine dendrimer for enhanced synergistic cancer therapy. *Acta Biomaterilia* **2019**, *84*, 367–377. [CrossRef]
74. Kitchens, K.M.; Kolhatkar, R.B.; Swaan, P.W.; Ghandehari, H. Endocytosis inhibitors prevent poly(amidoamine) dendrimer internalization and permeability across Caco-2 cells. *Mol. Pharm.* **2008**, *5*, 364–369. [CrossRef] [PubMed]
75. Chittasupho, C.; Anuchapreeda, S.; Sarisuta, N. CXCR4 targeted dendrimer for anti-cancer drug delivery and breast cancer cell migration inhibition. *Eur. J. Pharm. Biopharm.* **2017**, *119*, 310–321. [CrossRef] [PubMed]
76. Wang, M.; Li, Y.; HuangFu, M.; Xiao, Y.; Zhang, T.; Han, M.; Xu, D.; Li, F.; Ling, D.; Jin, Y.; et al. Pluronic-attached polyamidoamine dendrimer conjugates overcome drug resistance in breast cancer. *Nanomedicine* **2016**, *11*, 2917–2934. [CrossRef]
77. Kojima, C.; Suehiro, T.; Watanabe, K.; Ogawa, M.; Fukuhara, A.; Nishisaka, E.; Harada, A.; Kono, K.; Inui, T.; Magata, Y. Doxorubicin-conjugated dendrimer/collagen hybrid gels for metastasis-associated drug delivery systems. *Acta Biomater.* **2013**, *9*, 5673–5680. [CrossRef]
78. Kaminskas, L.M.; Kelly, B.D.; McLeod, V.M.; Sberna, G.; Owen, D.J.; Boyd, B.J.; Porter, C.J. Characterisation and tumour targeting of PEGylated polylysine dendrimers bearing doxorubicin via a pH labile linker. *J. Control. Release* **2011**, *152*, 241–248. [CrossRef]
79. Mehta, D.; Leong, N.; McLeod, V.M.; Kelly, B.D.; Pathak, R.; Owen, D.J.; Porter, C.J.; Kaminskas, L.M. Reducing dendrimer generation and PEG chain length increases drug release and promotes anticancer activity of PEGylated polylysine dendrimers conjugated with doxorubicin via a cathepsin-cleavable peptide linker. *Mol. Pharm.* **2018**, *15*, 4568–4576. [CrossRef] [PubMed]
80. Tacar, O.; Sriamornsak, P.; Dass, C.R. Doxorubicin: An update on anticancer molecular action, toxicity and novel drug delivery systems. *J. Pharm. Pharmacol.* **2013**, *65*, 157–170. [CrossRef]
81. Wang, P.; Zhao, X.; Wang, Z.; Meng, M.; Li, X.; Ning, Q. Generation 4 polyamidoamine dendrimers is a novel candidate of nano-carrier for gene delivery agents in breast cancer treatment. *Cancer Lett.* **2010**, *298*, 34–49. [CrossRef]
82. Chen, A.M.; Santhakumaran, L.M.; Nair, S.K.; Amenta, P.S.; Thomas, T.; He, H.; Thomas, T.J. Oligodeoxynucleotide nanostructure formation in the presence of polypropyleneimine dendrimers and their uptake in breast cancer cells. *Nanotechnology* **2006**, *17*, 5449–5460. [CrossRef]
83. Pourianazar, N.T.; Gunduz, U. CpG oligodeoxynucleotide-loaded PAMAM dendrimer-coated magnetic nanoparticles promote apoptosis in breast cancer cells. *Biomed. Pharmacother.* **2016**, *78*, 81–91. [CrossRef]
84. Xin, G.; Zhao, X.; Duan, X.; Ning, Q.; Meng, M.; Meng, D.; Liu, L. Antitumor Effect of a Generation 4 Polyamidoamine Dendrimer/Cyclooxygenase-2 Antisense Oligodeoxynucleotide Complex on Breast Cancer In Vitro and In Vivo. *Cancer Biother. Radiopharm.* **2012**, *27*, 77–87. [CrossRef] [PubMed]
85. Kulhari, H.; Pooja, D.; Shrivastava, S.; Kuncha, M.; Naidu, V.G.; Bansal, V.; Sistla, R.; Adams, D.J. Trastuzumab-grafted PAMAM dendrimers for the selective delivery of anticancer drugs to HER2-positive breast cancer. *Sci. Rep.* **2016**, *6*, 1–13. [CrossRef] [PubMed]
86. Miyano, T.; Wijagkanalan, W.; Kawakami, S.; Yamashita, F.; Hashida, M. Anionic Amino Acid Dendrimer–Trastuzumab Conjugates for Specific Internalization in HER2-Positive Cancer Cells. *Mol. Pharm.* **2010**, *7*, 1318–1327. [CrossRef] [PubMed]
87. Marcinkowska, M.; Stanczyk, M.; Janaszewska, A.; Sobierajska, E.; Chworos, A.; Klajnert-Maculewicz, B. Multicomponent conjugates of anticancer drugs and monoclonal antibody with PAMAM dendrimers to increase efficacy of HER-2 positive breast cancer therapy. *Pharm. Res.* **2019**, *36*, 154. [CrossRef]
88. Aleanizy, F.S.; Alqahtani, F.Y.; Seto, S.; Al Khalil, N.; Aleshaiwi, L.; Alghamdi, M.; Alquadeib, B.; Alkahtani, H.; Aldarwesh, A.; Alqahtani, Q.H.; et al. Trastuzumab Targeted Neratinib Loaded Poly-Amidoamine Dendrimer Nanocapsules for Breast Cancer Therapy. *Int. J. Nanomed.* **2020**, *15*, 5433. [CrossRef]

89. Chan, C.; Cai, Z.; Reilly, R.M. Trastuzumab Labeled to High Specific Activity with 111 In by Conjugation to G4 PAMAM Dendrimers Derivatized with Multiple DTPA Chelators Exhibits Increased Cytotoxic Potency on HER2-Positive Breast Cancer Cells. *Pharm. Res.* **2013**, *30*, 1999–2009. [CrossRef]
90. Oddone, N.; Lecot, N.; Fernández, M.; Rodriguez-Haralambides, A.; Cabral, P.; Cerecetto, H.; Benech, J.C. In vitro and in vivo uptake studies of PAMAM G4.5 dendrimers in breast cancer. *J. Nanobiotechnol.* **2016**, *14*, 45. [CrossRef]
91. Bielawski, K.; Bielawska, A.; Muszy, A.; Czarnomysy, R. Cytotoxic activity of G3 PAMAM-NH 2 dendrimer-chlorambucil conjugate in human breast cancer cells. *Environ. Toxicol. Pharmacol.* **2011**, *32*, 364–372. [CrossRef]
92. Kociecka, B.; Surazynski, A.; Miltyk, W.; Palka, J. The effect of telmisartan on collagen biosynthesis depends on the status of estrogen activation in breast cancer cells. *Eur. J. Pharmacol.* **2010**, *628*, 51–56. [CrossRef]
93. Abdel-Rahman, M.A.; Al-Abd, A.M. Thermoresponsive dendrimers based on oligoethylene glycols: Design, synthesis and cytotoxic activity against MCF-7 breast cancer cells. *Eur. J. Med. Chem.* **2013**, *69*, 848–854. [CrossRef]
94. Li, K.; Wen, S.; Larson, A.C.; Shen, M.; Zhang, Z.; Chen, Q.; Shi, X.; Zhang, G. Multifunctional dendrimer-based nanoparticles for in vivo MR/CT dual-modal molecular imaging of breast cancer. *Int. J. Nanomed.* **2013**, *8*, 2589–2600. [CrossRef]
95. Finlay, J.; Roberts, C.M.; Lowe, G.; Loeza, J.; Rossi, J.J.; Glackin, C.A. RNA-Based TWIST1 Inhibition via Dendrimer Complex to Reduce Breast Cancer Cell Metastasis. *BioMed Res. Int.* **2015**, *2015*. [CrossRef]
96. Wallerand, H.; Robert, G.; Pasticier, G.; Ravaud, A.; Ballanger, P.; Reiter, R.E.; Ferrière, J.M. September. The epithelial-mesenchymal transition-inducing factor TWIST is an attractive target in advanced and/or metastatic bladder and prostate cancers. *Urol. Oncol. Semin. Orig. Investig.* **2010**, *28*, 473–479.
97. Winnicka, K.; Bielawski, K.; Rusak, M.; Bielawska, A. The Effect of Generation 2 and 3 Poly (amidoamine) Dendrimers on Viability of Human Breast Cancer Cells. *J. Health Sci.* **2009**, *55*, 169–177. [CrossRef]
98. Debnath, S.; Saloum, D.; Dolai, S.; Sun, C.; Averick, S.; Raja, K.; Fata, J. Dendrimer-curcumin conjugate: A water soluble and effective cytotoxic agent against breast cancer cell lines. *Anti-Cancer Agents Med. Chem.* **2013**, *13*, 1531–1539. [CrossRef]
99. Yao, H.; Veine, D.M.; Fay, K.S.; Staszewski, E.D.; Zeng, Z.Z.; Livant, D.L. The PHSCN dendrimer as a more potent inhibitor of human breast cancer cell invasion, extravasation, and lung colony formation. *Breast Cancer Res. Treat.* **2011**, *125*, 363–375. [CrossRef]
100. Lozano-Cruz, T.; Gómez, R.; de la Mata, F.J.; Ortega, P. New bow-tie cationic carbosilane dendritic system with a curcumin core as an anti-breast cancer agent. *New J. Chem.* **2018**, *42*, 11732–11738. [CrossRef]
101. Winnicka, K.; Bielawski, K.; Bielawska, A. Synthesis and cytotoxic activity of G3 PAMAM-NH 2 dendrimer-modified digoxin and proscillaridin A conjugates in breast cancer cells. *Pharmacol. Rep.* **2010**, *62*, 414–423. [CrossRef]
102. Mei, M.; Ren, Y.; Zhou, X.; Yuan, X.B.; Li, F.; Jiang, L.H.; Kang, C.S.; Yao, Z. Suppression of breast cancer cells in vitro by polyamidoamine-dendrimer-mediated 5-fluorouracil chemotherapy combined with antisense micro-RNA 21 gene therapy. *J. Appl. Polym. Sci.* **2011**, *114*, 3760–3766. [CrossRef]
103. Zhang, J.; Liu, D.; Zhang, M.; Sun, Y.; Zhang, X.; Guan, G.; Zhao, X.; Qiao, M.; Chen, D.; Hu, H. The cellular uptake mechanism, intracellular transportation, and exocytosis of polyamidoamine dendrimers in multidrug-resistant breast cancer cells. *Int. J. Nanomed.* **2016**, *11*, 3677–3690. [CrossRef]
104. Zhang, C.; Pan, D.; Li, J.; Hu, J.; Bains, A.; Guys, N.; Zhu, H.; Li, X.; Luo, K.; Gong, Q.; et al. Enzyme-responsive peptide dendrimer-gemcitabine conjugate as a controlled-release drug delivery vehicle with enhanced antitumor efficacy. *Acta Biomater.* **2017**, *55*, 153–162. [CrossRef]
105. Matai, L.; Gopinath, P. Hydrophobic myristic acid modified PAMAM dendrimers augment the delivery of tamoxifen to breast cancer cells. *RSC Adv.* **2016**, *6*, 24808–24819. [CrossRef]
106. Zhou, X.; Zheng, Q.; Wang, C.; Xu, J.; Wu, J.P.; Kirk, T.B.; Ma, D.; Xue, W. Star-shaped amphiphilic hyperbranched polyglycerol conjugated with dendritic poly (L-lysine) for the codelivery of docetaxel and MMP-9 siRNA in cancer therapy. *ACS Appl. Mater. Interfaces* **2016**, *8*, 12609–12619. [CrossRef]
107. Kaminskas, L.M.; McLeod, V.M.; Porter, C.J.; Boyd, B.J. Association of chemotherapeutic drugs with dendrimer nanocarriers: An assessment of the merits of covalent conjugation compared to noncovalent encapsulation. *Mol. Pharm.* **2012**, *9*, 355–373. [CrossRef]

108. Bugno, J.; Hsu, H.J.; Hong, S. Tweaking dendrimers and dendritic nanoparticles for controlled nano-bio interactions: Potential nanocarriers for improved cancer targeting. *J. Drug Target.* **2015**, *23*, 642–650. [CrossRef] [PubMed]
109. Caminade, A.M.; Turrin, C.O. Dendrimers for drug delivery. *J. Mater. Chem. B* **2014**, *2*, 4055–4066. [CrossRef]
110. Labieniec-Watala, M.; Watala, C. PAMAM dendrimers: Destined for success or doomed to fail? Plain and modified PAMAM dendrimers in the context of biomedical applications. *J. Pharm. Sci.* **2015**, *104*, 2–14. [CrossRef] [PubMed]
111. Singh, J.; Jain, K.; Mehra, N.K.; Jain, N.K. Dendrimers in anticancer drug delivery: Mechanism of interaction of drug and dendrimers. *Artif. Cells Nanomed. Biotechnol.* **2016**, *44*, 1626–1634. [CrossRef]
112. Jones, C.F.; Campbell, R.A.; Franks, Z.; Gibson, C.C.; Thiagarajan, G.; Vieira-de-Abreu, A.; Sukavaneshvar, S.; Mohammad, S.F.; Li, D.Y.; Ghandehari, H.; et al. Cationic PAMAM dendrimers disrupt key platelet functions. *Mol. Pharm.* **2012**, *9*, 1599–1611. [CrossRef]
113. Lesniak, W.G.; Mishra, M.K.; Jyoti, A.; Balakrishnan, B.; Zhang, F.; Nance, E.; Romero, R.; Kannan, S.; Kannan, R.M. Biodistribution of fluorescently labeled PAMAM dendrimers in neonatal rabbits: Effect of neuroinflammation. *Mol. Pharm.* **2013**, *10*, 4560–4571. [CrossRef]
114. Valenzuela-Oses, J.K.; García, M.C.; Feitosa, V.A.; Pachioni-Vasconcelos, J.A.; Gomes-Filho, S.M.; Lourenço, F.R.; Cerize, N.N.P.; Bàsseres, D.S.; Rangel-Yagui, C.O. Development and characterization of miltefosine-loaded polymeric micelles for cancer treatment. *Mater. Sci. Eng. C* **2017**, *81*, 327–333. [CrossRef]
115. Mahmud, A.; Lavasanifar, A. The effect of block copolymer structure on the internalization of polymeric micelles by human breast cancer cells. *Colloids Surf. B Biointerfaces* **2005**, *45*, 82–89. [CrossRef]
116. Suroshe, S.; Nerkar, P.; Patil, K.; Chalikwar, S. Breast cancer: Recent review on micelles as nano-carriers for treatment. *Indo Am. J. Pharm. Res.* **2019**, *9*, 2231–6876.
117. Zhong, G.; Yang, C.; Liu, S.; Zheng, Y.; Lou, W.; Yng, J.; Bao, C.; Cheng, W.; Tan, J.P.K.; Gao, S.; et al. Polymers with distinctive anticancer mechanism that kills MDR cancer cells and inhibits tumor metastasis. *Biomaterials* **2019**, *199*, 76–87. [CrossRef]
118. Chen, T.; Tu, L.; Wang, G.; Qi, N.; Wu, W.; Zhang, W.; Feng, J. Multi-functional chitosan polymeric micelles as oral paclitaxel delivery systems for enhanced bioavailability and anti-tumor e fficacy. *Intern. J. Pharm.* **2020**, *578*, 119105. [CrossRef]
119. Wang, W.; Zhao, B.; Meng, X.; She, P.; Zhang, P.; Cao, Y.; Zhang, X. Preparation of dual-drug conjugated polymeric micelles with synergistic anti-cancer efficacy in vitro. *J. Drug Deliv. Sci. Technol.* **2018**, *43*, 388–396. [CrossRef]
120. Wei, X.; Liu, L.; Li, X.; Wang, Y.; Guo, X.; Zhao, J.; Zhou, S. Selectively targeting tumor-associated macrophages and tumor cells with polymeric micelles for enhanced cancer chemo-immunotherapy. *J. Control. Release* **2019**, *313*, 42–53. [CrossRef]
121. Senevirathne, S.A.; Washington, K.E.; Biewer, M.C.; Stefan, M.C. PEG based anti-cancer drug conjugated prodrug micelles for the delivery of anti-cancer agents. *J. Mater. Chem. B.* **2016**, *4*, 360–370. [CrossRef]
122. Guo, X.; Zhao, Z.; Chen, D.; Qiao, M.; Wan, F.; Cun, D.; Sun, Y.; Yang, M. Co-delivery of resveratrol and docetaxel via polymeric micelles to improve the treatment of drug-resistant tumors. *Asian J. Pharm. Sci.* **2019**, *14*, 78–85. [CrossRef]
123. Lang, T.; Dong, X.; Zheng, Z.; Liu, Y.; Wang, G.; Yin, Q.; Li, Y. Tumor microenvironment-responsive docetaxel-loaded micelle combats metastatic breast cancer. *Sci. Bull.* **2019**, *64*, 91–100. [CrossRef]
124. Logie, J.; Ganesh, A.N.; Aman, A.M.; Al-awar, R.S.; Shoichet, M.S. Preclinical evaluation of taxane-binding peptide-modified polymeric micelles loaded with docetaxel in an orthotopic breast cancer mouse model. *Biomaterials* **2017**, *123*, 39–47. [CrossRef] [PubMed]
125. Hu, Q.; Rijcken, C.J.; Bansal, R.; Hennink, W.E.; Storm, G.; Prakash, J. Complete regression of breast tumour with a single dose of docetaxel-entrapped core-cross-linked polymeric micelles. *Biomaterials* **2015**, *53*, 370–378. [CrossRef] [PubMed]
126. Li, W.; Peng, J.; Tan, L.; Wu, J.; Shi, K.; Qu, Y.; Wei, X.; Qian, Z. Mild photothermal therapy/photodynamic therapy/chemotherapy of breast cancer by Lyp-1 modi fi ed Docetaxel/IR820 Co-loaded micelles. *Biomaterials* **2016**, *106*, 119–133. [CrossRef]
127. Kutty, R.V.; Feng, S. Cetuximab conjugated vitamin E TPGS micelles for targeted delivery of docetaxel for treatment of triple negative breast cancers. *Biomaterials* **2013**, *34*, 10160–10171. [CrossRef] [PubMed]

128. Wang, Y.; Chen, L.; Tan, L.; Zhao, Q.; Luo, F.; Wei, Y.; Qian, Z. PEG-PCL based micelle hydrogels as oral docetaxel delivery systems for breast cancer therapy. *Biomaterials* **2014**, *35*, 6972–6985. [CrossRef]
129. Tan, L.; Ma, B.; Chen, L.; Peng, J.; Qian, Z. Toxicity evaluation and anti-tumor study of docetaxel loaded mPEG-polyester micelles for breast cancer therapy. *J. Biomed. Nanotechnol.* **2017**, *13*, 393–408. [CrossRef]
130. Li, Y.; Jin, M.; Shao, S.; Huang, W.; Yang, F.; Chen, W.; Zhang, S.; Xia, G.; Gao, Z. Small-sized polymeric micelles incorporating docetaxel suppress distant metastases in the clinically-relevant 4T1 mouse breast cancer model. *BMC Cancer* **2014**, *14*, 329. [CrossRef]
131. Raza, K.; Kumar, N.; Misra, C.; Kaushik, L.; Guru, S.K.; Kumar, P.; Malik, R.; Bhushan, S.; Katare, O.P. Dextran-PLGA-loaded docetaxel micelles with enhanced cytotoxicity and, better pharmacokinetic profile. *Int. J. Biol. Macromol.* **2016**, *88*, 206–212. [CrossRef]
132. Kutty, R.V.; Chia, S.L.; Setyawati, M.I.; Muthu, M.S.; Feng, S.; Leong, T.D. In vivo and ex vivo proofs of concept that cetuximab conjugated vitamin E TPGS micelles increases ef fi cacy of delivered docetaxel against triple negative breast cancer. *Biomaterials* **2015**, *63*, 58–69. [CrossRef]
133. Koo, A.N.; Min, K.H.; Lee, H.J.; Lee, S.; Kim, K.; Kwon, I.C.; Cho, S.H.; Jeong, S.Y.; Lee, S.C. Tumor accumulation and antitumor efficacy of docetaxel-loaded core-shell-corona micelles with shell-specific redox-responsive cross-links. *Biomaterials* **2012**, *33*, 1489–1499. [CrossRef]
134. Muthu, M.S.; Kutty, R.V.; Luo, Z.; Xie, J.; Feng, S. Theranostic vitamin E TPGS micelles of transferrin conjugation for targeted co-delivery of docetaxel and ultra bright gold nanoclusters. *Biomaterials* **2015**, *39*, 234–248. [CrossRef] [PubMed]
135. Tan, L.; Peng, J.; Zhao, Q.; Zhang, L.; Tang, X.; Chen, L.; Lei, M.; Qian, Z. A Novel MPEG-PDLLA-PLL Copolymer for Docetaxel Delivery in Breast Cancer Therapy. *Theranostics* **2017**, *7*, 2652–2672. [CrossRef]
136. Zhang, X.; Zeng, X.; Liang, X.; Yang, Y.; Li, X.; Chen, H.; Huang, L.; Mei, L.; Feng, S.-S. The chemotherapeutic potential of PEG-*b*-PLGA copolymer micelles that combine chloroquine as autophagy inhibitor and docetaxel as an anti-cancer drug. *Biomaterials* **2014**, *35*, 9144–9154. [CrossRef]
137. Jun, Y.J.; Jadhav, V.B.; Min, J.H.; Cui, J.X.; Chae, S.W.; Cjoi, J.M.; Kim, I.; Choi, S.; Lee, H.J.; Sohn, Y.S. Stable and efficient delivery of docetaxel by micelle-encapsulation using a tripodal cyclotriphosphazene amphiphile. *Int. J. Pharm.* **2012**, *422*, 374–380. [CrossRef] [PubMed]
138. Enteshari, S.; Varshosaz, J.; Minayian, M.; Hassanzadeh, F. Antitumor activity of raloxifene-targeted poly (styrene maleic loaded with docetaxel in breast cancer-bearing mice. *Investig. New Drugs* **2018**, *32*, 206–216. [CrossRef]
139. Varshosaz, J.; Dehkordi, A.J.; Setayesh, S. Magnetic polyvinyl caprolactam–polyvinyl acetate–polyethylene glycol micelles for docetaxel delivery in breast cancer: An in vitro study on two cell lines of breast cancer. *Pharm. Dev. Technol.* **2017**, *22*, 659–668. [CrossRef] [PubMed]
140. Zheng, C.; Zheng, M.; Gong, P.; Deng, J.; Yi, H.; Zhang, P.; Zhang, Y.; Liu, P.; Ma, Y.; Cai, L. Polypeptide cationic micelles mediated co-delivery of docetaxel and siRNA for synergistic tumor therapy. *Biomaterials* **2013**, *34*, 3431–3438. [CrossRef]
141. Tong, S.; Xiang, B.; Dong, D.; Qi, X. Enhanced antitumor efficacy and decreased toxicity by self-associated docetaxel in phospholipid-based micelles. *Int. J. Pharm.* **2012**, *434*, 413–419. [CrossRef]
142. Ho, M.Y.; Mackey, J.R. Presentation and management of docetaxel-related adverse effects in patients with breast cancer. *Cancer Manag. Res.* **2014**, *6*, 253–259. [CrossRef] [PubMed]
143. Esmaeli, B.; Valero, V. Epiphora and canalicular stenosis associated with adjuvant docetaxel in early breast cancer: Is excessive tearing clinically important? *J. Clin. Oncol.* **2013**, *31*, 2076–2077. [CrossRef] [PubMed]
144. Wakharde, A.A.; Awad, A.H.; Bhagat, A.; Karuppayil, S.M. Synergistic activation of doxorubicin against cancer: A review. *Am. J. Clin. Microbiol. Antimicrob.* **2018**, *1*, 1–6.
145. Zhao, N.; Woodle, M.C.; Mixson, A.J. Advances in delivery systems for doxorubicin. *J. Nanomed. Nanotechnol.* **2018**, *9*, 519. [CrossRef] [PubMed]
146. Gao, Q.; Zhang, C.; Zhang, E.; Chen, H.; Zhen, Y.; Zhang, S.; Zhang, S. Zwitterionic pH-responsive hyaluronic acid polymer micelles for delivery of doxorubicin. *Colloids Surf. B Biointerfaces* **2019**, *178*, 412–420. [CrossRef] [PubMed]
147. Gao, Z.; Tian, L.; Hu, J.; Park, I.; Bae, Y.H. Prevention of metastasis in a 4T1 murine breast cancer model by doxorubicin carried by folate conjugated pH sensitive polymeric micelles. *J. Control. Release* **2011**, *152*, 84–89. [CrossRef]

148. Zhao, Y.; Alakhova, D.Y.; Zhao, X.; Band, V.; Batrakova, E.V.; Kabanov, A.V. Eradication of cancer stem cells in triple negative breast cancer using doxorubicin/pluronic polymeric micelles. *Nanomed. Nanotechnol. Biol. Med.* **2020**, *24*, 102124. [CrossRef]
149. Bae, Y.; Diezi, T.A.; Zhao, A.; Kwon, G.S. Mixed polymeric micelles for combination cancer chemotherapy through the concurrent delivery of multiple chemotherapeutic agents. *J. Control. Release* **2007**, *122*, 324–330. [CrossRef]
150. Zhang, X.; Li, L.; Li, C.; Zheng, H.; Song, H.; Xiong, F.; Qiu, T.; Yang, J. Cisplatin-crosslinked glutathione-sensitive micelles loaded with doxorubicin for combination and targeted therapy of tumors. *Carbohydr. Polym.* **2017**, *155*, 407–415. [CrossRef]
151. Varshosaz, J.; Sadeghi-Aliabadi, H.; Ghasemi, S.; Behdadfar, B. Use of Magnetic Folate-Dextran-Retinoic Acid Micelles for Dual Targeting of Doxorubicin in Breast Cancer. *BioMed Res. Int.* **2013**, *2013*, 680712. [CrossRef]
152. Lv, L.; Qiu, K.; Yu, X.; Chen, C.; Qin, F.; Shi, Y.; Ou, J.; Zhang, T.; Zhu, H.; Wu, J.; et al. Amphiphilic copolymeric micelles for doxorubicin and curcumin co-delivery to reverse multidrug resistance in breast cancer. *J. Biomed. Nanotechnol.* **2016**, *12*, 973–985. [CrossRef]
153. Cuong, N.; Jiang, J.; Li, Y.; Chen, J.; Jwo, S.; Hsieh, M. Doxorubicin-Loaded PEG-PCL-PEG Micelle Using Xenograft Model of Nude Mice: Effect of Multiple Administration of Micelle on the Suppression of Human Breast Cancer. *Cancers* **2011**, *3*, 61–78. [CrossRef]
154. Yu, H.; Cui, Z.; Yu, P.; Guo, C.; Feng, B.; Jiang, T.; Wang, S.; Yin, Q.; Zhong, D.; Yang, X.; et al. pH and NIR light-responsive micelles with hyperthermia-triggered tumor penetration and cytoplasm drug release to reverse doxorubicin resistance in breast cancer. *Adv. Funct. Mater.* **2015**, *25*, 2489–2500. [CrossRef]
155. Lee, E.S.; Na, K.; Bae, Y.H. Doxorubicin loaded pH-sensitive polymeric micelles for reversal of resistant MCF-7 tumor. *J. Control. Release* **2005**, *103*, 405–418. [CrossRef] [PubMed]
156. Varshosaz, J.; Hassanzadeh, F.; Sadeghi-Aliabadi, H.; Larian, Z.; Rostami, M. Synthesis of Pluronic Ò F127-poly (methyl vinyl ether-alt-maleic acid) copolymer and production of its micelles for doxorubicin delivery in breast cancer. *Chem. Eng. J.* **2014**, *240*, 133–146. [CrossRef]
157. Sun, Y.; Zou, W.; Bian, S.; Huang, Y.; Tan, Y.; Liang, J.; Fan, Y.; Zhang, X. Bioreducible PAA-g-PEG graft micelles with high doxorubicin loading for targeted antitumor effect against mouse breast carcinoma. *Biomaterials* **2013**, *34*, 6818–6828. [CrossRef]
158. Shuai, X.; Ai, H.; Nasongkla, N.; Kim, S.; Gao, J. Micellar carriers based on block copolymers of poly (q-caprolactone) and poly (ethylene glycol) for doxorubicin delivery. *J. Control. Release* **2004**, *98*, 415–426. [CrossRef]
159. Cuong, N.V.; Li, Y.L.; Hsieh, M.F. Targeted delivery of doxorubicin to human breast cancers by folate-decorated. *J. Mater. Chem.* **2012**, *22*, 1006. [CrossRef]
160. Cuong, N.V.; Hsieh, M.F.; Chen, Y.T.; Liau, I. Doxorubicin-Loaded Nanosized Micelles of a Star-Shaped Poly (ε-Caprolactone)-Polyphosphoester Block Co-polymer for Treatment of Human Breast Cancer for Treatment of Human Breast Cancer. *J. Biomater. Sci. Polym. Ed.* **2012**, *22*, 1409–1426. [CrossRef]
161. Zhou, Y.; Wang, S.; Ying, X.; Wang, Y.; Geng, P.; Deng, A.; Yu, Z. Doxorubicin-loaded redox-responsive micelles based on dextran and indomethacin for resistant breast cancer. *Int. J. Nanomed.* **2017**, *12*, 6153–6168. [CrossRef]
162. Liao, C.; Sun, Q.; Liang, B.; Shen, J.; Shuai, X. Targeting EGFR-overexpressing tumor cells using Cetuximab-immunomicelles loaded with doxorubicin and superparamagnetic iron oxide. *Eur. J. Radiol.* **2011**, *80*, 699–705. [CrossRef]
163. Chen, C.; Cuong, N.Y.; Chen, Y.; So, R.C.; Liau, I.; Hsieh, M.F. Overcoming Multidrug Resistance of Breast Cancer Cells by the Micellar Doxorubicin Nanoparticles of mPEG-PCL-Graft-Cellulose. *J. Nanosci. Nanotechnol.* **2010**, *10*, 53–60. [CrossRef]
164. Zeng, X.; Zhang, Y.; Wu, Z.; Lundberg, P.; Malkoch, M.; Nystrom, A.M. Hyperbranched Copolymer Micelles as Delivery Vehicles of Doxorubicin in Breast Cancer Cells. *J. Polym. Sci. Part A Polym. Chem.* **2012**, *50*, 280–288. [CrossRef]
165. Cheng, Y.; Hao, J.; Lee, L.A.; Biewer, M.C.; Wang, Q.; Stefan, M.C. Thermally Controlled Release of Anticancer Drug from Self-Assembled β-Substituted Amphiphilic Poly (ε-caprolactone) Micellar Nanoparticles. *Biomacromolecules* **2012**, *13*, 2163–2173. [CrossRef] [PubMed]
166. Danhier, F.; Kouhé, T.T.; Duhem, N.; Ucakar, B.; Staub, A.; Draoui, N.; Feron, O.; Préat, V. Vitamin E-based micelles enhance the anticancer activity of doxorubicin. *Int. J. Pharm.* **2014**, *476*, 9–15. [CrossRef] [PubMed]

167. Liu, D.; Chen, Y.; Feng, X.; Deng, M.; Xie, G.; Wang, J.; Zhang, L.; Liu, Q.; Yuan, P. Micellar nanoparticles loaded with gemcitabine and doxorubicin showed synergistic effect. *Colloids Surf. B Biointerfaces* **2014**, *113*, 158–168. [CrossRef]
168. Cagel, M.; Bernabeu, E.; Gonzalez, L.; Lagomarsino, E.; Zubillaga, M.; Moretton, M.A.; Chiappetta, D.A. Mixed micelles for encapsulation of doxorubicin with enhanced in vitro cytotoxicity on breast and ovarian cancer cell lines versus Doxil®. *Biomed. Pharmacother.* **2017**, *95*, 894–903. [CrossRef]
169. Chen, Y.; Zhang, W.; Huang, Y.; Gao, F.; Sha, X.; Fang, X. Pluronic-based functional polymeric mixed micelles for co-delivery of doxorubicin and paclitaxel to multidrug resistant tumor. *Int. J. Pharm.* **2014**, *488*, 44–58. [CrossRef]
170. Wang, Y.; Ma, S.; Xie, Z.; Zhang, H. A synergistic combination therapy with paclitaxel and doxorubicin loaded micellar nanoparticles. *Colloids Surf. B Biointerfaces* **2014**, *116*, 41–48. [CrossRef]
171. Abu Samaan, T.M.; Samec, M.; Liskova, A.; Kubatka, P.; Büsselberg, D. Paclitaxel's Mechanistic and Clinical Effects on Breast Cancer. *Biomolecules* **2019**, *9*, 789. [CrossRef]
172. Barbuti, A.M.; Chen, Z.S. Paclitaxel through the ages of anticancer therapy: Exploring its role in chemoresistance and radiation therapy. *Cancers* **2015**, *7*, 2360–2371. [CrossRef]
173. Wang, X.; Guo, Y.; Qiu, L.; Wang, X.; Li, T.; Han, L. Preparation and evaluation of carboxymethyl chitosan-rhein polymeric micelles with synergistic antitumor effect for oral delivery of paclitaxel. *Carbohydr. Polym.* **2019**, *206*, 121–131. [CrossRef]
174. Zajdel, A.; Wilczok, A.; Jelonek, K.; Musiał-Kulik, M.; Foryś, A.; Li, S.; Kasperczyk, J. Cytotoxic effect of paclitaxel and lapatinib Co-delivered in polylactide-*co*-Poly (ethylene glycol) micelles on HER-2-Negative breast Cancer cells. *Pharmaceutics* **2019**, *11*, 169. [CrossRef]
175. Wu, D.; Zheng, Y.; Hu, X.; Fan, Z.; Jing, X. Anti-tumor activity of folate targeted biodegradable polymer—Paclitaxel conjugate micelles on EMT-6 breast cancer model. *Mater. Sci. Eng. C* **2015**, *53*, 68–75. [CrossRef]
176. Wang, Z.; Li, X.; Wang, D.; Zou, Y.; Qu, X.; He, C.; Deng, Y.; Jin, Y.; Zhou, Y.; Zhou, Y.; et al. Concurrently suppressing multidrug resistance and metastasis of breast cancer by co-delivery of paclitaxel and honokiol with pH-sensitive polymeric micelles. *Acta Biomater.* **2017**, *62*, 144–156. [CrossRef]
177. Oda, C.M.R.; Barros, A.L.B.; Farnandes, R.S.; Miranda, S.E.M.; Teixeira, X.M.; Cardoso, N.V.; Oliveira, C.M.; Leite, A.E. Freeze-dried diethylenetriaminepentaacetic acid-functionalized polymeric micelles containing paclitaxel: A kit formulation for theranostic application in cancer. *J. Drug Deliv. Sci. Technol.* **2018**, *46*, 182–187. [CrossRef]
178. Zhang, L.; He, Y.; Ma, G.; Song, C.; Sun, H. Paclitaxel-loaded polymeric micelles based on poly (ε-caprolactone)-poly (ethylene glycol)-poly (ε-caprolactone) triblock copolymers: In vitro and in vivo evaluation. *Nanomed. Nanotechnol. Biol. Med.* **2012**, *8*, 925–934. [CrossRef]
179. Zhang, Y.; Zhang, H.; Wang, X.; Wang, J.; Zhang, X.; Zhang, Q. The eradication of breast cancer and cancer stem cells using octreotide modified paclitaxel active targeting micelles and salinomycin passive targeting micelles. *Biomaterials* **2012**, *33*, 679–691. [CrossRef]
180. Yin, T.; Wang, L.; Yin, L.; Zhou, J.; Huo, M. Co-delivery of hydrophobic paclitaxel and hydrophilic AURKA specific siRNA by redox-sensitive micelles for effective treatment of breast cancer. *Biomaterials* **2015**, *61*, 10–25. [CrossRef]
181. Wang, Y.; Zhao, H.; Peng, J.; Chen, L.; Tan, L.; Huang, Y.; Qian, Z. Targeting therapy of neuropilin-1 receptors overexpressed breast cancer by paclitaxel-loaded CK3-conjugated polymeric micelles. *J. Biomed. Nanotechnol.* **2016**, *12*, 2097–2111. [CrossRef]
182. Kelishady, P.D.; Saadat, E.; Ravar, F.; Akbari, H.; Dorkoosh, F. Pluronic F127 polymeric micelles for co-delivery of paclitaxel and lapatinib against metastatic breast cancer: Preparation, optimization and in vitro evaluation. *Pharm. Dev. Technol.* **2014**, *7450*, 1009–1017.
183. Hou, J.; Sun, E.; Sun, C.; Wang, J.; Yang, L.; Jia, X.B.; Zhang, Z.H. Improved oral bioavailability and anticancer efficacy on breast cancer of paclitaxel via Novel Soluplus—Solutol 1 HS15 binary mixed micelles system. *Int. J. Pharm.* **2016**, *512*, 186–193. [CrossRef]
184. Zhong, Y.; Goltsche, K.; Cheng, L.; Xie, F.; Meng, F.; Deng, C.; Zhong, Z.; Haag, R. Hyaluronic acid-shelled acid-activatable paclitaxel prodrug micelles effectively target and treat CD44-overexpressing human breast tumor xenografts in vivo. *Biomaterials* **2016**, *84*, 250–261. [CrossRef]

185. Hasenstein, J.R.; Shin, H.; Kasmerchak, K.; Buehler, D.; Kwon, G.S.; Kozak, K.R. Antitumor Activity of Triolimus: A Novel Multidrug-Loaded Micelle Containing Paclitaxel, Rapamycin, and 17-AAG. *Mol. Cancer Ther.* **2012**, *11*, 2233–2243. [CrossRef]
186. Lee, K.S.; Chung, H.C.; Im, S.A.; Park, Y.H.; Kim, C.S.; Kim, S.B.; Rha, S.Y.; Lee, M.Y.; Ro, J. Multicenter phase II trial of Genexol-PM, a Cremophor-free, polymeric micelle formulation of paclitaxel, in patients with metastatic breast cancer. *Breast Cancer Res. Treat.* **2008**, *108*, 241–250. [CrossRef]
187. Mei, D.; Lin, Z.; Fu, J.; He, B.; Gao, W.; Ma, L.; Dai, W.; Zhang, H.; Wang, X.; Wang, J.; et al. The use of α-conotoxin ImI to actualize the targeted delivery of paclitaxel micelles to a 7 nAChR-overexpressing breast cancer. *Biomaterials* **2015**, *42*, 52–65. [CrossRef] [PubMed]
188. Liu, P.; Situ, J.Q.; Li, W.S.; Shan, C.L.; You, J.; Yuan, H.; Hu, F.Q.; Du, Y.Z. High tolerated paclitaxel nano-formulation delivered by poly (lactic-*co*-glycolic acid)-*g*-dextran micelles to efficient cancer therapy. *Nanomed. Nanotechnol. Biol. Med.* **2015**, *11*, 855–866. [CrossRef]
189. Yang, Z.; Sun, N.; Cheng, R.; Zhao, C.; Liu, Z.; Li, X.; Liu, J.; Tian, Z. pH multistage responsive micellar system with charge-switch and PEG layer detachment for co-delivery of paclitaxel and curcumin to synergistically eliminate breast cancer stem cells. *Biomaterials* **2017**, *147*, 53–67. [CrossRef] [PubMed]
190. Han, X.; Dong, X.; Li, J.; Wang, M.; Luo, L.; Li, Z.; Lu, X.; He, R.; Xu, R.; Gong, M. Free paclitaxel-loaded E-selectin binding peptide modified micelle self-assembled from hyaluronic acid-paclitaxel conjugate inhibit breast cancer metastasis in a murine model. *Int. J. Pharm.* **2017**, *258*, 33–46. [CrossRef]
191. Wang, T.; Petrenko, V.A.; Torchilin, V.P. Paclitaxel-loaded polymeric micelles modified with MCF-7 cell-specific phage protein: Enhanced binding to target cancer cells and increased cytotoxicity. *Mol. Pharm.* **2010**, *7*, 1007–1014. [CrossRef]
192. Bernabeu, E.; Gonzalez, L.; Cagel, M.; Gergic, E.P.; Moretton, M.A.; Chiappetta, D.A. Novel Soluplus®—TPGS mixed micelles for encapsulation of paclitaxel with enhanced in vitro cytotoxicity on breast and ovarian cancer cell lines. *Colloids Surf. B Biointerfaces* **2016**, *140*, 403–411. [CrossRef]
193. Chen, Y.; Yue, Q.; De, G.; Wang, J.; Li, Z.; Xiao, S.; Yu, H.; Ma, H.; Sui, F.; Zhao, Q. Inhibition of breast cancer metastasis by paclitaxel-loaded pH responsive poly (β-amino ester) copolymer micelles. *Nanomedicine* **2017**, *12*, 147–164. [CrossRef] [PubMed]
194. Wang, T.; Yang, S.; Mei, L.A.; Parmar, C.K.; Gillespie, J.W.; Praveen, K.P.; Petrenko, V.A.; Torchilin, V.P. Paclitaxel-Loaded PEG-PE—Based Micellar Nanopreparations Targeted with Tumor-Specific Landscape Phage Fusion Protein Enhance Apoptosis and efficiently Reduce Tumors. *Mol. Cancer Ther.* **2014**, *13*, 2864–2875. [CrossRef]
195. Wang, N.; Wang, Z.; Nie, S.; Song, L.; He, T.; Yang, S.; Yang, X.; Yi, C.; Wu, Q.; Gong, C. Biodegradable polymeric micelles coencapsulating paclitaxel and honokiol: A strategy for breast cancer therapy in vitro and in vivo. *Int. J. Nanomed.* **2017**, *12*, 1499–1514. [CrossRef]
196. Lang, T.; Dong, X.; Huang, Y.; Ran, W.; Yin, Q.; Zhang, P.; Zhang, Z.; Yu, H.; Li, Y. Ly6Chi Monocytes Delivering pH-Sensitive Micelle Loading Paclitaxel Improve Targeting Therapy of Metastatic Breast Cancer. *Adv. Funct. Mater.* **2017**, *27*, 3. [CrossRef]
197. Wang, Y.; Yu, L.; Han, L.; Sha, X.; Fang, X. Difunctional Pluronic copolymer micelles for paclitaxel delivery: Synergistic effect of folate-mediated targeting and Pluronic-mediated overcoming multidrug resistance in tumor cell lines. *Int. J. Pharm.* **2007**, *337*, 63–73. [CrossRef]
198. Lu, J.; Huang, Y.; Zhao, W.; Marquez, R.T.; Meng, X.; Li, J.; Gao, X.; Venkataramanan, R.; Wang, Z.; Li, S. PEG-derivatized embelin as a nanomicellar carrier for delivery of paclitaxel to breast and prostate cancers. *Biomaterials* **2013**, *34*, 1591–1600. [CrossRef]
199. Zhu, W.J.; Yang, C.X.S.; Zhu, Q.L.; Chen, W.L.; Li, F.; Yuan, Z.Q.; Liu, Y.; You, B.G.; Zhang, X.N. Low-density lipoprotein-coupled micelles with reduction and pH dual sensitivity for intelligent co-delivery of paclitaxel and siRNA to breast tumor. *Int. J. Nanomed.* **2017**, *12*, 3375–3393. [CrossRef]
200. Chen, W.; Li, L.; Zhang, X.; Liang, Y.; Pu, Z.; Wang, L.; Mo, J. Curcumin: A calixarene derivative micelle potentiates anti-breast cancer stem cells effects in xenografted, triple-negative breast cancer mouse models. *Drug Deliv.* **2017**, *24*, 1470–1481. [CrossRef]
201. Huang, S.; Liu, J.; Zhu, H.; Hussain, A.; Liu, Q.; Li, J.; Shen, Y.; Cheng, J.; Guo, S. PEGylated Doxorubicin Micelles Loaded with Curcumin Exerting Synergic Effects on Multidrug Resistant Tumor Cells. *J. Nanosci. Nanotechnol.* **2016**, *16*, 2873–2880. [CrossRef]

202. Jung, K.H.; Lee, J.H.; Park, J.W.; Kim, D.H.; Moon, S.H.; Cho, Y.S.; Lee, K.H. Targeted therapy of triple negative MDA-MB-468 breast cancer with curcumin delivered by epidermal growth factor—Conjugated phospholipid nanoparticles. *Oncol. Lett.* **2018**, *15*, 9093–9100. [CrossRef]
203. Medel, S.; Syrova, Z.; Kovacik, L.; Hrdy, J.; Hornacek, M.; Jager, E.; Hruby, M.; Lund, R.; Cmarko, D.; Stepanek, P.; et al. Curcumin-bortezomib loaded polymeric nanoparticles for synergistic cancer therapy. *Eur. Polym. J.* **2017**, *93*, 116–131. [CrossRef]
204. Liu, L.; Sun, L.; Wu, Q.; Guo, W.; Li, L.; Chen, Y.; Li, Y.; Gong, C.; Qian, Z.; Wei, Y. Curcumin loaded polymeric micelles inhibit breast tumor growth and spontaneous pulmonary metastasis. *Int. J. Pharm.* **2013**, *443*, 175–182. [CrossRef] [PubMed]
205. Wan, X.; Beaudoin, J.J.; Vinod, N.; Min, Y.; Makita, N.; Bludau, H.; Jordan, R.; Wang, A.; Sokolsky, M.; Kabanov, A.V. Co-delivery of paclitaxel and cisplatin in poly (2-oxazoline) polymeric micelles: Implications for drug loading, release, pharmacokinetics and outcome of ovarian and breast cancer treatments. *Biomaterials* **2019**, *192*, 1–14. [CrossRef] [PubMed]
206. Ahmad, Z.; Tang, Z.; Shah, A.; Lv, S.; Zhang, D.; Zhang, Y.; Chen, X. Cisplatin Loaded Methoxy Poly (ethylene glycol)-block-Poly (L-glutamic acid-co-L-Phenylalanine) Nanoparticles against Human Breast Cancer Cell. *Macromol. Biosci.* **2014**, *14*, 1337–1345. [CrossRef] [PubMed]
207. Wang, R.; Hu, X.; Wu, S.; Xiao, H.; Cai, H.; Xie, Z.; Huang, Y.; Jing, X. Biological Characterization of Folate-Decorated Biodegradable Polymer—Platinum(II) Complex Micelles. *Mol. Pharm.* **2012**, *9*, 3200–3208. [CrossRef]
208. He, S.; Yang, H.; Zhang, R.; Li, Y.; Duan, L. Preparation and in vitro–in vivo evaluation of teniposide nanosuspensions. *Int. J. Pharm.* **2015**, *478*, 131–137. [CrossRef]
209. Kubisz, P.; Seghier, F.; Dobrotora, M.; Stasko, J.; Cronberg, S. Influence of teniposide on platelet functions in vitro. *Thromb. Res.* **1995**, *77*, 145–148. [CrossRef]
210. Chu, B.; Shi, S.; Li, X.; Hu, L.; Shi, L.; Zhang, H.; Xu, Q.; Ye, L.; Lin, G.; Zhang, N.; et al. Preparation and evaluation of teniposide-loaded polymeric micelles for breast cancer therapy. *Int. J. Pharm.* **2016**, *513*, 118–129. [CrossRef]
211. Zhang, J.; Kinoh, H.; Hespel, L.; Liu, X.; Quader, S.; Martin, J.; Chida, T.; Cabral, H.; Kataoka, K. Effective treatment of drug resistant recurrent breast tumors harboring cancer stem-like cells by staurosporine/epirubicin co-loaded polymeric micelles. *J. Control. Release* **2017**, *264*, 127–135. [CrossRef] [PubMed]
212. Min, H.K.; Kim, J.; Bae, S.M.; Shin, H.; Kim, M.S.; Park, S.; Lee, H.; Park, R.; Kim, I.; Kim, K.; et al. Tumoral acidic pH-responsive MPEG-poly (β-amino ester) polymeric micelles for cancer targeting therapy. *J. Control. Release* **2010**, *144*, 259–266. [CrossRef]
213. Lee, E.S.; Gao, Z.; Kim, D.; Park, K.; Kwon, I.C.; Bae, Y.H. Super pH-sensitive multifunctional polymeric micelle for tumor pH(e) specific TAT exposure and multidrug resistance. *J. Control. Release* **2008**, *129*, 228–236. [CrossRef]
214. Sethuraman, V.A.; Na, K.; Bae, Y.H. pH-responsive sulfonamide/PEI system for tumor specific gene delivery: An in vitro study. *Biomacromolecules* **2006**, *7*, 64–70. [CrossRef] [PubMed]
215. Chida, T.; Miura, Y.; Cabral, H.; Nomoto, T.; Kataoka, K.; Nishiyama, N. Epirubicin-loaded polymeric micelles effectively treat axillary lymph nodes metastasis of breast cancer through selective accumulation and pH-triggered drug release. *J. Control. Release* **2018**, *292*, 130–140. [CrossRef]
216. Gener, P.; Montero, S.; Xandri-Monje, H.; Díaz-Riascos, Z.V.; Rafael, D.; Andrade, F.; Martínez-Trucharte, F.; González, P.; Seras-Franzoso, J.; Manzano, A.; et al. Zileuton TM loaded in polymer micelles effectively reduce breast cancer circulating tumor cells and intratumoral cancer stem cells. *Nanomed. Nanotechnol. Biol. Med.* **2020**, *24*, 102106. [CrossRef] [PubMed]
217. Lee, G.; Hall, R.R.; Ahmed, A.U. Cancer stem cells: Cellular plasticity, niche and its Clinical Relevance. *J. Stem Cell Res. Ther.* **2016**, *6*, 363. [CrossRef] [PubMed]
218. Lamch, L.; Bazyli, U.; Kulbacka, J.; Pietkiewicz, J.; Biezunska-Kusiak, K.; Wilk, K.A. Polymeric micelles for enhanced Photofrin II ®delivery, cytotoxicity and pro-apoptotic activity in human breast and ovarian cancer cells. *Photodiagnosis Photodyn. Ther.* **2014**, *11*, 570–585. [CrossRef]

219. Marcos, X.; Padilla-beltrán, C.; Bernad-bernad, M.J.; Rosales-hernández, M.C.; Pérez-casas, S.; Correa-basurto, J. Controlled release of N-(2-hydroxyphenyl)-2-propylpentanamide nanoencapsulated in polymeric micelles of P123 and F127 tested as anti- proliferative agents in MDA-MB-231 cells. *J. Drug Deliv. Sci. Technol.* **2018**, *48*, 403–413. [CrossRef]
220. Lu, H.; Blunden, B.M.; Scarano, W.; Lu, M.; Stenzel, M.H. Anti-metastatic effects of RAPTA-C conjugated polymeric micelles on multicellular tumor spheroids. *Acta Biomater.* **2016**, *32*, 68–76. [CrossRef]
221. Wu, B.; Ong, M.S.; Groessl, M.; Adhireksan, Z.; Hartinger, C.G.; Dyson, P.J.; Davey, C.A. A ruthenium antimetastasis agent forms specific histone protein adducts in the nucleosome core. *Chem. Eur. J.* **2011**, *17*, 3562–3566. [CrossRef]
222. Brinkman, A.M.; Chen, G.; Wang, Y.; Hedman, C.J.; Sherer, N.M.; Havighurst, T.C.; Gong, S.; Xu, W. Aminoflavone-loaded EGFR-targeted unimolecular micelle nanoparticles exhibit anti-cancer effects in triple negative breast cancer. *Biomaterials* **2016**, *101*, 20–31. [CrossRef]
223. Yang, Y.; Pearson, R.M.; Lee, O.; Lee, C.W.; Chatterton, J.R.T.; Khan, S.A.; Hong, S. Dendron-Based Micelles for Topical Delivery of Endoxifen: A Potential Chemo-Preventive Medicine for Breast Cancer. *Adv. Funct. Mater.* **2014**, *24*, 2442–2449. [CrossRef]
224. Zhong, P.; Gu, X.; Cheng, R.; Deng, C.; Meng, F.; Zong, Z. αvβ3 integrin-targeted micellar mertansine prodrug effectively inhibits triple-negative breast cancer in vivo. *Int. J. Nanomed.* **2017**, *12*, 7913. [CrossRef] [PubMed]
225. Lu, Y.; Zhang, E.; Yang, J.; Cao, Z. Strategies to improve micelle stability for drug delivery. *Nano Res.* **2018**, *11*, 4985–4998. [CrossRef] [PubMed]
226. Tang, L.; Yang, X.J.; Yin, Q.; Cai, K.M.; Wang, H.; Chaudhury, I.; Yao, C.; Zhou, Q.; Kwon, M.; Hartman, J.A. Investigating the optimal size of anticancer nanomedicine. *Proc. Natl. Acad. Sci. USA* **2014**, *111*, 15344–15349. [CrossRef]
227. Stirland, D.L.; Nichols, J.W.; Miura, S.; Bae, Y.H. Mind the gap: A survey of how cancer drug carriers are susceptible to the gap between research and practice. *J. Control. Release* **2013**, *172*, 1045–1064. [CrossRef] [PubMed]
228. Kim, S.; Shi, Y.; Kim, J.Y.; Park, K.; Cheng, J.X. Overcoming the barriers in micellar drug delivery: Loading efficiency, in vivo stability, and micelle-cell interaction. *Expert Opin. Drug Deliv.* **2010**, *7*, 49–62. [CrossRef] [PubMed]
229. Wakaskar, R. Polymeric Micelles and their Properties. *J. Nanomed. Nanotechnol.* **2017**, *8*. [CrossRef]
230. Yokoyama, M. Clinical Applications of Polymeric Micelle Carrier Systems in Chemotherapy and Image Diagnosis of Solid Tumors. *J. Exp. Clin. Med.* **2011**, *3*, 151–158. [CrossRef]
231. van Nostrum, C.F. Covalently cross-linked amphiphilic block copolymer micelles. *Soft Matter* **2011**, *7*, 3246–3259. [CrossRef]
232. Blanco, E.; Shen, H.F.; Ferrari, M. Principles of nanoparticle design for overcoming biological barriers to drug delivery. *Nat. Biotechnol.* **2015**, *33*, 941–951. [CrossRef]
233. Talelli, M.; Barz, M.; Rijcken, C.J.; Kiessling, F.; Hennink, W.E.; Lammers, T. Core-Crosslinked Polymeric Micelles: Principles, Preparation, Biomedical Applications and Clinical Translation. *Nano Today* **2015**, *10*, 93–117. [CrossRef]

Publisher's Note: MDPI stays neutral with regard to jurisdictional claims in published maps and institutional affiliations.

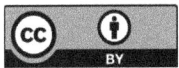

© 2020 by the authors. Licensee MDPI, Basel, Switzerland. This article is an open access article distributed under the terms and conditions of the Creative Commons Attribution (CC BY) license (http://creativecommons.org/licenses/by/4.0/).

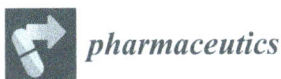

Article

Physicochemical, Pharmacokinetic, and Toxicity Evaluation of Soluplus® Polymeric Micelles Encapsulating Fenbendazole

Ik Sup Jin [1], Min Jeong Jo [1], Chun-Woong Park [1], Youn Bok Chung [1], Jin-Seok Kim [2] and Dae Hwan Shin [1,*]

1. College of Pharmacy, Chungbuk National University, Cheongju 28160, Korea; iksup0418@gmail.com (I.S.J.); cmj0310@naver.com (M.J.J.); cwpark@chungbuk.ac.kr (C.-W.P.); chungyb@chungbuk.ac.kr (Y.B.C.)
2. Drug Information Research Institute (DIRI), College of Pharmacy, Sookmyung Women's University, Cheongpa-ro 47-gil 100, Yongsan-gu, Seoul 04310, Korea; jsk9574@sookmyung.ac.kr
* Correspondence: dshin@chungbuk.ac.kr; Tel.: +82-43-261-2820; Fax: +82-43-268-2732

Received: 29 September 2020; Accepted: 19 October 2020; Published: 21 October 2020

Abstract: Fenbendazole (FEN), a broad-spectrum benzimidazole anthelmintic, suppresses cancer cell growth through various mechanisms but has low solubility and achieves low blood concentrations, which leads to low bioavailability. Solubilizing agents are required to prepare poorly soluble drugs for injections; however, these are toxic. To overcome this problem, we designed and fabricated low-toxicity Soluplus® polymeric micelles encapsulating FEN and conducted toxicity assays in vitro and in vivo. FEN-loaded Soluplus® micelles had an average particle size of 68.3 ± 0.6 nm, a zeta potential of −2.3 ± 0.2 mV, a drug loading of 0.8 ± 0.03%, and an encapsulation efficiency of 85.3 ± 2.9%. MTT and clonogenic assays were performed on A549 cells treated with free FEN and FEN-loaded Soluplus® micelles. The in vitro drug release profile showed that the micelles released FEN more gradually than the solution. Pharmacokinetic studies revealed lower total clearance and volume of distribution and higher area under the curve and plasma concentration at time zero of FEN-loaded Soluplus® micelles than of the FEN solution. The in vivo toxicity assay revealed that FEN-loaded Soluplus® micelle induced no severe toxicity. Therefore, we propose that preclinical and clinical safety and efficacy trials on FEN-loaded Soluplus® micelles would be worthwhile.

Keywords: fenbendazole; micelle solubilization; pharmacokinetics; Soluplus® polymeric micelles; toxicity test

1. Introduction

Certain cancers have high mortality rates in humans. Therefore, the development of safe anticancer drugs with few side effects is an important research objective in pharmaceutical science. Fenbendazole (FEN) is a broad-spectrum benzimidazole anthelmintic. It has been widely used in veterinary medicine and induces no significant side effects. The European Medicines Agency has not established a no observable adverse effects level (NOAEL) for single-dose FEN administration but recommended a NOAEL of 4 mg kg^{-1} BW d^{-1} for repeated FEN administration. Moreover, no significant side effects were observed in humans in response to the administration of the major FEN metabolite oxfendazole even at 60 mg kg^{-1} for 14 d [1]. Benzimidazole (BZD) anthelmintic agents have been studied in recent years for their anticancer effects [2,3]. Several papers have reported their modes of action and positive effects [4,5]. FEN suppresses cancer cell growth through various mechanisms. It inhibits proteasomal activity and induces endoplasmic reticulum stress and reactive oxygen species-dependent apoptosis [6]. Second, it has anti-tubulin efficacy [5]. Other BZDs arrest mitosis and promote apoptosis. Mebendazole displays anti-tubulin and antitumor efficacy in vivo [7]. However, FEN has low solubility and achieves only low blood concentrations [8,9]. The limited solubility makes it difficult to develop parenteral and even topical preparations. For these reasons, it has a low area under the curve (AUC) and poor bioavailability [10]. AUC is an intuitive indicator of how much body has been exposed to drugs and is also strongly related to drug efficacy and number of drug administration. Therefore, it is important to increase the solubility of FEN, which can lead to improved bioavailability [11,12]. Hence, injectable forms of FEN are preferable as they can bypass the various obstacles of the digestive tract. However, solubilizing agent is needed to prepare poorly soluble drugs for injections. Ethanol (EtOH) and Cremophor EL® increase paclitaxel solubility. However, Cremophor EL may induce peripheral neurotoxicity, neutropenia, and hypersensitivity reactions [13–15]. Another solubilizing agent, polysorbate 80 (Tween 80®), which exerts acute toxicity in an in vivo zebrafish model, is used in Taxotere®, an anticancer drug containing docetaxel [16]. Finally, dimethylacetamide (DMA), used in anticancer drug Vunom® containing teniposide, results in hepatic fatty infiltration, liver hypertrophy, and focal hepatic necrosis in animals, and acute hepatitis has been reported in humans [17–19]. There is a formulation technology using nanoparticles to replace such a solubilizing agent. Examples of nanoparticles include liposomes, microemulsions, and micelles [20–22]. We designed and tested various micelles composed of amphiphilic diblock copolymers to enhance FEN solubilization while mitigating the toxicity of the different excipients used for this purpose [23]. The enhanced permeability and retention (EPR) effect of nanomicelles increases their accumulation in cancer cells. The EPR effect is a phenomenon manifested by the peculiar pathophysiological characteristics of solid tumors. Nanoparticles are trapped in the solid tumors and stay longer for reasons such as hyper vasculature and impaired lymphatic drainage/recovery system [24]. In addition, polymeric micelles are biodegradable, biocompatible, have low toxicity, and may have nearly solid inner cores that can serve as drug carriers [25]. We found four suitable candidate polymers to fabricate the micelles. Each polymer has both specific and general nanoparticle advantages. The mPEG-*b*-PLA micelle can hold and carry multiple drugs [26]. This polymer can also remain in circulation for a long time and has low toxicity [27]. In cancer treatment, the occurrence of drug resistance owing to P-glycoprotein (P-gp) overexpression is a serious problem [28]. However, Soluplus® might be able to inhibit P-gp [29]. Paclitaxel encapsulated with Pluronic® F127 overcomes multidrug resistance (MDR) and has favorable pharmacokinetics. Intracellular ATP depletion and lowered mitochondrial potential are assumed to be involved in the modulation of MDR [30].

In this study, we selected the most suitable polymer and fabricated micelles using the freeze-drying method. This is advantageous for scaled-up production, easy storage, and cake-state distribution. Then, we evaluated the in vitro cytotoxicity, in vivo toxicity, in vitro release, and pharmacokinetic profile. Our findings will help to develop a potent and innovative injectable micellar formulation facilitating the clinical study and application of FEN for anticancer purposes (Figure 1).

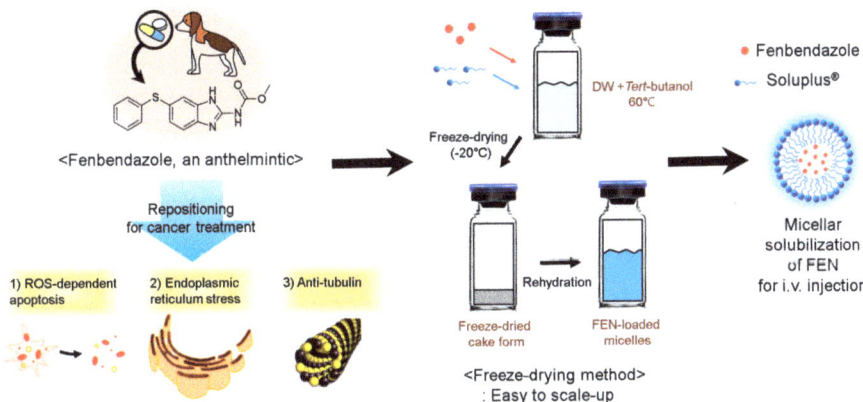

Figure 1. Schematic illustration of fenbendazole (FEN)-loaded Soluplus® micelle preparation for i.v. injection.

2. Materials and Methods

2.1. Materials and Reagents

Soluplus® (Polyvinyl caprolactam-polyvinyl acetate-polyethylene glycol graft copolymer (PCL-PVAc-PEG)), was kindly donated by BASF (Ludwigshafen, Rhineland-Palatinate, Germany). Methoxy poly(ethylene glycol)-b-poly(d,l-lactide) (mPEG [4000]-b-PLA [2200]) was purchased from Advanced Polymer Materials, Inc. (Montreal, QC, Canada). Poly(ethylene oxide-b-ε-caprolactone) (PEO[5000]-b-PCL[10000]) was purchased from Polymer Source, Inc. (Montreal, QC, Canada). Pluronic® F127 was purchased from Sigma-Aldrich Corp. (St. Louis, MO, USA). Dulbecco's phosphate-buffered saline (DPBS), and trypsin were purchased from Corning Inc. (Corning, NY, USA). EtOH and acetonitrile (ACN) were obtained from Thermo Fisher Scientific (Waltham, MA, USA). Distilled water (DW) was purchased from Tedia (Fairfield, OH, USA). FEN, Thiazolyl blue tetrazolium bromide (MTT), Dimethyl sulfoxide (DMSO), Polysorbate 80 (Tween 80®), DMA, and Cremophor EL® were purchased from Sigma-Aldrich Corp. (St. Louis, MO, USA). All other reagents were of at least analytical or HPCL grade.

2.2. Methods

2.2.1. Preparation of FEN-Loaded Polymeric Micelles

FEN-loaded polymeric micelles were prepared from four polymers by the freeze-drying method [31]. Briefly, 1 mg of FEN and 100 mg of polymers were dissolved in 1 mL of tert-butanol and stirred for 1 min in prewarmed water at 60 °C. Then 1 mL of DW was added and the mixture was vortexed for 1 min. The mixture was rapidly frozen at −70 °C for 1 h, placed in a freeze-dryer (Advantage Pro; SP Scientific, Warminster, PA, USA), and lyophilized for 24 h. Then, 1 mL of DW at 60 °C was added to hydrate the mixture. The solution was then centrifuged at 16,600× g at 4 °C (Hanil Science Inc., Gimpo, Korea) for 5 min to remove drug or polymer precipitates. A non-pyrogenic sterile syringe filter with 0.2 μm pore size (Corning, NY, USA) was used to further remove remaining debris and to make sterile condition [32,33].

2.2.2. High-Performance Liquid Chromatography (HPLC) Analysis

A HPLC system was used for the analysis of concentrations of FEN. All samples were obtained from the in vitro and in vivo assays through this study. The HPLC system consisted of Waters 2695 separation module and a Waters 2996 photodiode array detector (Waters, Milford, MA, USA). A Fortis C18 chromatography column (5 μm, 4.6 × 250 mm) (Fortis Technologies Ltd., Cheshire, UK) was run in a 30 °C environment. FEN and a genistein internal standard (IS) were eluted in the isocratic mode. The mobile phase consisted of water/ACN (30:70, v/v), and it was replaced and degassed for each run. The sample injection volume was 10 μL, and the mobile phase flow rate was 1.0 mL min^{-1}. The IS and FEN retention times were 3.4 and 5.4 min, respectively (Supplementary Materials Figure S1). The predetermined calibration curve was used to calculate the concentrations. The concentration was calculated by substituting the peak area of each sample into the calibration curve.

2.2.3. Physicochemical Micelle Characterization

A dynamic light scattering (DLS) device (Litesizer 500, Anton Paar, Graz, Austria) measured the FEN-loaded micelles zeta-potentials and particle sizes. The angle of measurement was automatically selected and used between side scatter (90°) and back scatter (175°). The FEN-loaded micelle encapsulation efficiency (EE, %) and drug loading (DL, %) were obtained by HPLC and calculated as follows:

$$DL\% = \text{weight of drug in micelles/weight of feeding polymer and drug} \times 100 \quad (1)$$

$$EE\% = \text{weight of drug in micelles/weight of feeding drug} \times 100 \quad (2)$$

The results of each sample analysis are expressed as the mean ± standard deviation of three separate experiments.

2.2.4. Transmission Electron Microscopy Study

Images of micelles were obtained using a transmission electron microscope (TEM) (JEM-2100 Plus, JEOL, Tokyo, Japan). Diluted micelle suspensions were dropped onto 200-mesh formvar-coated copper grids. After loaded, it was dried at 60 °C in a dry oven for 12 h. Finally, FEN-loaded Soluplus® micelles were measured using a TEM operated at 200 kV.

2.2.5. In Vitro Drug Release Assay

Dialysis with a phosphate-buffered saline (PBS, pH 7.4) medium was used to investigate the in vitro drug release patterns. In brief, FEN-loaded micelles and FEN solution were inserted into a dialysis membrane bag (molecular weight cut-off = 20 kDa), which was then tied and immersed in 2.0 L of medium maintained at 37 °C and stirred constantly with a magnetic bar at 200 rpm. The PBS medium was replaced after 8, 24, 72, 168, and 240 h to reproduce the sink condition [34]. For sample collection, 20-μL aliquots were collected at 0, 2, 4, 6, 8, 24, 48, 72, 168, 240 and 336 h. The samples were diluted 10× with ACN, and the FEN concentrations were calculated by HPLC. All experiments were performed in triplicate.

2.2.6. In Vitro Cytotoxicity Assay

The A549 human non-small cell lung cancer cell line was purchased from the American Type Culture Collection (Manassas, VA, USA). The media for growing cells consists of the following: Roswell Park Memorial Institute medium (RPMI 1640) with 1% (w/v) streptomycin/penicillin and 10% (v/v) fetal bovine serum. The cells were grown at 37 °C with a 5% CO_2 atmosphere conditions. A549 cells were seeded in 96-well plates at a density of 5000 cells per well. After 24 h, the cells were treated with free FEN drug (After dissolving in DMSO, it was diluted 1000 times with RPMI) or FEN-loaded micelles. The initial concentration of treated FEN-loaded soluplus® micelles are 205.5 μM, and the initial concentration of treated free FEN is 33.4 μM. Treatment was done by diluting 10 times from the initial concentration ($n = 6$). After 48 h of incubation, cell viability was assessed by the MTT assay. Microplate reader (Spectra Max ID3, Molecular Devices, San Jose, CA, USA) was used to measure the absorbance at 540 nm 4 h after MTT treatment. Data were handled and curves were fitted with GraphPad Prism v. 5 (GraphPad Software, La Jolla, CA, USA).

2.2.7. Clonogenic Assay

A549 cells were seeded in six-well plates at a density of 300 cells per well. After 24 h, the cells were treated with free FEN drug (After dissolving in DMSO, it was diluted 1000 times with RPMI) or FEN-loaded micelles. The treatments included three increasing concentrations and one control group. After 336 h of incubation, the colonies were stained with crystal violet (0.5% w/v). After 30 min, the crystal violet was gently washed away with water and the colonies were counted.

2.2.8. FEN-Loaded Micelle Stability Test

Stability tests were conducted at 4, 25 and 37 °C, representing cold chain management, room temperature, and human body temperature, respectively. Briefly, the micelles in water was incubated at 4 °C refrigerator, 25 °C room, and 37 °C water bath. At days 0, 1, 2, 5, 7 and 14, micelles were collected from each sample. Micelle size changes and poly-dispersity indices (PDI) were measured using a DLS device, and the experiment was conducted in triplicate.

2.2.9. Pharmacokinetic Study

All animal experiments conducted in this study were approved by the Institutional Animal Care and Use Committee of Chungbuk National University (No. CBNUR-1407-20; 23 July 23 2020). Male Sprague-Dawley rats (7 weeks old) were purchased from Orient Bio Inc. (Seongnam, Korea) and used in all animal experiments. The rats were maintained in ventilated plastic cages filled with aspen shaving and they were given enough water and food. The animals in each group were cannulated and intravenously injected with FEN (2 mg kg^{-1}) in 25% Cremophor EL®/EtOH (FEN solution) or FEN-loaded Soluplus® micelles. Blood was then collected at 2, 5, 15, 30, 60, 120, 240 and 480 min after drug administration and the samples were centrifuged at 3000 rpm for 5 min to obtain the plasma [35]. Heparin was used as an anticoagulant, and 400~450 µL of blood was collected through the femoral artery. The samples were immediately frozen at −70 °C and maintained in deep freeze until analysis. A non-compartmental model was used to calculate the relevant pharmacokinetic parameters for FEN including total clearance (CL$_t$), AUC, volume of distribution (V$_d$), and plasma concentration at time zero (C$_0$). The curve fitting for the calculation of pharmacokinetic parameters was carried out using the Sigma Plot V 10.0. (Systat Software, San Jose, CA, USA).

2.2.10. Biological Sample Pretreatment for HPLC Analysis

A 200-µL plasma supernatant sample was extracted with ACN and mixed with 20 µL of IS. The mixture was then centrifuged at 16,600× g at 4 °C for 5 min, and 10 µL of supernatant was injected into the HPLC system [35]. Biodistribution was determined by the homogenization method [36]. The sample tissues were homogenized in a glass Potter-Elvehjem-type homogenizer (Ultra Turrax T-25; IKA Works Inc., Staufen, Germany) with a Teflon pestle. The FEN concentration in the supernatant was determined as previously described in Section 2.2.2.

2.2.11. Biodistribution Study

A biodistribution study was performed on the rats after the intravenous injection of FEN solution or FEN-loaded micelles (2 mg kg^{-1}). The experiment was conducted twice to observe temporal changes (n = 3). The rats were euthanized using CO$_2$ gas 1 and 8 h after the first injection, and their kidneys, livers, hearts, spleens, and lungs were excised. The samples were washed with DPBS and stored at −70 °C until the subsequent analysis.

2.2.12. In Vivo Toxicity Assay

Five groups of rats ($n = 6$ per group) were used to assess in vivo toxicity. The rats were intravenously injected with 25% Cremophor EL®/EtOH solution containing 2 mg kg^{-1} FEN, 25% polysorbate 80 (Tween 80®) solution containing 2 mg kg^{-1} FEN, 25% DMA solution containing 2 mg kg^{-1} FEN, or FEN-loaded Soluplus® micelle solution containing 2 mg kg^{-1} FEN. Change in body weight was measured every 2 days for 14 days. Intravenous injections were performed on days 0, 4, and 8. Toxicity was defined as > 10% loss of total body weight, evidence of discomfort, abnormal behavior, or death. Body weight changes were normalized and displayed as percentages. The initial weight was taken to be 100%. The rats were euthanized in response to serious disability and at the end of the experiment [37].

2.2.13. Statistics

For statistical processing of all data used, Student's *t*-test or ANOVA of GraphPad Prism v 5.0 was used.

3. Results

3.1. Physicochemical Characterization of FEN-Loaded Micelles

The DL (%), EE (%), and particle sizes of the FEN-loaded micelles prepared with various polymers (Soluplus®, mPEG-*b*-PLA, Pluronic® F127, and mPEO-*b*-PCL) are listed in Table 1. After freeze-drying, the unincorporated drug or polymer was removed by centrifugation and passed through a 0.2-µm filter. As FEN has low water solubility, only small amounts of it would be present in the water. Hence, FEN would be well encapsulated in polymeric micelles [38,39]. DLS analysis revealed that the average particle size of the FEN-loaded Soluplus® micelles was 68.3 nm. In contrast, the other polymeric micelles prepared with mPEG-*b*-PLA, Pluronic® F127, and mPEO-*b*-PCL were much larger (Figure 2). Pluronic® F127 and mPEG-*b*-PLA did not have nano-particle attributes as they were > 300 nm in size. In addition, we confirmed the formation of Soluplus® micelles using TEM. The average particle size in TEM image measured by ImageJ software was 65.6 ± 26.2 nm.

Table 1. Characteristics of fenbendazole (FEN)-loaded micelles.

Polymer Amount Used (mg)	FEN Amount Used (mg)	Particle Size (nm)	Poly-Dispersity Index (PDI)	Zeta-Potential (mV)	Encapsulation Efficiency (EE %)	Drug Loading (DL %)
mPEO-*b*-PCL 100 mg	1.0	96.8 ± 3.8	0.14 ± 0.01	−0.4 ± 0.1	24.7 ± 2.0	0.2 ± 0.02
mPEG-*b*-PLA 100 mg	1.0	347.7 ± 40.4	0.26 ± 0.04	−9.5 ± 2.1	56.8 ± 2.8	0.6 ± 0.03
Pluronic F127® 100 mg	1.0	1566.5 ± 157.8	0.23 ± 0.09	−4.6 ± 0.1	N.D.[a]	N.D.[a]
Soluplus® 50 mg	1.0	65.4 ± 2.3	0.11 ± 0.03	−2.4 ± 0.2	58.3 ± 3.1	0.6 ± 0.03
Soluplus® 100 mg	1.0	68.3 ± 0.6	0.01 ± 0.02	−2.3 ± 0.2	85.3 ± 2.9	0.8 ± 0.03

[a] N.D., not detectable due to precipitation. ($n = 3$; mean ± SD).

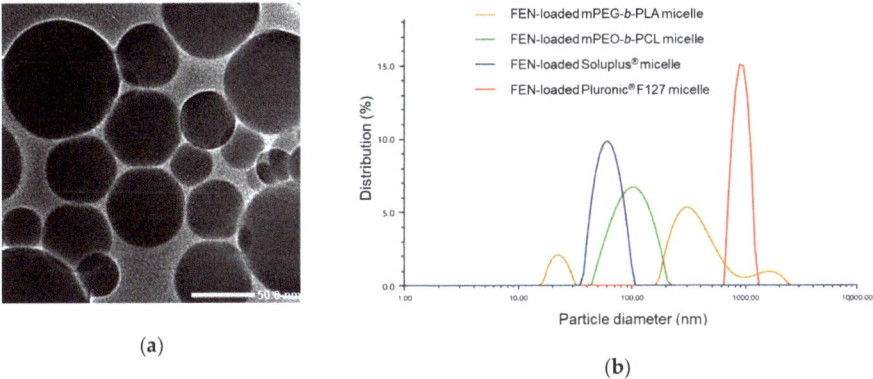

(a) (b)

Figure 2. Particle size analysis of the various formulations in this study. (**a**) Transmission electron microscopy (TEM) image of FEN-loaded Soluplus® micelles. (**b**) Size distribution of micelles made of four different polymers.

3.2. In Vitro Drug Release Profile

The in vitro drug release profiles of FEN-loaded Soluplus® micelle and FEN dissolved in 25% Cremophor EL®/EtOH solution are shown in Figure 3. After 6 h, the release rates were 12.9% for the micelle formulation and 46.3% for the solution. At ≤ 72 h, the release rates were 50.4% for the micelle and 75.1% for the solution. Over the first 168 h, the solution released FEN significantly faster than the micelle.

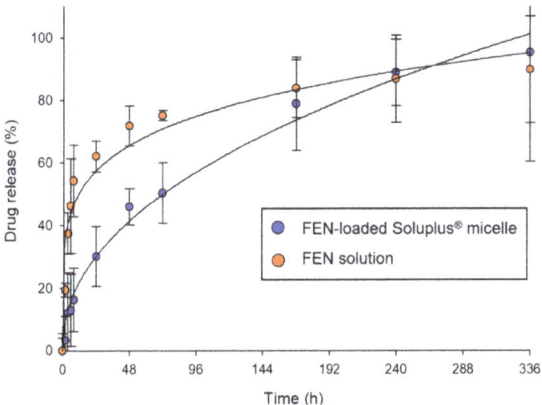

Figure 3. In vitro release profile of fenbendazole (FEN) from Soluplus® micelles and 25% Cremophor EL®/EtOH solution at 37 °C.

3.3. In Vitro Cytotoxicity Assay

The free FEN drug treatment IC_{50} = 2707 nM, whereas the FEN-loaded Soluplus® micelle treatment IC_{50} = 3070 nM (Figure 4).

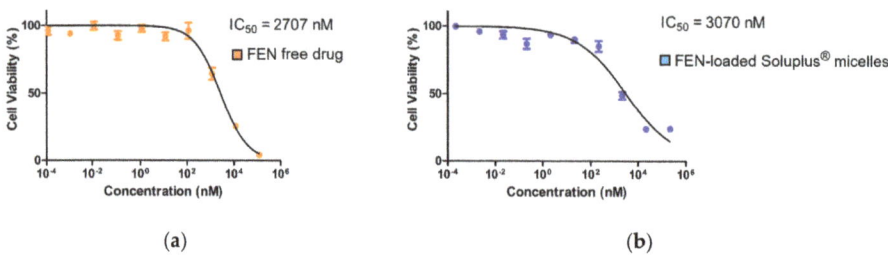

Figure 4. In vitro MTT assay results for the (**a**) free fenbendazole (FEN) drug and (**b**) FEN-loaded Soluplus® micelle treatments of the A549 human non-small cell lung cancer (NSCLC) cell line.

3.4. Clonogenic Assay

We performed a clonogenic assay to determine the long-term inhibitory efficacy of the treatments against cell reproduction. The cells formed no colonies at 1740 µM. Colony formation was slightly suppressed in the micelle-treated group at 174 µM. Above 17.4 µM, colony formation was not significantly inhibited (Figure 5).

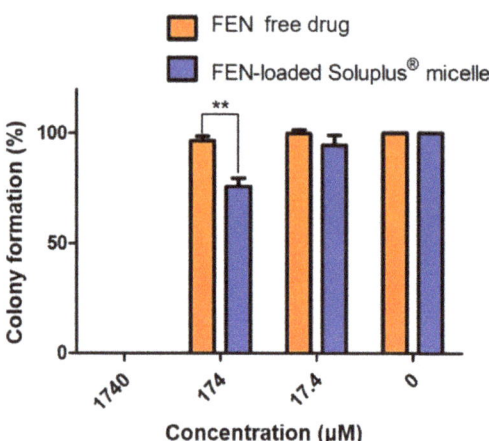

Figure 5. In vitro clonogenic assay of free fenbendazole (FEN)- and FEN-loaded Soluplus® micelle-treated A549 cell line, ** $p < 0.01$.

3.5. Stability Test of FEN-Loaded Soluplus® Micelles

FEN-loaded Soluplus® micelles were stable for 2 weeks at 4, 25, and 37 °C. In all cases, the size was ≤100 nm, and the PDI was ≤0.3 (Figure 6).

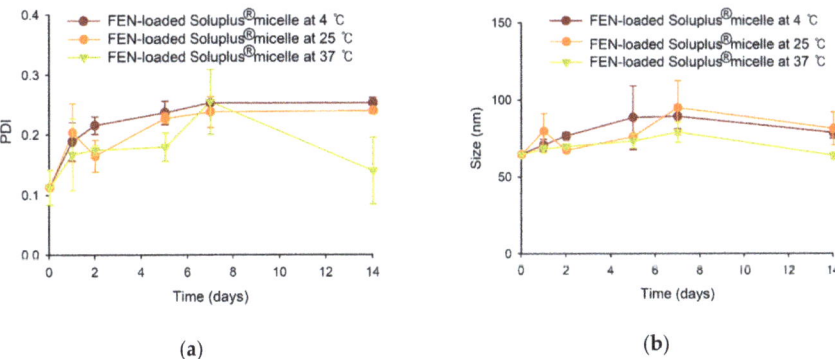

Figure 6. PDI (**a**) and size (**b**) changes of FEN-loaded Soluplus® micelles at various temperature.

3.6. Pharmacokinetics of FEN Solution and FEN-Loaded Soluplus® Micelles in Rats

The plasma concentration–time profiles of the FEN solution and FEN-loaded Soluplus® micelles are shown in Figure 7. The plasma FEN concentration rapidly decreased after the intravenous injection of FEN solution and FEN-loaded Soluplus® micelles. However, FEN-loaded Soluplus® micelles were detected 2 h after injection, whereas the FEN solution was detected within 1 h. At 2 h, no FEN solution was found as its concentration was below the limit of detection (LOD). The pharmacokinetic parameters (Table 2) were calculated assuming a non-compartment model. The AUC and C_0 were approximately 1.5-fold and more than 2-fold higher for the micelle formulation than for the solution, respectively. Moreover, the CL_t and V_d were 1.4-fold and more than 2-fold lower for the micelle formulation than for the solution, respectively.

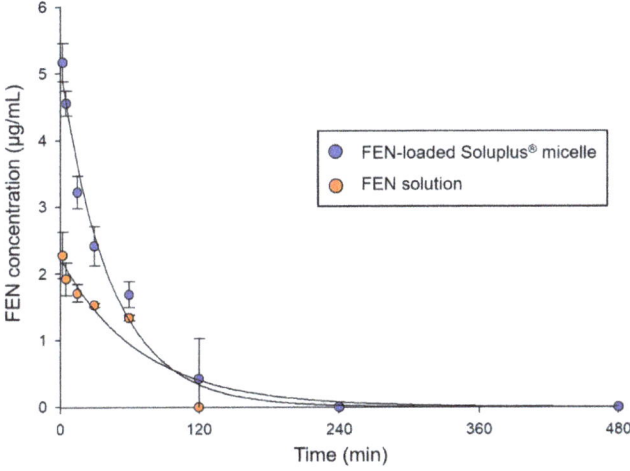

Figure 7. Plasma fenbendazole (FEN) concentration vs. time profile after intravenous injection of FEN-loaded Soluplus® micelles and FEN dissolved in 25% Cremophor EL®/EtOH solution.

Table 2. Pharmacokinetic parameters of fenbendazole (FEN) after intravenous injection of FEN-loaded Soluplus® micelles and FEN dissolved in 25% Cremophor EL®/EtOH solution.

Parameter	FEN Solution	FEN-Loaded Soluplus® Micelle
AUC [a] (min·µg·mL^{-1})	156 ± 2.6	234 ± 56.9
C_0 [b] (µg·mL^{-1})	2.2 ± 0.3	5.1 ± 0.2
CL_t [c] (mL·kg^{-1}·min)	12.8 ± 0.2	9.0 ± 1.9
Vd [d] (mL·kg^{-1})	906 ± 112	393 ± 12.9

[a] AUC, area under the curve; [b] C_0, plasma concentration at time zero; [c] CL_t, total clearance; [d] Vd, volume of distribution.

3.7. Biodistribution of FEN Solution and FEN-Loaded Soluplus® Micelles in Rats

Figure 8 shows the total drug distribution in each organ measured 1 and 8 h after the intravenous injection of FEN solution and FEN-loaded Soluplus® micelles. After 1 h, the organ distribution of the drug was lower in micelles than in solution in all other organs except the spleen. After 8 h, both the solution and the micelles were present below the LOD in all organs. In particular, a significantly higher amount of drug was detected in the lungs 1 h after the administration of the solution than 1 h after the administration of the micelles. Additionally, when organs were obtained, some hemolysis was observed in the lungs (data not shown).

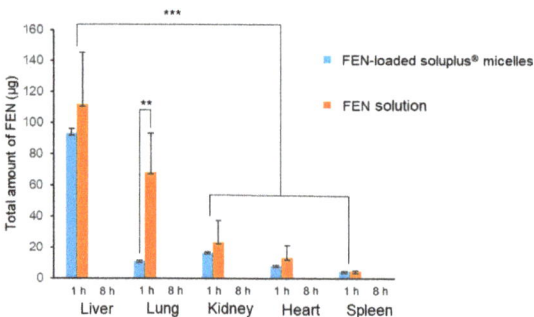

Figure 8. Total amount of fenbendazole (FEN) in each organ at 1 and 8 h after administration of FEN in 25% Cremophor EL®/EtOH solution and FEN-loaded Soluplus® micelles, ** $p < 0.01$, *** $p < 0.001$.

3.8. In Vivo Toxicity Assay

Figure 9 shows the total body weight changes and the survival rate after three injections of DPBS (control), FEN dissolved in 25% Cremophor EL®/EtOH, FEN dissolved in 25% DMA, FEN dissolved in 25% Tween 80®, or FEN-loaded Soluplus® micelles. Intravenous doses were administered on days 0, 4, and 8 of the experiment, and the survival rates and total body weights were measured. Compared with the control, the FEN-loaded Soluplus® micelle treatment group presented with 100% survival and higher body weight. One rat each in the Tween 80® and Cremophor EL®/EtOH groups died on day 6. In the DMA group, three rats died on day 10. After 2 weeks, half the rats in the DMA group, four rats in the Cremophor EL®/EtOH group, and one rat in the Tween 80® group survived. All animals in the micelle and control groups survived.

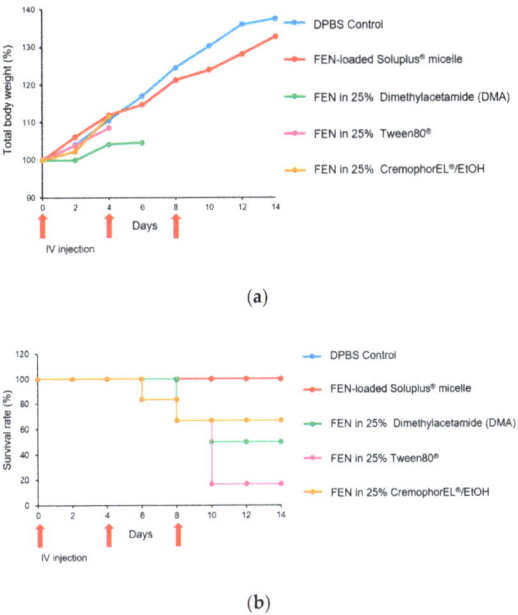

Figure 9. Relative rat body weight changes and survival rates after three intravenous injections of Dulbecco's phosphate-buffered saline (DPBS) control, fenbendazole (FEN) dissolved in 25% Cremophor EL®/EtOH, FEN dissolved in 25% dimethylacetamide (DMA), FEN dissolved in 25% Tween 80®, or FEN-loaded Soluplus® micelles on days 0, 4, and 8 (All doses are equal to 2 mgmL·kg^{-1}). (**a**) Relative daily body weight change. Missing data points indicate death of an animal. (**b**) Kaplan–Meier plot illustrating survival rates.

4. Discussion

FEN is a drug used as an anthelmintic. However, in recent years, the potential of the drug as an anticancer drug through various mechanisms and its few side effects are being revealed [5,6]. However, the low solubility and bioavailability poses an obstacle to its use [10]. To overcome this deficiency and obtain the advantages of micelles, we formulated, optimized, and tested polymeric FEN micelles. Here, we tested four different polymers and sought the optimal formulation. We compared their physicochemical properties, including particle size, poly-dispersity index, zeta-potential, and encapsulation efficiency. The present study showed that Soluplus® had the highest EE (%) and DL (%), the most appropriate size, and the lowest PDI. Nanoparticles < 200 nm have numerous drug delivery benefits and excellent micelle-forming ability. Small nanoparticles reduce the incidence of nonspecific interactions, including those that occur in the reticuloendothelial system. Secondly, the intravenous injection of micelles obviates the need for kidney excision and mitigates cancer accumulation via the EPR effect [40]. Also, by obtaining TEM data, we clearly showed that the nanoscale micelles we wanted were formed. All four polymers had negative zeta-potentials. Hence, they created electrostatic repulsion and remained safely within the physiological environment [41]. In vitro release profiles disclosed that the micelle formulation had 3-fold and 1.5-fold slower FEN release rates than the solution at 6 and 72 h, respectively. Micelle formulations can solubilize hydrophobic drugs and impede their rapid drug release, possibly because intermolecular interactions occur between the drug and the hydrophobic micelle core. The lipophilic moiety of Soluplus® consists of polyvinyl caprolactam-polyvinyl acetate, which should hydrophobically interact and form hydrogen bonds with FEN. The MTT assay confirmed the short-term (48 h) cytotoxicity of FEN. The difference between the IC$_{50}$ of free FEN and FEN-loaded Soluplus® micelles was ≈10% according to the MTT assay.

The IC$_{50}$ was slightly higher for the micelles than for the free drug as the former had a 48-h release rate of only 11.8%. Nevertheless, the micelles and their drug load were internalized, possibly through endocytosis [30,42]. Therefore, despite the low release rate, it is expected that the difference in effect was not large. The IC$_{50}$ for free FEN drug was 3070 nM (3.07 µM). Curcumin has an IC$_{50}$ range of 5.43–108.69 µM, and its anticancer action is downregulation of the BCL-2 family. 17-AAG has an IC$_{50}$ range of 0.1–2.37 µM, and its anticancer mechanism is the suppression of heat shock protein 90. Hence, the IC$_{50}$ of FEN indicates that the drug has sufficient anticancer efficacy [43–45]. The clonogenic assay confirmed the long-term inhibition of cell reproduction. It revealed that the FEN micellar formulation entirely inhibited colony formation at 1740 µM but was also effective at only 174 µM. Furthermore, both the size and PDI of the FEN-loaded Soluplus® micelles remained stable for two weeks at three temperatures. Therefore, this product is appropriate for long-term transport and storage in various situations. The FEN-loaded Soluplus® micelles also maintained stability at 37 °C. This is the temperature inside the body, and in terms of temperature, we may expect stability inside the body. The FEN-loaded Soluplus® micelles had superior pharmacokinetic parameters compared to the solution, including higher AUC and C$_0$. This is expected to be owing to the decrease in the volume of distribution and total clearance of FEN. Thus, FEN-loaded Soluplus® micelles may exhibit better bioavailability than the free FEN drug solution at equal doses. The biodistribution study indicated that lung damage could be responsible for the observed high pulmonary drug accumulation in the solution group. Cremophor EL® increased the total numbers of cells and macrophages in the lungs, which might suggest inflammation [46]. Therefore, the observed unknown lung injury may have induced localized FEN accumulation. For the in vivo toxicity assay, three commercially applied or extensively tested solubilizing agents were selected and compared against FEN-loaded Soluplus® micelles. However, all the products may induce side effects and could be hepatotoxic and/or neurotoxic. Here, the toxicity of these agents was adjudged by determining the reduction in body weight and survival rate in rats. In the solubilizing agent groups, ≥ 2 rats died. The tween80® group had the largest number of deaths with five. Three were killed in the DMA group and two in the Cremophor EL®/EtOH group. It is inferred that this death was caused by the toxicity of solubilizing agent. In contrast, none of the rats in the control and FEN-loaded Soluplus® micelles groups died and they presented with consistent weight gain. Therefore, the FEN-loaded Soluplus® micelles may be considered relatively low toxicity.

5. Conclusions

Here, we tested various excipients to solubilize the veterinary anthelmintic FEN. It was recently discovered that this drug also has anticancer efficacy. We selected the Soluplus® micelle by optimization experiments and evaluated its physicochemical properties including particle diameter, zeta-potential, encapsulation efficiency, and drug release. We also conducted pharmacokinetic and biodistribution studies on rats intravenously injected with FEN-loaded Soluplus® micelles. The micellar formulation had superior bioavailability compared to that of free FEN. The biodistribution results indicate that FEN solution is mainly distributed to the lungs and liver compared to other organs. In addition, FEN solution was more specifically distributed to the lungs than micelles. In vivo toxicity tests showed that the FEN-loaded Soluplus® micelle formulation was less toxic than FEN solubilized with other excipients. As FEN has already demonstrated anticancer efficacy, the nanoparticle formulation developed here merits further preclinical research. The ultimate objective is to conduct human clinical safety and efficacy trials on FEN-loaded Soluplus® micelles.

Supplementary Materials: The following are available online at http://www.mdpi.com/1999-4923/12/10/1000/s1, Figure S1: Representative chromatograms of fenbendazole (FEN) and genistein (internal standard [IS]) in stock solution and biological plasma sample.

Author Contributions: Conceptualization, I.S.J. and D.H.S.; methodology, I.S.J. and M.J.J.; software, I.S.J., M.J.J.; validation, I.S.J. and D.H.S.; formal analysis, I.S.J.; investigation, I.S.J.; resources, I.S.J.; data curation, I.S.J.; writing—original draft preparation, I.S.J.; writing—review and editing, I.S.J., M.J.J. and D.H.S. visualization, I.S.J.

and M.J.J.; supervision, C.-W.P., Y.B.C., J.-S.K.; project administration, I.S.J. and D.H.S. All authors have read and agreed to the published version of the manuscript.

Funding: This research was funded by the Basic Science Research Program through the National Research Foundation of Korea (NRF) funded by the Ministry of Education (NRF-2019R1C1C1009996).

Acknowledgments: The authors would like to thank Yu Jin lee, Moon Sup Yoon, Hee Ji Shin for their technical assistances.

Conflicts of Interest: The authors declare no conflict of interest.

References

1. An, G.; Murry, D.J.; Gajurel, K.; Bach, T.; Deye, G.; Stebounova, L.V.; Codd, E.E.; Horton, J.; Gonzalez, A.E.; Garcia, H.H.; et al. Pharmacokinetics, safety, and tolerability of oxfendazole in healthy volunteers: A randomized, placebo-controlled first-in-human single-dose escalation study. *Antimicrob. Agents Chemother.* **2019**, *63*, e02255-18. [CrossRef] [PubMed]
2. Duan, Q.; Liu, Y.; Rockwell, S. Fenbendazole as a potential anticancer drug. *Anticancer Res.* **2013**, *33*, 355–362. [PubMed]
3. Bai, R.-Y.; Staedtke, V.; Aprhys, C.M.; Gallia, G.L.; Riggins, G.J. Antiparasitic mebendazole shows survival benefit in 2 preclinical models of glioblastoma multiforme. *Neuro Oncol.* **2011**, *13*, 974–982. [CrossRef] [PubMed]
4. Gao, P.; Dang, C.V.; Watson, J. Unexpected antitumorigenic effect of fenbendazole when combined with supplementary vitamins. *J. Am. Assoc Lab. Anim. Sci.* **2008**, *47*, 37–40. [PubMed]
5. Lai, S.R.; Castello, S.A.; Robinson, A.C.; Koehler, J.W. In vitro anti-tubulin effects of mebendazole and fenbendazole on canine glioma cells. *Vet. Comp. Oncol.* **2017**, *15*, 1445–1454. [CrossRef] [PubMed]
6. Dogra, N.; Mukhopadhyay, T. Impairment of the ubiquitin-proteasome pathway by methyl N-(6-phenylsulfanyl-1H-benzimidazol-2-yl)carbamate leads to a potent cytotoxic effect in tumor cells: A novel antiproliferative agent with a potential therapeutic implication. *J. Biol. Chem.* **2012**, *287*, 30625–30640. [CrossRef] [PubMed]
7. Sasaki, J.-i.; Ramesh, R.; Chada, S.; Gomyo, Y.; Roth, J.A.; Mukhopadhyay, T. The anthelmintic drug mebendazole induces mitotic arrest and apoptosis by depolymerizing tubulin in non-small cell lung cancer cells. *Mol. Cancer Ther.* **2002**, *1*, 1201–1209.
8. Short, C.R.; Barker, S.A.; Hsieh, L.C.; Ou, S.-P.; McDowell, T. Disposition of fenbendazole in the rabbit. *Vet. Sci. Res. J.* **1988**, *44*, 215–219. [CrossRef]
9. Mckellar, Q.A.; Harrison, P.; Galbraith, E.A.; Inglis, H. Pharmacokinetics of fenbendazole in dogs. *J. Vet. Pharmacol. Ther.* **1990**, *13*, 386–392. [CrossRef]
10. Petersen, M.B.; Friis, C. Pharmacokinetics of fenbendazole following intravenous and oral administration to pigs. *Am. J. Vet. Res.* **2000**, *61*, 573–576. [CrossRef]
11. Amidon, G.L.; Lennernas, H.; Shah, V.P.; Crison, J.R. A theoretical basis for a biopharmaceutic drug classification: The correlation of in vitro drug product dissolution and in vivo bioavailability. *Pharm. Res.* **1995**, *12*, 413–420. [CrossRef] [PubMed]
12. Lipinski, C. Poor aqueous solubility—An industry wide problem in drug discovery. *Am. Pharm. Rev.* **2002**, *5*, 82–85.
13. Weiss, R.B.; Donehower, R.C.; Wiernik, P.H.; Ohnuma, T.; Gralla, R.J.; Trump, D.L.; Baker, J.R., Jr.; Van Echo, D.A.; Von Hoff, D.D.; Leyland-Jones, B. Hypersensitivity reactions from taxol. *Clin. Oncol.* **1990**, *8*, 1263–1268. [CrossRef] [PubMed]
14. Scripture, C.D.; Figg, W.D.; Sparreboom, A. Peripheral neuropathy induced by paclitaxel: Recent insights and future perspectives. *Curr. Neuropharmacol.* **2006**, *4*, 165–172. [CrossRef] [PubMed]
15. Dorr, R.T. Pharmacology and toxicology of cremophor EL diluent. *Ann. Pharmacother.* **1994**, *28*, S11–S14. [CrossRef]
16. Sun, H.; Yang, R.; Wang, J.; Yang, X.; Tu, J.; Xie, L.; Li, C.; Lao, Q.; Sun, C. Component-based biocompatibility and safety evaluation of polysorbate 80. *RSC Adv.* **2017**, *7*, 15127–15138. [CrossRef]
17. Craig, D.K.; Weir, R.J.; Wagner, W.; Groth, D. Subchronic Inhalation toxicity of dimethylformamide in rats and mice. *Drug Chem. Toxicol.* **1984**, *7*, 551–571. [CrossRef]

18. Baum, S.L.; Suruda, A.J. Toxic hepatitis from dimethylacetamide. *Int. J. Occup. Environ. Health* **1997**, *3*, 1–4. [CrossRef]
19. Horn, H.J. Toxicology of dimethylacetamide. *Toxicol. Appl. Pharmacol.* **1961**, *3*, 12–24. [CrossRef]
20. Mohammed, A.R.; Weston, N.; Coombes, A.G.A.; Fitzgerald, M.; Perrie, Y. Liposome formulation of poorly water soluble drugs: Optimisation of drug loading and ESEM analysis of stability. *Int. J. Pharm.* **2004**, *285*, 23–34. [CrossRef]
21. Kawakami, K.; Yoshikawa, T.; Moroto, Y.; Kanaoka, E.; Takahashi, K.; Nishihara, Y.; Masuda, K. Microemulsion formulation for enhanced absorption of poorly soluble drugs: I. Prescription design. *J. Control. Release* **2002**, *81*, 65–74. [CrossRef]
22. Cho, H.; Lai, T.C.; Tomoda, K.; Kwon, G.S. Polymeric micelles for multi-drug delivery in cancer. *AAPS PharmSciTech.* **2015**, *16*, 10–20. [CrossRef] [PubMed]
23. Zhao, J.; Xu, Y.; Wang, C.; Ding, Y.; Chen, M.; Wang, Y.; Peng, J.; Li, L.; Lv, L. Soluplus/TPGS mixed micelles for dioscin delivery in cancer therapy. *Drug Dev. Ind. Pharm.* **2017**, *43*, 1197–1204. [CrossRef] [PubMed]
24. Fang, J.; Nakamura, H.; Maeda, H. The EPR effect: Unique features of tumor blood vessels for drug delivery, factors involved, and limitations and augmentation of the effect. *Adv. Drug Deliv. Rev.* **2011**, *63*, 136–151. [CrossRef]
25. Kwon, G.S.; Okano, T. Polymeric micelles as new drug carriers. *Adv. Drug Deliv. Rev.* **1996**, *21*, 107–116. [CrossRef]
26. Shin, H.-C.; Alani, A.W.G.; Rao, D.A.; Rockich, N.C.; Kwon, G.S. Multi-drug loaded polymeric micelles for simultaneous delivery of poorly soluble anticancer drugs. *J. Control. Release* **2009**, *140*, 294–300. [CrossRef]
27. Jo, M.J.; Jo, Y.H.; Lee, Y.J.; Park, C.W.; Kim, J.S.; Hong, J.T.; Chung, Y.B.; Lee, M.K.; Shin, D.H. Physicochemical, pharmacokinetic, and toxicity evaluation of methoxy poly(ethylene glycol)-*b*-poly(d,l-lactide) polymeric micelles encapsulating alpinumisoflavone extracted from unripe Cudrania tricuspidata fruit. *Pharmaceutics* **2019**, *11*, 366. [CrossRef]
28. Thomas, H.; Coley, H.M. Overcoming multidrug resistance in cancer: An update on the clinical strategy of inhibiting P-glycoprotein. *Cancer Control.* **2003**, *10*, 159–165. [CrossRef]
29. Jin, X.; Zhou, B.; Xue, L.; San, W. Soluplus micelles as a potential drug delivery system for reversal of resistant tumor. *Biomed. Pharmacother.* **2015**, *69*, 388–395. [CrossRef]
30. Zhang, W.; Shi, Y.; Chen, Y.; Yu, S.; Hao, J.; Luo, J.; Sha, X.; Fang, X. Enhanced antitumor efficacy by paclitaxel-loaded pluronic P123/F127 mixed micelles against non-small cell lung cancer based on passive tumor targeting and modulation of drug resistance. *Eur. J. Pharm. Biopharm.* **2010**, *75*, 341–353. [CrossRef]
31. Miyata, K.; Kakizawa, Y.; Nishiyama, N.; Yamasaki, Y.; Watanabe, T.; Kohara, M.; Kataoka, K. Freeze-dried formulations for in vivo gene delivery of PEGylated polyplex micelles with disulfide crosslinked cores to the liver. *J. Control. Release* **2005**, *109*, 15–23. [CrossRef] [PubMed]
32. Tam, Y.T.; Repp, L.; Ma, Z.-X.; Feltenberger, J.B.; Kwon, G.S. Oligo(lactic acid)8-rapamycin prodrug-loaded poly(ethylene glycol)-block-poly(lactic acid) micelles for injection. *Pharm. Res.* **2019**, *36*, 70. [CrossRef]
33. Cho, H.; Lai, T.C.; Kwon, G.S. Poly(ethylene glycol)-block-poly(ε-caprolactone) micelles for combination drug delivery: Evaluation of paclitaxel, cyclopamine and gossypol in intraperitoneal xenograft models of ovarian cancer. *J. Control. Release* **2013**, *166*, 1–9. [CrossRef] [PubMed]
34. Tam, Y.T.; Shin, D.H.; Chen, K.E.; Kwon, G.S. Poly(ethylene glycol)-block-poly(d,l-lactic acid) micelles containing oligo(lactic acid)8-paclitaxel prodrug: In vivo conversion and antitumor efficacy. *J. Control. Release* **2019**, *298*, 186–193. [CrossRef]
35. Kim, H.J.; Shin, D.H.; Lim, E.A.; Kim, J.-S. Sustained-release formulation of sarpogrelate hydrochloride. *Arch. Pharmacal Res.* **2015**, *38*, 35–41. [CrossRef]
36. Shin, D.H.; Park, S.H.; Jeong, S.W.; Park, C.-W.; Han, K.; Chung, Y.B. Hepatic uptake of epirubicin by isolated rat hepatocytes and its biliary excretion after intravenous infusion in rats. *Arch. Pharm. Res.* **2014**, *37*, 1599–1606. [CrossRef] [PubMed]
37. Toth, L.A. Defining the moribund condition as an experimental endpoint for animal research. *ILAR J.* **2000**, *41*, 72–79. [CrossRef]
38. Shin, D.H.; Kwon, G.S. Epothilone B-based 3-in-1 polymeric micelle for anticancer drug therapy. *Int. J. Pharm.* **2017**, *518*, 307–311. [CrossRef] [PubMed]
39. Forrest, M.L.; Won, C.-Y.; Malick, A.W.; Kwon, G.S. In vitro release of the mTOR inhibitor rapamycin from poly(ethylene glycol)-*b*-poly(ε-caprolactone) micelles. *J. Control. Release* **2006**, *110*, 370–377. [CrossRef]

40. Maeda, H.; Wu, J.; Sawa, T.; Matsumura, Y.; Hori, K. Tumor vascular permeability and the EPR effect in macromolecular therapeutics: A review. *J. Control. Release* **2000**, *65*, 271–284. [CrossRef]
41. Qin, Z.; Chen, T.; Teng, W.; Jin, Q.; Ji, J. Mixed-charged zwitterionic polymeric micelles for tumor acidic environment responsive intracellular drug delivery. *Langmuir ACS J. Surf. Colloids* **2019**, *35*, 1242–1248. [CrossRef] [PubMed]
42. Liu, Z.; Liu, D.; Wang, L.; Zhang, J.; Zhang, N. Docetaxel-loaded pluronic p123 polymeric micelles: In vitro and in vivo evaluation. *Int. J. Mol. Sci.* **2011**, *12*, 1684–1696. [CrossRef] [PubMed]
43. Kuttan, G.; Kumar, K.B.; Guruvayoorappan, C.; Kuttan, R. Antitumor, anti-invasion, and antimetastatic effects of curcumin. *Adv. Exp. Med. Biol.* **2007**, *595*, 173–184. [PubMed]
44. Ui, T.; Morishima, K.; Saito, S.; Sakuma, Y.; Fujii, H.; Hosoya, Y.; Ishikawa, S.; Aburatani, H.; Fukayama, M.; Niki, T.; et al. The HSP90 inhibitor 17-N-allylamino-17-demethoxy geldanamycin (17-AAG) synergizes with cisplatin and induces apoptosis in cisplatin-resistant esophageal squamous cell carcinoma cell lines via the Akt/XIAP pathway. *Oncol. Rep.* **2014**, *31*, 619–624. [CrossRef]
45. Shin, D.H.; Kwon, G.S. Pre-clinical evaluation of a themosensitive gel containing epothilone B and mTOR/Hsp90 targeted agents in an ovarian tumor model. *J. Control. Release* **2017**, *268*, 176–183. [CrossRef]
46. Luo, T.; Loira-Pastoriza, C.; Patil, H.P.; Ucakar, B.; Muccioli, G.G.; Bosquillon, C.; Vanbever, R. PEGylation of paclitaxel largely improves its safety and anti-tumor efficacy following pulmonary delivery in a mouse model of lung carcinoma. *J. Control. Release* **2016**, *239*, 62–71. [CrossRef]

Publisher's Note: MDPI stays neutral with regard to jurisdictional claims in published maps and institutional affiliations.

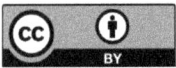

© 2020 by the authors. Licensee MDPI, Basel, Switzerland. This article is an open access article distributed under the terms and conditions of the Creative Commons Attribution (CC BY) license (http://creativecommons.org/licenses/by/4.0/).

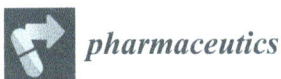

Review

Nanodelivery Systems Targeting Epidermal Growth Factor Receptors for Glioma Management

Sathishbabu Paranthaman [1], Meghana Goravinahalli Shivananjegowda [1], Manohar Mahadev [1], Afrasim Moin [2], Shivakumar Hagalavadi Nanjappa [3], Nandakumar Dalavaikodihalli Nanjaiyah [4], Saravana Babu Chidambaram [5] and Devegowda Vishakante Gowda [1,*]

[1] Department of Pharmaceutics, JSS College of Pharmacy, JSS Academy of Higher Education and Research, Mysuru 570015, India; psathishbabu@jssuni.edu.in (S.P.); gsmeghana@jssuni.edu.in (M.G.S.); mmanohar@jssuni.edu.in (M.M.)
[2] Department of Pharmaceutics, Hail University, Hail PO BOX 2440, Saudi Arabia; a.moinuddin@uoh.edu.sa
[3] Department of Pharmaceutics, KLE College of Pharmacy, Bangalore 590010, India; shivakumarhn@gmail.com
[4] Department of Neurochemistry, National Institute of Mental Health and Neuroscience, Bangalore 560029, India; nandakumardn@nimhans.ac.in
[5] Department of Pharmacology, JSS College of Pharmacy, JSS Academy of Higher Education and Research, Mysuru 570015, India; saravanababu.c@jssuni.edu.in
* Correspondence: dvgowda@jssuni.edu.in; Tel.: +91-9663162455

Received: 30 September 2020; Accepted: 18 October 2020; Published: 10 December 2020

Abstract: A paradigm shift in treating the most aggressive and malignant form of glioma is continuously evolving; however, these strategies do not provide a better life and survival index. Currently, neurosurgical debulking, radiotherapy, and chemotherapy are the treatment options available for glioma, but these are non-specific in action. Patients invariably develop resistance to these therapies, leading to recurrence and death. Receptor Tyrosine Kinases (RTKs) are among the most common cell surface proteins in glioma and play a significant role in malignant progression; thus, these are currently being explored as therapeutic targets. RTKs belong to the family of cell surface receptors that are activated by ligands which in turn activates two major downstream signaling pathways via Rapidly Accelerating Sarcoma/mitogen activated protein kinase/extracellular-signal-regulated kinase (Ras/MAPK/ERK) and phosphatidylinositol 3-kinase/a serine/threonine protein kinase/mammalian target of rapamycin (PI3K/AKT/mTOR). These pathways are critically involved in regulating cell proliferation, invasion, metabolism, autophagy, and apoptosis. Dysregulation in these pathways results in uncontrolled glioma cell proliferation, invasion, angiogenesis, and cancer progression. Thus, RTK pathways are considered a potential target in glioma management. This review summarizes the possible risk factors involved in the growth of glioblastoma (GBM). The role of RTKs inhibitors (TKIs) and the intracellular signaling pathways involved, small molecules under clinical trials, and the updates were discussed. We have also compiled information on the outcomes from the various endothelial growth factor receptor (EGFR)–TKIs-based nanoformulations from the preclinical and clinical points of view. Aided by an extensive literature search, we propose the challenges and potential opportunities for future research on EGFR–TKIs-based nanodelivery systems.

Keywords: glioblastoma; receptor tyrosine kinases; epidermal growth factor receptor; small molecule inhibitors; nanoformulations

1. Introduction

Gliomas are the most common and lethal solid brain tumors and are known to affect about 0.02% of the worldwide population [1]. The occurrence of malignant gliomas and the frequency of cancer deaths have increased at an amplified rate across the world [2]. More than 330,000 new Central Nervous system (CNS) tumor cases and 227,000 brain cancer-related deaths were documented globally in the Global Burden of Disease (GBD) 2016 tumor database [3]. Despite the increase in cancer awareness programs, advancement in diagnostic tools, and treatment strategies in the United States, the prevalence of gliomas has been unstoppable [4–6].

Based on the molecular characteristics and origin of apparent cell types, the CNS tumors were classified using I to IV grade criteria by the World Health Organization (WHO) in 2007 and 2016 [7]. Accordingly, Grade, I, II, III, and IV are pilocytic astrocytomas, gliomas including diffuse astrocytomas, anaplastic astrocytomas, and glioblastoma multiforme (GBM), respectively [8,9]. The current standard treatment approaches across the world are dependent on surgery, radiotherapy, and chemotherapeutic drugs, i.e., temozolomide (TMZ), which resulted in the average survival rate of about 14 months [10–12]. Therefore, there is a definite need for understanding the molecular pathways and mechanisms involved in GBM pathology and thereby determine better management [13].

Generally, Receptor Tyrosine Kinase (RTKs) are commonly identified cell surface receptors that are considered to be pivotal regulators of critical cellular processes (epidermal growth factor receptor (EGFR) and vascular endothelial growth factor receptor (VEGFR)). EGFR is a transmembrane receptor tyrosine kinase that controls cancer cell proliferation, migration, differentiation, and homeostasis [14]. Nearly 50–60% of GBMs have EGFR genetic variants, with mutations, readjustments, selective linking, and amplification [15].

Over the past decades, many investigators have hundreds of designs and synthesized small molecular drugs as RTK inhibitors with extensive research. The Food and Drug Administration (FDA) has approved a few medications as first-line therapy for various forms of cancer (Table 1) [16]. However, the significant development of anti-cancer components has developed new problems [17]. For example, clinical studies that were conducted for the first and second generation of anti-EGFR drugs on the inhibition of cell growth, angiogenesis, and proliferation were found to be of no therapeutic benefit in GBM treatment. Many researchers also reported significant limitations such as low solubility, poor oral bioavailability, and severe adverse effects in the existing EGFR–TKIs drugs. In addition, the gradual rise of drug resistance during therapy instantly needs to be addressed [18]. The third generation of EGFR–TKIs drug (AZD9291) was developed recently and confirmed to have an effective preclinical investigation in GBM the in vitro and in vivo models' above-listed drawbacks [15]. The advantages of nanotechnology offer a potential drug delivery approach with apparent benefits of nanoformulations such as lesser particle size, bulky surface area, excellent surface reactivity, active sites, and appropriate adsorption ability. Nano particles (NPs) applied as drug transporters have the potential to increase drug absorption and bioavailability, enrich effective targeting delivery, prolong the circulation time, and limit the dangerous side effects on healthy tissues [19].

In the present review, the authors have summarized epidemiology and risk factors associated with GBM, RTKs, and their inhibitors of intracellular signaling pathways in glioma, the clinical profile of small molecule inhibitors (EGFR–TKIs) drugs, and the associated multiple failures/resistance. In addition, the current progressive research of various nanopreparations for EGFR–TKIs and the combination of chemotherapeutic drugs to target GBM have been discussed. Aided by an extensive literature search and review, the authors have also proposed the possibilities and challenges for upcoming research on EGFR-TKIs and other chemotherapeutic agents.

Table 1. Approved small molecular tyrosine kinase inhibitors for cancer therapy [16,19].

Drugs	IC_{50} (nmol/L)	Targeting Receptor	Disease
Gefitinib (Iressa®)	14.6	EGFR	NSCLC, pancreatic cancer
Erlotinib (Tarceva®)	2		
Icotinib (Conmana®)	45		
Lapatinib (Tykerb®)	10.8, 9.2	EGFR, HER2	Breast cancer
Neratinib (Nerlynx®)	92, 59	EGFR, HER2	NSCLC, breast cancer
Afatinib (Gilotrif®)	0.5	EGFR, HER2 14	NSCLC, breast cancer, squamous cell carcinoma of the head and neck
Imatinib (Glivec®, Gleevec®)	600, 100	Abl, PDGFR, Kit SRC, PDGFR	CML, CMML, GIST
Dasatinib (Sprycel®)	<10		CML resistant to imatinib
Nilotinib (Tasigna®)	<30		CML resistant to imatinib
Sunitinib (Sutent®)	<100	VEGFR1-3, PDGFR, Kit FLT3, RET, CSF1R GIST, BRAF	Advanced RCC, CML resistant to imatinib, Hepatocellular carcinoma
Sorafenib (Nexavar®)	<100		
Pazopanib (Votrient®)	<150		

2. Molecular Pathology of Glioma

Different genetic investigations determine various noteworthy biomarkers. Many of these were utilized in neuro-oncology to identify glioma patients, specifically the combined losses of the chromosome arms 1p and 19q in oligodendroglial cancer. Then, the methylation status of O-6 methylguanine–DNA methyltransferase gene promoter and modifications in the EGFR pathway in GBM, isocitrate dehydrogenase 1 (IDH1) and IDH2 gene mutations in diffuse gliomas, as well as B-Raf status in pilocytic astrocytomas. These groups are associated with different prognosis, germline variants, and the median age at diagnosis, highlighting different pathogenic mechanisms [20]. Although most GBM patients receive standard treatments, significant variations in clinical outcomes are often seen due to the heterogeneity of the tumors [21,22]. Hence, it is essential to determine more significant and practical biomarkers for analyzing the prognosis in GBM patients. Inflammation and immunity are critically involved in glioma initiation and progression [23,24], and various study reports suggested that inflammatory response cells such as neutrophils [25], lymphocytes [26], and platelets [27] are associated with the prognosis of cancer patients. In recent years, the prognostic value of preoperative hematological markers, such as albumin-to-globulin ratio (AGR), monocyte-to-lymphocyte ratio (MLR), median platelet volume (MPV), neutrophil-to-lymphocyte ratio (NLR), platelet distribution width (PDW), and platelet-to-lymphocyte ratio (PLR), have been investigated in several cancers, including gliomas [28–32]. However, there were no scientific investigations to the prognostic value of hematological biomarkers in a cohort of gliomas, mainly in relation to the various molecular classes. Therefore, a study examined the predictive value of preoperative hematological biomarkers (AGR, MLR, MPV, NLR, PDW, and PLR) alone and in combination with the five glioma molecular groups on the clinical trial results of a comparatively great cohort (n = 592) of Grade II–IV GBM patients. Based on these results, we suggest an analytical model for Grade II–IV GBM based on molecular pathology and NLR, and identify for lower-grade gliomas (LGG) four risk groups with distinct overall survival [33].

3. Epidemiology and Risk Factors of Glioma

In the past few decades, the investigation of adult glioma was prioritized because of a lesser global incidence of GBM, i.e., 10 per 100,000 people. Due to the lack of new and efficient diagnostic strategies, the survival rate (SR) of 15 months after diagnosis creates a critical public health problem [2,34,35]. GBM accounts for 50% of all gliomas in various age groups [36]. Although the peak incidence is between 55 and 60 years of age, GBM could occur at any age, with a mortality rate of 2.5% of the worldwide cancer death toll. GBM accounts for the third foremost cause of deaths due to cancer in patients from 15 to 34 years [37,38]. The GBM incidence ratio was more in men when compared to females [39]. The Western world reported a higher incidence of gliomas than less developed countries, which could be recognized as due to under-recording glioma cases, narrow contact to health care, and alterations in diagnostic practices [40–42]. A few studies showed that blacks were less prone to GBM. Further, the incidence of GBM was reported to be higher in Asians, Latinos, and Whites [43].

The current global standard for the catalog and identification of gliomas is as per WHO classification. WHO categorizes gliomas as Grade I to IV based on malignancy level, which is committed by the histopathological measures. Class I to III gliomas relay to abrasions with less proliferative potential and can be managed surgically with chemo and/or radiotherapy. In contrast, Grade IV gliomas are highly malignant and invasive. GBM is the utmost aggressive, offensive, and identical type of cancer and was labeled as Grade IV [44].

A positive family history, absence of atrophic conditions, longer length of leukocyte telomere, and risk alleles at more than twenty genetic loci are a few of the endogenous factors that enhance glioma risk. A high dose of ionizing radiation is also one of the environmental factors attributed to a higher risk of glioma [45]. Identifying modifiable factors that would enable primary prevention approaches remain the quintessential goal of glioma epidemiologic research.

Several studies on the allergic and nutritional epidemiology of glioma showed an inverse association between allergy and gliomas but did not provide any causal relationship between them [46]. The nutritional epidemiology studies suggested that various food groups and nutrients were associated with glioma risk; the results were inconclusive and not replicable in subsequent research [24,47]. The results of epidemiological analysis also suggested the presence of an inverse association between cancer and certain neurological conditions, mainly age-related neurodegenerative diseases [48]. In recent research, a potent negative association was observed between the expression levels of microRNAs in GBM than Alzheimer's disease (AD), suggesting that although the molecular pathways behind the development of these two pathologies are the same, they appear to be inversely controlled by microRNAs [49]. Another epidemiological study indicated that the patients suffering from AD have a lower risk of developing lung cancer (LC) and suggest a higher risk of developing GBM [50].

4. Receptors Tyrosine Kinase (RTK) and Their Inhibitors of Intracellular Signaling Pathways in Glioma

RTKs belong to the family of cell surface receptors and are receptors for hormones, growth factors, neurotrophic factors, cytokines, and extracellular signaling molecules. The tyrosine kinase (TK) comprises the intracellular TK domain, extracellular ligand-binding domain, and a hydrophobic transmembrane domain. The domains as mentioned above get activated upon binding of the ligand, leading to the TK domain's autophosphorylation and dimerization. This receptor, when activated by ligands in turn, activates two downstream signaling pathways, Rapidly Accelerating Sarcoma/mitogen activated protein kinase/extracellular-signal-regulated kinase (Ras/MAPK/ERK) and phosphatidylinositol 3-kinase/a serine/threonine protein kinase/mammalian target of rapamycin (PI3K/AKT/mTOR) [51] (Figure 1), which play a prominent role in cell differentiation, survival, proliferation, and angiogenesis. Thus, RTKs and their ligands were proven to be promising targets in the treatment of GBM. Among the several receptors belonging to the RTK group in human glioma, the signaling pathways such as EGFR and VEGF receptor mutations have played a significant role in GBM described below in detail [52].

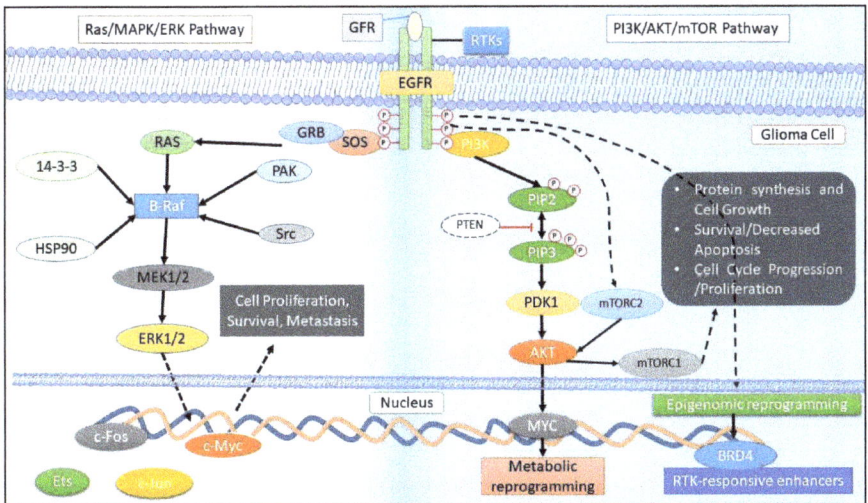

Figure 1. Schematic representation of Receptor Tyrosine Kinases (RTK) activation and the downstream signaling. RTKs, particularly epidermal growth factor receptors (EGFR), are amplified in glioblastoma, which significantly alters the nutrient uptake and utilization. The Rapidly Accelerating Sarcoma/mitogen activated protein kinase/extracellular-signal-regulated kinase (Ras/MAPK/ERK) and phosphatidylinositol 3-kinase/a serine/threonine protein kinase/mammalian target of rapamycin (PI3K/AKT/mTOR) pathways get activated through the stimulation by growth factor receptor (GFR). Physiologically, these two pathways orchestrate to execute cell proliferation, survival, motility, adhesion, and angiogenesis. Any deregulation in these pathways leads to an activation of oncogenic signaling cascades causing glioma.

4.1. EGFR Family and Its Mutations

RTKs that generally control the proliferation, migration, and differentiation of neural progenitors via signaling EGFR and its downstream MAPK and PI3K/AKT/mTOR pathways (Figure 1) [17]. EGFR, a member of the ErbB family, is commonly expressed in neural progenitors during brain growth and initiated stem cell astrocytes and transit-amplifying cells in the adult rodent subventricular zone (SVZ) [53,54]. Among 45–57% of GBM patients, the mutation and amplification in EGFR ErbB1 (EGFR, HER1) were detected, which indicated its major role in the pathogenesis of GBM [55,56]. In addition, about 8–41% of GBM patients showed mutations in erythroblastic oncogenic B/human epidermal growth factor receptor (ErbB2/HER-2) [55,57]. Its expression reduces significantly in the adult human cortex (Cx) and white matter (WM) under non-reactive conditions but is retained within the adult human SVZ astrocyte ribbon. The mechanisms maintaining more EGFR expression in human neural growth and its silencing upon difference are not well understood and not have been investigated before at the epigenetic level [58]. Excitingly, the most diffuse gliomas of LGG and high-grade glioma (HGG) have shown the pathological expression of EGFR. Generally, EGFR overexpression in gliomas has been mainly recognized to gene amplification, the activating mutation EGFRvIII, and gene fusion events, which overall comprise approximately half of GBM and are rarely observed in LGG [59,60]. EGFRvIII, a truncated species, is often expressed in GBM and independently activated by a ligand, resulting in cell survival and proliferation. Despite the growth-enhancing properties of the EGFRvIII, its expression has been linked to the increasing overall survival of patients. Furthermore, EGFRvIII, being a neoantigen, equally elicits an immune response [60,61]. Recent investigations have started to explore EGFR overexpression mechanisms in gliomas outside of genetic alterations, including the role of epigenetics. Still, there is no study that has analyzed the EGFR promoter in human glioma samples.

4.2. VEGF Family and Its Mutations

VEGF, a potent angiogenic protein, is known to enhance vascular permeability. Although VEGF has a role in normal tissues, malignant transformation has been shown to induce VEGF expression—especially under hypoxic conditions inducing the transcription factors (HIF1α and HIF1β) to translocate to the nucleus, thereby activating the VEGF gene [61] (Figure 1). Upon activation of the VEGF gene, angiogenesis is enhanced to neutralize the hypoxia. GBM tumors enhanced the expression of VEGF and hypoxia, which in turn caused irregular vasculature [62]. The enhanced expression of VEGF in GBM tissues was due to the up-regulation of the VEGF receptor, VEGFR2, which acted by RAS (Rapidly Accelerating Sarcoma) or PI3K (phosphatidylinositol 3-kinase) or the PLCγ–PKC–MAPK pathway in contrast to RTKs [63]. VEGFR3 operates similarly to TK activities. The PKC and RAS pathway is known to be stimulated by lymphangiogenesis in VEGFR-3. VEGF was also shown to play a vital role in vascularization and endothelial cells' neoplastic growth [64].

5. Molecular Drug Therapy Targets and Its Clinical Profile of EGFR Family in Glioma

5.1. Small-Molecule Kinase Inhibitors

Various active components prevent the EGFR activity, and its ligands have been under progress since the starting of this era. Small molecular EGFR protein tyrosine kinase inhibitors (EGFR–TKIs) have become the most innovative active component in anti-cancer management [52]. EGFR–TKIs are a 4-anilinoquinazoline structure that could covalently link with the ATP binding site of the RTK to procedure the dynamic conformation. The initiation loop was phosphorylated and consequently inhibited the phosphorylation of TK (Figure 2) [65].

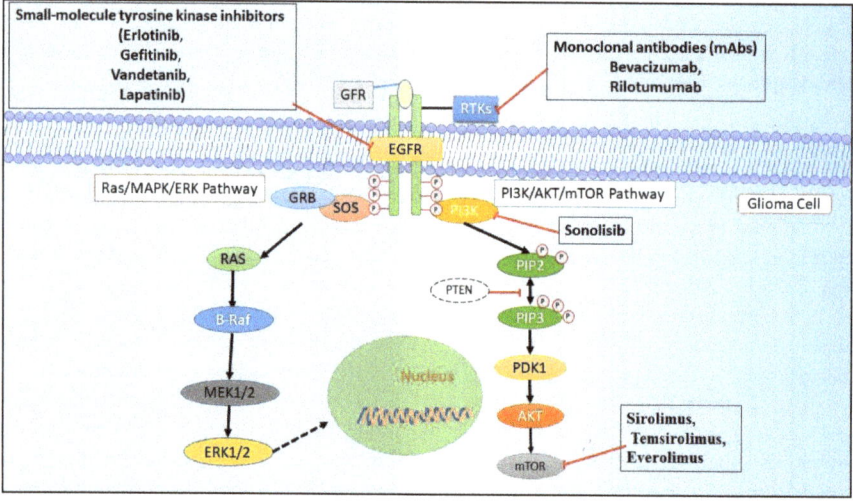

Figure 2. RTKs (EGFR) signal transduction and are a target site for small molecule and monoclonal antibody in glioma treatment. Small-molecule tyrosine kinase inhibitors block the downstream signaling by competing for ATP at the catalytic site of the kinase domain whilst the monoclonal antibodies (mAbs), which have an outstanding degree of specificity, block downstream signaling by binding to the leucine-rich and cysteine-rich ectodomains. Compounds that inhibit mammalian target of rapamycin (mTOR), a downstream signal in the EGFR pathway, facilitate the autophagic clearance of cancerous cells.

Erlotinib, an EGFR-TKI drug, prevents the phosphorylation of the TK intracellular domain of EGFR [66]. Several phase II studies for GBM were not efficient in recurrent GBM [67] patients. In contrast,

Erlotinib's combination therapy with temozolamide was well tolerated and enhanced the survival rate in the newly diagnosed GBM patients [68,69]. Gefitinib (ZD1839/Iressa®), another EGFR–TKI, radio sensitized U251 GBM cells in vitro [70]. Still, there was no improvement in the survival rate shown in the phase II clinical trial with newly diagnosed GBM patients [71]. AEE788 and Vandetanib inhibited both EGFR and VEGFR TK (Table 2), but when tested on GBM, patients showed lesser efficacy or enhanced toxicity. AEE788, in a phase I clinical trial, exhibited less efficacy and higher toxicity in treating recurrent GBM patients [72]. Although AEE788 showed very little efficacy in an in vitro GBM cell line, it decreased cell proliferation in vitro when administered in combination with histone deacetylase inhibitors (HDACIs) [73]. In a phase II trial, when incorporated into the standard regimen (surgery + chemotherapy + radiotherapy), AEE788 showed no/little effects, due to which the study was terminated [74].

Lapatinib, an inhibitor of both EGFR and HER2 TKs, showed little effect in a phase I/II clinical trial [75], but in combination therapy with CUDC-101, an HDAC inhibitor, it enhanced the radiosensitivity of the GBM cell line in vitro [76]. Few VEGFR–TKIs such as vatalanib (PTK787), sorafenib, and tivozanib showed lesser efficacy when individually administered (Table 2). Vatalanib and tivozanib did not affect the tumor volume; however, they were well tolerated in a phase II trial [77,78]. Sorafenib's combination therapy with the standard regimen had little effect on recurrent GBM patients in a phase II trial [79]. A phase III trial of Cediranib (AZD2171), another VEGFR–TKI, failed to improve the progression-free survival, both in monotherapy and lomustine recurrent GBM patients [80].

5.2. Targeting Extracellular Domain of RTKs through Antibody Therapies

Among the various therapies targeted toward the kinase domains of RTK, the extracellular domain also served as a probable target for antibody therapy. The antibodies antagonized the ligand-binding site of RTKs, preventing the ligand binding and thereby activating the kinase domains [81]. An EGFR targeting the antibody cetuximab showed antagonistic activity by inhibiting the activation of RTKs, which in turn inhibited the tumor malignancy [82]. The antibody was used as rescue therapy in patients who have not responded to standard treatment. In addition, cetuximab monotherapy was well tolerated, and minimal recurrence of GBM was reported by a phase II clinical trial [83]. Another monoclonal antibody (mAb), ornartuzumab, targeting the hepatocyte growth factor receptor/tyrosine-protein kinase Met (HGFR/c-MET) receptor's extracellular domain was reported to prevent the cancer growth in orthotopic U87 GBM xenograft. MK-0646 (H7C10/F50035/dalotuzumab), a humanized monoclonal insulin-like growth factor receptor type 1 (IGF-1R) antibody, was shown to be an antagonist that decreased cell proliferation and induced apoptosis [84].

The antibody therapies are still in the preliminary stages of investigation and are promising therapeutic targets for GBM compared to the small molecule kinase inhibitors [85,86]. In addition, the primary constraint faced in the antibody therapy was the Blood Brain Barrier (BBB) penetrability and the large size of molecules, which could be overcome by engineered antibodies capable of penetrating the BBB [87]. Antibodies binding with the transferrin receptors were used to cross the BBB in both murine and primate models. On the other hand, using Ommaya reservoirs or during surgery, the antibodies could directly be delivered to the brain, bypassing the BBB [88].

Table 2. Ongoing trials targeting the EGFR in glioblastoma (GBM).

Drug	GBM	Phase	Characteristics	NCT No.
Small-Molecule Kinase Inhibitors and/or Combination with Other Therapy				
GC1118	R	II	Focuses on overall response rate and exploration of predictive/prognostic biomarkers	NCT03618667
Osimertinib Fludeoxyglucose F-18 (FDG)	R	II	Studied the intra-patient variability of tumor FDG uptake, which was determined using double baseline FDG PET prior to osimertinib exposure	NCT03732352
EGFR BATs with SOC RT and TMZ	R	I	Immune measures in blood anti-GBM cytotoxicity of peripheral blood mononuclear cells directed at GBM cell lines	NCT03344250
Dacomitinib	C	II	Progression-free survival (PFS) at six months (PFS6m) and Safety and tolerability of oral administration of PF-00299804.	NCT01520870
Temozolomide, ABT-414, Radiation	A, NR	II III	Overall Survival (OS)	NCT02573324
EGFR(V)-EDV-Dox	R	I	Overall Survival (OS) and identification of recommended phase 2 dose of EGFR(V)-EDV-Dox in subjects with recurrent GBM	NCT02766699
C225-ILs-dox	R	I	Tumor response achieved in the treatment phase was assessed as per RANO criteria	NCT03603379
Protein expression analysis	C	-	Overall survival and the free survival was predicted based on the molecular characteristics	NCT00897663
EGFRvIII-CARs	R	I	Assessment of T cell trafficking within the brain tumor	NCT03283631
EGFRBi Armed Autologous T Cells	W	I II	Overall survival, change of cytokine profile, incident toxicity, and the overall survival was assessed as per the National Cancer Institute Common Terminology Criteria for Adverse Events Version 4.0	NCT02521090
Erlotinib hydrochloride	T	II	Disease response measured objectively by MRI of brain duration of progression-free survival (PFS)	NCT00387894
Radiation, temozolomide depatuxizumab mafodotin	A, NR	III	Cumulative dose of depatuxizumab mafodotin	NCT03419403
Gefitinib + Radiation therapy	C	I II	Overall survival by EGFR status	NCT00052208
Cetuximab, Mannitol	R	I II	Composite overall response rate was assessed through RANO	NCT02861898
AMG 596	R	I	Number of subject with treatment-emergent adverse events	NCT03296696
AMG 596	C	I	Overall survival and anti-AMG 595 antibody formation	NCT01475006

Table 2. Cont.

Drug	GBM	Phase	Characteristics	NCT No.
PI3K/ART/mTOR				
PX-866	C	II	Measurement of progression and response of brain tumor using MRI or CT scan	NCT01259869
INC280	T	I, II	Number of Patients Reporting Dose Limiting Toxicities (DLTs) in Phase 1 and Phase II Surgical Arm: Concentrations of INC280 and Buparlisib in Tumor	NCT01870726
XL765 (SAR 245409) + XL147 (SAR 245408)	C	I	To assess the biological effect and PI3K/mTOR modulations of XL 765 and XL 147 in GBM tissue	NCT01240460
BKM120 + Surgery	C	II	BKM120 brain plasma ratio at time of surgery	NCT01339052
MK-3475 + PI3K/AKT Inhibitors	#	I, II	Progression-free survival	NCT02430363
GDC-0084 + Radio Therapy	R	I	To estimate the maximum tolerated dose (MTD) or RP2D of GDC-0084 after radiation therapy (RT)	NCT03696355
AZD2014	A, NR	I	Recommended phase II dose (RP2D) of AZD2014	NCT02619864
GDC-0084	R	II	Dose-limiting toxicities (DLTs)	NCT03522298
AZD8055	C	I	Establishment of MTD of AZD8055 with recurrent gliomas	NCT01316809
GDC-0084 + Radiation Therapy	R	I	To estimate the MTD or RP2D of GDC-0084 after RT	NCT03696355
CC-115	A, NR	I	To determine the MTD, Non-tolerated dose and Dose-Limiting Toxicity	NCT01353625

R—Recruiting, C—Completed, A—Active, NR—Not Recruiting, T—Terminated, W—Withdrawn, and #—Study has passed its completion date and status has not been verified in more than two years.

5.3. Therapies Directed at RTK Ligands

Antibodies not only bind to the extracellular domains but also are capable of trapping the ligands that activate the RTK signaling pathways [89]. Targeting the ligands might serve as an attractive means for GBM therapy. However, the usage of antibody was reduced due to various factors such as mutations in EGFRvIII and the inability to cross the BBB, which limited the tumor penetration and efficacy of the therapy. Bevacizumab, a humanized murine mAb, was reported to bind to VEGF and prevent it from binding to the receptor [90]. Bevacizumab was granted accelerated approval by the FDA in 2009; however, the drug demonstrated reduced efficacy against the newly diagnosed GBM and had no benefit on the patient's overall survival [91]. Aflibercept, another trap for VEGF, prevented its binding to the receptor, and recurrent GBM patients were proven to have only 7.7% of participants resulting in progression-free survival rates after six months in a phase II trial. Rilotumumab (AMG102), an anti-HGF mAb, was shown to bind to HGF, thus preventing the binding to the HGFR/c-MET and thereby activating downstream targets. In combination with temozolomide in vitro, rilotumumab was shown to inhibit the growth of U87MG glioblastoma cells. The combination showed only minimal effects on GBM in the phase II clinical trial [18].

5.4. Targeting Downstream Pathway of EGFR

A comprehensively studied downstream pathway of EGFR is the PI3K/AKT/mTOR, which is critically involved in regulating cell apoptosis, autophagy, proliferation, and metabolism. Dysregulation of the pathway, as mentioned earlier, played a prominent role in various cancers [92,93]. Therapeutic strategies targeting PI3K/AKT in GBM have given promising results in the in vitro and in vivo xenograft models; however, clinical safety and efficacy need to be proven. Sonolisib (PX-866), an irreversible PI3K inhibitor, inhibited the angiogenesis and invasion of GBM cells in vitro but did not induce the apoptosis of GBM cells; nevertheless, the drug caused cell cycle arrest. Sonolisib was well tolerated but showed disease progression in almost 73% of recurrent GBM patients in the phase II clinical trial [94]. Various other inhibitors such as XL765 (SAR245409) and GDC-0084, both PI3K and mTOR inhibitors, showed efficacy against GBM in the in vitro and in vivo models. However, the results as mentioned above lack the support from relevant clinical data [95].

Sirolimus (rapamycin), temsirolimus (CCI-779), and everolimus (RAD001), the mTOR inhibitors were evaluated in the various clinical phases and showed little efficacy in treating GBM patients. Everolimus showed very little effectiveness and a low survival rate in monotherapy and combination with temozolomide radiotherapy in a phase II clinical trial [96]. Sirolimus monotherapy and in combination with erlotinib [97] and temsirolimus [98] failed to show any effect in the treatment of GBM patients in a phase II clinical trial.

Other inhibitors such as vistusertib (AZD2014), palomid 529, and mTOR kinase inhibitor (CC-223) were dual inhibitors of mTORC1 and mTORC2. Vistusertib showed radiosensitization in GBM cell lines both in the in vitro and in vivo models, due to which the participants were recruited to phase I and II clinical trials [99] (clinical trial ID: NCT02619864). In a GBM xenograft model (U87MG cells), CC-223 exhibited an anti-tumor effect, while Palomid 529 exhibited anti-tumor activity in the orthotopic murine tumor model [100].

6. Mechanism of Drug Resistance to EGFR–TKIs in Glioma

Although the mechanism of drug resistance to EGFR–TKI in GBM remain unclear, few reports discussed the possible mechanisms in this regard. The absence of mutation in exons 19 and 21 of the TK domain was reported, especially in first-line EGFR-TKIs such as erlotinib and gefitinib. Their pharmacological actions were dependent on the modifications, as mentioned above [101]. Another possible mechanism mentioned was an alternative activating signal that compensated for the inactivation of EGFR signaling by EGFR–TKIs. In addition, the absence of EGFRvIII and loss of phosphatase and tensin homolog (PTEN) were the other determinants of resistance in certain studies [102].

The inhibition of mTOR, a downstream molecule of the PI3K/PTEN/AKT pathway, promoted the response of glioma cells to EGFR-TKIs in vitro [103,104]. Conversely, there was no responsiveness to erlotinib and no expression of EGFRvIII and PTEN in the phase II clinical trial with relapsed GBM patients [105]. In addition, a combination of the mTOR and EGFR–TKIs inhibitors (sirolimus) did not improve the patients' responsiveness in recurrent GBM patients [106]. On the other hand, erlotinib inhibited EGFR in EGFRvIII expressing U87 GBM cells and enhanced the expression of PDGFRα, thereby compensating the signaling pathway inhibited by erlotinib [97].

Despite the numerous studies on GBM treatment targeting EGFR, no therapeutic efficacy has been reported [107,108]. The therapeutic efficacy was minimal or nil in the case of first and second-generation EGFR inhibitors for the treatment of recurrent GBM [109,110]. The primary reasons for the above drugs' failure were their inability to cross the BBB and the requirement of a relatively high amount of drug concentrations in the brain [92], which in turn limited their usage. By overcoming the above-said limitations, effective therapy for GBM could be discovered [92].

7. Current Pharmaceutical Drug Targets in Glioma

Despite the great activity of EGFR–TKIs, mAb, and chemotherapeutic agents, the therapeutic outcomes limited by BBB penetration in both preclinical and clinical studies have urged the thought of using TKIs-loaded nanoformulations in the management of GBM [111]. For example, lipophobic and less molecular weight drugs could not achieve specific delivery in tumor tissues and were characterized by a short circulation half-life [112]. Furthermore, compared to the other cancer types harboring EGFR amplification, clonal resistance was not observed in GBM after the EGFR inhibitor treatment. However, multiple failures and/or resistance such as the absence of exons 19 and 21 of the TK domain, an alternative activation of signals, rapid adaptive responses due to EGFR inhibitors, and the lesser ability of EGFR–TKI drugs to cross the BBB were reported in various studies [113].

Consequently, the novel drug delivery systems (NDDS) were employed for the specific delivery of FDA-approved drugs to increase its therapeutic outcomes and reduce the adverse effects during GBM treatment. Among the above-mentioned NDDS, the NPs (Figure 3) with various structures and properties to serve as the desirable carriers for anti-cancer drugs were invented [114,115]. In addition, the systems appear to be promising approaches to solve the existing problems in the management of GBM [114]. NPs-based systems have many unique benefits. Firstly, NPs can be loaded with the hydrophilic and hydrophobic drugs simultaneously, which results in an enhanced solubility and anti-cancer effect when employed with the suitable combinations of medicines in carriers. Secondly, the uniform particle size distribution and surface modifications enabled passive or active cancer targeting and resulted in improved drug availability in the tumor region. Lastly, the NPs as drug carriers also aided the sustained and controlled drug release at a specific region. The augmented drug release profiles with extended circulation time permitted improved pharmacokinetics and decreased the dose-dependent toxicity of therapeutic agents [116,117]. Hence, the subsequent portion reviews the benefits of various classes of NPs used in EGFR-targeted drug delivery to manage glioma.

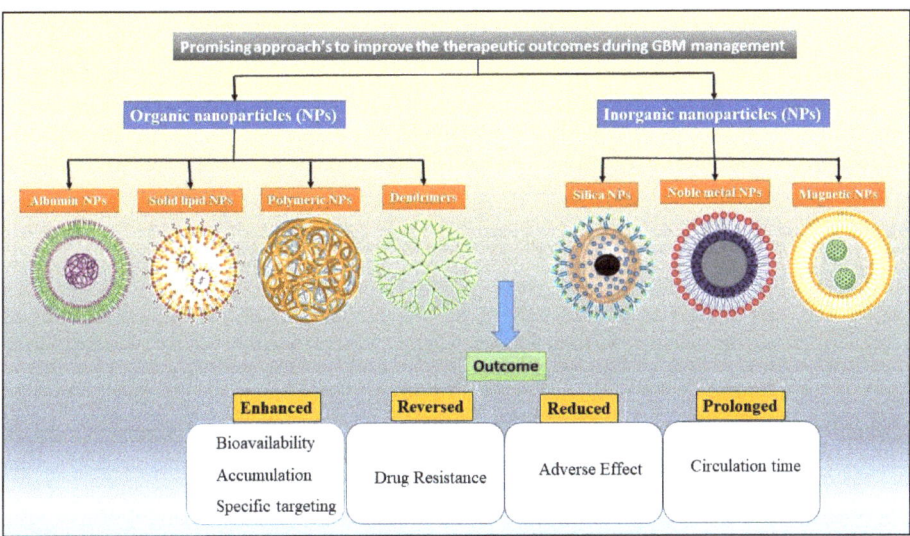

Figure 3. Different nanodelivery systems that facilitate BBB penetration and target-specific action in glioma.

7.1. Organic Nanoparticles

7.1.1. Albumin Nanoparticles

Due to the greater biodegradability and low immunogenicity of serum albumin, it has been identified as a suitable nanocarrier for the cancer management in recent years. In addition, the ability of binding or absorbent proteins around the NPs was showcased as the foremost prominent factor for prolonged circulation time and phagocytosis [118]. As an endogenous substance, albumin might inhibit therapeutics drugs from unnecessary stability interaction and targeting efficiency. The human serum albumin-based paclitaxel (PTX) nanoparticles exhibited superior anti-tumor activity by the prolongation of survival and pro-apoptotic effect, as depicted by terminal deoxynucleotidyl transferase dUTP nick end labeling (TUNEL) analysis, thereby serving as a novel strategy for treating GBM (Figure 4A,B) [119]. Furthermore, radioiodine cross-linking anti-EGFR (cetuximab) and bovine serum albumin (BSA) polycaprolactone (PCL) nanoparticles were also useful to induce tumor regression, which in turn enhanced the cytotoxicity on tumor cells and limited the adverse effects of chemical agents [120]. Thus, it can be stated that albumin NPs exhibited an improvement in therapeutic outcomes.

Tsutsui et al. demonstrated bio-nano capsules (BNCs) as an efficient way to deliver drugs to brain tumors in Gli36 cell lines. BNCs are composed of a hepatitis B surface antigen, small interfering ribonucleic acid (siRNA), genes, chemical components, and proteins that selectively target brain tumors. BNCs, when conjugated with an EGFR antibody, were capable of recognizing EGFRvIII, which in turn was overexpressed in various human malignancies. EGFRvIII was reported to be overexpressed in the variability of human malignancies of epithelial origin, particularly in gliomas. As mentioned above, the reports indicated BNC's potential as a means to achieve tumor targeting delivery [121].

The intravenous (i.v.) administration of T7 peptide modified core–shell NPs (T7-LPC/siRNA NPs) consisting of protamine/chondroitin sulfate/siRNA/cationic liposomes assembled layer by layer followed by modification using T7 peptide resulted in siRNA targeted delivery. T7-LPC/siRNA NPs, when compared with PEG-LPC/siRNA NPs, showed increased fluorescence intensity in microvascular endothelial cells of the brain (BMVECs) and U87 glioma cell lines. The NPs resulted in the downregulation of expression of EGFR protein in U87 glioma cells in vitro. The accumulation of NPs was more specific to the tumor tissues and penetrated the deep region ascertained by the co-culture model of BMVECs and U87 cells and in vivo imaging. The reports also confirmed that the NPs demonstrated the most prolonged survival period and highest down-regulated expression of EGFR, thereby showing the potential of siRNA delivery for the targeted therapy of GBM [122].

7.1.2. Immunoliposomes (IL) and Solid Lipid Nanoparticles (SLNs)

The sustained and targeted drug release profiles of the immunoliposomes (ILs) and solid lipid nanoparticles (SLNs) nanosystems enabled the enhanced cancer cell inhibition and decreased the adverse effects throughout the tumor therapy [123]. Lipids (phospholipids) were utilized to manufacture NPs due to their safety and biocompatibility [124]. The dual targeting SLN loaded with etoposide (ETP) containing mAb for insulin receptors and anti-EGFR was used to treat GBM. The dual-functionalized SLNs crossed the BMVECs/HA (human astrocytes), which is an in vitro model for BBB, and showed enhanced cytotoxicity against U87MG cells [125], thus proving its potential against GBM. In another study, the Cetuximab (C225)-immunoliposomes (ILs) encapsulating boron anion were constructed by using novel maleimido–Polyethylene Glycol (PEG)–cholesterol for the targeted delivery of boron compounds to EGFR (+) glioma cells for boron neutron capture therapy (BNCT). It was concluded that the prepared ILs could serve as an efficient delivery vehicle for the BNCT of glioma [126].

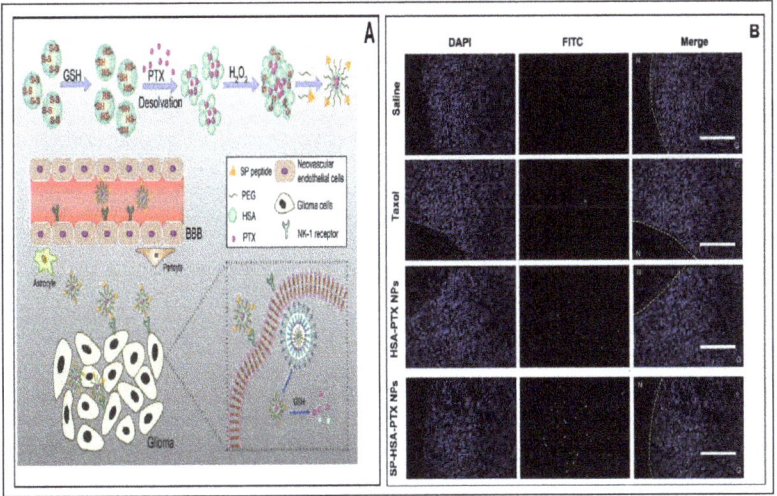

Figure 4. (**A**) Schematic representation of preparation and mechanism of action of albumin nanoparticles (NPs); (**B**) Fluorescent microscopic terminal deoxynucleotidyl transferase dUTP nick end labeling (TUNEL) assay images of in vivo anti-cancer efficacy of SP–HSA–PTX NPs (Green: TUNEL-stained apoptosis cells. Blue: 4′,6-diamidino-2-phenylindole (DAPI)-labeled nucleus, Yellow dashed lines: boundary between (N) normal brain and (G) glioma section). Reprinted with permission from [119], Elsevier, 2018.

Quantum dot immunoliposome (QD-IL), a hybrid nanoparticle, was targeted toward EGFR to treat GBM. QD-ILs were taken up efficiently by the malignant cells. In addition, QD-ILs served as imaging methods proven in both the in vitro and in vivo models. Furthermore, the NPs were also employed in ligand-directed delivery that allowed targeted drug delivery to the desired site to achieve efficient treatment for GBM [127]. Moreover, the anti-tumor effect of the combination of bevacizumab (Bev) and gemcitabine (GM) loaded IL (Bev-GM-IL) in a xenograft mice model (XMM) showed that the combinational therapy is better than monotherapy. This is due to the synergistic activity of two different drugs on GBM stem cells. Likewise, the combinational treatment extended the mean survival time of XMM. Altogether, the above results suggested that the combination of Bev-GM-IL offered promising outcomes in the treatment of GBM [128].

In another study, doxorubicin (DOX) and vincristine (VCR) were loaded with T7 and ^{D}A7R dual peptides-modified liposomes (T7/^{D}A7R-Ls) to treat glioma. The in vivo (Figure 5) results of T7/^{D}A7R-Ls showed improved glioma localization compared with mono ligand-modified liposomes or the free drug. In conclusion, the dual-targeting, co-delivery approach delivered a potential method for successful brain drug delivery in the glioma treatment [129].

7.1.3. Polymeric Nanoparticles

The comparative evaluation of the other conventional nanocarriers, the polymeric NPs, exhibited promising benefits in the biomedical applications due to their improved solubility, biocompatibility, and biodegradability. The biodegradation through circulation in vivo can be eluded efficiently, and the elimination half-life of the drugs is also prolonged after polymeric NPs encapsulation [130]. Additionally, the polymeric NPs with an applicable particle size distribution could passively help accumulate medicines in the tumor region by improved permeability and retention time [131,132]. Moreover, the retention time of encapsulated drugs in the tumor region could also be precisely regulated by various strategies [133]. For all of these advantages, the surface of polymeric NPs could be altered by selecting specific ligands to achieve active targeting delivery [134]. A study demonstrated the delivery of curcumin using poly (D, L-lactic-co-glycolic acid) (PLGA) NPs tagged with an EGFRvIII, which was internalized by EGFRvIII overexpressed GBM cells leading to the enhanced photodynamic toxicity of curcumin [135].

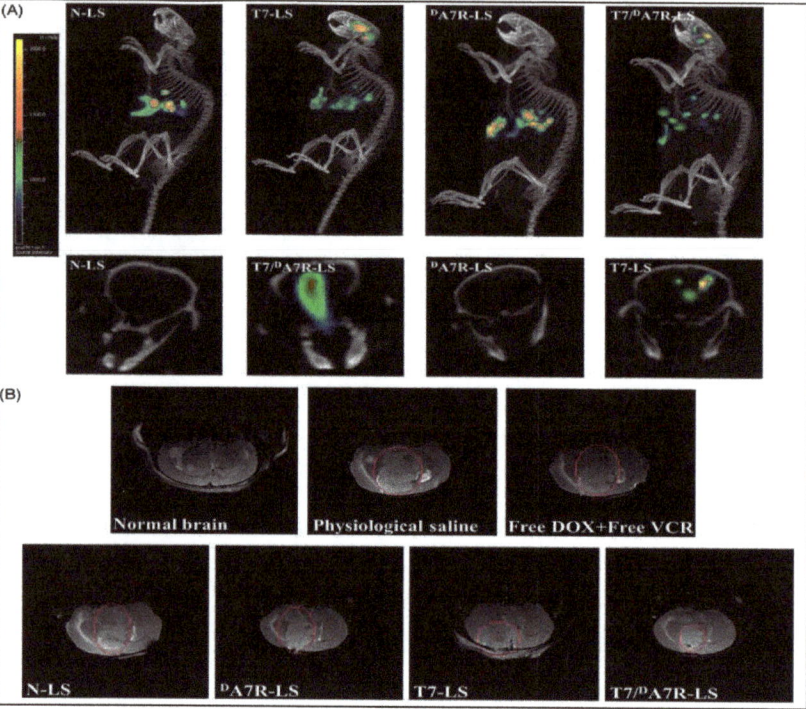

Figure 5. In vivo anti-glioma effect of doxorubicin (DOX) and vincristine (VCR)-loaded T7/^{D}A7R-LS immunoliposomes. (**A**) Distribution of Cy5.5 in the mice brain bearing intracranial C6 glioma determined by a CLSM; (**B**) MRI of normal and pathological brains at 16 d after inoculation. Reprinted from [129], Taylor and Fransis Group, 2017.

Lei Wang et al. (2015) prepared the angiopep-2 (ANG)-modified PLGA/DOX/siRNA NPs, which inhibited the cells by inducing apoptosis and silenced the EGFR pathway in U87MG cells. The NPs were capable of penetrating the BBB, thus resulting in the enhanced accumulation of drugs in brain in vivo. Animal studies not only demonstrated the co-delivery of DOX and EGFR SiRNA but also prolonged the life span of GBM-bearing mice [136]. Chengkun et al. (2019) utilized the Golgi phosphoprotein 3 (GOLPH3) nanobody to construct an angiopep-2 (A2)-modified cationic lipid PLGA NPs (A2-N) targeting the Ge and GOLPH3 siRNA (siGOLPH3). The NPs not only penetrated the BBB but also silenced the expression of GOLPH3 mRNA and enhanced the expression of EGFR and pEGFR upon entering glioma cells. In addition, the above-mentioned NPs acted as a combinational anti-tumor therapy in vitro and in vivo [137]. In vivo imaging revealed that the T7-LPC/siRNA NPs penetrated the deeper regions of the tumor. Furthermore, the accumulation was more in the brain, which was an added advantage compared to PEG-LPC/siRNA NPs. The group also demonstrated the enhanced survival period by down-regulating the expression of EGFR in mice, and therefore, it can serve as a potential target for treating GBM [119]. In another study, C225 was conjugated to TMZ-loaded PLGA NPs (C225–TMZ–PLGA–NPs) by cross-linking chemistry to target the EGFR receptor. Furthermore, in vitro cellular uptake and the in vivo evaluation of PLGA–NPs, TMZ–PLGA–NPs, and C225–TMZ–PLGA–NPs were conducted. In addition, the results of cell cytotoxicity, apoptosis in U-87MG, SW480, and SK-Mel 28 cancer cell lines confirmed that the C225-PLGA-NPs can be utilized as a versatile nanocarrier for the management of EGFR overexpressing cancers [138].

7.1.4. Dendrimers

The dendrimers are hyper-branched macromolecules that exhibit advantages over the conventional carriers (liposome, polymeric NPs etc.) such as enhanced stability in the blood circulation and ability to accommodate various ligands due to its chemosynthetic approach rather than self-assembly through non-covalent interaction [139,140]. In addition, the structure, size, and molecular weight of dendrimer have resemblance with bio-structures and proteins (insulin, hemoglobin and cytochrome), which makes them employable in various fields as gene delivery, immunodiagnosis, and encapsulation of drugs [141,142]. Dendrimer-based drug delivery employing polyamidoamine (PAMAM) was also explored for its application in GBM therapy [143,144].

An antisense oligonucleotide (ASODN) delivery of conjugates of folate–PAMAM (FA-PAMAM) inhibited the C6 cell growth in glioma. The coupling of folic acid to the surface amino groups of PAMAM dendrimers and ASODNs (ASODN: FA-PAMAM) corresponded to rat EGFR in the ratio of 16:1. The ASODN:FA-PAMAM combination suppressed EGFR and C6 cell growth expression, thus enhancing the survival time [145].

Cetuximab (C225) could be covalently linked to methotrexate (MTX) by the 5th generation (G5) of PAMAM dendrimers via its fragment crystallizable (Fc) region (C225–G5–MTX) to target EGFR and EGFR variant III (EGFRvIII). Competitive binding assay (CBA) demonstrated that C225–G5–MTX exhibited a higher affinity for the EGFR-expressing rat glioma cell line (F98$_{EGFR}$) than the wild-type rat glioma cell line (F98$_{WT}$). Subsequently, the improved distribution of ^{125}I bio-conjugate of C225-G5-MTX noticed in F98$_{EGFR}$ was six-fold greater than F98$_{WT}$ cells, thereby contributing to specific molecular targeting the GBM treatment. The animal models that received C225-G5-MTX and C-225 or MTX exhibited 15- and 19.5-day survival rates, respectively. Correspondingly, the results were non-significant between the control and test animals [146].

PAMAM dendrimer and Tat peptide were fabricated to bacterial magnetic NPs (Tat–BMPs–PAMAM), which were then complexed with the siRNA expression plasmid of human EGFR (psiRNA–EGFR) through electrostatic interplay (Tat–BMPs–PAMAM/psiRNA-EGFR). The conjugate offered promising results in reducing tumor growth and suppressing the expression of oncoproteins. In addition, the conjugate could serve as a possible targeted gene delivery for GBM [147].

Recently, an angiopeptide-2 (Ang2) and low-density lipoprotein receptor-relative protein-1 (LRP1) was conjugated with PAMAM to improve BBB penetration glioma sites. Furthermore, PAMAM was concurrently functionalized with an EGFR-targeting peptide (EP-1) to achieve specificity and improved affinity to target EGFR. The above results showed the potential of the dual drug-loaded PAMAM in the treatment of gliomas by improving BBB penetration and specific EGFR targeting efficiency, both in vitro and in vivo (Figure 6) [148].

All the above-mentioned experiments concluded that the dendrimer-based NPs could be utilized as extensive drug delivery carriers to target and treat various CNS cancer cells by BBB penetration with the backing of targeting ligands.

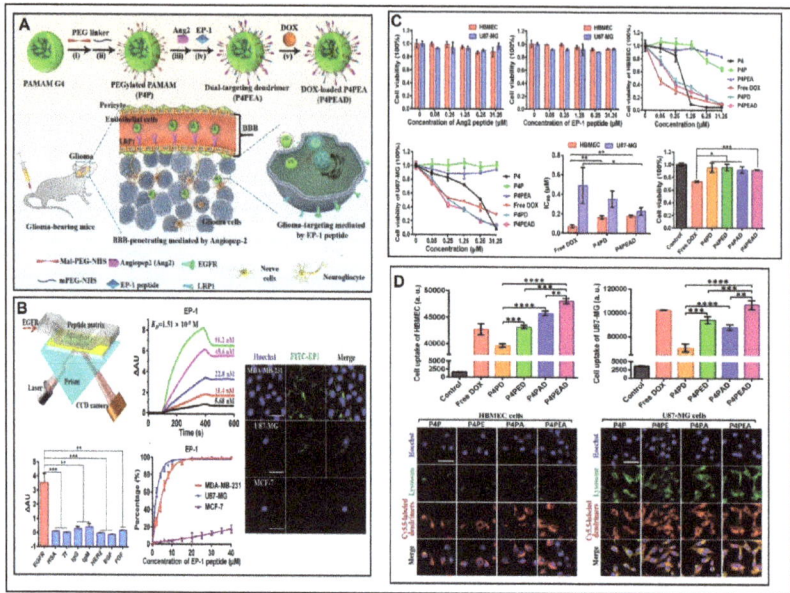

Figure 6. (**A**) Schematic representation of fabrication of the dual drug loaded polyamidoamine (PAMAM) dendrimers in the treatment of gliomas by improving BBB penetration; (**B**) Assessment of the affinity and specificity of peptide EP-1 toward EGFR; (**C**) In vitro evaluation of biocompatibility and anti-tumor efficacy of the dual drug-loaded PAMAM dendrimers; (**D**) Flow cytometry evaluation for intracellular uptake of different DOX-loaded dendrimers. Reprinted from [148] Ivyspring International Publisher, 2020. * $p < 0.1$, ** $p < 0.01$, *** $p < 0.001$, **** $p < 0.0001$ (Student's t-test).

7.2. Inorganic Nanoparticles (NPs)

7.2.1. Silica NPs

The mesoporous silica nanoparticles (MS-NPs) are frequently employed as multifunctional nanocarriers to treat cancer cells owing to its mesoporous structure and enormous surface area. As a result, the active components can be dumped in the porous structure of NPs to obtain the maximum amount of drug-loading, and the surface modification of MS-NPs could also increase the intracellular uptake. Additionally, the alteration of carriers' particle size, surface charge, and shape could increase the biocompatibility and minimize the cytotoxicity of MS-NPs [149]. In addition, MS-NPs could be encapsulated with contrast agents for MRI imaging. Hence, MS-NPs exhibit a chance to improve the solubility and stability of anti-EGFR drugs by being deposited in the porous structure.

Furthermore, prolonged drug release profiles resulted in decreased cytotoxicity in long-period cancer therapy [150,151]. The properties mentioned above were ensured by developing DOX magnetic (Fe_3O_4) NPs, encapsulated in polyethylene glycol (PEG), to functionalize the porous silica shell and treat cancer cells [152]. Likewise, multi-targeted oleic acid (OA)–MNPs were developed. Reports confirmed promising outcomes about the in vitro and in vivo efficacy in treating human cancer cells (HeLa). The study results stated that the MS-NPs formulations were more predominant than the placebo or free drugs and could overcome the drawbacks mentioned above of the conventional treatment approaches [153]. The synthesized and functionalized DOX magnetic MS-NPs were fabricated with PF-127 and then conjugated with transferrin (Tf) to enhance BBB penetration and achieve sustained release at the specific site. The Tf-loaded NPs resulted in improved BBB permeability (Figure 7). Thus, the prepared Tf nanocarriers could be considered as potential candidates in the treatment of brain tumors [154].

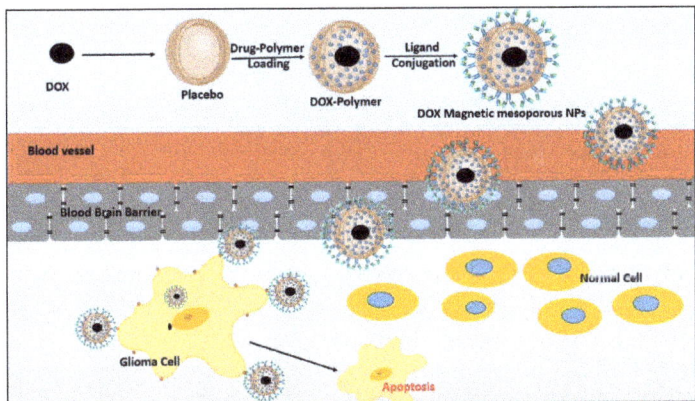

Figure 7. Synthesis of magnetic mesoporous nanoparticles using polymer and subsequently conjugated with ligands to achieve the sustained release of the drug at the specific targeted site.

7.2.2. Magnetic Nanoparticles (MNPs)

Magnetic nanoparticles (MNPs) specifically created an interest in the biomedical application and research due to various advantages: separation of molecules, gene/drug delivery, magnetic resonance imaging (MRI), and hyperthermic tumor treatment [155]. Among the several magnetic nanocarriers, super-paramagnetic iron oxide (SPIO) has been commonly utilized owing to its promising biocompatibility and magnetic properties. For example, an improved survival rate was noticed in animal models with C225-IONPs compared to pure C225 in the treatment of GBM [156]. In addition, SPIO and peptide nanoprobe were effectively combined and demonstrated for specific molecular MRI and sensitive optical imaging (SOI). Both in vitro and in vivo MRI and SOI showed that the nanoprobe was useful for targeting GBM with desirable biosafety [157]. In another study, MNPs were employed by convection-enhanced delivery (CED) in the brain to target the EGFRvIII xenografts GBM model. Then, MRI was conducted to evaluate brain targeting and the delivery of conjugated MNPs after CED. The accomplishment of a human clinical trial containing a direct injection of MNPs into recurrent GBM for thermotherapy proved the safety, efficacy, and feasibility in the patients [158]. In a recent report, pazopanib was loaded in MNPs, which stimulated the ultrasound's drug release. The enhanced drug distribution in the non-small cell lung cancer (NSCLC) region resulted in improved therapeutic outcomes [159].

7.2.3. Noble Metal Nanoparticles (NM-NPs)

Commonly, the Gold (Au) NPs are known as noble metal NPs, which were comprehensively studied for biomedical applications due to their lower toxicity, distinctive electronic, and optic properties that prompted cellular destruction with an application of radiation [160] or light [161]. In addition, AuNPs could be loaded with organic molecules (antibodies), which enhanced the accumulation of AuNPs within specific cancer tissues or lesions [162]. AuNPs were loaded with malondialdehyde-modified low-density lipoprotein (MDA-LDL) antibodies by distinct chemistries for drug recognition and capture from the biological system [163]. Furthermore, 40 nm AuNPs with mAb targeting the EGFR acted by random adsorption to treat oral squamous cancer. The antibody-loaded AuNPs accumulation into the tumor region enhanced cancer cell death by photothermal therapy [161]. In addition, the 5 nm AuNPs were surface modified with EGFR antibodies and functionalized using GM for targeting GBM cells [164]. In another study, Au nanocubes (AuNCs) with pH or temperature sensitivity were prepared for erlotinib or DOX encapsulation. Firstly, the drug-loaded AuNCs could accumulate more at the cancer tissue; the particular acidic microenvironment of cancer initiated erlotinib's release, precisely. Finally, the controlled release of DOX by near-infrared (NIR) laser irradiation improved the therapeutic effect of AuNCs-based nano carrier in A431 cancer cell lines [165]. In addition, the in vivo activity of the Au–C225 conjugate resulted in a similar effect compared to free C225, concluding that the site-specific conjugation to the AuNP did not affect the biological action of the EGFR antibody, thereby signifying the value of the intended functionalization approach. The opportunity to yield accurate AuNP–Immunoglobuin G (IgG) conjugates creates novel paths to assay the Au–C225 conjugate for cancer therapy, either for sensitizing tumor cells to external radiation [166]. Based on the promising results of the developed NM-NPs provided a novel way for the delivery of chemotherapeutic and TKIs drugs.

8. Current Clinical Studies of Nanoformulations

After promising results of preclinical investigations, the organic and inorganic nanoformulations have entered the clinical trials to assess the tolerability, safety, pharmacokinetics, and efficacy for the treatment of GBM [167]. Table 3 summarizes the list of current clinical trials on EGFR loaded nanoformulation for the treatment of GBM. Firstly, the researchers have a newly developed EnGeneIC delivery vehicle (EDV). This inorganic nanocarrier exploits antibody-targeted, transporting active anti-cancer drugs into EGFR-expressing cancer cells (EnGeneIC, Lane Cove West, Australia). In a phase I/II study, the recurrent GBM adult patients were dosed of up to 5×10^9 to determine the safety and possible dose of EGFR–EDV–DOX (NCT02766699) [168]. The effect of anti-EGFR targeted DOX loaded into C225-decorated Immunoliposomes (ILs) (C225–ILs–Dox) is being evaluated in a phase I clinical trial (NCT03603379) [169]. Analogously, DOX–trastuzumab consisting of PEGylated liposomes has completed a phase I/II clinical trial (NCT01386580). The phase I clinical study of cationic liposomes loaded with cancer suppressor gene p53 and TMZ (SGT–53–TMZ) was conducted to observe minimal side effects with a 6-month progression-free survival (PFS) and overall survival (OS) rate in patients with advanced solid tumors (NCT02340156) [170]. The phase I/II clinical trial was conducted to estimate side effects and a suitable dose of EGFR-bispecific antibody armed T cells (EGFR-Bi-T) in GBM patients' treatment. In phase I trials, the patients received EGFR-Bi-T intrathecal (IT) injection twice per week for four weeks to determine the efficacy and toxicity profile. In phase II trials, the patients received EGFR-Bi-T IT twice weekly for four weeks and then i.v. over 15–30 min twice weekly for two weeks (NCT02521090).

Table 3. List of Current Clinical Studies of Nanoformulations.

Nano Carriers	Drug	Phase	Outcome Measures	NCT Number	Reference
EnGeneIC delivery vehicle (EDV)	EGFR-EDV-DOX	I	Determination of a possible phase II dose of drug for recurrent GBM.	NCT02766699	[168]
ILs	C225-IL-DOX	I	Determination of a suitable ratio of C225–IL–DOX concentration.	NCT03603379	[169]
PEGylated Liposoomes	DOX-Trastuzumab	I/II	To determine the safety and tolerability of i.v. administration of the PEGylated liposomes	NCT01386580	NA
Albumin NPs	Rapamycin + Avastin + Radiation	II	To determine progression-free survival (PFS) and overall survival (OS) rate according to response assessment in neuro-oncology (RANO) criteria	NCT03463265	[171]
Cationic Liposoomes	SGT-53 + TMZ	II	To determine six-month PFS and OS, anti-cancer activity, safety, and efficacy of NPs.	NCT02340156	[170]
enzyme-linked immune spots	EGFR-Bi-T	I/II	To determine the maximum tolerated dose (MTD) for eight intrathecal (IT) injections	NCT02521090	NA

9. Future Perspectives

The results of EGFR–TKIs drugs in clinical research showed that the molecularly targeted medicines combined chemotherapy could achieve the highest therapeutic outcome compared to free active components. However, the low specific inhibition and drug resistance during treatment were difficulties in developing targeted molecular active agents. Novel signaling transduction anti-cancer drugs based on modified therapy could minimize or overcome drug resistance. Remarkably, nanotechnology's benefits for the currently available chemotherapeutic and TKI agents provided alternative strategies for improving therapeutic results: low solubility and BBB penetration, and prolonging the drug accumulation in the cancer region, decreasing the side effects triggered by non-specific distribution. The nanocarriers' design has been moved forward via its technological upgradations, yet the nanoplatform fails to attain comprehensive clinical interpretation. Thus, the nanocarrier delivery approach is intended to assure better chances of success in a clinical trial [172].

Moreover, the clinical trial evidence (Table 3) was intended to determine the safety and efficacy of nanoformulations for the GBM treatment that have been happening since the beginning of the twenty-first century. Hence, the results of clinical studies have not yet been published, which contribute to paving the way for the clinical interpretation of nanotherapies for GBM. The researchers have recently considered utilizing natural compounds such as polyphenols and cannabinoids to target EGFR and its downstream pathway in various cancer cell lines [173–178]. The brain's microenvironment, prominently advanced as per our understanding, targeting GBM cells with Janus kinases/signal transducer and activator of transcription proteins (JAK/STAT) inhibitors via combinational approaches could boost immunity with the reduced oncogenic effect of the GBM cancer cells [179,180].

10. Conclusions

The clinical trials of the nano-based formulations of chemotherapeutic and/or TKI drugs in combination are awaited. After an extensive literature search, it could be stated that novel approaches to treat GBM using mono or combinational therapy of polyphenols and anti-EGFR drugs to target multi signaling pathways (EGFR, JAK/STAT, and PI3K/AKT/mTOR) would help overcome the multiple failures of EGFR–TKI drug trials. Furthermore, the novel nano-based combinational therapy might positively reverse chemotherapeutic and TKI drug-induced resistance.

Author Contributions: Conceptualization, S.P., D.V.G. and S.B.C.; methodology, S.P., D.V.G. and S.B.C.; software, S.P., M.G.S., A.M. and M.M.; validation, D.V.G., S.B.C., N.N. and S.H.N.; formal analysis, S.P.; investigation, D.V.G., S.B.C.; resources, S.P.; data curation, S.P., writing—original draft preparation, S.P., writing—review and editing, S.P., M.G.S. and M.M.; visualization, D.V.G.; supervision, D.V.G. and S.B.C.; project administration, D.V.G. All authors have read and agreed to the published version of the manuscript.

Funding: This work received no external funding.

Acknowledgments: This work was supported by JSS Academy of Higher Education and Research, Mysore, Karnataka, India. S.P. is thankful to Department of Biotechnology (DBT), India for providing Junior Research Fellowship for his research work. Authors are thankful to Edit n Stat for Proofreading this Manuscript.

Conflicts of Interest: The authors declare no conflicts of interest.

References

1. Ersoz, M.; Erdemir, A.; Duranoglu, D.; Uzunoglu, D.; Arasoglu, T.; Derman, S.; Mansuroglu, B. Comparative evaluation of hesperetin loaded nanoparticles for anticancer activity against C6 glioma cancer cells. *Artif. Cells Nanomed. Biotechnol.* **2019**, *47*, 319–329. [CrossRef] [PubMed]
2. Hanif, F.; Muzaffar, K.; Perveen, K.; Malhi, S.M.; Simjee, S.U. Glioblastoma multiforme: A review of its epidemiology and pathogenesis through clinical presentation and treatment. *Asian Pac. J. Cancer Prev.* **2017**, *18*, 3–9.

3. Patel, A.P.; Fisher, J.L.; Nichols, E.; Abd-Allah, F.; Abdela, J.; Abdelalim, A.; Abraha, H.N.; Agius, D.; Alahdab, F.; Alam, T.; et al. Global, regional, and national burden of brain and other CNS cancer, 1990–2016: A systematic analysis for the Global Burden of Disease Study 2016. *Lancet Neurol.* **2019**, *18*, 376–393. [CrossRef]
4. Ferlay, J.; Colombet, M.; Soerjomataram, I.; Mathers, C.; Parkin, D.M.; Piñeros, M.; Znaor, A.; Bray, F. Estimating the global cancer incidence and mortality in 2018: GLOBOCAN sources and methods. *Int. J. Cancer* **2019**, *144*, 1941–1953. [CrossRef] [PubMed]
5. Bray, F.; Ferlay, J.; Soerjomataram, I.; Siegel, R.L.; Torre, L.A.; Jemal, A. Global cancer statistics 2018: GLOBOCAN estimates of incidence and mortality worldwide for 36 cancers in 185 countries. *CA Cancer J. Clin.* **2018**, *68*, 394–424. [CrossRef] [PubMed]
6. Piñeros, M.; Sierra, M.S.; Izarzugaza, M.I.; Forman, D. Descriptive epidemiology of brain and central nervous system cancers in Central and South America. *Cancer Epidemiol.* **2016**, *44*, S141–S149. [CrossRef]
7. Louis, D.N.; Perry, A.; Reifenberger, G.; Von Deimling, A.; Figarella-Branger, D.; Cavenee, W.K.; Ohgaki, H.; Wiestler, O.D.; Kleihues, P.; Ellison, D.W. The 2016 World Health Organization Classification of Tumors of the Central Nervous System: A summary. *Acta Neuropathol.* **2016**, *131*, 803–820. [CrossRef]
8. Jooma, R.; Waqas, M.; Khan, I. Diffuse low-grade glioma–Changing concepts in diagnosis and management: A review. *Asian J. Neurosurg.* **2019**, *14*, 356. [CrossRef]
9. Louis, D.N.; Ohgaki, H.; Wiestler, O.D.; Cavenee, W.K.; Burger, P.C.; Jouvet, A.; Scheithauer, B.W.; Kleihues, P. The 2007 WHO classification of tumours of the central nervous system. *Acta Neuropathol.* **2007**, *114*, 97–109. [CrossRef]
10. Roy, S.; Lahiri, D.; Maji, T.; Biswas, J. Recurrent Glioblastoma: Where we stand. *South Asian J. Cancer* **2015**, *4*, 163. [CrossRef]
11. Carlsson, S.K.; Brothers, S.P.; Wahlestedt, C. Emerging treatment strategies for glioblastoma multiforme. *EMBO Mol. Med.* **2014**, *6*, 1359–1370. [CrossRef] [PubMed]
12. Tom, M.C.; Cahill, D.P.; Buckner, J.C.; Dietrich, J.; Parsons, M.W.; Yu, J.S. Management for Different Glioma Subtypes: Are All Low-Grade Gliomas Created Equal? *Am. Soc. Clin. Oncol. Educ. B* **2019**, 133–145. [CrossRef] [PubMed]
13. Fung, N.H.; Grima, C.A.; Widodo, S.S.; Kaye, A.H.; Whitehead, C.A.; Stylli, S.S.; Mantamadiotis, T. Understanding and exploiting cell signalling convergence nodes and pathway cross-talk in malignant brain cancer. *Cell. Signal.* **2019**, *57*, 2–9. [CrossRef] [PubMed]
14. Westover, D.; Zugazagoitia, J.; Cho, B.; Lovly, C.M.; Paz-Ares, L. Mechanisms of acquired resistance to first-and second-generation EGFR tyrosine kinase inhibitors. *Ann. Oncol.* **2018**, *29*, i10–i19. [CrossRef]
15. Liu, X.; Chen, X.; Shi, L.; Shan, Q.; Cao, Q.; Yue, C.; Li, H.; Li, S.; Wang, J.; Gao, S.; et al. The third-generation EGFR inhibitor AZD9291 overcomes primary resistance by continuously blocking ERK signaling in glioblastoma. *J. Exp. Clin. Cancer Res.* **2019**, *38*, 1–14. [CrossRef] [PubMed]
16. Falzone, L.; Salomone, S.; Libra, M. Evolution of cancer pharmacological treatments at the turn of the third millennium. *Front. Pharmacol.* **2018**, *9*, 1300. [CrossRef]
17. An, Z.; Aksoy, O.; Zheng, T.; Fan, Q.W.; Weiss, W.A. Epidermal growth factor receptor and EGFRvIII in glioblastoma: Signaling pathways and targeted therapies. *Oncogene* **2018**, *37*, 1561–1575. [CrossRef]
18. Taylor, O.G.; Brzozowski, J.S.; Skelding, K.A. Glioblastoma multiforme: An overview of emerging therapeutic targets. *Front. Oncol.* **2019**, *9*, 963. [CrossRef]
19. Yin, Y.; Yuan, X.; Gao, H.; Yang, Q. Nanoformulations of small molecule protein tyrosine kinases inhibitors potentiate targeted cancer therapy. *Int. J. Pharm.* **2020**, *573*, 118785. [CrossRef]
20. Eckel-Passow, J.E.; Lachance, D.H.; Molinaro, A.M.; Walsh, K.M.; Decker, P.A.; Sicotte, H.; Pekmezci, M.; Rice, T.; Kosel, M.L.; Smirnov, I.V.; et al. Glioma Groups Based on 1p/19q, *IDH*, and *TERT* Promoter Mutations in Tumors. *N. Engl. J. Med.* **2015**, *372*, 2499–2508. [CrossRef]
21. Aum, D.J.; Kim, D.H.; Beaumont, T.L.; Leuthardt, E.C.; Dunn, G.P.; Kim, A.H. Molecular and cellular heterogeneity: The hallmark of glioblastoma. *Neurosurg. Focus* **2014**, *37*, E11. [CrossRef] [PubMed]
22. Silantyev, A.S.; Falzone, L.; Libra, M.; Gurina, O.I.; Kardashova, K.S.; Nikolouzakis, T.K.; Nosyrev, A.E.; Sutton, C.W.; Mitsias, P.D.; Tsatsakis, A. Current and Future Trends on Diagnosis and Prognosis of Glioblastoma: From Molecular Biology to Proteomics. *Cells* **2019**, *8*, 863. [CrossRef] [PubMed]
23. Michelson, N.; Rincon-Torroella, J.; Quiñones-Hinojosa, A.; Greenfield, J.P. Exploring the role of inflammation in the malignant transformation of low-grade gliomas. *J. Neuroimmunol.* **2016**, *297*, 132–140. [CrossRef] [PubMed]

24. Kuan, A.S.; Green, J.; Kitahara, C.M.; De González, A.B.; Key, T.; Reeves, G.K.; Floud, S.; Balkwill, A.; Bradbury, K.; Liao, L.M.; et al. Diet and risk of glioma: Combined analysis of 3 large prospective studies in the UK and USA. *Neuro-Oncology* **2019**, *21*, 944–952. [CrossRef]
25. Galdiero, M.R.; Bonavita, E.; Barajon, I.; Garlanda, C.; Mantovani, A.; Jaillon, S. Tumor associated macrophages and neutrophils in cancer. *Immunobiology* **2013**, *218*, 1402–1410. [CrossRef]
26. Santoiemma, P.P.; Powell, D.J. Tumor infiltrating lymphocytes in ovarian cancer. *Cancer Biol. Ther.* **2015**, *16*, 807–820. [CrossRef]
27. Franco, A.T.; Corken, A.; Ware, J. Platelets at the interface of thrombosis, inflammation, and cancer. *Blood* **2015**, *126*, 582–588. [CrossRef]
28. Wang, P.-F.; Song, H.-W.; Cai, H.-Q.; Kong, L.-W.; Yao, K.; Jiang, T.; Li, S.-W.; Yan, C.-X.; Wang, P.-F.; Song, H.-W.; et al. Preoperative inflammation markers and IDH mutation status predict glioblastoma patient survival. *Oncotarget* **2017**, *8*, 50117–50123. [CrossRef]
29. Hu, H.; Yao, X.; Xie, X.; Wu, X.; Zheng, C.; Xia, W.; Ma, S. Prognostic value of preoperative NLR, dNLR, PLR and CRP in surgical renal cell carcinoma patients. *World J. Urol.* **2017**, *35*, 261–270. [CrossRef]
30. Xia, W.-K.; Liu, Z.-L.; Shen, D.; Lin, Q.-F.; Su, J.; Mao, W.-D. Prognostic performance of pre-treatment NLR and PLR in patients suffering from osteosarcoma. *World J. Surg. Oncol.* **2016**, *14*, 127. [CrossRef]
31. Hochberg, F.H.; Atai, N.A.; Gonda, D.; Hughes, M.S.; Mawejje, B.; Balaj, L.; Carter, R.S. Glioma diagnostics and biomarkers: An ongoing challenge in the field of medicine and science. *Expert Rev. Mol. Diagn.* **2014**, *14*, 439–452. [CrossRef] [PubMed]
32. Szopa, W.; Burley, T.A.; Kramer-Marek, G.; Kaspera, W. Diagnostic and therapeutic biomarkers in glioblastoma: Current status and future perspectives. *BioMed Res. Int.* **2017**, *2017*. [CrossRef] [PubMed]
33. Zhang, Z.-Y.; Zhan, Y.-B.; Zhang, F.-J.; Yu, B.; Ji, Y.-C.; Zhou, J.-Q.; Bai, Y.-H.; Wang, Y.-M.; Wang, L.; Jing, Y.; et al. Prognostic value of preoperative hematological markers combined with molecular pathology in patients with diffuse gliomas. *Aging* **2019**, *11*, 6252–6272. [CrossRef] [PubMed]
34. Davis, M.E. Glioblastoma: Overview of disease and treatment. *Clin. J. Oncol. Nurs.* **2016**, *20*, 1–8. [CrossRef]
35. Tamimi, A.F.; Juweid, M. Epidemiology and outcome of glioblastoma. In *Glioblastoma*; De Vleeschouwer, S., Ed.; Codon Publications: Brisbane, Australia, 2017. [CrossRef]
36. Perkins, A.; Physician, G.L. Primary brain tumors in adults: Diagnosis and treatment. *Am. Fam. Physician* **2016**, *93*, 211–217.
37. Ladomersky, E.; Scholtens, D.M.; Kocherginsky, M.; Hibler, E.A.; Bartom, E.T.; Otto-Meyer, S.; Zhai, L.; Lauing, K.L.; Choi, J.; Sosman, J.A.; et al. The coincidence between increasing age, immunosuppression, and the incidence of patients with glioblastoma. *Front. Pharmacol.* **2019**, *10*, 200. [CrossRef]
38. Thakkar, J.P.; Dolecek, T.A.; Horbinski, C.; Ostrom, Q.T.; Lightner, D.D.; Barnholtz-Sloan, J.S.; Villano, J.L. Epidemiologic and molecular prognostic review of glioblastoma. *Cancer Epidemiol. Biomark. Prev.* **2014**, *23*, 1985–1996. [CrossRef]
39. Tian, M.; Ma, W.; Chen, Y.; Yu, Y.; Zhu, D.; Shi, J.; Zhang, Y. Impact of gender on the survival of patients with glioblastoma. *Biosci. Rep.* **2018**, *38*. [CrossRef]
40. Bell, J.S.; Koffie, R.M.; Rattani, A.; Dewan, M.C.; Baticulon, R.E.; Qureshi, M.M.; Wahjoepramono, E.J.; Rosseau, G.; Park, K.; Nahed, B.V. Global incidence of brain and spinal tumors by geographic region and income level based on cancer registry data. *J. Clin. Neurosci.* **2019**, *66*, 121–127. [CrossRef]
41. Gupta, T.; Achari, R.; Chatterjee, A.; Chen, Z.P.; Mehta, M.; Bouffet, E.; Jalali, R. Comparison of epidemiology and outcomes in neuro-oncology between the east and the west: Challenges and opportunities. *Clin. Oncol.* **2019**, *31*, 539–548. [CrossRef]
42. Werlenius, K.; Fekete, B.; Blomstrand, M.; Carén, H.; Jakola, A.S.; Rydenhag, B.; Smits, A. Patterns of care and clinical outcome in assumed glioblastoma without tissue diagnosis: A population-based study of 131 consecutive patients. *PLoS ONE* **2020**, *15*, e0228480. [CrossRef] [PubMed]
43. Bohn, A.; Braley, A.; De La Vega, P.R.; Carlos Zevallos, J.; Barengo, N.C. The association between race and survival in glioblastoma patients in the US: A retrospective cohort study. *PLoS ONE* **2018**, *13*, e0198581. [CrossRef] [PubMed]
44. Komori, T. The 2016 WHO classification of tumours of the central nervous system: The major points of revision. *Neurol. Med. Chir.* **2017**, *57*, 301–311. [CrossRef] [PubMed]

45. Ostrom, Q.T.; Bauchet, L.; Davis, F.G.; Deltour, I.; Fisher, J.L.; Langer, C.E.; Pekmezci, M.; Schwartzbaum, J.A.; Turner, M.C.; Walsh, K.M.; et al. Response to "The epidemiology of glioma in adults: A 'state of the science' review". *Neuro-Oncology* **2015**, *17*, 624–626. [CrossRef]
46. Costanza, M.; Finocchiaro, G. Allergic Signs in Glioma Pathology: Current Knowledge and Future Perspectives. *Cancers* **2019**, *11*, 404. [CrossRef]
47. Reblin, M.; Sahebjam, S.; Peeri, N.C.; Martinez, Y.C.; Thompson, Z.; Egan, K.M. Medical cannabis use in glioma patients treated at a comprehensive cancer center in Florida. *J. Palliat. Med.* **2019**, *22*, 1202–1207. [CrossRef]
48. Driver, J.A. Inverse association between cancer and neurodegenerative disease: Review of the epidemiologic and biological evidence. *Biogerontology* **2014**, *15*, 547–557. [CrossRef]
49. Candido, S.; Lupo, G.; Pennisi, M.; Basile, M.S.; Anfuso, C.D.; Petralia, M.C.; Gattuso, G.; Vivarelli, S.; Spandidos, D.A.; Libra, M.; et al. The analysis of miRNA expression profiling datasets reveals inverse microRNA patterns in glioblastoma and Alzheimer's disease. *Oncol. Rep.* **2019**, *42*, 911–922. [CrossRef]
50. Sánchez-Valle, J.; Tejero, H.; Ibáñez, K.; Portero, J.L.; Krallinger, M.; Al-Shahrour, F.; Tabarés-Seisdedos, R.; Baudot, A.; Valencia, A. A molecular hypothesis to explain direct and inverse co-morbidities between Alzheimer's Disease, Glioblastoma and Lung cancer. *Sci. Rep.* **2017**, *7*, 1–12. [CrossRef]
51. Regad, T. Targeting RTK signaling pathways in cancer. *Cancers* **2015**, *7*, 1758–1784. [CrossRef]
52. Metibemu, D.S.; Akinloye, O.A.; Akamo, A.J.; Ojo, D.A.; Okeowo, O.T.; Omotuyi, I.O. Exploring receptor tyrosine kinases-inhibitors in Cancer treatments. *Egypt. J. Med. Hum. Genet.* **2019**, *20*, 1–16. [CrossRef]
53. Romano, R.; Bucci, C. Role of EGFR in the Nervous System. *Cells* **2020**, *9*, 1887. [CrossRef] [PubMed]
54. Galvez-Contreras, A.Y.; Quiñones-Hinojosa, A.; Gonzalez-Perez, O. The role of EGFR and ErbB family related proteins in the oligodendrocyte specification in germinal niches of the adult mammalian brain. *Front. Cell. Neurosci.* **2013**, *7*, 258. [CrossRef] [PubMed]
55. Hatanpaa, K.J.; Burma, S.; Zhao, D.; Habib, A.A. Epidermal growth factor receptor in glioma: Signal transduction, neuropathology, imaging, and radioresistance1. *Neoplasia* **2010**, *12*, 675–684. [CrossRef] [PubMed]
56. Zhang, Y.J.; Xu, Z.G.; Li, S.Q.; He, L.J.; Tang, Y.; Chen, Z.Z.; Yang, D.L. Benzimidazoisoquinoline derivatives inhibit glioblastoma cell proliferation through down-regulating Raf/MEK/ERK and PI3K/AKT pathways. *Cancer Cell Int.* **2018**, *18*, 90. [CrossRef] [PubMed]
57. Connell, C.M.; Doherty, G.J. Activating HER2 mutations as emerging targets in multiple solid cancers. *ESMO Open* **2017**, *2*, e000279. [CrossRef] [PubMed]
58. Erfani, P.; Tome-Garcia, J.; Canoll, P.; Doetsch, F.; Tsankova, N.M. EGFR promoter exhibits dynamic histone modifications and binding of ASH2L and P300 in human germinal matrix and gliomas. *Epigenetics* **2015**, *10*, 496–507. [CrossRef]
59. Chen, R.; Smith-Cohn, M.; Cohen, A.L.; Colman, H. Glioma Subclassifications and Their Clinical Significance. *Neurotherapeutics* **2017**, *14*, 284–297. [CrossRef]
60. Rutkowska, A.; Stoczyńska-Fidelus, E.; Janik, K.; Włodarczyk, A.; Rieske, P. EGFRvIII: An Oncogene with Ambiguous Role. *J. Oncol.* **2019**, 10922587. [CrossRef]
61. Chistiakov, D.A.; Chekhonin, I.V.; Chekhonin, V.P. The EGFR variant III mutant as a target for immunotherapy of glioblastoma multiforme. *Eur. J. Pharmacol.* **2017**, *810*, 70–82. [CrossRef]
62. Weathers, S.P.; de Groot, J. VEGF manipulation in glioblastoma. *Oncology* **2015**, *29*, 720–727. [PubMed]
63. Soubéran, A.; Brustlein, S.; Gouarné, C.; Chasson, L.; Tchoghandjian, A.; Malissen, M.; Rougon, G. Effects of VEGF blockade on the dynamics of the inflammatory landscape in glioblastoma-bearing mice. *J. Neuroinflamm.* **2019**, *16*, 191. [CrossRef] [PubMed]
64. Shibuya, M. Vascular Endothelial Growth Factor (VEGF) and Its Receptor (VEGFR) Signaling in Angiogenesis: A Crucial Target for Anti- and Pro-Angiogenic Therapies. *Genes Cancer* **2011**, *2*, 1097–1105. [CrossRef] [PubMed]
65. Jiao, Q.; Bi, L.; Ren, Y.; Song, S.; Wang, Q.; Wang, Y.S. Advances in studies of tyrosine kinase inhibitors and their acquired resistance. *Mol. Cancer* **2018**, *17*, 1–12. [CrossRef] [PubMed]
66. Thomas, R.; Weihua, Z. Rethink of EGFR in cancer with its kinase independent function on board. *Front. Oncol.* **2019**, *9*, 800. [CrossRef]

67. Kim, Y.; Apetri, M.; Luo, B.B.; Settleman, J.E.; Anderson, K.S. Differential effects of tyrosine kinase inhibitors on normal and oncogenic EGFR signaling and downstream effectors. *Mol. Cancer Res.* **2015**, *13*, 765–774. [CrossRef]
68. Raizer, J.J.; Abrey, L.E.; Lassman, A.B.; Chang, S.M.; Lamborn, K.R.; Kuhn, J.G.; Yung, W.K.A.; Gilbert, M.R.; Aldape, K.A.; Wen, P.Y.; et al. A phase II trial of erlotinib in patients with recurrent malignant gliomas and nonprogressive glioblastoma multiforme postradiation therapy. *Neuro-Oncology* **2010**, *12*, 95–103. [CrossRef]
69. Gallego, O. Nonsurgical treatment of recurrent glioblastoma. *Curr. Oncol.* **2015**, *22*, e273–e281. [CrossRef]
70. Stea, B.; Falsey, R.; Kislin, K.; Patel, J.; Glanzberg, H.; Carey, S.; Ambrad, A.A.; Meuillet, E.J.; Martinez, J.D. Time and dose-dependent radiosensitization of the glioblastoma multiforme U251 cells by the EGF receptor tyrosine kinase inhibitor ZD1839 ('Iressa'). *Cancer Lett.* **2003**, *202*, 43–51. [CrossRef]
71. Uhm, J.H.; Ballman, K.V.; Wu, W.; Giannini, C.; Krauss, J.C.; Buckner, J.C.; James, C.D.; Scheithauer, B.W.; Behrens, R.J.; Flynn, P.J.; et al. Phase II evaluation of gefitinib in patients with newly diagnosed grade 4 astrocytoma: Mayo/north central cancer treatment group study n0074. *Int. J. Radiat. Oncol. Biol. Phys.* **2011**, *80*, 347–353. [CrossRef]
72. Reardon, D.A.; Conrad, C.A.; Cloughesy, T.; Prados, M.D.; Friedman, H.S.; Aldape, K.D.; Mischel, P.; Xia, J.; DiLea, C.; Huang, J.; et al. Phase i study of AEE788, a novel multitarget inhibitor of ErbB- and VEGF-receptor-family tyrosine kinases, in recurrent glioblastoma patients. *Cancer Chemother. Pharmacol.* **2012**, *69*, 1507–1518. [CrossRef] [PubMed]
73. Jane, E.P.; Premkumar, D.R.; Addo-Yobo, S.O.; Pollack, I.F. Abrogation of mitogen-activated protein kinase and akt signaling by vandetanib synergistically potentiates histone deacetylase inhibitor-induced apoptosis in human glioma cells. *J. Pharmacol. Exp. Ther.* **2009**, *331*, 327–337. [CrossRef] [PubMed]
74. Lee, E.Q.; Kaley, T.J.; Duda, D.G.; Schiff, D.; Lassman, A.B.; Wong, E.T.; Mikkelsen, T.; Purow, B.W.; Muzikansky, A.; Ancukiewicz, M.; et al. A multicenter, phase II, randomized, noncomparative clinical trial of radiation and temozolomide with or without vandetanib in newly diagnosed glioblastoma patients. *Clin. Cancer Res.* **2015**, *21*, 3610–3618. [CrossRef] [PubMed]
75. Thiessen, B.; Stewart, C.; Tsao, M.; Kamel-Reid, S.; Schaiquevich, P.; Mason, W.; Easaw, J.; Belanger, K.; Forsyth, P.; McIntosh, L.; et al. A phase I/II trial of GW572016 (lapatinib) in recurrent glioblastoma multiforme: Clinical outcomes, pharmacokinetics and molecular correlation. *Cancer Chemother. Pharmacol.* **2010**, *65*, 353–361. [CrossRef] [PubMed]
76. Schlaff, C.D.; Arscott, W.T.; Gordon, I.; Camphausen, K.A.; Tandle, A. Human EGFR-2, EGFR and HDAC triple-inhibitor CUDC-101 enhances radiosensitiviy of GBM cells. *Biomed. Res. J.* **2015**, *2*, 105–119.
77. Gerstner, E.R.; Eichler, A.F.; Plotkin, S.R.; Drappatz, J.; Doyle, C.L.; Xu, L.; Duda, D.G.; Wen, P.Y.; Jain, R.K.; Batchelor, T.T. Phase I trial with biomarker studies of vatalanib (PTK787) in patients with newly diagnosed glioblastoma treated with enzyme inducing anti-epileptic drugs and standard radiation and temozolomide. *J. Neurooncol.* **2011**, *103*, 325–332. [CrossRef]
78. Kalpathy-Cramer, J.; Chandra, V.; Da, X.; Ou, Y.; Emblem, K.E.; Muzikansky, A.; Cai, X.; Douw, L.; Evans, J.G.; Dietrich, J.; et al. Phase II study of tivozanib, an oral VEGFR inhibitor, in patients with recurrent glioblastoma. *J. Neurooncol.* **2017**, *131*, 603–610. [CrossRef]
79. Hainsworth, J.D.; Ervin, T.; Friedman, E.; Priego, V.; Murphy, P.B.; Clark, B.L.; Lamar, R.E. Concurrent radiotherapy and temozolomide followed by temozolomide and sorafenib in the first-line treatment of patients with glioblastoma multiforme. *Cancer* **2010**, *116*, 3663–3669. [CrossRef]
80. Batchelor, T.T.; Mulholland, P.; Neyns, B.; Nabors, L.B.; Campone, M.; Wick, A.; Mason, W.; Mikkelsen, T.; Phuphanich, S.; Ashby, L.S.; et al. Phase III randomized trial comparing the efficacy of cediranib as monotherapy, and in combination with lomustine, versus lomustine alone in patients with recurrent glioblastoma. *J. Clin. Oncol.* **2013**, *31*, 3212–3218. [CrossRef]
81. Fauvel, B.; Yasri, A. Antibodies directed against receptor tyrosine kinases: Current and future strategies to fight cancer. *MAbs* **2014**, *6*, 838–851. [CrossRef]
82. Belda-Iniesta, C.; Carpeño, J.D.C.; Saenz, E.C.; Gutiérrez, M.; Perona, R.; Barón, M.G. Long term responses with cetuximab therapy in glioblastoma multiforme. *Cancer Biol. Ther.* **2006**, *5*, 912–914. [CrossRef]
83. Neyns, B.; Sadones, J.; Joosens, E.; Bouttens, F.; Verbeke, L.; Baurain, J.F.; D'Hondt, L.; Strauven, T.; Chaskis, C.; In't Veld, P.; et al. Stratified phase II trial of cetuximab in patients with recurrent high-grade glioma. *Ann. Oncol.* **2009**, *20*, 1596–1603. [CrossRef]

84. Martens, T.; Schmidt, N.O.; Eckerich, C.; Filibrandt, R.; Merchant, M.; Schwall, R.; Westphal, M.; Lamszus, K. A novel one-armed anti-c-Met antibody inhibits glioblastoma growth in vivo. *Clin. Cancer Res.* **2006**, *12*, 6144–6152. [CrossRef]
85. Park, T.E.; Mustafaoglu, N.; Herland, A.; Hasselkus, R.; Mannix, R.; FitzGerald, E.A.; Prantil-Baun, R.; Watters, A.; Henry, O.; Benz, M.; et al. Hypoxia-enhanced Blood-Brain Barrier Chip recapitulates human barrier function and shuttling of drugs and antibodies. *Nat. Commun.* **2019**, *10*, 1–12. [CrossRef]
86. Yu, Y.J.; Watts, R.J. Developing Therapeutic Antibodies for Neurodegenerative Disease. *Neurotherapeutics* **2013**, *10*, 459–472. [CrossRef]
87. Brinkmann, U.; Kontermann, R.E. The making of bispecific antibodies. *MAbs* **2017**, *9*, 182–212. [CrossRef]
88. Razzak, R.A.; Florence, G.J.; Gunn-Moore, F.J. Approaches to CNS drug delivery with a focus on transporter-mediated transcytosis. *Int. J. Mol. Sci.* **2019**, *20*, 3108. [CrossRef]
89. Kong, D.H.; Kim, M.R.; Jang, J.H.; Na, H.J.; Lee, S. A review of anti-angiogenic targets for monoclonal antibody cancer therapy. *Int. J. Mol. Sci.* **2017**, *18*, 1786. [CrossRef]
90. Castro, B.A.; Aghi, M.K. Bevacizumab for glioblastoma: Current indications, surgical implications, and future directions. *Neurosurg. Focus* **2014**, *37*, E9. [CrossRef]
91. De Groot, J.F.; Lamborn, K.R.; Chang, S.M.; Gilbert, M.R.; Cloughesy, T.F.; Aldape, K.; Yao, J.; Jackson, E.F.; Lieberman, F.; Robins, H.I.; et al. Phase II study of aflibercept in recurrent malignant glioma: A North American brain tumor consortium study. *J. Clin. Oncol.* **2011**, *29*, 2689–2695. [CrossRef]
92. Wang, X.; Yeo, R.X.; Hogg, P.J.; Goldstein, D.; Crowe, P.; Dilda, P.J.; Yang, J.L. The synergistic inhibitory effect of combining therapies targeting EGFR and mitochondria in sarcomas. *Oncotarget* **2020**, *11*, 46–61. [CrossRef] [PubMed]
93. Zhou, X.Y.; Liu, H.; Ding, Z.B.; Xi, H.P.; Wang, G.W. lncRNA SNHG16 promotes glioma tumorigenicity through miR-373/EGFR axis by activating PI3K/AKT pathway. *Genomics* **2020**, *112*, 1021–1029. [CrossRef] [PubMed]
94. Zhao, H.F.; Wang, J.; Shao, W.; Wu, C.P.; Chen, Z.P.; To, S.S.T.; Li, W.P. Recent advances in the use of PI3K inhibitors for glioblastoma multiforme: Current preclinical and clinical development. *Mol. Cancer* **2017**, *16*, 1–16. [CrossRef]
95. Pearson, J.R.; Regad, T. Targeting cellular pathways in glioblastoma multiforme. *Nat. Publ. Gr.* **2017**, *2*. [CrossRef] [PubMed]
96. Ma, D.J.; Galanis, E.; Anderson, S.K.; Schiff, D.; Kaufmann, T.J.; Peller, P.J.; Giannini, C.; Brown, P.D.; Uhm, J.H.; McGraw, S.; et al. A phase II trial of everolimus, temozolomide, and radiotherapy in patients with newly diagnosed glioblastoma: NCCTG N057K. *Neuro-Oncology* **2015**, *17*, 1261–1269. [CrossRef]
97. Reardon, D.A.; Desjardins, A.; Vredenburgh, J.J.; Gururangan, S.; Friedman, A.H.; Herndon, J.E.; Marcello, J.; Norfleet, J.A.; McLendon, R.E.; Sampson, J.H.; et al. Phase 2 trial of erlotinib plus sirolimus in adults with recurrent glioblastoma. *J. Neurooncol.* **2010**, *96*, 219–230. [CrossRef]
98. Chang, S.M.; Wen, P.; Cloughesy, T.; Greenberg, H.; Schiff, D.; Conrad, C.; Fink, K.; Robins, H.I.; De Angelis, L.; Raizer, J.; et al. Phase II study of CCI-779 in patients with recurrent glioblastoma multiforme. *Investig. New Drugs* **2005**, *23*, 357–361. [CrossRef]
99. Kahn, J.; Hayman, T.J.; Jamal, M.; Rath, B.H.; Kramp, T.; Camphausen, K.; Tofilon, P.J. The mTORC1/mTORC2 inhibitor AZD2014 enhances the radiosensitivity of glioblastoma stem-like cells. *Neuro-Oncology* **2014**, *16*, 23–37. [CrossRef]
100. Lin, F.; Buil, L.; Sherris, D.; Beijnen, J.H.; Van Tellingen, O. Dual mTORC1 and mTORC2 inhibitor Palomid 529 penetrates the Blood-Brain Barrier without restriction by ABCB1 and ABCG2. *Int. J. Cancer* **2013**, *133*, 1222–1233. [CrossRef]
101. Huang, L.; Fu, L. Mechanisms of resistance to EGFR tyrosine kinase inhibitors. *Acta Pharm. Sin. B* **2015**, *5*, 390–401. [CrossRef]
102. Bianco, R.; Shin, I.; Ritter, C.A.; Yakes, F.M.; Basso, A.; Rosen, N.; Tsurutani, J.; Dennis, P.A.; Mills, G.B.; Arteaga, C.L. Loss of PTEN/MMAC1/TEP in EGF receptor-expressing tumor cells counteracts the antitumor action of EGFR tyrosine kinase inhibitors. *Oncogene* **2003**, *22*, 2812–2822. [CrossRef] [PubMed]
103. Fan, Q.W.; Cheng, C.K.; Nicolaides, T.P.; Hackett, C.S.; Knight, Z.A.; Shokat, K.M.; Weiss, W.A. A dual phosphoinositide-3-kinase α/mTOR inhibitor cooperates with blockade of epidermal growth factor receptor in PTEN-mutant glioma. *Cancer Res.* **2007**, *67*, 7960–7965. [CrossRef] [PubMed]

104. Gallego, O.; Cuatrecasas, M.; Benavides, M.; Segura, P.P.; Berrocal, A.; Erill, N.; Colomer, A.; Quintana, M.J.; Balaña, C.; Gil, M.; et al. Efficacy of erlotinib in patients with relapsed gliobastoma multiforme who expressed EGFRVIII and PTEN determined by immunohistochemistry. *J. Neurooncol.* **2014**, *116*, 413–419. [CrossRef] [PubMed]
105. Groot, J.F.; Gilbert, M.R.; Aldape, K.; Hess, K.R.; Hanna, T.A.; Ictech, S.; Groves, M.D.; Conrad, C.; Colman, H.; Puduvalli, V.K.; et al. Phase II study of carboplatin and erlotinib (Tarceva, OSI-774) in patients with recurrent glioblastoma. *J. Neurooncol.* **2008**, *90*, 89–97. [CrossRef]
106. Akhavan, D.; Pourzia, A.L.; Nourian, A.A.; Williams, K.J.; Nathanson, D.; Babic, I.; Villa, G.R.; Tanaka, K.; Nael, A.; Yang, H.; et al. De-repression of PDGFRβ transcription promotes acquired resistance to EGFR tyrosine kinase inhibitors in glioblastoma patients. *Cancer Discov.* **2013**, *3*, 534–547. [CrossRef]
107. Thorne, A.H.; Zanca, C.; Furnari, F. Epidermal growth factor receptor targeting and challenges in glioblastoma. *Neuro-Oncology* **2016**, *18*, 914–918. [CrossRef]
108. Brandes, A.A.; Franceschi, E.; Tosoni, A.; Hegi, M.E.; Stupp, R. Epidermal growth factor receptor inhibitors in neuro-oncology: Hopes and disappointments. *Clin. Cancer Res.* **2008**, *14*, 957–960. [CrossRef]
109. Reardon, D.A.; Nabors, L.B.; Mason, W.P.; Perry, J.R.; Shapiro, W.; Kavan, P.; Mathieu, D.; Phuphanich, S.; Cseh, A.; Fu, Y.; et al. Phase I/randomized phase II study of afatinib, an irreversible ErbB family blocker, with or without protracted temozolomide in adults with recurrent glioblastoma. *Neuro-Oncology* **2015**, *17*, 430–439. [CrossRef]
110. Sathornsumetee, S.; Desjardins, A.; Vredenburgh, J.J.; McLendon, R.E.; Marcello, J.; Herndon, J.E.; Mathe, A.; Hamilton, M.; Rich, J.N.; Norfleet, J.A.; et al. Phase II trial of bevacizumab and erlotinib in patients with recurrent malignant glioma. *Neuro-Oncology* **2010**, *12*, 1300–1310. [CrossRef]
111. Nam, L.; Coll, C.; Erthal, L.C.S.; de la Torre, C.; Serrano, D.; Martínez-Máñez, R.; Santos-Martínez, M.J.; Ruiz-Hernández, E. Drug delivery nanosystems for the localized treatment of glioblastoma multiforme. *Materials* **2018**, *11*, 378. [CrossRef]
112. Mahmoud, B.S.; AlAmri, A.H.; McConville, C. Polymeric nanoparticles for the treatment of malignant gliomas. *Cancers* **2020**, *12*, 175. [CrossRef] [PubMed]
113. Westphal, M.; Maire, C.L.; Lamszus, K. EGFR as a Target for glioblastoma treatment: An unfulfilled promise. *CNS Drugs* **2017**, *31*, 723–735. [CrossRef] [PubMed]
114. Rizvi, S.A.A.; Saleh, A.M. Applications of nanoparticle systems in drug delivery technology. *Saudi Pharm. J.* **2018**, *26*, 64–70. [CrossRef] [PubMed]
115. Senapati, S.; Mahanta, A.K.; Kumar, S.; Maiti, P. Controlled drug delivery vehicles for cancer treatment and their performance. *Signal Transduct. Target. Ther.* **2018**, *3*, 1–19. [CrossRef]
116. Zhao, Z.; Ukidve, A.; Krishnan, V.; Mitragotri, S. Effect of physicochemical and surface properties on in vivo fate of drug nanocarriers. *Adv. Drug Deliv. Rev.* **2019**, *143*, 3–21. [CrossRef]
117. Donahue, N.D.; Acar, H.; Wilhelm, S. Concepts of nanoparticle cellular uptake, intracellular trafficking, and kinetics in nanomedicine. *Adv. Drug Deliv. Rev.* **2019**, *143*, 68–96. [CrossRef]
118. Nguyen, V.H.; Lee, B.J. Protein corona: A new approach for nanomedicine design. *Int. J. Nanomed.* **2017**, *12*, 3137–3151. [CrossRef]
119. Ruan, C.; Liu, L.; Lu, Y.; Zhang, Y.; He, X.; Chen, X.; Zhang, Y.; Chen, Q.; Guo, Q.; Sun, T.; et al. Substance P-modified human serum albumin nanoparticles loaded with paclitaxel for targeted therapy of glioma. *Acta Pharm. Sin. B* **2018**, *8*, 85–96. [CrossRef]
120. Li, C.; Tan, J.; Chang, J.; Li, W.; Liu, Z.; Li, N.; Ji, Y. Radioiodine-labeled anti-epidermal growth factor receptor binding bovine serum albumin-polycaprolactone for targeting imaging of glioblastoma. *Oncol. Rep.* **2017**, *38*, 2919–2926. [CrossRef]
121. Tsutsui, Y.; Tomizawa, K.; Nagita, M.; Michiue, H.; Nishiki, T.I.; Ohmori, I.; Seno, M.; Matsui, H. Development of bionanocapsules targeting brain tumors. *J. Control. Release* **2007**, *122*, 159–164. [CrossRef]
122. Wei, L.; Guo, X.Y.; Yang, T.; Yu, M.Z.; Chen, D.W.; Wang, J.C. Brain tumor-targeted therapy by systemic delivery of siRNA with Transferrin receptor-mediated core-shell nanoparticles. *Int. J. Pharm.* **2016**, *510*, 394–405. [CrossRef] [PubMed]
123. Kulkarni, A.A.; Vijaykumar, V.E.; Natarajan, S.K.; Sengupta, S.; Sabbisetti, V.S. Sustained inhibition of cMET-VEGFR2 signaling using liposome-mediated delivery increases efficacy and reduces toxicity in kidney cancer. *Nanomed. Nanotechnol. Biol. Med.* **2016**, *12*, 1853–1861. [CrossRef] [PubMed]

124. Zhao, X.; Li, F.; Li, Y.; Wang, H.; Ren, H.; Chen, J.; Nie, G.; Hao, J. Co-delivery of HIF1α siRNA and gemcitabine via biocompatible lipid-polymer hybrid nanoparticles for effective treatment of pancreatic cancer. *Biomaterials* **2015**, *46*, 13–25. [CrossRef] [PubMed]
125. Kuo, Y.C.; Lee, C.H. Dual targeting of solid lipid nanoparticles grafted with 83-14 MAb and anti-EGF receptor for malignant brain tumor therapy. *Life Sci.* **2016**, *146*, 222–231. [CrossRef] [PubMed]
126. Pan, X.; Wu, G.; Yang, W.; Barth, R.F.; Tjarks, W.; Lee, R.J. Synthesis of cetuximab-immunoliposomes via a cholesterol-based membrane anchor for targeting of EGFR. *Bioconjug. Chem.* **2007**, *18*, 101–108. [CrossRef]
127. Weng, K.C.; Hashizume, R.; Noble, C.O.; Serwer, L.P.; Drummond, D.C.; Kirpotin, D.B.; Kuwabara, A.M.; Chao, L.X.; Chen, F.F.; James, C.D.; et al. Convection-enhanced delivery of targeted quantum dot-immunoliposome hybrid nanoparticles to intracranial brain tumor models. *Nanomedicine* **2013**, *8*, 1913–1925. [CrossRef]
128. Shin, D.H.; Lee, S.J.; Kim, J.S.; Ryu, J.H.; Kim, J.S. Synergistic effect of immunoliposomal gemcitabine and bevacizumab in glioblastoma stem cell-targeted therapy. *J. Biomed. Nanotechnol.* **2015**, *11*, 1989–2002. [CrossRef]
129. Zhang, Y.; Zhai, M.; Chen, Z.; Han, X.; Yu, F.; Li, Z.; Xie, X.Y.; Han, C.; Yu, L.; Yang, Y.; et al. Dual-modified liposome codelivery of doxorubicin and vincristine improve targeting and therapeutic efficacy of glioma. *Drug Deliv.* **2017**, *24*, 1045–1055. [CrossRef]
130. Naahidi, S.; Jafari, M.; Edalat, F.; Raymond, K.; Khademhosseini, A.; Chen, P. Biocompatibility of engineered nanoparticles for drug delivery. *J. Control. Release* **2013**, *166*, 182–194. [CrossRef]
131. Alves Rico, S.R.; Abbasi, A.Z.; Ribeiro, G.; Ahmed, T.; Wu, X.Y.; De Oliveira Silva, D. Diruthenium (II, III) metallodrugs of ibuprofen and naproxen encapsulated in intravenously injectable polymer-lipid nanoparticles exhibit enhanced activity against breast and prostate cancer cells. *Nanoscale* **2017**, *9*, 10701–10714. [CrossRef]
132. Ni, X.L.; Chen, L.X.; Zhang, H.; Yang, B.; Xu, S.; Wu, M.; Liu, J.; Yang, L.L.; Chen, Y.; Fu, S.Z.; et al. In vitro and in vivo antitumor effect of gefitinib nanoparticles on human lung cancer. *Drug Deliv.* **2017**, *24*, 1501–1512. [CrossRef] [PubMed]
133. Hu, C.; Cun, X.; Ruan, S.; Liu, R.; Xiao, W.; Yang, X.; Yang, Y.; Yang, C.; Gao, H. Enzyme-triggered size shrink and laser-enhanced NO release nanoparticles for deep tumor penetration and combination therapy. *Biomaterials* **2018**, *168*, 64–75. [CrossRef] [PubMed]
134. Zhu, H.; Cheng, P.; Chen, P.; Pu, K. Recent progress in the development of near-infrared organic photothermal and photodynamic nanotherapeutics. *Biomater. Sci.* **2018**, *6*, 746–765. [CrossRef] [PubMed]
135. Jamali, Z.; Khoobi, M.; Hejazi, S.M.; Eivazi, N.; Abdolahpour, S.; Imanparast, F.; Moradi-Sardareh, H.; Paknejad, M. Evaluation of targeted curcumin (CUR) loaded PLGA nanoparticles for in vitro photodynamic therapy on human glioblastoma cell line. *Photodiagn. Photodyn. Ther.* **2018**, *23*, 190–201. [CrossRef] [PubMed]
136. Wang, L.; Hao, Y.; Li, H.; Zhao, Y.; Meng, D.; Li, D.; Shi, J.; Zhang, H.; Zhang, Z.; Zhang, Y. Co-delivery of doxorubicin and siRNA for glioma therapy by a brain targeting system: Angiopep-2-modified poly(lactic-co-glycolic acid) nanoparticles. *J. Drug Target.* **2015**, *23*, 832–846. [CrossRef] [PubMed]
137. Ye, C.; Pan, B.; Xu, H.; Zhao, Z.; Shen, J.; Lu, J.; Yu, R.; Liu, H. Co-delivery of GOLPH3 siRNA and gefitinib by cationic lipid-PLGA nanoparticles improves EGFR-targeted therapy for glioma. *J. Mol. Med.* **2019**, *97*, 1575–1588. [CrossRef] [PubMed]
138. Duwa, R.; Banstola, A.; Emami, F.; Jeong, J.H.; Lee, S.; Yook, S. Cetuximab conjugated temozolomide-loaded poly (lactic-co-glycolic acid) nanoparticles for targeted nanomedicine in EGFR overexpressing cancer cells. *J. Drug Deliv. Sci. Technol.* **2020**, *60*, 101928. [CrossRef]
139. Yu, F.; Asghar, S.; Zhang, M.; Zhang, J.; Ping, Q.; Xiao, Y. Local strategies and delivery systems for the treatment of malignant gliomas. *J. Drug Target.* **2019**, *27*, 367–378. [CrossRef]
140. Sherje, A.P.; Jadhav, M.; Dravyakar, B.R.; Kadam, D. Dendrimers: A versatile nanocarrier for drug delivery and targeting. *Int. J. Pharm.* **2018**, *548*, 707–720. [CrossRef]
141. Márquez-Miranda, V.; Camarada, M.B.; Araya-Durán, I.; Varas-Concha, I.; Almonacid, D.E.; González-Nilo, F.D. Biomimetics: From Bioinformatics to Rational Design of Dendrimers as Gene Carriers. *PLoS ONE* **2015**, *10*, e0138392. [CrossRef]
142. Svenson, S.; Tomalia, D.A. Dendrimers in biomedical applications-Reflections on the field. *Adv. Drug Deliv. Rev.* **2005**, *57*, 2106–2129. [CrossRef] [PubMed]

143. Madaan, K.; Kumar, S.; Poonia, N.; Lather, V.; Pandita, D. Dendrimers in drug delivery and targeting: Drug-dendrimer interactions and toxicity issues. *J. Pharm. Bioallied Sci.* **2014**, *6*, 139–150. [CrossRef] [PubMed]
144. Kesharwani, P.; Iyer, A.K. Recent advances in dendrimer-based nanovectors for tumor-targeted drug and gene delivery. *Drug Discov. Today* **2015**, *20*, 536–547. [CrossRef] [PubMed]
145. Kang, C.; Yuan, X.; Li, F.; Pu, P.; Yu, S.; Shen, C.; Zhang, Z.; Zhang, Y. Evaluation of folate-PAMAM for the delivery of antisense oligonucleotides to rat C6 glioma cells in vitro and in vivo. *J. Biomed. Mater. Res. Part A* **2010**, *93*, 585–594. [CrossRef]
146. Wu, G.; Barth, R.F.; Yang, W.; Kawabata, S.; Zhang, L.; Green-Church, K. Targeted delivery of methotrexate to epidermal growth factor receptor-positive brain tumors by means of cetuximab (IMC-C225) dendrimer bioconjugates. *Mol. Cancer Ther.* **2006**, *5*, 52–59. [CrossRef]
147. Gajbhiye, V.; Jain, N.K. The treatment of Glioblastoma Xenografts by surfactant conjugated dendritic nanoconjugates. *Biomaterials* **2011**, *32*, 6213–6225. [CrossRef]
148. Liu, C.; Zhao, Z.; Gao, H.; Rostami, I.; You, Q.; Jia, X.; Wang, C.; Zhu, L.; Yang, Y. Research paper enhanced blood-brain-barrier penetrability and tumor-targeting efficiency by peptide-functionalized poly(Amidoamine) dendrimer for the therapy of gliomas. *Nanotheranostics* **2019**, *3*, 311–330. [CrossRef]
149. Mekaru, H.; Lu, J.; Tamanoi, F. Development of mesoporous silica-based nanoparticles with controlled release capability for cancer therapy. *Adv. Drug Deliv. Rev.* **2015**, *95*, 40–49. [CrossRef]
150. Zhou, Y.; Quan, G.; Wu, Q.; Zhang, X.; Niu, B.; Wu, B.; Huang, Y.; Pan, X.; Wu, C. Mesoporous silica nanoparticles for drug and gene delivery. *Acta Pharm. Sin. B* **2018**, *8*, 165–177. [CrossRef]
151. Narayan, R.; Nayak, U.Y.; Raichur, A.M.; Garg, S. Mesoporous silica nanoparticles: A comprehensive review on synthesis and recent advances. *Pharmaceutics* **2018**, *10*, 118. [CrossRef]
152. Chen, F.H.; Zhang, L.M.; Chen, Q.T.; Zhang, Y.; Zhang, Z.J. Synthesis of a novel magnetic drug delivery system composed of doxorubicin-conjugated Fe3O4 nanoparticle cores and a PEG-functionalized porous silica shell. *Chem. Commun.* **2010**, *46*, 8633–8635. [CrossRef] [PubMed]
153. Guan, Y.Q.; Zheng, Z.; Huang, Z.; Li, Z.; Niu, S.; Liu, J.M. Powerful inner/outer controlled multi-target magnetic nanoparticle drug carrier prepared by liquid photo-immobilization. *Sci. Rep.* **2014**, *4*, 4990. [CrossRef] [PubMed]
154. Heggannavar, G.B.; Hiremath, C.G.; Achari, D.D.; Pangarkar, V.G.; Kariduraganavar, M.Y. Development of doxorubicin-loaded magnetic silica-pluronic F-127 nanocarriers conjugated with transferrin for treating glioblastoma across the blood-brain barrier using an in vitro model. *ACS Omega* **2018**, *3*, 8017–8026. [CrossRef] [PubMed]
155. Bharde, A.A.; Palankar, R.; Fritsch, C.; Klaver, A.; Kanger, J.S.; Jovin, T.M.; Arndt-Jovin, D.J. Correction: Magnetic nanoparticles as mediators of ligand-free activation of EGFR signaling. *PLoS ONE* **2013**, *8*. [CrossRef]
156. Kaluzova, M.; Bouras, A.; Machaidze, R.; Hadjipanayis, C.G. Targeted therapy of glioblastoma stem-like cells and tumor nonstem cells using cetuximab-conjugated iron-oxide nanoparticles. *Oncotarget* **2015**, *6*, 8788–8806. [CrossRef] [PubMed]
157. Wankhede, M.; Bouras, A.; Kaluzova, M.; Hadjipanayis, C.G. Magnetic nanoparticles: An emerging technology for malignant brain tumor imaging and therapy. *Expert Rev. Clin. Pharmacol.* **2012**, *5*, 173–186. [CrossRef]
158. Liu, X.; Du, C.; Li, H.; Jiang, T.; Luo, Z.; Pang, Z.; Geng, D.; Zhang, J. Engineered superparamagnetic iron oxide nanoparticles (SPIONs) for dual-modality imaging of intracranial glioblastoma via EGFRvIII targeting. *Beilstein J. Nanotechnol.* **2019**, *10*, 1860–1872. [CrossRef]
159. Hamarat Şanlıer, Ş.; Ak, G.; Yılmaz, H.; Ünal, A.; Bozkaya, Ü.F.; Tanıyan, G.; Yıldırım, Y.; Yıldız Türkyılmaz, G. Development of ultrasound-triggered and magnetic-targeted nanobubble system for dual-drug delivery. *J. Pharm. Sci.* **2019**, *108*, 1272–1283. [CrossRef]
160. Chattopadhyay, N.; Cai, Z.; Kwon, Y.L.; Lechtman, E.; Pignol, J.P.; Reilly, R.M. Molecularly targeted gold nanoparticles enhance the radiation response of breast cancer cells and tumor xenografts to X-radiation. *Breast Cancer Res. Treat.* **2013**, *137*, 81–91. [CrossRef]

161. El-Sayed, I.H.; Huang, X.; El-Sayed, M.A. Selective laser photo-thermal therapy of epithelial carcinoma using anti-EGFR antibody conjugated gold nanoparticles. *Cancer Lett.* **2006**, *239*, 129–135. [CrossRef]
162. Nie, S. Understanding and overcoming major barriers in cancer nanomedicine. *Nanomedicine* **2010**, *5*, 523–528. [CrossRef] [PubMed]
163. Haller, E.; Lindner, W.; Lämmerhofer, M. Gold nanoparticle-antibody conjugates for specific extraction and subsequent analysis by liquid chromatography-tandem mass spectrometry of malondialdehyde-modified low density lipoprotein as biomarker for cardiovascular risk. *Anal. Chim. Acta* **2015**, *857*, 53–63. [CrossRef] [PubMed]
164. Patra, C.R.; Bhattacharya, R.; Wang, E.; Katarya, A.; Lau, J.S.; Dutta, S.; Muders, M.; Wang, S.; Buhrow, S.A.; Safgren, S.L.; et al. Targeted delivery of gemcitabine to pancreatic adenocarcinoma using cetuximab as a targeting agent. *Cancer Res.* **2008**, *68*, 1970–1978. [CrossRef] [PubMed]
165. Feng, Y.; Cheng, Y.; Chang, Y.; Jian, H.; Zheng, R.; Wu, X.; Xu, K.; Wang, L.; Ma, X.; Li, X.; et al. Time-staggered delivery of erlotinib and doxorubicin by gold nanocages with two smart polymers for reprogrammable release and synergistic with photothermal therapy. *Biomaterials* **2019**, *217*, 119327. [CrossRef]
166. Groysbeck, N.; Stoessel, A.; Donzeau, M.; Da Silva, E.C.; Lehmann, M.; Strub, J.M.; Cianferani, S.; Dembélé, K.; Zuber, G. Synthesis and biological evaluation of 2.4 nm thiolate-protected gold nanoparticles conjugated to Cetuximab for targeting glioblastoma cancer cells via the EGFR. *Nanotechnology* **2019**, *30*, 184005. [CrossRef]
167. Anselmo, A.C.; Mitragotri, S. Nanoparticles in the clinic: An update. *Bioeng. Transl. Med.* **2019**, *4*. [CrossRef]
168. Kwan, K.; Schneider, J.R.; Kobets, A.; Boockvar, J.A. Targeting epidermal growth factor receptors in recurrent glioblastoma via a novel epithelial growth factor receptor-conjugated nanocell doxorubicin delivery system. *Clin. Neurosurg.* **2018**, *82*, N23–N24. [CrossRef]
169. Mamot, C.; Ritschard, R.; Wicki, A.; Stehle, G.; Dieterle, T.; Bubendorf, L.; Hilker, C.; Deuster, S.; Herrmann, R.; Rochlitz, C. Tolerability, safety, pharmacokinetics, and efficacy of doxorubicin-loaded anti-EGFR immunoliposomes in advanced solid tumours: A phase 1 dose-escalation study. *Lancet Oncol.* **2012**, *13*, 1234–1241. [CrossRef]
170. Senzer, N.; Nemunaitis, J.; Nemunaitis, D.; Bedell, C.; Edelman, G.; Barve, M.; Nunan, R.; Pirollo, K.F.; Rait, A.; Chang, E.H. Phase i study of a systemically delivered p53 nanoparticle in advanced solid tumors. In *Proceedings of the Molecular Therapy*; Nature Publishing Group: Edinburgh, UK, 2013; pp. 1096–1103.
171. Kesari, S.; Juarez, T.; Carrillo, J.; Truong, J.; Nguyen, M.; Heng, A.; Gill, J.; Nguyen, H.; Nomura, N.; Grigorian, B.; et al. A phase 2 trial with Abi-009 (nab-sirolimus) as single-agent and combinations in recurrent high-grade glioma (RHGG) and in newly diagnosed glioblastoma (ndGBM). *Neuro-Oncology* **2019**, *21*, vi218–vi219. [CrossRef]
172. Balasubramanian, K.; Rajakani, M. Problems in cryptography and cryptanalysis. In *Algorithmic Strategies for Solving Complex Problems in Cryptography*; IGI Global: Hershey, PA, USA, 2017; pp. 23–38. [CrossRef]
173. Palko-Labuz, A.; Sroda-Pomianek, K.; Uryga, A.; Kostrzewa-Suslow, E.; Michalak, K. Anticancer activity of baicalein and luteolin studied in colorectal adenocarcinoma LoVo cells and in drug-resistant LoVo/Dx cells. *Biomed. Pharmacother.* **2017**, *88*, 232–241. [CrossRef]
174. Stompor, M.; Podgórski, R.; Kubrak, T. Combined effect of flavonoid compounds and cytostatics in cancer treatment. *Eur. J. Clin. Exp. Med.* **2017**, *15*, 157–164. [CrossRef]
175. Sharma, N.; Dobhal, M.; Joshi, Y.; Chahar, M. Flavonoids: A versatile source of anticancer drugs. *Pharmacogn. Rev.* **2011**, *5*, 1. [CrossRef] [PubMed]
176. Chae, H.S.; Xu, R.; Won, J.Y.; Chin, Y.W.; Yim, H. Molecular targets of genistein and its related flavonoids to exert anticancer effects. *Int. J. Mol. Sci.* **2019**, *20*, 2420. [CrossRef] [PubMed]
177. Kashyap, D.; Garg, V.K.; Tuli, H.S.; Yerer, M.B.; Sak, K.; Sharma, A.K.; Kumar, M.; Aggarwal, V.; Sandhu, S.S. Fisetin and quercetin: Promising flavonoids with chemopreventive potential. *Biomolecules* **2019**, *9*, 174. [CrossRef] [PubMed]
178. Martín, V.; Herrera, F.; García-Santos, G.; Antolín, I.; Rodriguez-Blanco, J.; Rodriguez, C. Signaling pathways involved in antioxidant control of glioma cell proliferation. *Free Radic. Biol. Med.* **2007**, *42*, 1715–1722. [CrossRef] [PubMed]

179. Nicolas, C.S.; Amici, M.; Bortolotto, Z.A.; Doherty, A.; Csaba, Z.; Fafouri, A.; Dournaud, P.; Gressens, P.; Collingridge, G.L.; Peineau, S. The role of JAK-STAT signaling within the CNS. *Jak-Stat* **2013**, *2*, e22925. [CrossRef] [PubMed]
180. Swiatek-Machado, K.; Kaminska, B. STAT Signaling in Glioma Cells. *Adv. Exp. Med. Biol.* **2013**, *1202*, 189–208. [CrossRef]

Publisher's Note: MDPI stays neutral with regard to jurisdictional claims in published maps and institutional affiliations.

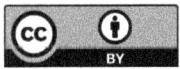 © 2020 by the authors. Licensee MDPI, Basel, Switzerland. This article is an open access article distributed under the terms and conditions of the Creative Commons Attribution (CC BY) license (http://creativecommons.org/licenses/by/4.0/).

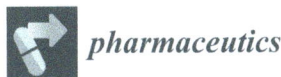

Article

Deep Tumor Penetration of Doxorubicin-Loaded Glycol Chitosan Nanoparticles Using High-Intensity Focused Ultrasound

Yongwhan Choi [1,2], Hyounkoo Han [2,3], Sangmin Jeon [2], Hong Yeol Yoon [2], Hyuncheol Kim [3], Ick Chan Kwon [1,2,*] and Kwangmeyung Kim [1,2,*]

1. KU-KIST Graduate School of Converging Science and Technology, Korea University, 145 Anam-ro, Seongbuk-gu, Seoul 02841, Korea; 113377@kist.re.kr
2. Center for Theragnosis, Biomedical Research Institute, Korea Institute of Science and Technology (KIST), Seoul 02792, Korea; zingouki@gmail.com (H.H.); jeon@kist.re.kr (S.J.); seerou@kist.re.kr (H.Y.Y.)
3. Department of Chemical & Biomolecular Engineering, Sogang University, Shinsu-dong, Mapo-gu, Seoul 121-742, Korea; hyuncheol@sogang.ac.kr
* Correspondence: ikwon@kist.re.kr (I.C.K.); kim@kist.re.kr (K.K.); Tel.: +82-2-958-5916 (K.K.)

Received: 8 September 2020; Accepted: 14 October 2020; Published: 15 October 2020

Abstract: The dense extracellular matrix (ECM) in heterogeneous tumor tissues can prevent the deep tumor penetration of drug-loaded nanoparticles, resulting in a limited therapeutic efficacy in cancer treatment. Herein, we suggest that the deep tumor penetration of doxorubicin (DOX)-loaded glycol chitosan nanoparticles (CNPs) can be improved using high-intensity focused ultrasound (HIFU) technology. Firstly, we prepared amphiphilic glycol chitosan-5β-cholanic acid conjugates that can self-assemble to form stable nanoparticles with an average of 283.7 ± 5.3 nm. Next, the anticancer drug DOX was simply loaded into the CNPs via a dialysis method. DOX-loaded CNPs (DOX-CNPs) had stable nanoparticle structures with an average size of 265.9 ± 35.5 nm in aqueous condition. In cultured cells, HIFU-treated DOX-CNPs showed rapid drug release and enhanced cellular uptake in A549 cells, resulting in increased cytotoxicity, compared to untreated DOX-CNPs. In ECM-rich A549 tumor-bearing mice, the tumor-targeting efficacy of intravenously injected DOX-CNPs with HIFU treatment was 1.84 times higher than that of untreated DOX-CNPs. Furthermore, the deep tumor penetration of HIFU-treated DOX-CNPs was clearly observed at targeted tumor tissues, due to the destruction of the ECM structure via HIFU treatment. Finally, HIFU-treated DOX-CNPs greatly increased the therapeutic efficacy at ECM-rich A549 tumor-bearing mice, compared to free DOX and untreated DOX-CNPs. This deep penetration of drug-loaded nanoparticles via HIFU treatment is a promising strategy to treat heterogeneous tumors with dense ECM structures.

Keywords: glycol chitosan nanoparticle; high-intensity focused ultrasound; deep tumor penetration; dense ECM; cancer treatment

1. Introduction

Anticancer drug-loaded nanoparticles have been used extensively in cancer treatment. This is because drug-loaded nanoparticles can be efficiently localized at targeted tumor tissues via nanoparticle-derived enhanced permeation and retention (EPR) effects in many pre-clinical tests [1–3]. The rapid growth of tumor tissues can cause a leaky vasculature as well as a suppression of lymphatic drainage, resulting in making different characteristics from those of the normal vasculature. In particular, since nanoparticles can extravasate into tumor tissues efficiently via the EPR effect, the EPR effect is regarded as the golden standard in designing nanoparticles for drug delivery [4,5]. Therefore, various nanosized materials, such as liposomes, polymeric nanoparticles, metal nanoparticles, and inorganic nanoparticles have been used in tumor-targeting delivery systems [6–9]. However, challenges remain to further improve the therapeutic efficacy of drug-loaded nanoparticles in heterogeneous tumors [10–12]. In particular, the delivery efficacy of drug-loaded nanoparticles is hampered greatly by limited deep tumor penetration in the complex tumor microenvironment [13–15]. It has been known that heterogeneous tumors differ in their vascular structure and perfusion rate [16,17]. Moreover, the thick extracellular matrix (ECM) which consists of collagen and hyaluronan (HA) in the tumor tissue can inhibit the deep tissue penetration of drug-loaded nanoparticles [18,19]. This is because the dense ECM can act as a physical barrier to the accumulation and deep tissue penetration of drug-loaded nanoparticles [15,20]. Thus, the development of a way to ensure a deep penetration of drug-loaded nanoparticles into tumor tissue is an essential challenge to improve the therapeutic efficacy of nanoparticle-based drug delivery systems in cancer treatment.

Many researchers have tried to improve the delivery efficiency of drug-loaded nanoparticles through the remodeling of the ECM in the tumor microenvironment [21,22]. Enzyme-conjugated nanoparticles have been used to increase the deep tissue penetration of nanoparticles through deconstructing the ECM structure, resulting in improvements in the therapeutic efficacy of the tumor. For example, matrix metalloprotease (MMP)-conjugated nanoparticles could break down the ECM structure, resulting in an improved delivery efficiency into deep tumor tissue and the therapeutic efficacy of drug-loaded nanoparticles [23]. Nevertheless, the applications of enzyme-conjugated nanoparticles is still limited due to the complex chemical reactions that bind the enzyme to the nanoparticle surface [24,25]. More practically, high-intensity focused ultrasound (HIFU) technology has been used to break down physically the dense ECM structure in the tumor microenvironment without any toxicity in normal organs. HIFU-mediated drug delivery systems could improve the delivery of high-molecular-weight antibodies and nanoparticles to tumor tissue, due to the successful destruction of the ECM barrier in tumor tissues [26,27]. In our previous report, we reported the exact mechanism of the HIFU-mediated deep tumor penetration of nanoparticles in heterogeneous tumor models [28,29]. Many human solid tumors express high levels of collagen and hyaluronan matrixes that can acts as physical barriers for inhibiting the deep tumor penetration of antibodies and high molecular anticancer drugs [30]. In particular, these EMC-rich tumor tissues composed of highly expressed collagen and hyaluronan matrixes can affect the accessibility and deep tumor penetration of nanosized drug delivery systems in pre-clinical tests [31]. Interestingly, the dense ECM structure of tumor tissues was successfully destroyed by non-invasive pulsed-HIFU exposure. Furthermore, the interstitial flow pressure (IFP) in the tumor tissue was reduced by normalizing the tumor vessels in ECM-rich tumors. Surprisingly, intravenously injected nanosized nanoparticles could be successfully accumulated at in ECM-rich tumors exposed to non-invasive HIFU treatments. These overall results demonstrate that ECM remodeling by HIFU treatment is a promising strategy to enhance the deep tumor penetration and enhanced tumor targeting of drug-loaded nanoparticles in solid tumors.

Glycol chitosan is a natural polysaccharide which is derived from chitosan, it has biocompatibility, non-toxicity, biodegradability, and easy fabrication properties [32]. Notably, a large number of reactive functional groups (primary amine and hydroxyl group) on the glycol chitosan backbone can be modified with cholanic acids, hydrotropic oligomer, photosensitizers, and fullerene, resulting in the formulation of nanomedicines for chemotherapy, gene therapy, and photodynamic therapy [33]. Among them, hydrophobically modified glycol chitosan can form self-assembled nanoparticles due to its amphiphilic structure. In particular, the hydrophobic inner cores of glycol chitosan nanoparticles can be used to deliver theranostic agents such as paclitaxel, docetaxel, and iron oxide nanoparticles via the EPR effect in tumor tissue, resulting in an improved drug delivery efficiency as well as tumor-specific imaging in pre-clinical mice tumor models [34–36].

Herein, we evaluate the drug delivery efficacy and therapeutic efficacy of HIFU-triggered drug-loaded nanoparticles at ECM-rich tumor models, wherein the ECM-rich tumor tissues were treated with HIFU to destroy the dense ECM structure at A549 tumor tissues (Figure 1a). First, we prepared doxorubicin-loaded glycol chitosan nanoparticles as model drug-loaded nanoparticles. We expect that doxorubicin (DOX)-chitosan nanoparticles (CNPs) are very suitable as model drug delivery systems, due to their high-tumor-targeting ability and low systemic toxicity in vivo [37]. The biodegradable and hydrophilic glycol chitosan polymers were modified hydrophobic 5β-cholanic acid and the conjugates were self-assembled to form glycol chitosan nanoparticles (CNPs). Next, the anticancer drug doxorubicin (DOX) was loaded into CNPs via a simple dialysis method, resulting in DOX-loaded CNPs (DOX-CNPs). The in vitro drug release, cellular uptake and cytotoxicity of HIFU-triggered DOX-CNPs were characterized in cultured cells. Finally, the deep tumor penetration and therapeutic efficacy of HIFU-triggered DOX-CNPs were carefully examined in an ECM-rich A549 tumor animal model, compared to free DOX and untreated DOX-CNPs.

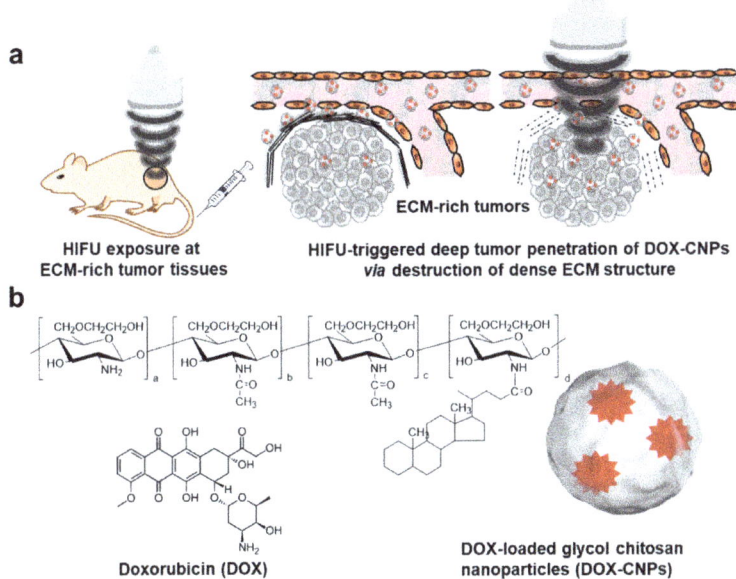

Figure 1. (a) High-intensity focused ultrasound (HIFU) treatment of doxorubicin (DOX)-loaded glycol chitosan nanoparticles (CNPs) (DOX-CNPs) to increase their deep tumor penetration in extracellular matrix (ECM)-rich tumor models. (b) Schematic illustration of glycol chitosan-5β-cholanic acid conjugate. The glycol chitosan-5β-cholanic acid conjugates form self-assembled nanoparticles in aqueous condition. The anticancer drug of DOX can be loaded into CNPs via a dialysis method, resulting in DOX-CNPs.

2. Materials and Methods

2.1. Materials

Glycol chitosan (MW = 250 kDa; degree of deacetylation > 60%), doxorubicin hydrochloride (DOX-HCl), 5β-cholanic acid, 1-ethyl-3-(3-dimethylaminopropyl)-carbodiimide hydrochloride (EDC), N-hydroxysuccinimide (NHS), triethylamine (TEA), anhydrous methanol and anhydrous dimethyl sulfoxide (DMSO) were purchased from Sigma-Aldrich (Merck, Darmstadt, Germany). A fluorescent molecule, Cy5.5-NHS ester, was purchased from Lumiprobe Corporation (Hunt Valley, MD, USA). All other chemicals were purchased as reagent grade and used without further purification or modification.

2.2. Synthesis and Characterization of Doxorubicin-Loaded Glycol Chitosan Nanoparticles (DOX-CNPs)

To prepare glycol chitosan nanoparticles (CNPs), hydrophobic 5β-cholanic acid was chemically conjugated to the hydrophilic glycol chitosan through amide linkage formation in the presence of EDC and NHS [15,38]. Briefly, 150 mg of 5β-cholanic acid was dissolved in 120 mL of methanol and mixed with EDC (120 mg) and NHS (72 mg). A total of 500 mg of glycol chitosan was dissolved in 120 mL of methanol/deionized distilled water solution (1:1 v/v), followed by slow mixing with 5β-cholanic acid solution. The mixture was vigorously stirred at room temperature for 24 h, and then purified by dialysis against distilled water/methanol (1:1 and 1:0 v/v) using a Spectra/Por®4 dialysis membrane (MWCO = 12–14 kDa, Repligen Corporation, Waltham, MA, USA). The resulting solution was lyophilized to obtain a white powder of CNPs. For the in vitro and in vivo fluorescence monitoring of CNPs, CNPs were chemically modified with near-infrared fluorescence (NIRF) dye, Cy5.5. In brief, 100 mg of CNPs were dissolved in 40 mL of DMSO, followed by mixing with 1 mL of DMSO containing 1 mg of Cy5.5-NHS. The mixture was stirred for 12 h at room temperature. Subsequently, the mixture was purified by dialysis against distilled water for 2 days using a Spectra/Por® 4 dialysis membrane (MWCO = 12–14 kDa, Repligen Corporation, Waltham, MA, USA). The resulting solution was lyophilized to obtain Cy5.5-conjugated CNPs.

To prepare DOX-encapsulated CNPs (DOX-CNPs), DOX-HCl was physically encapsulated into CNPs using a simple dialysis method. In brief, 50 mg of CNPs was dissolved in 10 mL of DMSO/distilled water (1:1 v/v). A total of 21.4 mg of DOX-HCl was dissolved in 2 mL of DMSO/distilled water (1:1 v/v). Then, the DOX-HCl solution was treated 10.8 µL of TEA for desalting, followed by mixing with CNP solution. The mixture was purified by a dialysis against distilled water for 12 h using a Spectra/Por® 4 dialysis membrane (MWCO = 12–14 kDa, Repligen Corporation, Waltham, MA, USA). The resulting solution was filtered using 0.8 µm syringe filter, followed by lyophilizing to obtain DOX-CNPs.

To confirm the hydrodynamic diameter of CNPs and DOX-CNPs, 1 mg of CNPs and DOX-CNPs were dispersed into 1 mL of PBS (pH 7.4) using a probe-type sonicator (Amp 21%, 1 min, VCX-750, Sonics and Materials, Newtown, CT, USA). The volume-weighted size distribution and zeta potential of CNPs and DOX-CNPs were measured using dynamic light scattering (DLS, Nano ZS, Malvern Panalytical Ltd., Grovewood Road, Malvern, UK) at 25 °C. The size stability and volume-weighted size distribution of CNPs and DOX-CNPs were monitored in both PBS (pH 7.4) and 1% FBS-containing PBS (pH 7.4) conditions using DLS. The morphologies of CNPs and DOX-CNPs were observed using transmission electron microscopy (TEM, CM30 Electron Microscope, Philips, CA, USA) at 200 eKV of an accelerating voltage. For TEM images, CNPs and DOX-CNPs were dispersed in distilled water and 5 µL of CNPs or DOX-CNPs solution was dropped on a 200 mesh carbon-coated copper grid, followed by negative staining using 2% uranyl acetate solution. Based on TEM images ($n = 10$), size distribution of CNPs and DOX-CNPs were determined using Image Pro Plus4.5 5 software (Media Cybernetics, Bethesda, Rockville, MD, USA).

2.3. In Vitro Release Profile of HIFU-Triggered DOX-CNPs

An in vitro DOX release from DOX-CNPs was observed in 37 °C PBS (pH 7.4) containing 0.1% of Tween 80. To observe the HIFU-triggered DOX-release, 10 mg of DOX-CNPs was dispersed in PBS (2 mL) and placed in a dialysis membrane (MWCO = 100 kDa, Repligen Corporation, Waltham, MA, USA) ($n = 3$). The membrane was transferred into a 50 mL conical tube filled with 10 mL of PBS (pH 7.4) containing 0.1% of Tween 80. The conical tubes were placed in a 37 °C water bath then shaken horizontally (100 rpm). The dialysis membrane was treated with HIFU in destruction mode for 5 min (power: 10 MHz, mechanical index: 0.235) using a High-Resolution Micro-Imaging System (Vevo 770, Visualsonics, Toronto, ON, Canada). The amount of DOX released from CNPs at a pre-determined time point was determined using an absorbance at 490 nm measured by the UV–Vis spectrometer (G1103A, Agilent, Santa Clara, CA, USA).

2.4. Cellular Uptake Behavior of HIFU-Triggered DOX-CNPs

Human non-small cell lung tumor cells, A549, was cultured in Roswell Park Memorial Institute (RPMI) 1640 media (Welgene, Daegu, Korea) containing 10% fetal bovine serum (FBS) and 1% penicillin/streptomycin at 37 °C in a 5% CO_2 incubator. To demonstrate the cellular uptake of DOX-CNPs, A549 cancer cells (1×10^4 cells) were seeded onto 35 mm glass bottom dish and incubated for 24 h. After 24 h post-incubation, the medium was replaced with 1 mL of FBS-free RPMI-containing Cy5.5-labeled DOX-CNPs (1 μg/mL of DOX, 1 mL). To characterize the cellular uptake mechanism of the HIFU-triggered cellular uptake mechanism of DOX-CNPs, DOX-CNP-treated A549 cells were treated with HIFU in destruction mode (power: 10 MHz, mechanical index: 0.235) for 5 min and then incubated for pre-determined time. DOX-CNP-treated A549 cells were washed twice using Dulbecco's Phosphate Buffered Saline (DPBS) and fixed with a 4% paraformaldehyde solution for 10 min. The nuclei of A549 cells was stained with DAPI for 5 min at room temperature. The fluorescence from A549 cells was visualized using confocal laser scanning microscopy (Leica TCS SP8, Wetzlar, Land Hessen, Germany) equipped with 405-diode (405 nm), Ar (488 nm), and HeNe-Red (633 nm) lasers. Tumor tissue fluorescence images were acquired using LAS X software (Leica Microsystems, Wetzlar, Land Hessen, Germany). The fluorescence of DOX and CNP was measured using Image Pro Plus 4.5 5 image analysis software (Media Cybernetics, Bethesda, Rockville, MD, USA).

2.5. In Vitro Cytotoxicity Test of HIFU-Triggered DOX-CNPs

The A549 tumor cells (5×10^3 cells/well) were seeded onto 96-well plates and stabilized for 12 h. The A549 cells were then incubated with various concentrations (0, 0.1, 1, 10, 100 and 500 μg/mL of DOX) of free DOX, CNPs and DOX-CNPs for 24 h. To measure cell viability, 10% (v/v) CCK-8 solution was added to each well, followed by further incubation for 1 h at 37 °C. The absorbance at 450 nm was measured using a microplate reader (VERSAmax™, Molecular Devices Corp., Sunnyvale, CA, USA).

To analyze the cell viability after HIFU treatment, A549 cells were incubated with CNPs and DOX-CNPs (100 μg/mL of DOX) for 24 h. These A549 cells were exposed to HFU in destruction mode (power: 10 MHz, mechanical index: 0.235) for 5 min, followed by further incubation for 24 h at 37 °C in a 5% CO_2 incubator. Finally, the A549 cells were washed twice with DPBS. Subsequently, 10% (v/v) CCK-8 solution was added to each well, followed by further incubating for 1 h at 37 °C. The absorbance at 450 nm was measured using a microplate reader (VERSAmax™, Molecular Devices Corp., Sunnyvale, CA, USA).

2.6. In Vivo Biodistribution of HIFU-Triggered DOX-CNPs in A549 Tumor-Bearing Mice

All animal experiments were performed in compliance with the guidelines of the Institutional Animal Care and Use Committee (IACUC) in the Research Animal Resource Center of Korea Institute of Science and Technology (approved number: 2017-109). To establish A549 tumor-bearing mice, 1×10^7 cells of A549 cells were inoculated in the left flank of male Balb-c/nude mice (4 weeks old, ORIENT BIO Inc., Gyeonggi-do, Korea). When the tumor volume reached approximately 250 ± 50 mm^3, Cy5.5-labeled DOX-CNPs (20 mg/kg, 100 μL) was injected through the tail vein. HIFU (VIFU 2000, ALPINION, Gyeonggi-do, Korea) was applied at the tumor site for 5 min simultaneously with an intravenous injection of Cy5.5-DOX-CNPs as pre-set conditions (intensity: 5 W/cm^2, frequency: 1.5 MHz, duty cycle: 10%, pulse repetition frequency: 1 Hz, time per spot: 30 s, interval: 2 mm). Near infrared fluorescence (NIRF) images of mice animal models were carried out through IVIS SPECTRUM (Xenogen, Alameda, CA, USA). To compare the tumor and organ distributions of Cy5.5-labeled DOX-CNPs, the mice were sacrificed 24 h post-injection. Tumor, liver, lung, spleen, kidney, and heart were dissected from mice, and then NIRF images were obtained via IVIS SPECTRUM.

To observe the deep tissue penetration of Cy5.5-labeled DOX-CNPs, tumor tissues were excised 24 h post-injection of Cy5.5-labeled DOX-CNPs. Excised tumor tissues were embedded in an optimum cutting temperature tissue compound (OCT compound, Sakura Finetek, Chuo-ku, Tokyo, Japan), followed by a transfer to a refrigerator at under −20 °C for 24 h. The tumor tissue blocks were sectioned with a 10 μm thickness with a cryostat (Leica, Bannockburn, IL, USA). The tumor tissue slides were washed with distilled water twice to remove the OCT compound, followed by nuclei staining using DAPI solution for about 10 min. After being washed three times with DPBS, tumor tissue slides were fixed using mounting solution (Vectashield, Vector Laboratories Inc., Burlingame, CA, USA). The fluorescence of the tumor tissue was observed using a fluorescence microscopy (OLYMPUS, Tokyo, Japan).

2.7. Antitumor Efficacy of DOX-CNPs with HIFU Treatment

To evaluate antitumor efficacy in animal models, 1×10^7 cells of A549 cells were inoculated in the left flank of male Balb-c/nude mice (4 weeks old, ORIENT BIO Inc., Gyeonggi-do, Korea). When the tumor volume reached approximately 60 ± 5 mm^3, saline, DOX (2 mg/kg), DOX-CNPs (2 mg/kg of DOX) were injected into the A549 tumor-bearing mice through the tail vein. At 1, 3, 5 and 7 days post-injection, the tumor tissues were treated with HIFU for 5 min as pre-set conditions (intensity: 5 W/cm^2, frequency: 1.5 MHz, duty cycle: 10%, pulse repetition frequency: 1 Hz, time per spot: 30 s, interval: 2 mm). Tumor volume and survival rate were monitored for 22 days to evaluate the antitumor efficacy of each group.

2.8. Histological Analysis

To observe the ECM-rich structure of A549 tumor tissue, collagen in murine squamous cell carcinoma (SCC7) and A549 tumor tissues were stained using Masson's trichrome staining method [28].

In brief, 1×10^6 cells of SCC7 cells and 1×10^7 cells of A549 cells were inoculated in the left flank of male Balb-c/nude mice (4 weeks old, ORIENT BIO Inc., Gyeonggi-do, Korea). When SCC7 and A549 tumor tissues grew to 250 ± 50 mm^3, both tumors were excised and fixed in 4% formalin solution. The tumor tissues were then embedded in paraffin after dehydration. Paraffin-embedded tumor tissues were cut to 6 μm thick and tissue slides were stained with Masson's trichrome staining solution.

Furthermore, ECM structure changes of A549 tumor tissues after HIFU treatment were observed using Masson's trichrome staining method. In brief, 1×10^7 cells of A549 cells were inoculated in the left flank of male Balb-c/nude mice (4 weeks old, ORIENT BIO Inc., Gyeonggi-do, Korea). When A549 tumor tissues grew to 250 ± 50 mm^3, the tumor tissues were treated with HIFU for 5 min as pre-set conditions (intensity: 5 W/cm^2, frequency: 1.5 MHz, duty cycle: 10%, pulse repetition frequency: 1 Hz, time per spot: 30 s, interval: 2 mm). The tumor tissues were then excised and embedded in paraffin after dehydration. Paraffin-embedded tumor tissues were cut to 6 μm thick and tissue slides were stained with Masson's trichrome staining solution. Blue-stained collagen in the tumor tissue slides were observed using a light microscope (Olympus, Tokyo, Japan). For the quantification of blue-stained collagen areas, they were measured using Image Pro Plus 4.5 5 image analysis software (Media Cybernetics, Bethesda, Rockville, MD, USA).

To observe the organ toxicity of DOX-CNPs according to HIFU exposure, the liver and kidneys were excised from the A549 tumor-bearing mice at 24 h post-injection of DOX-CNPs with HIFU exposure. The excised liver and kidneys were fixed using 4% formaldehyde solution, followed by embedding in paraffin after dehydration. The paraffin-embedded tissues were cut into 6 μm-thick sections and were stained with hematoxylin and eosin (H&E).

To observe morphological changes in the tumor tissues, tumor tissues were excised from the A549 tumor-bearing mice at 22 days post-treatment. The excised tumor tissues were fixed using 4% formaldehyde solution, followed by embedding in paraffin after dehydration. The paraffin-embedded tissues were cut into 6 μm-thick sections and were stained with hematoxylin and eosin (H&E). All histological analysis images were acquired through a light microscope (Olympus, Tokyo, Japan).

2.9. Statistical Analysis

In this study, the statistical differences between each group were analyzed through a one-way ANOVA in the Origin 2020 software (OriginLab Corporation, Northampton, MA, USA). The significant difference was marked with an asterisk (*) in the figures.

3. Results and Discussion

3.1. In Vitro Characterization of DOX-Loaded Glycol Chitosan Nanoparticles (DOX-CNPs)

The amphiphilic glycol chitosan-5β-cholanic acid conjugates were prepared by direct coupling between hydrophobic 5β-cholanic acid and hydrophilic glycol chitosan, resulting in the formation of nanoparticles in an aqueous condition (Figure 1b). The glycol chitosan-5β-cholanic acid conjugates contained 162 ± 6.5 molecules of 5β-cholanic acid per glycol chitosan backbone, confirmed by a colloidal titration method [39,40]. For the in vitro and in vivo near-infrared fluorescence (NIRF) imaging, 3.9 molecules of Cy5.5 were chemically conjugated to glycol chitosan-5β-cholanic acid conjugates. Next, the anticancer drug, DOX, was encapsulated into the hydrophobic cores of CNPs via a dialysis method. The amount of DOX in DOX-CNPs was 10 ± 1.5 wt%, calculated by the DOX-standard curve measured at 490 nm in the UV–Vis spectrum. The sizes of CNPs and DOX-CNPs in the aqueous solution measured by DLS were 283.7 ± 5.3 nm and 265.9 ± 35.5 nm. The volume-weighted distribution of CNPs and DOX-CNPs ranged from 260 to 300 nm and 140 to 300 nm, respectively, showing a wider size distribution after DOX encapsulation (Figure 2a). Additionally, the TEM images showed that CNPs and DOX-CNPs had spherical nanoparticle structures with diameters of 262 ± 12 nm and 250 ± 17 nm, respectively (Figure 2b). The size histogram from the TEM images of CNPs and DOX-CNPs showed 200 to 260 nm of distribution, resulting in the similar size distribution of CNPs and DOX-CNPs (Figure S1a and S1b). The surface charges of CNPs and DOX-CNPs were measured to +15.45 ± 0.90 mV and +15.3 ± 0.45 mV, indicating that the surface of CNPs and DOX-CNPs were covered with positively charged glycol chitosan polymers (Figure 2c). Although CNPs and DOX-CNPs had a positive surface, the volume-weighted size distribution of CNPs and DOX-CNPs showed no changes in the size distribution under 1% FBS-containing medium (Figure S1c and S1d). Furthermore, the size of CNPs and DOX-CNPs was stable for 3 days in both PBS (pH 7.4) and 1% FBS-containing PBS (pH 7.4) conditions (Figure 2d). This is because glycol moiety can act as poly(ethylene glycol) (PEG), resulting in the inhibition of size changes by interrupting protein adsorption [41]. This biocompatible glycol chitosan polymer outer surface of CNPs and DOX-CNPs could prevent the adsorption of non-specific proteins in vivo and enables high accumulation at targeted tumor tissues through EPR in vivo [37]. Based on these characterization results, we expect that CNPs can sufficiently encapsulate the anticancer drug DOX into the hydrophobic inner cores of 5β-cholanic acid. Prior to the in vivo study of the DOX-CNPs, in vitro drug release profiles were evaluated. In the case of DOX-CNPs without ultrasound treatment, it was confirmed that the drug was released gradually up to 24 h, but 5 min of HIFU treatment (destruction mode, power: 10 MHz, mechanical index: 0.235) substantially increased the drug release amount by 1.6 and 2.2 times after 30 min or 1 h post-incubation in PBS at 37 °C, compared to untreated DOX-CNPs, due to the ultrasound-triggered rapid drug release from DOX-CNPs (Figure 2e).

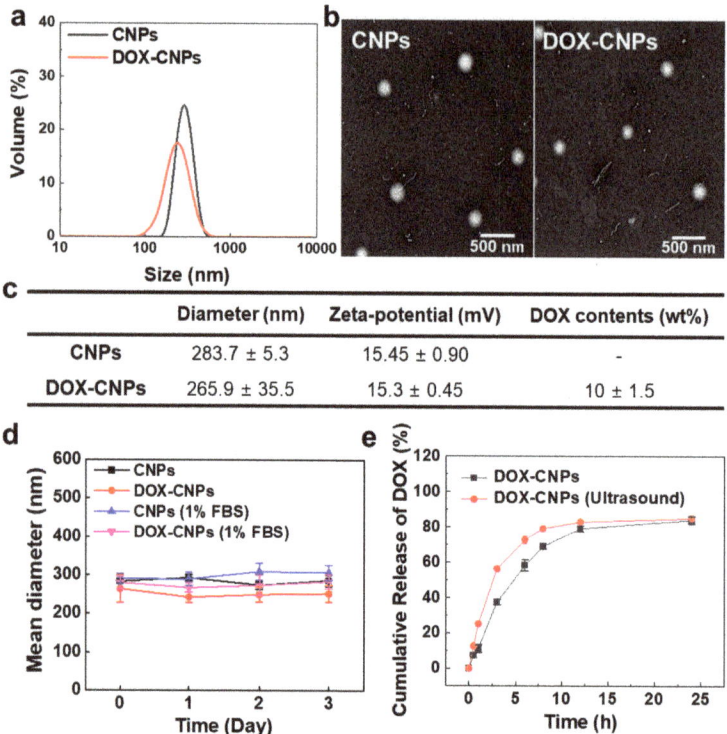

Figure 2. Physicochemical properties of DOX-CNPs in vitro. (**a**) The volume-weighted size distribution of CNPs and DOX-CNPs (1 mg/mL) in PBS (pH 7.4), measured using dynamic light scattering. (**b**) TEM image of CNPs and DOX-CNPs. (**c**) Characteristic table of CNPs and DOX-CNPs summarized diameter, zeta potential, and DOX contents. (**d**) Size stability of CNPs and DOX-CNPs in PBS (pH 7.4) and 1% FBS-containing PBS (pH 7.4) for 3 days. (**e**) In vitro release behavior of DOX from the DOX-CNPs (mean ± SD, $n = 5$). HIFU treatment was carried out for 5 min.

3.2. In Vitro Cellular Uptake and Cytotoxicity of HIFU-Triggred DOX-CNPs

To observe the cellular uptake of HIFU-triggered Cy5.5-labeled DOX-CNPs, A549 cells were treated with 100 µg of DOX-CNPs and the cells were exposed to HIFU in destruction mode (power: 10 MHz and mechanical index: 0.235) for 5 min and the cellular uptake of HIFU-triggered Cy5.5-labeled DOX-CNPs were visualized with confocal microscopy (Figure 3a). In the control, without HIFU exposure, Cy5.5-labeled DOX-CNPs (red colors) slowly bound to cell membranes after 10 min post-incubation and then they were internalized into the cytoplasm at up to 30 min, wherein the bright red colors of Cy5.5-labeled DOX-CNPs were clearly observed in the cytoplasm compartment of A549 cells. It is reported that CNPs show a fast uptake into cancer cells via diverse nanoparticle-derived endocytic pathways [42–44]. Interestingly, the HIFU-triggered cellular uptake of Cy5.5-labeled DOX-CNPs (red color) was clearly observed after 5 min of HIFU pre-treatment (destruction mode; power: 10 MHz, mechanical index: 0.235), compared to untreated Cy5.5-labeled DOX-CNPs. After 10 min post-incubation, a large amount of Cy5.5-labeled DOX-CNPs in the cell membrane and cytoplasm were observed in A547 cells. Furthermore, most DOX-CNPs were rapidly internalized into the cytoplasm compartment of A549 cells after 30 min post-incubation, due to the HIFU-triggered rapid cellular uptake mechanism. More importantly, the rapid cellular uptake of DOX (green color) in CNPs was clearly observed via the HIFU-triggered fast cellular uptake of DOX-CNPs, compared to free DOX. In the case of HIFU exposure, the cellular uptake of Cy5.5-labeled DOX-CNPs increased by 1.6 and 2.0 times after 10 and 30 min post-incubation, compared to untreated DOX-CNPs (Figure S2). Finally, after 30 min post-incubation, the cellular uptake of DOX molecules in CNPs increased by 5.1 times via the HIFU-triggered cellular uptake of DOX-CNPs, compared to free DOX. This is because HIFU exposure to live cells can increase the permeability of nanoparticles into cell membranes via the sonoporation effect as well as the mechanical effects of ultrasound [45–47].

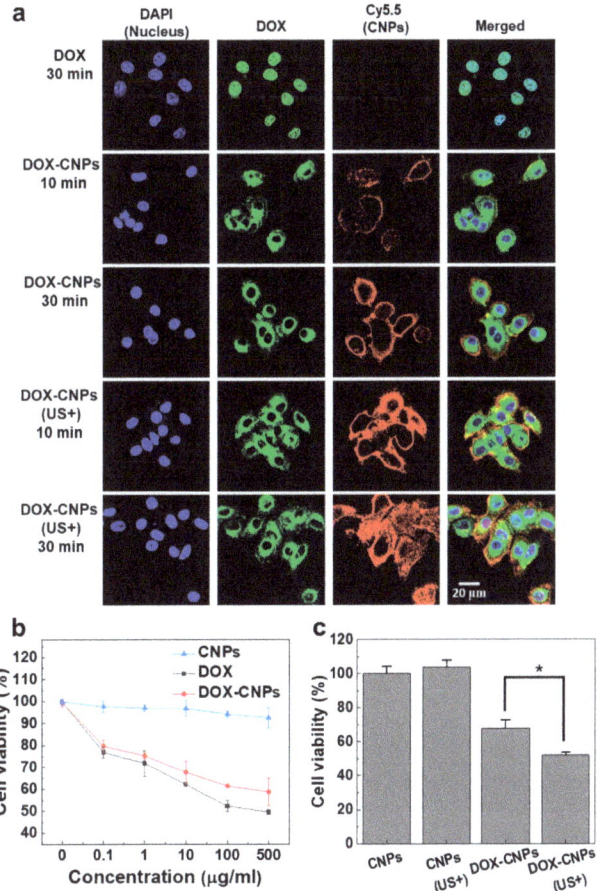

Figure 3. In vitro cellular uptake and cell viability of DOX-CNPs in cultured cells. (**a**) HIFU-triggered (US+) cellular uptake mechanism of DOX-CNPs. A549 cancer cells were incubated with free DOX (1 µg/mL), DOX-CNPs (10 µg/mL) and HIFU-triggered (US+) DOX-CNPs (10 µg/mL) for 10 min and 30 min. DOX-CNP-treated A549 cells were exposed to HIFU in destruction mode (power: 10 MHz, mechanical index: 0.235) for 5 min. (**b**) Cell viability of free DOX, CNPs and DOX-CNPs in cultured A549 cells (mean ± SD, n = 5). (**c**) Cell viability of HIFU-triggered DOX-CNPs (10 µg/mL) in A549 cells. CNPs (US+) and DOX-CNPs (US+) groups were treated with HIFU in destruction mode (power: 10 MHz, mechanical index: 0.235) for 5 min and the cell viability was measured 24 h post-incubation (mean ± SD, n = 5). (*) indicates difference at the $p < 0.05$ significance level.

To evaluate the cytotoxicity of DOX-CNPs in A549 tumor cells, the cell viability of A549 cells was assayed using cell counting kit-8 (CCK-8) at various concentrations of free DOX, CNPs, and DOX-CNPs. CNPs did not show severe cytotoxicity at a high concentration (500 µg/mL) in culture media. However, the cell viability of DOX-CNPs-treated A549 cells gradually decreased, due to the release of free DOX from DOX-CNPs (Figure 3b). Furthermore, the cell viability of free DOX-treated A549 cells decreased in a DOX concentration-dependent manner. Interestingly, HIFU exposure could increase the cytotoxicity of DOX-CNPs in cultured cells, compared to untreated DOX-CNPs (Figure 3c). When the A549 cells were treated with 100 µg of DOX-CNPs (10 µg of DOX) for 24 h, the cell viability was measured at 67.68 ± 5.07%. However, after HIFU exposure for 5 min, the cell viability of DOX-CNP-treated A549 decreased to 51.99 ± 1.79%. It is deduced that the rapid cellular uptake and the rapid drug release of HIFU-triggered DOX-CNPs could increase the cytotoxicity of drug-loaded nanoparticles in cultured cells, compared to untreated DOX-CNPs.

3.3. In Vivo Biodistribution and Therapeutic Efficacy of HIFU-Triggered DOX-CNPs

The in vivo biodistribution of Cy5.5-labeled DOX-CNPs without or with HIFU treatment was monitored in ECM-rich A549 tumor-bearing mice. This is because A549 tumor tissues with stiff ECMs composed of dense collagen and hyaluronan could prevent the deep tissue penetration of nanosized drug carriers [15,28]. Prior to monitor-targeted tumor accumulation, we firstly confirmed the collagen contents of tumor tissues using A549 and SCC7 tumor-bearing mice. When the tumor volume reached to 250 ± 50 mm^3, tumor tissues were excised from the mice, followed by staining using Masson's trichrome staining solution. Compared to SCC7 tumor tissue images, A549 tumor tissue images showed a widely dispersed collagen area which was blue-stained by Masson's trichrome staining solution (Figure S3a). Furthermore, the blue-colored collagen fibers were intricately connected to each other throughout A549 tumor tissues, indicating ECM-rich tumor tissues. However, in the case of SCC7 tumor tissues, almost no collagen fibers were seen in ECM-less tumor tissues. In particular, the amount of collagen fibers in A549 tumor tissues was eight times higher than that of SCC7 tumor tissues (Figure S3b).

Next, we confirmed a tumor tissue collagen destruction effect by HIFU treatment. The A549 tumor model was established by a subcutaneous injection of 1×10^7 cells into the Balb-c/nude mice. When the tumor was grew up 250 ± 50 mm^3, A549 tumor tissues were treated with HIFU (intensity: 5 W/cm^2, frequency: 1.5 MHz, duty cycle: 10%, pulse repetition frequency: 1 Hz, and time per spot: 30 s) for 5 min. Then, A549 tumor tissues were excised from the mice, followed by staining using Masson's trichrome staining solution. A549 tumor tissue images showed a widely dispersed blue-stained collagen area whereas the blue-stained collagen area was dramatically reduced after HIFU treatment (Figure S4a). Furthermore, the blue-stained collagen area of the HIFU-treated A549 tumor tissue observed was six times lower than that of the A549 tumor tissue, resulting in a significant reduction in collagen in the tumor tissue by HIFU treatment (Figure S4b).

To monitor the targeted tumor accumulation of DOX-CNPs, the A549 tumor model was made by a subcutaneous injection of 1×10^7 cells into the Balb-c/nude mice. When the tumor volume reached 250 ± 50 mm^3, Cy5.5-DOX-CNPs (20 µg/kg, 100 µL) were intravenously injected into the A549 tumor-bearing mice ($n = 3$). After an intravenous injection of Cy5.5-DOX-CNPs, the tumor was treated with HIFU (intensity: 5W/cm^2, frequency: 1.5 MHz, duty cycle: 10%, pulse repetition frequency: 1 Hz, and time per spot: 30 s) for 5 min and the tumor-targeting ability of Cy5.5-DOX-CNPs were visualized using non-invasive NIRF imaging. As we expect, 6 h post-injection, HIFU-treated groups showed a high NIRF intensity of Cy5.5-labeled DOX-CNPs at targeted tumor tissues (white dotted circle), compared to untreated DOX-CNP groups (Figure 4a). The tumor accumulation of HIFU-treated DOX-CNPs groups increased noticeably via the nanoparticle-derived EPR effect for 24 h, whereas untreated DOX-CNP groups slightly accumulated at targeted tumor tissues up to 24 h post-incubation, due to the dense ECM structure of A549 tumor tissues. To observe ex vivo NIRF images, the tumor tissues and the major organs, including liver, lung, spleen, kidney, and heart, were excised from the tumor-bearing mice at 24 h post-injection (Figure 4b). The bright NIRF signal of HIFU-treated DOX-CNPs was clearly observed at targeted tumor tissues. In the control, both DOX-CNPs without and with HIFU treatment showed the similar non-specific accumulations in normal tissues, such as liver, lung, and kidney. In the HIFU-treated groups, the NIRF signal intensity of Cy5.5-labeled DOX-CNPs in the tumor tissue was 1.84 times higher than that of the untreated groups (Figure 4c). It is deduced that HIFU treatment at targeted tumor tissues could destroy dense ECMs composed of collagen and hyaluronan, resulting in the deep tumor penetration of DOX-CNPs at ECM-rich A549 tumor tissues [28,48]. Surprisingly, intravenously injected DOX-CNPs could be successfully accumulated at in ECM-rich tumors exposed to HIFU treatments. Lastly, the excised tumor tissues were further observed using fluorescence microscopy. The NIRF microscopic images showed that untreated DOX-CNPs mainly localized in the boundary region of ECM-rich tumor tissues, indicating that dense ECM structures inhibited the deep tumor penetration of drug-loaded nanoparticles (Figure 4d). However, HIFU-treated DOX-CNPs localized substantially in the deep inner part of ECM-rich tumor tissues via the HIFU-derived destruction of the dense ECM structure. These results indicate that HIFU treatment on ECM-rich tumor tissues helped the deep tumor penetration of DOX-CNPs in vivo.

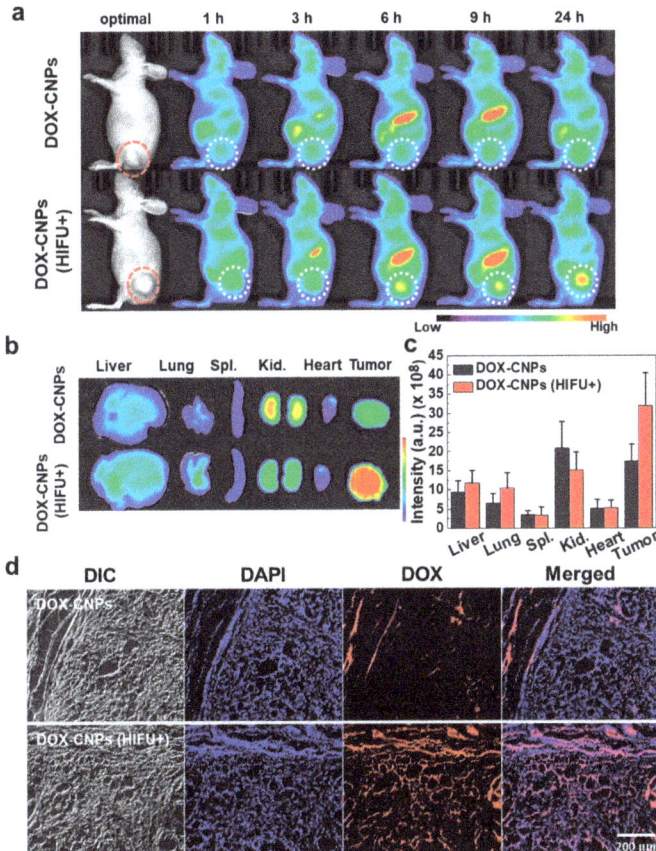

Figure 4. In vivo near-infrared fluorescence (NIRF) imaging of Cy5.5-labeled DOX-CNPs in ECM-rich A549 tumor animal model. (**a**) Biodistribution of Cy5.5-labeled DOX-CNPs without and with HIFU treatment (intensity: 5 W/cm^2, frequency: 1.5 MHz, duty cycle: 10%, pulse repetition frequency: 1 Hz, time per spot: 30 s, interval: 2 mm, expose time: 5 min). The red and white dot circles indicate tumor site. (**b**) Ex vivo NIRF imaging of liver, lung, spleen, kidney, heart, and tumor at 24 h post-injection. (**c**) Mean NIRF signal intensity of ex vivo NIRF image (Spl.; spleen, Kid.; kidney). (**d**) Ex vivo NIRF microscopic images of deep tumor penetration of untreated Cy5.5-labeled DOX-CNPs and HIFU-treated Cy5.5-labeled DOX-CNPs in ECM-rich tumor tissues.

3.4. In Vivo Therapeutic Efficacy Using HIFU-Triggered DOX-CNPs in A549 Tumor-Bearing Mice

The in vivo therapeutic efficacy of HIFU-triggered DOX-CNPs in tumors was monitored up to 24 days. When tumors grew to approximately 60 ± 5 mm^3, saline, DOX (2 mg/kg), DOX-CNPs (2 mg/kg of DOX) were injected into the A549 tumor-bearing mice through the tail vein. At 1, 3, 5 and 7 days after injection, tumor tissues were treated with HIFU (+HIFU) (intensity: 5 W/cm^2, frequency: 1.5 MHz, duty cycle: 10%, pulse repetition frequency: 1 Hz, and time per spot: 30 s) for 5 min. In the control, saline-injected mice without and with HIFU treatment did not show any therapeutic efficacy during the experiment. However, free DOX, DOX (+HIFU), DOX-CNPs showed a mild inhibitory effect on tumor growth, indicating free DOX was not enough to kill A549 tumor cells. Moreover, DOX-CNPs did not present an enhanced therapeutic efficacy of drug-loaded nanoparticles in ECM-rich tumor tissues due to the limited deep tumor penetration effect. In particular, HIFU-treated DOX-CNPs showed an improved therapeutic efficacy, compared to free DOX and DOX-CNPs without HIFU treatment. At 22 days post-treatment, the mean tumor volumes of DOX-CNPs (+HIFU) were greatly suppressed to 110.46 ± 18.52 mm^3, compared to free DOX (+HIFU) (197.01 ± 21.22 mm^3) and DOX-CNPs without HIFU treatment (187.77 ± 18.30 mm^3) (Figure 5a). To demonstrate the organ toxicity of DOX-CNPs after HIFU treatment, H&E-stained tissue images of liver and kidney after 22 days post-injection confirmed that there was no organ toxicity (Figure S5). Furthermore, all animal groups showed no changes in survival rate during the treatment (Figure 5b). These results indicate that the HIFU treatment of DOX-CNPs could greatly increase the antitumor efficacy in ECM-rich tumor models, resulting in the deep tumor penetration of drug-loaded nanoparticles at targeted tumor tissues.

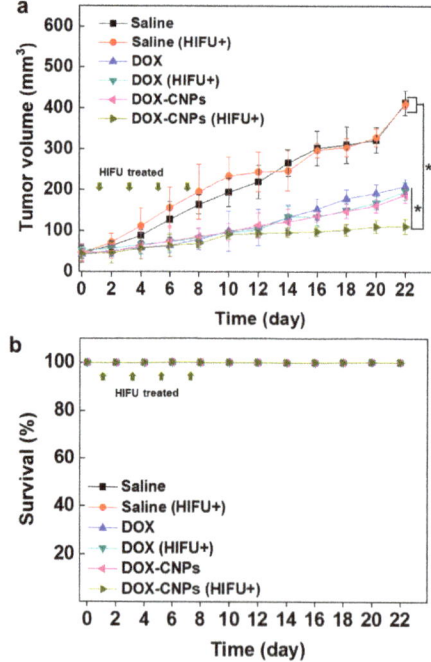

Figure 5. In vivo therapeutic efficacy of HIFU-triggered DOX-CNPs in ECM-rich A549 tumor-bearing mice. (**a**) Antitumor efficacy of DOX-CNPs with HIFU treatment (n = 5 per group). The arrows indicate DOX-CNP injection and HIFU treatment (intensity: 5 W/cm^2, frequency: 1.5 MHz, duty cycle: 10%, pulse repetition frequency: 1 Hz, time per spot: 30 s, interval: 2 mm, expose time: 5 min). (*) indicates difference at the $p < 0.05$ significance level. (**b**) Survival rate of A549 tumor-bearing mice treated with saline, saline (HIFU+), DOX, DOX (HIFU+), DOX-CNPs, and DOX-CNPs (HIFU+). The arrows indicate HIFU treatment.

4. Conclusions

We studied the drug delivery efficacy and therapeutic efficacy of HIFU-triggered drug-loaded nanoparticles on ECM-rich tumor models. Doxorubicin-loaded glycol chitosan nanoparticles (DOX-CNPs) could be well accumulated in ECM-rich tumor tissues through HIFU treatment. The in vitro HIFU-triggered DOX-CNPs showed enhanced cellular uptake and rapid drug release from drug-loaded nanoparticles in cultured cells, resulting in increased cytotoxicity, compared to DOX-CNPs without HIFU treatment. In addition, when ECM-rich A549 tumor tissues were treated with HIFU, DOX-CNP could be effectively accumulated at targeted tumor tissues via deep tumor penetration, wherein the dense ECM is broken by external HIFU. Based on these results, HIFU treatment on ECM-rich tumor tissues could increase the accumulation efficiency of DOX-CNPs and inhibit efficiently tumor growth. Therefore, the improved antitumor efficacy of HIFU-triggered DOX-CNPs can be successfully applied to heterogeneous cancer treatments.

Supplementary Materials: The following are available online at http://www.mdpi.com/1999-4923/12/10/974/s1, Figure S1: TEM size histogram and volume-weighted size distribution of CNPs and DOX-CNPs, Figure S2: Quantitative analysis of cellular uptake of free DOX and Cy5.5-labeled DOX-CNPs in A549 cancer cells, Figure S3: Collagen matrix in SCC7 and A549 tumor tissues that were stained with Masson's trichrome staining, Figure S4: Masson's trichrome staining images of A549 tumor tissues without or without HIFU treatment, Figure S5: Liver and kidney H&E staining images to demonstrate organ toxicity of DOX-CNPs after HIFU treatment.

Author Contributions: Conceptualization, H.Y.Y., H.K. and K.K.; methodology, Y.C. and H.H.; validation, Y.C. and H.H.; formal analysis, S.J. and H.Y.Y.; resources, H.K. and K.K.; data curation, S.J. and H.Y.Y.; writing—original draft, Y.C. and S.J.; writing—review and editing, H.Y.Y.; supervision, K.K.; project administration, H.K., I.C.K. and K.K.; funding acquisition, K.K. All authors have read and agreed to the published version of the manuscript.

Funding: This work was supported by grants from the National Research Foundation (NRF) of Korea, funded by the Ministry of Science (NRF-2019R1A2C3006283), the KU-KIST Graduate School of Converging Science and Technology (Korea University) and the Intramural Research Program of KIST.

Conflicts of Interest: The authors declare no conflict of interest.

References

1. Kim, K.; Kim, J.H.; Park, H.; Kim, Y.S.; Park, K.; Nam, H.; Lee, S.; Park, J.H.; Park, R.W.; Kim, I.S.; et al. Tumor-homing multifunctional nanoparticles for cancer theragnosis: Simultaneous diagnosis, drug delivery, and therapeutic monitoring. *J. Control. Release* **2010**, *146*, 219–227. [CrossRef] [PubMed]
2. Maeda, H. The enhanced permeability and retention (EPR) effect in tumor vasculature: The key role of tumor-selective macromolecular drug targeting. *Adv. Enzym. Regul.* **2001**, *41*, 189–207. [CrossRef]
3. Bazak, R.; Houri, M.; Achy, S.E.; Hussein, W.; Refaat, T. Passive targeting of nanoparticles to cancer: A comprehensive review of the literature. *Mol. Clin. Oncol.* **2014**, *2*, 904–908. [CrossRef] [PubMed]
4. Nel, A.; Ruoslahti, E.; Meng, H. *New Insights into "Permeability" as in the Enhanced Permeability and Retention Effect of Cancer Nanotherapeutics*; ACS Publications: Washington, DC, USA, 2017.
5. Fang, J.; Nakamura, H.; Maeda, H. The EPR effect: Unique features of tumor blood vessels for drug delivery, factors involved, and limitations and augmentation of the effect. *Adv. Drug Deliv. Rev.* **2011**, *63*, 136–151. [CrossRef] [PubMed]
6. Chen, Z.J.; Yang, S.C.; Liu, X.L.; Gao, Y.H.; Dong, X.; Lai, X.; Zhu, M.H.; Feng, H.Y.; Zhu, X.D.; Lu, Q.; et al. Nanobowl-Supported Liposomes Improve Drug Loading and Delivery. *Nano Lett.* **2020**, *20*, 4177–4187. [CrossRef] [PubMed]
7. Jeon, S.; Ko, H.; Rao, N.V.; Yoon, H.Y.; You, D.G.; Han, H.S.; Um, W.; Saravanakumar, G.; Park, J.H. A versatile gold cross-linked nanoparticle based on triblock copolymer as the carrier of doxorubicin. *RSC Adv.* **2015**, *5*, 70352–70360. [CrossRef]
8. Jeon, S.; Park, B.C.; Lim, S.; Yoon, H.Y.; Jeon, Y.S.; Kim, B.S.; Kim, Y.K.; Kim, K. Heat-Generating Iron Oxide Multigranule Nanoclusters for Enhancing Hyperthermic Efficacy in Tumor Treatment. *ACS Appl. Mater. Interfaces* **2020**, *12*, 33483–33491. [CrossRef]
9. Zabielska-Koczywąs, K.; Lechowski, R. The Use of Liposomes and Nanoparticles as Drug Delivery Systems to Improve Cancer Treatment in Dogs and Cats. *Molecules* **2017**, *22*, 2167. [CrossRef]

10. Denison, T.A.; Bae, Y.H. Tumor heterogeneity and its implication for drug delivery. *J. Control. Release* **2012**, *164*, 187–191. [CrossRef]
11. Rosenblum, D.; Joshi, N.; Tao, W.; Karp, J.M.; Peer, D. Progress and challenges towards targeted delivery of cancer therapeutics. *Nat. Commun.* **2018**, *9*, 1–12. [CrossRef]
12. Fisher, R.; Pusztai, L.; Swanton, C. Cancer heterogeneity: Implications for targeted therapeutics. *Br. J. Cancer* **2013**, *108*, 479–485. [CrossRef]
13. Yuan, F.; Leunig, M.; Huang, S.K.; Berk, D.A.; Papahadjopoulos, D.; Jain, R.K. Microvascular permeability and interstitial penetration of sterically stabilized (stealth) liposomes in a human tumor xenograft. *Cancer Res.* **1994**, *54*, 3352–3356. [PubMed]
14. Jain, R.K. Delivery of molecular and cellular medicine to solid tumors. *Adv. Drug Deliv. Rev.* **2001**, *46*, 149–168. [CrossRef]
15. Yhee, J.Y.; Jeon, S.; Yoon, H.Y.; Shim, M.K.; Ko, H.; Min, J.; Na, J.H.; Chang, H.; Han, H.; Kim, J.H.; et al. Effects of tumor microenvironments on targeted delivery of glycol chitosan nanoparticles. *J. Control. Release* **2017**, *267*, 223–231. [CrossRef]
16. Chauhan, V.P.; Jain, R.K. Strategies for advancing cancer nanomedicine. *Nat. Mater.* **2013**, *12*, 958–962. [CrossRef]
17. Junttila, M.R.; de Sauvage, F.J. Influence of tumour micro-environment heterogeneity on therapeutic response. *Nature* **2013**, *501*, 346–354. [CrossRef]
18. Simonsen, T.G.; Gaustad, J.V.; Leinaas, M.N.; Rofstad, E.K. High Interstitial Fluid Pressure Is Associated with Tumor-Line Specific Vascular Abnormalities in Human Melanoma Xenografts. *PLoS ONE* **2012**, *7*, e40006. [CrossRef] [PubMed]
19. Netti, P.A.; Berk, D.A.; Swartz, M.A.; Grodzinsky, A.J.; Jain, R.K. Role of extracellular matrix assembly in interstitial transport in solid tumors. *Cancer Res.* **2000**, *60*, 2497–2503.
20. Song, G.N.; Darr, D.B.; Santos, C.M.; Ross, M.; Valdivia, A.; Jordan, J.L.; Midkiff, B.R.; Cohen, S.; Nikolaishvili-Feinberg, N.; Miller, C.R.; et al. Effects of Tumor Microenvironment Heterogeneity on Nanoparticle Disposition and Efficacy in Breast Cancer Tumor Models. *Clin. Cancer Res.* **2014**, *20*, 6083–6095. [CrossRef]
21. Wong, C.; Stylianopoulos, T.; Cui, J.A.; Martin, J.; Chauhan, V.P.; Jiang, W.; Popovic, Z.; Jain, R.K.; Bawendi, M.G.; Fukumura, D. Multistage nanoparticle delivery system for deep penetration into tumor tissue. *Proc. Natl. Acad. Sci. USA* **2011**, *108*, 2426–2431. [CrossRef]
22. Hong, Y.; Nam, G.H.; Koh, E.; Jeon, S.; Kim, G.B.; Jeong, C.; Kim, D.H.; Yang, Y.; Kim, I.S. Exosome as a Vehicle for Delivery of Membrane Protein Therapeutics, PH20, for Enhanced Tumor Penetration and Antitumor Efficacy. *Adv. Funct. Mater.* **2018**, *28*, 1703074. [CrossRef]
23. Parodi, A.; Haddix, S.G.; Taghipour, N.; Scaria, S.; Taraballi, F.; Cevenini, A.; Yazdi, I.K.; Corbo, C.; Palomba, R.; Khaled, S.Z.; et al. Bromelain Surface Modification Increases the Diffusion of Silica Nanopartides in the Tumor Extracellular Matrix. *ACS Nano* **2014**, *8*, 9874–9883. [CrossRef] [PubMed]
24. Yao, Q.; Kou, L.F.; Tu, Y.; Zhu, L. MMP-Responsive 'Smart' Drug Delivery and Tumor Targeting. *Trends Pharm. Sci.* **2018**, *39*, 766–781. [CrossRef] [PubMed]
25. Talbert, J.N.; Goddard, J.M. Enzymes on material surfaces. *Colloids Surf. B* **2012**, *93*, 8–19. [CrossRef] [PubMed]
26. Oh, K.S.; Han, H.; Yoon, B.D.; Lee, M.; Kim, H.; Seo, D.W.; Seo, J.H.; Kim, K.; Kwon, I.C.; Yuk, S.H. Effect of HIFU treatment on tumor targeting efficacy of docetaxel-loaded Pluronic nanoparticles. *Colloids Surf. B* **2014**, *119*, 137–144. [CrossRef] [PubMed]
27. Wang, S.; Shin, I.S.; Hancock, H.; Jang, B.S.; Kim, H.S.; Lee, S.M.; Zderic, V.; Frenkel, V.; Pastan, I.; Paik, C.H.; et al. Pulsed high intensity focused ultrasound increases penetration and therapeutic efficacy of monoclonal antibodies in murine xenograft tumors. *J. Control. Release* **2012**, *162*, 218–224. [CrossRef] [PubMed]
28. Lee, S.; Han, H.; Koo, H.; Na, J.H.; Yoon, H.Y.; Lee, K.E.; Lee, H.; Kim, H.; Kwon, I.C.; Kim, K. Extracellular matrix remodeling in vivo for enhancing tumor-targeting efficiency of nanoparticle drug carriers using the pulsed high intensity focused ultrasound. *J. Control. Release* **2017**, *263*, 68–78. [CrossRef]
29. You, D.G.; Yoon, H.Y.; Jeon, S.; Um, W.; Son, S.; Park, J.H.; Kwon, I.C.; Kim, K. Deep tissue penetration of nanoparticles using pulsed-high intensity focused ultrasound. *Nano Converg.* **2017**, *4*, 30. [CrossRef]
30. Doherty, G.J.; Tempero, M.; Corrie, P.G. HALO-109-301: A Phase III trial of PEGPH20 (with gemcitabine and nab-paclitaxel) in hyaluronic acid-high stage IV pancreatic cancer. *Future Oncol.* **2018**, *14*, 13–22. [CrossRef]
31. Wilhelm, S.; Tavares, A.J.; Dai, Q.; Ohta, S.; Audet, J.; Dvorak, H.F.; Chan, W.C. Analysis of nanoparticle delivery to tumours. *Nat. Rev. Mater.* **2016**, *1*, 1–12. [CrossRef]

32. Knight, D.K.; Shapka, S.N.; Amsden, B.G. Structure, depolymerization, and cytocompatibility evaluation of glycol chitosan. *J. Biomed. Mater. Res. Part A Off. J. Soc. Biomater. Jpn. Soc. Biomater. Aust. Soc. Biomater. Korean Soc. Biomater.* **2007**, *83*, 787–798. [CrossRef] [PubMed]
33. Kim, S.E.; Kim, H.-J.; Rhee, J.-K.; Park, K. Versatile chemical derivatizations to design glycol chitosan-based drug carriers. *Molecules* **2017**, *22*, 1662. [CrossRef] [PubMed]
34. Kim, J.-H.; Kim, Y.-S.; Kim, S.; Park, J.H.; Kim, K.; Choi, K.; Chung, H.; Jeong, S.Y.; Park, R.-W.; Kim, I.-S. Hydrophobically modified glycol chitosan nanoparticles as carriers for paclitaxel. *J. Control. Release* **2006**, *111*, 228–234. [CrossRef] [PubMed]
35. Hwang, H.-Y.; Kim, I.-S.; Kwon, I.C.; Kim, Y.-H. Tumor targetability and antitumor effect of docetaxel-loaded hydrophobically modified glycol chitosan nanoparticles. *J. Control. Release* **2008**, *128*, 23–31. [CrossRef] [PubMed]
36. Key, J.; Cooper, C.; Kim, A.Y.; Dhawan, D.; Knapp, D.W.; Kim, K.; Park, J.H.; Choi, K.; Kwon, I.C.; Park, K. In vivo NIRF and MR dual-modality imaging using glycol chitosan nanoparticles. *J. Control. Release* **2012**, *163*, 249–255. [CrossRef]
37. Yoon, H.Y.; Son, S.; Lee, S.J.; You, D.G.; Yhee, J.Y.; Park, J.H.; Swierczewska, M.; Lee, S.; Kwon, I.C.; Kim, S.H. Glycol chitosan nanoparticles as specialized cancer therapeutic vehicles: Sequential delivery of doxorubicin and Bcl-2 siRNA. *Sci. Rep.* **2014**, *4*, 1–12. [CrossRef]
38. Park, K.; Kim, J.H.; Nam, Y.S.; Lee, S.; Nam, H.Y.; Kim, K.; Park, J.H.; Kim, I.S.; Choi, K.; Kim, S.Y.; et al. Effect of polymer molecular weight on the tumor targeting characteristics of self-assembled glycol chitosan nanoparticles. *J. Control. Release* **2007**, *122*, 305–314. [CrossRef]
39. Kwon, S.; Park, J.H.; Chung, H.; Kwon, I.C.; Jeong, S.Y.; Kim, I.S. Physicochemical characteristics of self-assembled nanoparticles based on glycol chitosan bearing 5 beta-cholanic acid. *Langmuir* **2003**, *19*, 10188–10193. [CrossRef]
40. Na, J.H.; Lee, S.Y.; Lee, S.; Koo, H.; Min, K.H.; Jeong, S.Y.; Yuk, S.H.; Kim, K.; Kwon, I.C. Effect of the stability and deformability of self-assembled glycol chitosan nanoparticles on tumor-targeting efficiency. *J. Control. Release* **2012**, *163*, 2–9. [CrossRef]
41. Na, J.H.; Koo, H.; Lee, S.; Han, S.J.; Lee, K.E.; Kim, S.; Lee, H.; Lee, S.; Choi, K.; Kwon, I.C.; et al. Precise Targeting of Liver Tumor Using Glycol Chitosan Nanoparticles: Mechanisms, Key Factors, and Their Implications. *Mol. Pharm.* **2016**, *13*, 3700–3711. [CrossRef]
42. Nam, H.Y.; Kwon, S.M.; Chung, H.; Lee, S.Y.; Kwon, S.H.; Jeon, H.; Kim, Y.; Park, J.H.; Kim, J.; Her, S.; et al. Cellular uptake mechanism and intracellular fate of hydrophobically modified glycol chitosan nanoparticles. *J. Control. Release* **2009**, *135*, 259–267. [CrossRef] [PubMed]
43. Park, S.; Lee, S.J.; Chung, H.; Her, S.; Choi, Y.; Kim, K.; Choi, K.; Kwon, I.C. Cellular Uptake Pathway and Drug Release Characteristics of Drug-Encapsulated Glycol Chitosan Nanoparticles in Live Cells. *Microsc. Res. Tech.* **2010**, *73*, 857–865. [CrossRef]
44. Yhee, J.Y.; Yoon, H.Y.; Kim, H.; Jeon, S.; Hergert, P.; Im, J.; Panyam, J.; Kim, K.; Nho, R.S. The effects of collagen-rich extracellular matrix on the intracellular delivery of glycol chitosan nanoparticles in human lung fibroblasts. *Int. J. Nanomed.* **2017**, *12*, 6089–6105. [CrossRef]
45. Mitragotri, S. Innovation—Healing sound: The use of ultrasound in drug delivery and other therapeutic applications. *Nat. Rev. Drug Discov.* **2005**, *4*, 255–260. [CrossRef] [PubMed]
46. Karshafian, R.; Bevan, P.D.; Williams, R.; Samac, S.; Burns, P.N. Sonoporation by Ultrasound-Activated Microbubble Contrast Agents: Effect of Acoustic Exposure Parameters on Cell Membrane Permeability and Cell Viability. *Ultrasound Med. Biol.* **2009**, *35*, 847–860. [CrossRef]
47. Borden, M.A.; Zhang, H.; Gillies, R.J.; Dayton, P.A.; Ferrara, K.W. A stimulus-responsive contrast agent for ultrasound molecular imaging. *Biomaterials* **2008**, *29*, 597–606. [CrossRef]
48. Frenkel, V. Ultrasound mediated delivery of drugs and genes to solid tumors. *Adv. Drug Deliv. Rev.* **2008**, *60*, 1193–1208. [CrossRef] [PubMed]

Publisher's Note: MDPI stays neutral with regard to jurisdictional claims in published maps and institutional affiliations.

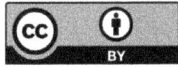

© 2020 by the authors. Licensee MDPI, Basel, Switzerland. This article is an open access article distributed under the terms and conditions of the Creative Commons Attribution (CC BY) license (http://creativecommons.org/licenses/by/4.0/).

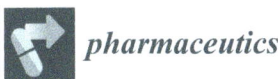

Article

Low-Intensity Sonoporation-Induced Intracellular Signalling of Pancreatic Cancer Cells, Fibroblasts and Endothelial Cells

Ragnhild Haugse [1,2,3], Anika Langer [3], Elisa Thodesen Murvold [4,5], Daniela Elena Costea [3,5], Bjørn Tore Gjertsen [3,6], Odd Helge Gilja [5,7], Spiros Kotopoulis [5,7,8,†], Gorka Ruiz de Garibay [3,†] and Emmet McCormack [1,2,3,4,9,*,†]

1. Centre for Pharmacy, Department of Clinical Science, The University of Bergen, Jonas Lies vei 65, 5021 Bergen, Norway; ragnhild.haugse@uib.no
2. Department of Quality and Development, Hospital Pharmacies Enterprise in Western Norway, Møllendalsbakken 9, 5021 Bergen, Norway
3. Centre for Cancer Biomarkers CCBIO, Department of Clinical Science, The University of Bergen, Jonas Lies vei 65, 5021 Bergen, Norway; Anika.Langer@uib.no (A.L.); Daniela.Costea@uib.no (D.E.C.); bjorn.gjertsen@uib.no (B.T.G.); gorka.garibay@uib.no (G.R.d.G.)
4. KinN Therapeutics AS, Jonas Lies vei 91B, 5021 Bergen, Norway; ethode12@gmail.com
5. Department of Clinical Medicine, The University of Bergen, Jonas Lies vei 65, 5021 Bergen, Norway; Odd.Gilja@uib.no (O.H.G.); spiros.kotopoulis@uib.no (S.K.)
6. Department of Internal Medicine, Hematology Section, Haukeland University Hospital, Jonas Lies vei 65, 5021 Bergen, Norway
7. National Centre for Ultrasound in Gastroenterology, Haukeland University Hospital, Jonas Lies vei 65, 5021 Bergen, Norway
8. EXACT Therapeutics AS, Ullernchausseen 64, 0379 Oslo, Norway
9. Department of Clinical Science, The University of Bergen, Jonas Lies vei 65, 5021 Bergen, Norway
* Correspondence: Emmet.Mc.Cormack@uib.no
† These authors contribute equally to this paper.

Received: 29 September 2020; Accepted: 3 November 2020; Published: 6 November 2020

Abstract: The use of ultrasound (US) and microbubbles (MB), usually referred to as sonoporation, has great potential to increase the efficacy of chemotherapy. However, the molecular mechanisms that mediate sonoporation response are not well-known, and recent research suggests that cell stress induced by US + MBs may contribute to the treatment benefit. Furthermore, there is a growing understanding that the effects of US + MBs are beyond only the cancer cells and involves the tumour vasculature and microenvironment. We treated pancreatic cancer cells (MIA PaCa-2) and stromal cells, fibroblasts (BJ) and human umbilical vein endothelial cells (HUVECs), with US ± MB, and investigated the extent of uptake of cell impermeable dye (calcein, by flow cytometry), viability (cell count, Annexin/PI and WST-1 assays) and activation of a number of key proteins in important intracellular signalling pathways immediately and 2 h after sonoporation (phospho flow cytometry). Different cell types responded differently to US ± MBs in all these aspects. In general, sonoporation induces immediate, transient activation of MAP-kinases (p38, ERK1/2), and an increase in phosphorylation of ribosomal protein S6 together with dephosphorylation of 4E-BP1. The sonoporation stress-response resembles cellular responses to electroporation and pore-forming toxins in membrane repair and restoring cellular homeostasis, and may be exploited therapeutically. The stromal cells were more sensitive to sonoporation than tumoural cells, and further efforts in optimising sonoporation-enhanced therapy should be targeted at the microenvironment.

Keywords: sonoporation; microbubbles; ultrasound; intracellular signaling; phosphorylation; ultrasound contrast agents; drug delivery; cellular stress; pancreatic cancer; tumour microenvironment

1. Introduction

The use of ultrasound (US) and microbubbles (MB) in combination with chemotherapy to increase the efficacy of cancer therapy has gained interest in the last 20 years. The term "sonoporation", is often used to describe this phenomenon. The term describes the formation of pores that occur when cells come into contact with MBs oscillating in an US field [1], hypothesised to enhance uptake for co-administered chemotherapeutics [2]. However, there is still no consensus on what the exact mechanisms underlying US + MBs enhanced cancer therapy are. Furthermore, the cellular stress induced by US + MBs themselves has been proposed to contribute to the anti-cancer effects [3,4].

Despite the insufficient mechanistic understanding, substantial in vitro [5–13] and in vivo research [5–9,14–17] has shown that US + MBs-enhanced cancer therapy is beneficial for cancer therapy. In 2016, results from the first Phase 1 human clinical trial using US + MBs in combination with chemotherapy to treat pancreatic ductal adenocarcinoma (PDAC) were published [18]. PDAC is a deadly cancer, with less than an 8% five-year overall survival [19], which requires better treatment options. The clinical trial demonstrated that the use of US + MBs is safe, and a secondary endpoint indicated that sonoporation + chemotherapy (gemcitabine) may increase survival of patients. PDAC is characterised by extensive desmoplastic stroma, thought to originate from cancer-associated fibroblasts (CAFs), and a complex hypoxic tumour microenvironment, which are major contributors to resistance to chemotherapy [19,20]. Some hypothesised effects of sonoporation on the tumour microenvironment are increased drug extravasation from the blood vessels or destruction of tumour vasculature [2], but the relevance of microenvironmental effects for the clinical efficacy of sonoporation remains largely unknown.

In vitro sonoporation research has typically focused on cancer cell lines, evaluating the sonoporation efficacy either by uptake of cell impermeable dyes [5,8,9,21] and/or by evaluation of the viability of cells exposed to sonoporation [21] or sonoporation in combination with drugs [5–9,22]. Based on the fact that MBs are usually injected into the vasculature, in vitro studies have also addressed the effects of sonoporation on endothelial cells, showing increased permeability both in the cellular membrane [23,24] and interendothelial openings between cells [25–28].

Our previous study [4] using leukemic cells as a model system of cancer compared to healthy peripheral blood cells demonstrated that different cell types have different sensitivities to sonoporation in terms of molecular uptake, effect on viability and intracellular signalling. This was a simplified system compared to solid tumours, which consist of the complex tumour microenvironment with stromal cells, immune cells, fibroblasts, blood vessels and extracellular matrix (ECM) in addition to, and supporting, the cancer cells [29]. The observed difference in sonoporation sensitivity raises the question of whether the cell types within a solid tumour may also respond differently, meaning that treatment of the cancer cells might not be the most important sonoporation effect in the enhancement of chemotherapeutic efficacy. Investigations on the cellular responses to US + MBs should, therefore, be carried out in cell types relevant for the tumour microenvironment.

In this study, we aim to improve our understanding of how sonoporation may affect pancreatic cancer by evaluating the effects on the uptake of cell impermeable dye, viability and intracellular signalling response in PDAC, endothelial and fibroblast cell types. The results from this study will help expand our understanding of how the different cell types respond to sonoporation, which is needed for the development of better in vitro and in vivo models for sonoporation, the optimisation of sonoporation parameters and the choice of drugs. In fact, the results indicate that the cancer cells are not the most sensitive to sonoporation in terms of uptake of cell-impermeable molecule, reduction in viability or intracellular signalling response (phosphorylation of p38, ERK1/2, ribosomal protein S6 and 4E-BP1), further suggesting that cells in the tumour microenvironment may be relevant for sonoporation efficacy.

2. Materials and Methods

2.1. Chemicals

All chemicals were purchased from Merck KGaA (Darmstadt, Germany) unless otherwise stated.

2.2. Maintenance Cell Culture

Pancreatic ductal adenocarcinoma cell line MIA PaCa-2 (ATCC® CRM-CRL-1420™, kindly donated by Professor Anders Molven, University of Bergen, Bergen, Norway) was cultured in high-glucose Dulbecco's modified Eagle's medium (DMEM #5671) supplemented with 10% foetal bovine serum (FBS), 2% L-glutamine, 1 mM sodium pyruvate and 2.5% horse serum. Human foreskin fibroblasts (BJ, ATCC® CRL-2522™, kindly donated by professor Donald Gullberg, University of Bergen, Bergen, Norway) were cultured in high-glucose DMEM #5671 supplemented with 10% FBS, 1% L-glutamine and 50 U/mL Penicillin/50 U/mL Streptomycin. Single-donor lot human umbilical vein endothelial cells (HUVECs) (Cat#CC-2517, Lonza, Basel, Switzerland, kindly donated by Prof. Jim Lorens, University of Bergen, Bergen, Norway) were cultured in EGM™-2 medium supplemented with EGM™-2 Endothelial Cell Growth Medium-2 BulletKit™ (Lonza). Cell culture medium was changed on the HUVECs every second day according to suppliers' recommendations, except when cultured in Petaka G3 LOT® (Celartia Ltd., Powell, OH, USA) [c.f. Section 2.4]. HUV-EC-Cs (ATCC® CRL-1730™) were cultured in F12-K medium (ATCC, Manassas, VA, USA) supplemented with endothelial growth supplement from bovine neural tissue (#E2759) and 10% FBS. All cells were cultured in a 5% CO_2 humidified atmosphere at 37 °C.

2.3. Isolation of Cancer-Associated Fibroblasts (CAFs)

CAFs were isolated from cancer tissue biopsies of PDAC patients with primary lesions after informed consent, and in accordance with the Declaration of Helsinki and approval by the Ethics Committee (REK 2013/1772). In brief, tissues were collected and washed in Dulbecco's modified Eagle's medium (DMEM #6429) supplemented with 2% antibiotic-antimycotic (AB/AM), 100 U/mL penicillin, 100 µg/mL Streptomycin and 25 ng/mL Amphotericin B (Thermo Fischer Scientific, Waltham, MA, USA). Bleeding and necrotic areas of the tissues were cut out using a sterile scalpel and washed thoroughly. Tumour tissues were then cut into approximately 2–4 mm^2 tissue bits and then transferred onto a 10 cm culture dish, slightly air-dried (approximately 2 min) to allow explants to attach on the growth surface of the dish, and incubated in FAD medium (DMEM/Nutrient Mixture F-12 Ham supplemented with 10% FBS, 0.4 mg/mL hydrocortisone, 1% Insulin-Transferrin-Selenium, 50 mg/mL L-ascorbic acid, 10 ng/mL epidermal growth factor and 1% AB/AM). Explants with an outgrowth of cells with fibroblast morphology were trypsinized in a clonal ring placed around the respective explant and fixed on the bottom of the dish with sterile vaseline and placed in 6-well plates. Isolated fibroblasts were further characterised for lineage-specific markers: ESA, CD31, CD45 and CD140b for epithelial, endothelial, blood-borne and mesenchymal origin, respectively. CAFs were further cultured in DMEM (#6429) supplemented with 10% FBS and without AB/AM.

2.4. Cell Culture for Experiments

Three days prior to experiments, 26 mL of cell suspension was injected in Petaka G3 LOT® (low oxygen transport) cell culture chambers (Figure 1a referred to as Petaka herein). A suitable number of cells were injected to achieve confluency at the time of US/MB exposure. To avoid the influx of air, the air valve on the Petakas was sealed with tape, and they were cultured in the horizontal position for a minimum of 24 h to allow for cells to adhere to the plastic surface. The Petaka chambers are designed for cell culture within a limited gas exchange and a gradually decreasing oxygen concentration [30], which is closer to pO_2 ("physioxia") found in living tissue compared to the "normoxic" conditions at atmospheric O_2 pressure commonly used in vitro [31].

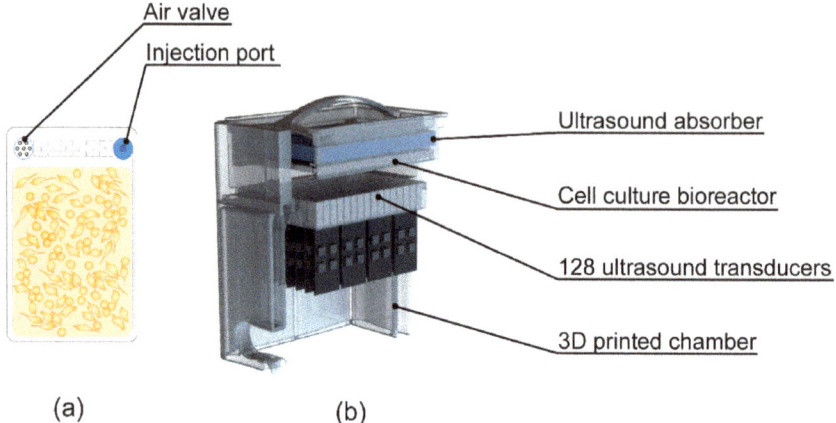

Figure 1. (a) Drawing of cell culture bioreactor (Petaka) used for culturing of cells prior to ultrasound (US) treatment; (b) cutaway of custom-made US treatment chamber used for US treatment of cells (adapted from [22], Pharmaceutics, 2020).

2.5. Microbubbles

Sonazoid™ (GE Healthcare, Little Chalfont, UK) was reconstituted by adding 2 mL NaCl 9 mg/mL (B Braun, Melsungen, Germany) and gently agitated for 30 s. MBs were aspirated via a 19 G needle and transferred to an eppendorf tube. A 19 G venting needle was used to avoid a pressure drop in the vial. To ensure that the reconstituted bubbles were stable, Sonazoid™ bubbles were used within 1 h of reconstitution. A 60 µL volume of reconstituted Sonazoid™ (1.2×10^9 bubbles/mL) was diluted in NaCl 9 mg/mL to a total volume of 1 mL and injected into the Petaka immediately prior to US exposure, giving a concentration of 2.8×10^6 bubbles/mL in the Petaka. In the untreated sample, and US alone controls, 1 mL of NaCl 9 mg/mL was added to Petaka. The Petakas were gently rolled in all directions to ensure a homogenous distribution of MBs and NaCl.

2.6. In Vitro Treatment with Ultrasound and Microbubbles

The cells were exposed to US using a custom-made US treatment chamber (Figure 1), based on a previous design [32] and previously used in [22], suited for US exposure of adherent cells when cultured in Petakas.

The US system consisted of 128, 9×6 mm PZ26 elements firing upwards as a plane-wave into the Petaka, ensuring US treatment of the entire cell-covered surface in the Petaka. The US transducers were driven by a custom Open Ultrasound system (Lecoeur Electronique, Chuelles, France). The acoustic field had been calibrated in three axes using a 200 µm needle hydrophone (Precision acoustics Ltd., Dorset, UK) in the fully assembled US chamber, and the Petaka was placed at the acoustic focus.

Before US treatment, air pockets were removed from the Petaka. To ensure that the floating MBs would come into contact with the cells, the Petaka was placed in the US treatment chamber (Figure 1) with the cell-covered side on top, closest to the US absorber. A low-Mechanical Index (MI) (<0.01) B-mode scan was performed before treatment with US ± MB to detect air pockets in the US bath between the water medium and the Petaka. Air pockets, if present, were removed before US treatment. The US conditions used were based on a previous study [22] and referred to as "Medium US" or "High US" (see Table 1 for details). As untreated control, a Petaka, containing cells but no MBs, was placed in the US treatment chamber for 5 min without application of US. All experiments were performed in triplicate at minimum, except CAFs, where sonoporation experiments were only performed once and only treated with "High US", due to limited material availability. Imaging of cells was performed immediately after sonoporation with 10× magnification using a Nikon Eclipse E200 microscope equipped with a Lumenera Infinity 1 camera.

Table 1. US parameters (5 min treatment with US ± microbubbles (MBs)).

Name	Frequency (MHz)	No. of Cycles	Duty Cycle (%)	Pulse Repetition Frequency (kHz)	MI	Intensity	
						I_{SPTA} (mW/cm^2)	I_{SPPA} (W/cm^2)
Medium	2.00	80	1.8	22	0.2	50	2.7
High	2.00	160	3.6	22	0.378	358	9.64

2.7. Calcein Uptake

To assess if the cell membrane had been permeabilised, a nontoxic cell-impermeable fluorescent dye, calcein, was added during treatment with US ± MB. A 50 mg/mL calcein stock solution in 1 M NaOH was kept at 2–8 °C protected from light. Immediately prior to treatment with US ± MB, calcein was mixed with NaCl 9 mg/mL ± MBs in the 1 mL that was injected into the Petaka. A concentration of 6 μM calcein was used in all experiments.

After treatment with US ± MB, the cells were incubated for 1 h to allow for cell membrane pores to re-seal [4,33], flushed twice with phosphate-buffered saline (PBS), detached using trypsin-EDTA 0.05% and harvested from the Petaka. Following centrifugation and resuspension in PBS, the cells were analysed by flow cytometry on an Accuri C6 flow cytometer (BDBioscience, Franklin Lakes, NJ, USA). Data collected from Acurri C6 were gated in FlowJo®, and the uptake of calcein was measured as a percentage of calcein-positive cells. The gating strategy is shown in Supplementary Figure S1. The median fluorescence intensity (MFI) of the cells in the calcein-positive population was also recorded.

2.8. Viability Analysis: Apoptosis and Cell Death

Cells were treated with US ± MBs and cultured in Petaka placed in a 5% CO_2 humidified atmosphere at 37 °C for 24 h. Following incubation, the medium from the Petaka was collected, cells were flushed with phosphate-buffered saline (PBS) and the cells were detached from the plastic using Accutase®. Harvested medium and cell suspension were combined, and cells were counted using a haemocytometer (later referred to as cell count 24 h). Trypan Blue® (Thermo Fischer Scientific, Waltham, MA, USA) was added to identify dead cells. Apoptosis was assessed by staining with Annexin V antibody and propidium iodide (PI) using Dead cell Apoptosis kit with Annexin V Alexa Fluor™ 488 and Propidium Iodide *(PI)* (Invitrogen, Catalog #V12341, Thermo Fischer Scientific, Waltham, MA, USA). The assay was performed in accordance with the manufacturer's protocol with two exceptions: Half the concentration of Annexin V antibody and of PI were used, based on titration, and PI was added shortly before flow cytometry analysis. Data were collected on an Acurri C6 flow cytometer and gated in FlowJo®. The gating strategy is shown in Figure S2.

To assess cell loss during US exposure (e.g., due to cell detachment or destruction), the cell count per Petaka was counted using a haemocytometer at 0 h (as described in Section 2.10). As mentioned above, cells were also counted after 24 h to assess sonoporation effects on viability. CAFs could not be reliably counted in the haemocytometer, due to low cell concentration. CAFs were counted 24 h after US exposure by analysis of a fixed volume of cell suspension (300 μL) using an Accuri C6 flow cytometer.

2.9. Viability Analysis: Growth Potential and Metabolic Activity

Cells harvested from the Petaka 24 h post-sonoporation were used to assess their proliferative capacity after re-seeding. Live cells (Trypan blue® negative) were seeded on 96-well cell culture plates (MIA PaCa-2: 3000 cells, fibroblasts: 6000 cells, HUVEC: 3000 cells), and their metabolic activity was assessed after 24, 48 and 72 h by addition of WST-1 reagent (Roche Diagnostics GmbH, Mannheim, Germany). WST-1 was added 2 h before detection on a multiwell spectrophotometer in accordance to the manufacturer's protocol. Live cells were also seeded on 24-well plates (MIA PaCa-2: 30,000 cells, fibroblasts: 60,000 cells, HUVEC: 30,000 cells), and the cells were detached using Accutase®, diluted in cell culture medium, and counted after 24, 48 and 72 h using a haemocytometer.

2.10. Sample Preparation for Phosphospecific Flow Cytometry

To investigate changes in intracellular signalling events, cells were harvested from separate Petakas as soon as possible after sonoporation and after 2 h of incubation. Timepoints were selected based on a previous study [4]. Cells cultured in separate Petakas were treated with 1 µM A23187 (calcium ionophore) + 100 nM phorbol myristate acetate (PMA: PKC activator) for 30 min as positive controls for intracellular signalling. Cells were detached from the Petaka using the cold trypsin method [34,35], i.e. with ice-cold 2.5% trypsin not containing ethylenediaminetetraacetic acid (EDTA). Prior to cell detachment, the medium was harvested, the Petaka was flushed once with ice-cold PBS, and the collected cell culture medium and PBS were placed on ice during detachment of cells. Ice-cold 2.5% trypsin was added to the Petaka and subsequently placed on ice during the detachment time. In all experiments, the cell detachment on ice started within 1–3 min after US exposure. Cell detachment time varied between cell lines, as shown in Figure S3. Cell culture medium, PBS, and cells were collected and fixed by adding 16% paraformaldehyde (PFA, Alfa Aesar, Haverhill, MA, USA) directly to yield a final concentration of 2%, incubated for 15 min at room temperature and permeabilised by adding ice-cold methanol [4,36]. Before addition of PFA, a sample was taken for cell count (later referred to as cell count 0 h) and counted using a haemocytometer.

2.11. Barcoding

To reduce antibody staining variability, the samples were barcode-stained. The six individual cell samples were stained with unique signatures of succinimidylesters of Pacific Blue and Pacific Orange (barcoding) for multiplex flow cytometry [37]. After barcode-staining, the samples were washed in PBS containing 1% bovine serum albumin and 2 mM EDTA, then pooled prior to antibody staining. A graphical depiction of barcoding/sample preparation is shown in Figure S4: One barcode represents all five samples from one timepoint in each experiment (Untreated cells, Medium US, High US, Medium US + MBs, High US + MBs) and a positive control. Pooled cells were split into different tubes and each tube was stained with an antibody panel. Each panel consisted of a combination of two antibodies conjugated to either Alexa Fluor® 488 or 647 (Table S1). The panels of markers were based on our previous study [4]: Mitogen-activated protein kinase (MAPK; p38 and extracellular regulated kinase 1/2 (ERK1/2), cAMP response element-binding element (CREB), protein kinase A (PKA), signal transducer and activator of transcription 3 (STAT3; 727 epitope), phosphoinositide 3-kinase (PI3K), Akt and mammalian target of rapamycin (mTOR) pathway proteins (ribosomal protein S6) and eukaryotic translation initiation factor 4E-binding protein (4E-BP1). The panel was extended to include focal adhesion kinase (FAK) and Src, based on studies on mechanotransduction in response to US [38–40]. Samples were analysed on an LSR Fortessa flow cytometer (BD Bioscience, Franklin Lakes, NJ, USA).

2.12. Data Analysis of Phosphospecific Flow Cytometry

Data collected on the LSR Fortessa were compensated, gated and de-barcoded in DIVA software. The gating strategy is shown in Figure S5. Analysis of median fluorescence intensity (MFI) was performed in Cytobank (Cytobank Inc., Santa Clara, CA, USA). The MFI of each sample was corrected for autofluorescence of the cells and the barcode staining by subtraction of MFI of the corresponding barcoded cells unstained with antibody. The arcsinh ratio (arcsinh (treated/5)−arcsinh (control/5)) was calculated in Microsoft Excel to depict changes in phosphorylation.

2.13. Statistical Analysis

Statistical comparisons were performed in GraphPad Prism 8 (San Diego, CA, USA). A Shapiro-Wilk normality test was performed on all datasets to determine if the data were normally distributed. As over 95% of the datasets passed the normality tests, a repeated-measures one-way Analysis of Variance (ANOVA) with Holm–Sidak's multiple comparison test of the sample MFI versus the untreated samples was used. In addition, an ordinary ANOVA was used for statistical comparisons of calcein uptake and viability (treated cells versus untreated cells; medium US + MBs vs. high US + MBs only for % calcein-positive cells). Significance level was set at p-value 0.05.

3. Results

3.1. Direct Effects of Sonoporation: Uptake of Cell Impermeable Dye and Cell Lysis (Cell Count)

In all cell types, uptake of calcein was only observed when MBs were added, suggesting that increased uptake only occurs after sonoporation. The lowest uptake was observed in MIA PaCa-2, 12% of cells at Medium US + MBs and 25% at High US + MBs (Figure 2a). In HUVECs, the percentage of cells taking up calcein was high (70%) at both Medium and High US + MBs (Figure 2b). The percentage of cells taking up calcein was even higher in fibroblasts, and increased with US intensity from Medium US (79%) to High US (90%) (Figure 2c). The increase in US parameters from medium US to high US had a significant effect on uptake in MIA PaCa-2 and fibroblasts ($p < 0.001$ and $p < 0.01$, respectively (statistic not displayed in Figure 2)).

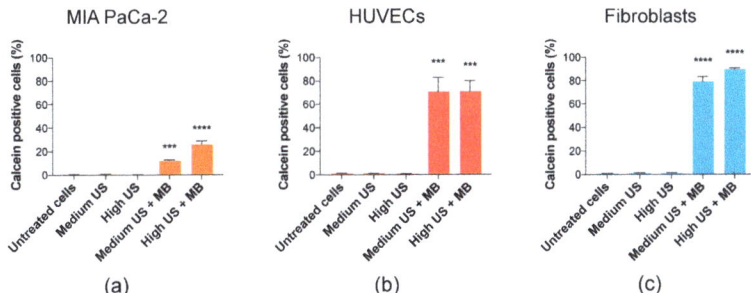

Figure 2. The percentage of cells taking up calcein. Addition of MBs was necessary for increased uptake in cells. (**a**) In MIA PaCa-2, increased US intensity increased the percentage of calcein-positive cells. (**b**) In human umbilical vein endothelial cells (HUVECs), increased US intensity was not important for percentage of calcein-positive cells. (**c**) In fibroblasts, increased US intensity resulted in a small increase in percentage of calcein-positive cells. Mean ± SEM; *** $p < 0.001$, **** $p < 0.0001$ (treated vs. untreated cells).

The sonoporation parameters used in this study did not induce a reduction of cells (cell lysis) in any of the cell lines used (Figure 3).

3.2. Cellular Viability upon Sonoporation

Sonoporation may induce apoptosis [41–44] and reduce proliferation of cells [4]. Sonoporation at the US intensities in this study had minimal negative effects on the viability of MIA PaCa-2, HUVECs and fibroblasts. In MIA PaCa-2, no increase in percentage of apoptotic cells were observed by Annexin/PI staining (Figure 4a), although a small increase in dead cells at High US ($p < 0.05$) was observed by Trypan Blue staining in samples taken directly after collecting cells and medium (Figure S6). In HUVECs, apoptosis measured by Annexin V/PI staining increased with increasing US + MBs, but this was not statistically significant (Figure 4b). The uptake of Trypan Blue in HUVECs at these parameters was significantly different from untreated cells ($p < 0.01$) (Figure S6). In fibroblasts, a very small, but statistically significant ($p < 0.05$), increase in cell count was observed after 24 h of culturing after sonoporation with Medium US + MBs (Figure 4c).

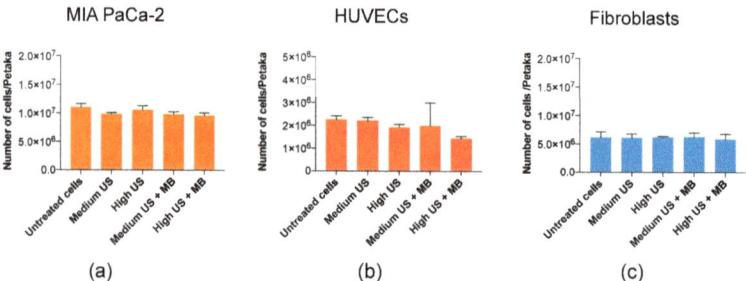

Figure 3. Cell count immediately (0 h) after sonoporation. Cell count (0 h) indicated no mechanical destruction of cells in (**a**) MIA PaCa-2 and (**c**) fibroblasts, while a minor and nonsignificant reduction was observed in (**b**) HUVECs. Mean ± SEM.

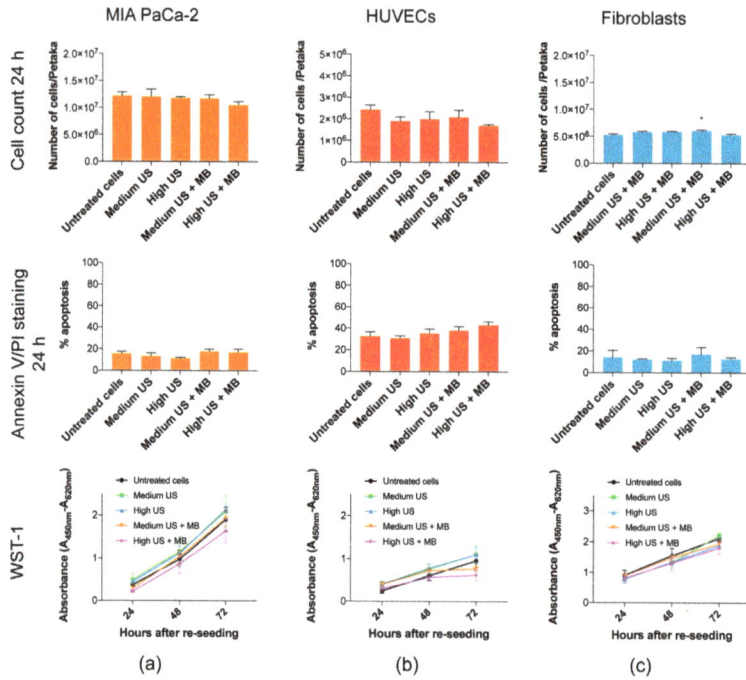

Figure 4. Viability of cells harvested after 24 h of incubation in Petaka. (**a**) No significant reduction in the cell count or increase in apoptotic AnnexinV/PI-stained cells of MIA PaCa-2 was observed. The metabolic activity (WST-1) after re-seeding was not affected by US + MB. (**b**) Cell count 24 h post-sonoporation of HUVECs is slightly, but not significantly, decreased in treated samples. Percentage of apoptotic cells 24 h post-sonoporation by AnnexinV/PI staining was increased, and also not statistically significant. No significant change was observed in the metabolic activity (WST-1) of the cells after re-seeding of the cells, although some reduction in metabolic activity was observed in cells exposed to US + MBs. (**c**) No significant reduction in the cell count, increase in apoptotic AnnexinV/PI stained cells or reduced metabolic activity (WST-1) after re-seeding of fibroblasts was observed. Mean ± SEM. * $p < 0.05$ (treated vs. untreated cells).

The long-term viability after the re-seeding of cells was not significantly reduced in any of the cell types (WST-1 in Figure 4, confirmed by cell counts in Figure S6). In HUVECs, there is a trend towards reduced cell metabolic activity and growth after 48 h in cells treated with US + MBs, although this was not significant.

3.3. Sonoporation Induced Changes in Intracellular Signalling

Sonoporation induced phosphorylation of MAP-kinases p38 T180/Y182 and ERK1/2 T202/Y204 in all three cell types, but with different magnitudes and timings (Figure 5a). The most pronounced activation was observed in fibroblasts immediately after sonoporation, while the activation on MIA PaCa-2 and HUVECs was weaker or delayed. In MIA PaCa-2, an immediate, weak activation of both p38 T180/Y182 (Medium and High US + MBs; $p = 0.15$ (ns) and $p < 0.05$, respectively) and ERK1/2 T202/Y204 (Medium and High US + MBs, $p < 0.05$ and $p = 0.15$ (ns), respectively) was observed in cells treated with the combination of US + MBs (Figure 5a). p38 was still significantly activated 2 h after sonoporation, but very weakly. In HUVECs, phosphorylation of p38 T180/Y182 was moderately increased in cells treated with US both with and without MBs immediately after sonoporation, although this effect was only significant in cells treated without MBs ($p < 0.05$) (Figure 5a). After 2 h, p38 T180/Y182 phosphorylation was still elevated, but lower than that at 0 h, in HUVECs treated without bubbles (ns). In HUVECs treated with US + MBs, phosphorylation of p38 T180/Y182 was further increased 2 h after sonoporation (Medium US and High US + MBs; $p < 0.01$ and $p = 0.08$ (ns), respectively). ERK1/2 T202/Y204 phosphorylation was unchanged in HUVECs immediately after sonoporation, but a small insignificant increase was observed 2 h after sonoporation in cells treated with US + MBs. In fibroblasts, US + MBs induced significant, immediate changes in the phosphorylation level of MAP-kinases p38 T180/Y182 ($p < 0.05$) and ERK1/2 T202/Y204 ($p < 0.01$) In response to both Medium and High US (Figure 5a). Two hours after sonoporation, the phosphorylation level was returned to the basal level. The phosphorylation of downstream target STAT3 S727 was not significantly changed in any of the cell types, although STAT3 S727 was weakly increased immediately and 2 h after sonoporation in fibroblasts.

In the mTOR pathway, 2 h after sonoporation, phosphorylation of ribosomal protein S6 was increased in MIA PaCa-2 at the S240 epitope and in fibroblasts at both the S240 and the S235/236 epitopes (Figure 5b). However, phosphorylation of S6 was not statistically significant and varied between experiments (Figure S7). Unlike the other cell lines, phosphorylation of ribosomal protein S6 was not increased at 2 h in HUVECs.

In general, sonoporation caused dephosphorylation of 4E-BP1 T36/45, particularly when MBs were added (Figure 5b). In MIA PaCa-2, 4E-BP1 T36/45 was significantly dephosphorylated 2 h after sonoporation using Medium US and Medium/High US + MBs ($p < 0.05$). Phosphorylation of 4E-BP1 T36/45 in HUVECs was decreased immediately using Medium US and High US + MBs ($p < 0.05$ and $p = 0.09$ (ns), respectively), and at 2 h after using sonoporation High US + MBs ($p < 0.05$). In fibroblasts, the dephosphorylation of 4E-BP1 T36/45 was most pronounced immediately after sonoporation MB (Medium and High US + MBs; $p < 0.001$ and $p < 0.0001$, respectively). 4E-BP1 T36/45 was also dephosphorylated in the fibroblasts in response to US without MBs, immediately after sonoporation using Medium US ($p < 0.05$) and 2 h after using Medium and High US ($p < 0.01$ and $p < 0.05$, respectively).

The only statistically significant change in phosphorylation of Akt S473 was observed in MIA PaCa-2, 2 h after sonoporation, but this effect was very small ($p < 0.05$) (Figure 5b). Changes in phosphorylation of CREB, PKA, Src and FAK, together with all experiments with CAFs, were nonsignificant, and are presented in Supplementary data (Figures S8–S10).

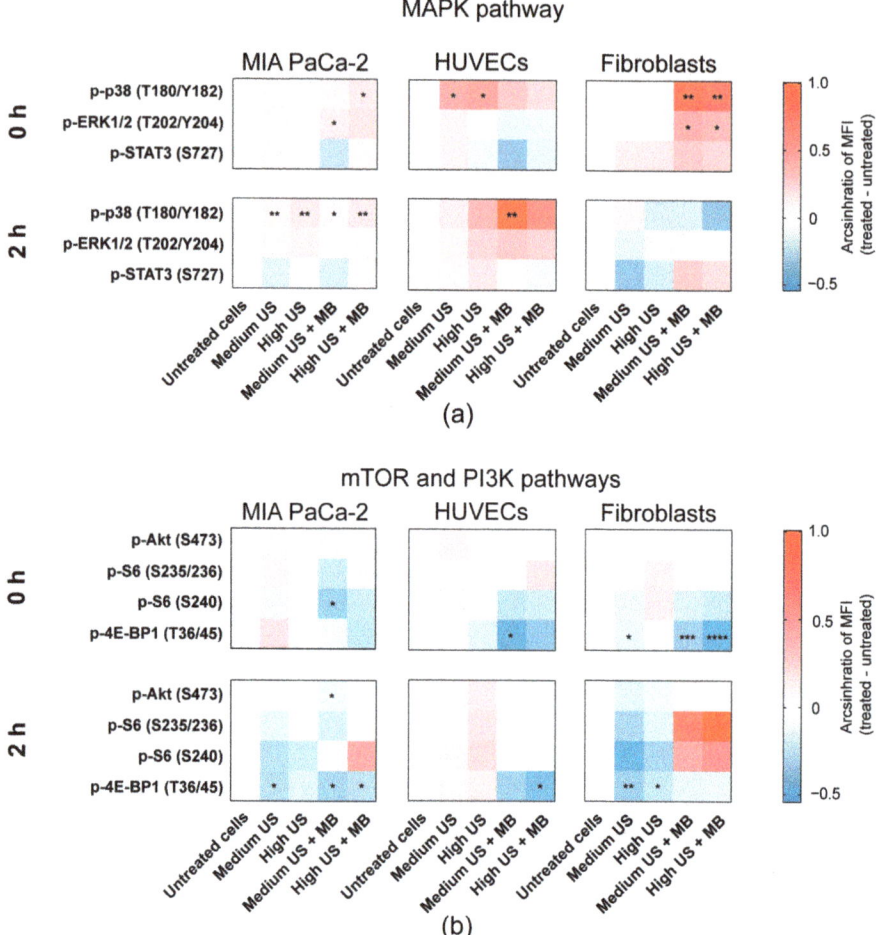

Figure 5. Intracellular signalling induced by sonoporation. Heatmaps displaying changes in phosphorylation status (shown as arcsinh ratio) of the chosen range of proteins in response to treatment with US with and without Sonazoid™ MBs. Phosphorylation status was detected immediately (0 h) and 2 h post-sonoporation. Different phosphorylation profiles were observed in the (**a**) MAP-kinase pathway (p38, ERK1/2 and downstream target STAT3 S727), and (**b**) mTOR (ribosomal protein S6 and 4E-BP1) and PI3K pathways (Akt). Mean ± SEM. * $p < 0.05$, ** $p < 0.01$, *** $p < 0.001$, **** $p < 0.0001$ (treated vs. untreated cells).

3.4. Induction of Apoptosis by Inhibition of MEK/ERK in Combination with Sonoporation

The role of the ERK1/2 activation in response to sonoporation is not yet known, but has been shown to be important for cellular recovery in cells exposed to pore-forming toxins through an intracellular mechanism involving p38 and ERK1/2 (similar to observations in fibroblasts in Figure 5) [45]. Similar to Cabezas et al. [45], we treated cells with MEK/ERK inhibitor U0126 prior to sonoporation, which increased the percentage of apoptotic fibroblasts (from 13% to 26%) and the percentage of apoptotic HUVECs from 43% to 51% (Figure 6), but not at all in MIA PaCa-2. However, the increases were only significant in HUVECs ($p < 0.05$).

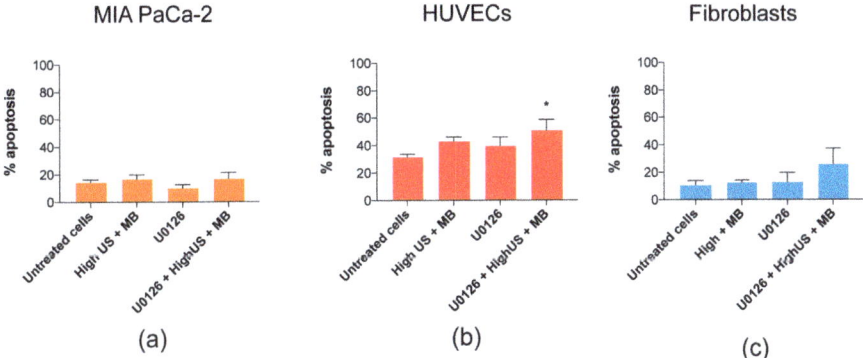

Figure 6. Inhibition of MEK/ERK with U0126 in combination with high US + MBs increased the percentage of apoptotic (**b**) HUVECs ($p < 0.05$) and (**c**) fibroblasts, but not (**a**) MIA PaCa-2. Mean ± SEM, * $p < 0.05$ (treated vs. untreated cells).

4. Discussion

4.1. Sensitivity to Sonoporation

In this work, we aimed to compare the sonoporation efficacy and intracellular signalling responses to sonoporation in a selection of cell lines representative of the cellular diversity present in solid tumours. The uptake of calcein and other cell-impermeable dyes is commonly used in sonoporation research as a measure of cell permeabilization and successful drug uptake [5,8,41,46–49]. The dye uptake may be measured both as a percentage of stained cells and sonoporation efficiency (amount of molecules taken up, measured as fluorescence intensity). In previous studies, the percentage of stained cells and sonoporation efficiency followed the same trend [4,33], but contrary to expectations, opposite trends were observed in percentage and efficiency (MFI) between the cell types in this study (Figure 2 and Supplemental Figure S11). For the purpose of this discussion, we have focussed on percentage calcein-stained cells (Figure 2), which is the most commonly used measure. Furthermore, this measurement followed similar trends as the observed changes in intracellular signalling.

Interestingly, the cancerous MIA PaCa2 cells experienced a considerably lower percentage of calcein-positive cells in both the medium and high US settings (12%/25%) compared to HUVECs (70%/70%) and fibroblasts (79%/90%). Whilst high US + MB was shown to be most efficient in sonoporation, the higher ultrasound intensity might lead to cell damage. However, the low-intensity US regimen used in this study did not have a major impact on cell viability. It has previously been concluded that cancerous cells may be more sensitive to US ± MB, both in terms of viability [50,51], or viability and uptake of cell-impermeable dye [4], but the current results indicate that sonoporation efficacy is not really a question of healthy versus cancer cells. In addition, different PDAC cancer cell lines have different sensitivities to sonoporation, as shown by Bjånes et al. (Supplementary Data) [22].

Sonoporation efficacy has been associated with multiple factors. While larger cells have a greater likelihood of interaction with microbubbles, additional factors might be more relevant [51]. This is supported by our results on sonoporation efficacy in small HUVECs versus larger HUV-EC-C cells (HUVEC cell line) (Figure S12) where the difference in uptake was not significant, and a larger difference was actually observed between HUVECs and MIA PaCa-2 despite their similarity in cell size (Figure S13). Cell membrane stiffness is also proposed to influence sonoporation [52], which should be explored in further studies.

4.2. Induction of Sonoporation Signalling

Activation of intracellular signalling follows a similar pattern as observed in our previous study on a leukemic cell line and peripheral mononuclear blood cells (PBMCs) [4], suggesting a general mechanism across cell types and irrespective of differences in the culturing of suspension and adherent cell lines. In both studies, the magnitude of activation follows the trend of calcein uptake (i.e. extent of permeabilisation). The most important pathways involved were activation of the MAP-kinases p38 and ERK1/2 (and CREB, STAT3, Akt in [4]), and activation of either 4E-BP1 or eIF2α [4], and ribosomal protein S6 2 h post-sonoporation. Just as in MIA PaCa-2, the changes in intracellular signalling previously observed were overall weaker in PBMCs [4], where a lower proportion of cells were sonoporated.

No major impact on cell viability was observed in this study, except a small increase in apoptotic fibroblasts and HUVECs when MEK/ERK was inhibited using U0126. The activation of MAP-kinase (p38, ERK) and dephosphorylation of 4E-BP1 in response to sonoporation resembles signalling related to membrane repair following pore formation and osmotic stress in cells exposed to pore-forming toxins [45,53] and electroporation [54,55]. The similarity was most pronounced in fibroblasts, which may explain why viability was not affected in the fibroblasts in spite of the high rate of sonoporation (calcein uptake). The mechanism for repair of sonoporation-induced pores, i.e. repairable sonoporation [56], is still not yet fully known but has also been compared by others to membrane repair in cells exposed to pore-forming toxins [57]. The relationship between pore formation (by sonoporation, pore-forming toxins, electroporation), signalling events and membrane repair requires further evidence in future studies.

Dephosphorylation of 4E-BP1 is most commonly known to suppress protein synthesis through inhibition of cap-dependent protein translation [58,59], which under stressful conditions, may be regulated though the unfolded protein response (UPR) to restore cellular homeostasis [60]. However, the sonoporation-inhibition of 4E-BP1 may itself contribute to the anti-cancer effects of sonoporation. In PDAC therapy, inhibition of 4E-BP1 in cancer-associated fibroblasts was found to repress secretion of proteins involved in chemoresistance, and to improve the efficacy of chemotherapy (gemcitabine) by acting as a stroma-targeted therapy [61].

Together with dephosphorylation of 4E-BP1, sonoporation induced a paradoxical phosphorylation of ribosomal protein S6 in the mTOR signalling pathway. The role of S6 activation in response to sonoporation is not yet known, but we observed this activation to be absent under conditions where cellular viability was decreased by sonoporation in our previous study on leukemic cells too [4]. Typically, activation of ribosomal protein S6 stimulates cap-dependent protein translation downstream of mTOR [62]. The activation may imply that cellular homeostasis is restored, resulting in stimulated protein synthesis, but further studies are required to confirm this.

4.3. Limitations of This Study and Future Perspectives

Whilst the effects of sonoporation on cancer cells have been extensively studied and, to some extent, also on HUVECs, the effects on fibroblasts, cancer-associated fibroblasts and other cells of the tumour microenvironment are less known. As these results show that the different cell types respond differently to sonoporation, it is important to include the cells of the tumour microenvironment in future studies. This study was limited by the inclusion of only one cell line for each cell type and only one cancer cell line. Based on differences in sonoporation efficacy between PDAC cell lines [22] differences in magnitude of signalling changes may be anticipated.

The main limitations are that each cell type was studied separately and cultured as a monolayer on a plastic surface with no regulation of liquid flow, temperature or gas saturation. Cells were cultured in Petaka G3 LOT cell culture chambers. Even though these are designed to regulate gas exchange, pO_2 depends on the cell line and cell counts, and a limitation in these experiments is that pO_2 was not monitored, as this parameter may affect both the physical properties of microbubbles and viability/responses of the cells.

Recent studies on interendothelial openings between cells [25–27] suggest that the effects of sonoporation are beyond the simple formation of pores in cancer cells interacting with bubbles in an US field. However, this was also studied on monolayers of endothelial cells alone. The term "sonopermeation" has been introduced to cover the broader range of effects leading to increased delivery of drugs, including endocytosis, opening of cellular junctions and changes in vessels and the stromal compartment [63], but actual determinations of the role of different cell types and the mechanism of sonoporation require more advanced organoid models or preclinical studies with humanised immune systems and tumours. Furthermore, as the results in all cell lines in this study confirm that MBs are essential for sonoporation, more advanced models are also required to assess if MBs only affect the endothelium or if the reduced viability and opening of junctions between endothelial cells can lead to interaction with the tumour microenvironment and cancer cells.

The majority of these studies have been performed in triplicate due to the complexity of the technical process required to obtain results. This may impact the statistical analysis and potential conclusions that can be drawn from this study. Further work and additional repetitions should be performed to independently validate these results.

5. Conclusions

Different cell types respond differently to US + MBs, in terms of uptake of cell-impermeable dye, reduction in viability and intracellular signalling. Sonoporation is associated with activation of the MAP-kinases p38 and ERK, and increase in the phosphorylation of ribosomal protein S6 together with dephosphorylation of 4E-BP1. This may be a stress-response for cells to survive and repair the cell membrane after sonoporation, resembling cellular responses to electroporation and pore-forming toxins, and are potential drug targets enhancing the efficacy of sonoporation in cancer therapy. As cell types in the tumour microenvironment are more sensitive to sonoporation, further efforts in optimising sonoporation-enhanced therapy should be targeted at the microenvironment.

Supplementary Materials: The following are available online at http://www.mdpi.com/1999-4923/12/11/1058/s1, Table S1: Antibody panels for phospho-flow cytometry; Figure S1: Gating strategy of flow cytometric data to identify calcein-positive cells; Figure S2: Gating strategy of flow cytometric data to identify cells stained with AnnexinV and propidium iodide (PI); Figure S3: Time for detachment of cells using cold-trypsinization; Figure S4: Sample processing for phospho-flow cytometry; Figure S5: Gating strategy for identification of each individually stained sample in the barcode (de-barcoding); Figure S6: Supplemental data on viability of cells harvested after 24 h incubation in Petaka G3 LOT®; Figure S7: Increase in ribosomal protein S6 phosphorylation was variable between experiments; Figure S8: Changes in phosphorylation of CREB and PKA was low; Figure S9: Changes in phosphorylation of FAK and Src; Figure S10: Treatment of cancer associated fibroblasts (CAFs) with US + MBs resulted in extensive uptake of the cell impermeable dye (calcein), a large reduction in cell viability and changes in intracellular signalling is observed in the cells that survived sonoporation; Figure S11: Median fluorescence intensity (MFI) of calcein-positive cells; Figure S12: The percentage of cells taking up calcein in HUVEC and HUV-EC-C cell lines; Figure S13: Images of sonoporated cells.

Author Contributions: Conceptualization, R.H., A.L., B.T.G., S.K., G.R.d.G. and E.M.; data curation, R.H. and E.T.M.; formal analysis, R.H. and S.K.; funding acquisition, R.H., B.T.G., O.H.G., S.K. and E.M.; investigation, R.H. and E.T.M.; methodology, R.H., A.L., E.T.M., D.E.C., S.K. and G.R.d.G.; software, E.T.M. and S.K.; supervision, S.K. and E.M.; visualization, R.H.; writing—original draft, R.H., A.L. and S.K.; writing—review and editing, R.H., A.L., E.T.M., D.E.C., B.T.G., O.H.G., S.K., G.R.d.G. and E.M. All authors have read and agreed to the published version of the manuscript.

Funding: This study was funded by the Western Health Board of Norway (Grant numbers 911779, 911182 and 912035), by the Norwegian Cancer Society (6833652, 182735) and by the Norwegian Research Council (SonoCURE grant no. 250317). This work was supported in part by the National Institutes of Health grant R01CA199646. This work was also supported by "Apoteker Morten Nyegaard og hustru Katrine Nygaards legat" awarded from the Norwegian Association of Pharmacists.

Acknowledgments: Flow cytometry was performed at the Flow Core Facility, Department of Clinical Science, University of Bergen. We want to thank Brith Bergum at the Core facility for technical assistance, and Brith Bergum, Jørn Skavland and Stein-Erik Gullaksen for valuable advice and discussions on flow cytometry and barcoding. We also thank Monica Hellesøy for advice on the flow cytometry of adherent cells.

Conflicts of Interest: The authors declare no conflict of interest. S.K. is currently a full-time employee of EXACT Therapeutics AS. EXACT Therapeutics AS did not have any influence in any part of this article but provided Sonazoid™ as a generous gift. KinN Therapeutics declares no conflict of interest.

References

1. Postema, M.; Kotopoulis, S.; Delalande, A.; Gilja, O.H. Sonoporation: Why Microbubbles Create Pores. *Ultraschall Med.* **2012**, *11*, 97–98.
2. Qin, J.; Wang, T.-Y.; Willmann, J.K. Sonoporation: Applications for Cancer Therapy. *Retin. Degener. Dis.* **2016**, *880*, 263–291. [CrossRef]
3. Chen, X.; Wan, J.M.; Yu, A.C.H. Sonoporation as a Cellular Stress: Induction of Morphological Repression and Developmental Delays. *Ultrasound Med. Biol.* **2013**, *39*, 1075–1086. [CrossRef] [PubMed]
4. Haugse, R.; Langer, A.; Gullaksen, S.-E.; Sundøy, S.M.; Gjertsen, B.T.; Kotopoulis, S.; McCormack, E. Intracellular Signaling in Key Pathways Is Induced by Treatment with Ultrasound and Microbubbles in a Leukemia Cell Line, but Not in Healthy Peripheral Blood Mononuclear Cells. *Pharmaceutics* **2019**, *11*, 319. [CrossRef] [PubMed]
5. Watanabe, Y.; Aoi, A.; Horie, S.; Tomita, N.; Mori, S.; Morikawa, H.; Matsumura, Y.; Vassaux, G.; Kodama, T. Low-intensity ultrasound and microbubbles enhance the antitumor effect of cisplatin. *Cancer Sci.* **2008**, *99*, 2525–2531. [CrossRef] [PubMed]
6. Matsuo, M.; Yamaguchi, K.; Feril, L.B.; Endo, H.; Ogawa, K.; Tachibana, K.; Nakayama, J. Synergistic inhibition of malignant melanoma proliferation by melphalan combined with ultrasound and microbubbles. *Ultrason. Sonochem.* **2011**, *18*, 1218–1224. [CrossRef] [PubMed]
7. Iwanaga, K.; Tominaga, K.; Yamamoto, K.; Habu, M.; Maeda, H.; Akifusa, S.; Tsujisawa, T.; Okinaga, T.; Fukuda, J.; Nishihara, T. Local delivery system of cytotoxic agents to tumors by focused sonoporation. *Cancer Gene Ther.* **2007**, *14*, 354–363. [CrossRef] [PubMed]
8. Sorace, A.G.; Warram, J.M.; Umphrey, H.; Hoyt, K. Microbubble-mediated ultrasonic techniques for improved chemotherapeutic delivery in cancer. *J. Drug Target.* **2012**, *20*, 43–54. [CrossRef]
9. Bressand, D.; Novell, A.; Girault, A.; Raoul, W.; Fromont-Hankard, G.; Escoffre, J.-M.; LeComte, T.; Bouakaz, A. Enhancing Nab-Paclitaxel Delivery Using Microbubble-Assisted Ultrasound in a Pancreatic Cancer Model. *Mol. Pharm.* **2019**, *16*, 3814–3822. [CrossRef] [PubMed]
10. Escoffre, J.M.; Piron, J.; Novell, A.; Bouakaz, A. Doxorubicin Delivery into Tumor Cells with Ultrasound and Microbubbles. *Mol. Pharm.* **2011**, *8*, 799–806. [CrossRef]
11. Lammertink, B.; Bos, C.; Van Der Wurff-Jacobs, K.M.; Storm, G.; Moonen, C.T.; Deckers, R. Increase of intracellular cisplatin levels and radiosensitization by ultrasound in combination with microbubbles. *J. Control. Release* **2016**, *238*, 157–165. [CrossRef]
12. Mariglia, J.; Momin, S.; Coe, I.; Karshafian, R. Analysis of the cytotoxic effects of combined ultrasound, microbubble and nucleoside analog combinations on pancreatic cells in vitro. *Ultrasonics* **2018**, *89*, 110–117. [CrossRef] [PubMed]
13. Heath, C.H.; Sorace, A.; Knowles, J.; Rosenthal, E.; Hoyt, K. Microbubble therapy enhances anti-tumor properties of cisplatin and cetuximab in vitro and in vivo. *Otolaryngol. Neck Surg.* **2012**, *146*, 938–945. [CrossRef] [PubMed]
14. Hirabayashi, F.; Iwanaga, K.; Okinaga, T.; Takahashi, O.; Ariyoshi, W.; Suzuki, R.; Sugii, M.; Maruyama, K.; Tominaga, K.; Nishihara, T. Epidermal growth factor receptor-targeted sonoporation with microbubbles enhances therapeutic efficacy in a squamous cell carcinoma model. *PLoS ONE* **2017**, *12*, e0185293. [CrossRef] [PubMed]
15. Zhao, Y.-Z.; Lu, C.-T.; Zhou, Z.-C.; Jin, Z.; Zhang, L.; Sun, C.-Z.; Xu, Y.-Y.; Gao, H.-S.; Tian, J.-L.; Gao, F.-H.; et al. Enhancing chemotherapeutic drug inhibition on tumor growth by ultrasound: An in vivo experiment. *J. Drug Target.* **2010**, *19*, 154–160. [CrossRef]
16. Kotopoulis, S.; Delalande, A.; Popa, M.; Mamaeva, V.; Dimcevski, G.; Gilja, O.H.; Postema, M.; Gjertsen, B.T.; McCormack, E. Sonoporation-Enhanced Chemotherapy Significantly Reduces Primary Tumour Burden in an Orthotopic Pancreatic Cancer Xenograft. *Mol. Imaging Biol.* **2013**, *16*, 53–62. [CrossRef]

17. Kotopoulis, S.; Stigen, E.; Popa, M.; Safont, M.M.; Healey, A.; Kvåle, S.; Sontum, P.; Gjertsen, B.T.; Gilja, O.H.; McCormack, E. Sonoporation with Acoustic Cluster Therapy (ACT®) induces transient tumour volume reduction in a subcutaneous xenograft model of pancreatic ductal adenocarcinoma. *J. Control. Release* **2017**, *245*, 70–80. [CrossRef]
18. Dimcevski, G.; Kotopoulis, S.; Bjånes, T.; Hoem, D.; Schjøtt, J.; Gjertsen, B.T.; Biermann, M.; Molven, A.; Sorbye, H.; McCormack, E.; et al. A human clinical trial using ultrasound and microbubbles to enhance gemcitabine treatment of inoperable pancreatic cancer. *J. Control. Release* **2016**, *243*, 172–181. [CrossRef]
19. Orth, M.; Metzger, P.; Gerum, S.; Mayerle, J.; Schneider, G.; Belka, C.; Schnurr, M.; Lauber, K. Pancreatic ductal adenocarcinoma: Biological hallmarks, current status, and future perspectives of combined modality treatment approaches. *Radiat. Oncol.* **2019**, *14*, 1–20. [CrossRef]
20. Grasso, C.; Jansen, G.; Giovannetti, E. Drug resistance in pancreatic cancer: Impact of altered energy metabolism. *Crit. Rev. Oncol.* **2017**, *114*, 139–152. [CrossRef]
21. Ward, M.; Wu, J.; Chiu, J.-F. Ultrasound-induced cell lysis and sonoporation enhanced by contrast agents. *J. Acoust. Soc. Am.* **1999**, *105*, 2951–2957. [CrossRef]
22. Bjånes, T.; Kotopoulis, S.; Murvold, E.T.; Kamčeva, T.; Gjertsen, B.T.; Gilja, O.H.; Schjøtt, J.; Riedel, B.; McCormack, E. Ultrasound- and Microbubble-Assisted Gemcitabine Delivery to Pancreatic Cancer Cells. *Pharmaceutics* **2020**, *12*, 141. [CrossRef]
23. Van Wamel, A.; Kooiman, K.; Emmer, M.; Cate, F.T.; Versluis, A.M.; De Jong, N. Ultrasound microbubble induced endothelial cell permeability. *J. Control. Release* **2006**, *116*, e100–e102. [CrossRef]
24. Park, J.; Fan, Z.; Kumon, R.E.; El-Sayed, M.E.H.; Deng, C.X. Modulation of Intracellular Ca^{2+} Concentration in Brain Microvascular Endothelial Cells in vitro by Acoustic Cavitation. *Ultrasound Med. Biol.* **2010**, *36*, 1176–1187. [CrossRef]
25. Helfield, B.; Chen, X.; Watkins, S.C.; Villanueva, F.S. Biophysical insight into mechanisms of sonoporation. *Proc. Natl. Acad. Sci. USA* **2016**, *113*, 9983–9988. [CrossRef]
26. Beekers, I.; Vegter, M.; Lattwein, K.R.; Mastik, F.; Beurskens, R.; Van Der Steen, A.F.; De Jong, N.; Verweij, M.D.; Kooiman, K. Opening of endothelial cell–cell contacts due to sonoporation. *J. Control. Release* **2020**, *322*, 426–438. [CrossRef]
27. Helfield, B.; Chen, X.; Watkins, S.C.; Villanueva, F.S. Transendothelial Perforations and the Sphere of Influence of Single-Site Sonoporation. *Ultrasound Med. Biol.* **2020**, *46*, 1686–1697. [CrossRef]
28. Juffermans, L.J.; Van Dijk, A.; Jongenelen, C.A.; Drukarch, B.; Reijerkerk, A.; De Vries, H.E.; Kamp, O.; Musters, R.J. Ultrasound and Microbubble-Induced Intra- and Intercellular Bioeffects in Primary Endothelial Cells. *Ultrasound Med. Biol.* **2009**, *35*, 1917–1927. [CrossRef] [PubMed]
29. Thomas, D.; Radhakrishnan, P. Tumor-stromal crosstalk in pancreatic cancer and tissue fibrosis. *Mol. Cancer* **2019**, *18*, 1–15. [CrossRef]
30. Herrera, G.; Díaz, L.; Barberá-Guillem, E.; O'connor, J. E Novel hermetic cell culture containers (Petaka") and cytomic assays for testing sustained in vitro toxicity and general cell biological research. *Toxicol. Lett.* **2010**, *196*, S147. [CrossRef]
31. Carreau, A.; El Hafny-Rahbi, B.; Matejuk, A.; Grillon, C.; Kieda, C. Why is the partial oxygen pressure of human tissues a crucial parameter? Small molecules and hypoxia. *J. Cell. Mol. Med.* **2011**, *15*, 1239–1253. [CrossRef] [PubMed]
32. Yddal, T.; Cochran, S.; Gilja, O.H.; Postema, M.; Kotopoulis, S. Open-source, high-throughput ultrasound treatment chamber. *Biomed. Tech. Eng.* **2015**, *60*, 77–87. [CrossRef] [PubMed]
33. Zeghimi, A.; Eescoffre, J.-M.; Bouakaz, A. Role of endocytosis in sonoporation-mediated membrane permeabilization and uptake of small molecules: A electron microscopy study. *Phys. Biol.* **2015**, *12*, 066007. [CrossRef]
34. Abrahamsen, I.; Lorens, J.B. Evaluating Extracellular Matrix influence on adherent cell signaling by Cold Trypsin Phosphorylation-specific Flow Cytometry. *BMC Cell Biol.* **2013**, *14*, 36. [CrossRef]
35. Hellesøy, M.; Lorens, J.B. Cellular context–mediated Akt dynamics regulates MAP kinase signaling thresholds during angiogenesis. *Mol. Biol. Cell* **2015**, *26*, 2698–2711. [CrossRef]
36. Krutzik, P.O.; Nolan, G.P. Intracellular phospho-protein staining techniques for flow cytometry: Monitoring single cell signaling events. *Cytometry* **2003**, *55*, 61–70. [CrossRef]
37. Krutzik, P.; Nolan, G.P. Fluorescent cell barcoding in flow cytometry allows high-throughput drug screening and signaling profiling. *Nat. Methods* **2006**, *3*, 361–368. [CrossRef] [PubMed]

38. Whitney, N.P.; Lamb, A.C.; Louw, T.; Subramanian, A. Integrin-Mediated Mechanotransduction Pathway of Low-Intensity Continuous Ultrasound in Human Chondrocytes. *Ultrasound Med. Biol.* **2012**, *38*, 1734–1743. [CrossRef]
39. Sato, M.; Nagata, K.; Kuroda, S.; Horiuchi, S.; Nakamura, T.; Karima, M.; Inubushi, T.; Tanaka, E. Low-Intensity Pulsed Ultrasound Activates Integrin-Mediated Mechanotransduction Pathway in Synovial Cells. *Ann. Biomed. Eng.* **2014**, *42*, 2156–2163. [CrossRef] [PubMed]
40. Zhou, S.; Schmelz, A.; Seufferlein, T.; Li, Y.; Zhao, J.; Bachem, M.G. Molecular Mechanisms of Low Intensity Pulsed Ultrasound in Human Skin Fibroblasts. *J. Biol. Chem.* **2004**, *279*, 54463–54469. [CrossRef]
41. Zhong, W.; Chen, X.; Jiang, P.P.; Wan, J.M.; Qin, P.; Yu, A.C.H. Induction of Endoplasmic Reticulum Stress by Sonoporation: Linkage to Mitochondria-Mediated Apoptosis Initiation. *Ultrasound Med. Biol.* **2013**, *39*, 2382–2392. [CrossRef]
42. Ando, H.; Feril, L.B.; Kondo, T.; Tabuchi, Y.; Ogawa, R.; Zhao, Q.-L.; Cui, Z.-G.; Umemura, S.-I.; Yoshikawa, H.; Misaki, T. An echo-contrast agent, Levovist, lowers the ultrasound intensity required to induce apoptosis of human leukemia cells. *Cancer Lett.* **2006**, *242*, 37–45. [CrossRef]
43. Honda, H.; Kondo, T.; Zhao, Q.-L.; Feril, L.B.; Kitagawa, H. Role of intracellular calcium ions and reactive oxygen species in apoptosis induced by ultrasound. *Ultrasound Med. Biol.* **2004**, *30*, 683–692. [CrossRef]
44. Feril, L.B.; Kondo, T.; Cui, Z.-G.; Tabuchi, Y.; Zhao, Q.-L.; Ando, H.; Misaki, T.; Yoshikawa, H.; Umemura, S.-I. Apoptosis induced by the sonomechanical effects of low intensity pulsed ultrasound in a human leukemia cell line. *Cancer Lett.* **2005**, *221*, 145–152. [CrossRef] [PubMed]
45. Cabezas, S.; Ho, S.; Ros, U.; Lanio, M.E.; Álvarez, C.; Van Der Goot, F.G. Damage of eukaryotic cells by the pore-forming toxin sticholysin II: Consequences of the potassium efflux. *Biochim. Biophys. Acta (BBA) Biomembr.* **2017**, *1859*, 982–992. [CrossRef] [PubMed]
46. Guzmaán, H.R.; Nguyen, D.X.; Khan, S.; Prausnitz, M.R. Ultrasound-mediated disruption of cell membranes. I. Quantification of molecular uptake and cell viability. *J. Acoust. Soc. Am.* **2001**, *110*, 588–596. [CrossRef]
47. Guzman, H.R.; Nguyen, D.X.; Khan, S.; Prausnitz, M.R. Ultrasound-mediated disruption of cell membranes. II. Heterogeneous effects on cells. *J. Acoust. Soc. Am.* **2001**, *110*, 597–606. [CrossRef]
48. Guzmán, H.R.; McNamara, A.J.; Nguyen, D.X.; Prausnitz, M.R. Bioeffects caused by changes in acoustic cavitation bubble density and cell concentration: A unified explanation based on cell-to-bubble ratio and blast radius. *Ultrasound Med. Biol.* **2003**, *29*, 1211–1222. [CrossRef]
49. Kinoshita, M.; Hynynen, K. Key factors that affect sonoporation efficiency in in vitro settings: The importance of standing wave in sonoporation. *Biochem. Biophys. Res. Commun.* **2007**, *359*, 860–865. [CrossRef] [PubMed]
50. Lejbkowicz, F.; Salzberg, S. Distinct sensitivity of normal and malignant cells to ultrasound in vitro. *Environ. Health Perspect.* **1997**, *105*, 1575–1578. [CrossRef]
51. Trendowski, M.; Wong, V.; Zoino, J.N.; Christen, T.D.; Gadeberg, L.; Sansky, M.; Fondy, T.P. Preferential enlargement of leukemia cells using cytoskeletal-directed agents and cell cycle growth control parameters to induce sensitivity to low frequency ultrasound. *Cancer Lett.* **2015**, *360*, 160–170. [CrossRef]
52. Fan, P.; Zhang, Y.; Guo, X.; Cai, C.; Wang, M.; Yang, D.; Li, Y.; Tu, J.; Crum, L.A.; Wu, J.; et al. Cell-cycle-specific Cellular Responses to Sonoporation. *Theranostics* **2017**, *7*, 4894–4908. [CrossRef] [PubMed]
53. Porta, H.; Cancino-Rodezno, A.; Soberón, M.; Bravo, A. Role of MAPK p38 in the cellular responses to pore-forming toxins. *Peptides* **2011**, *32*, 601–606. [CrossRef]
54. Morotomi-Yano, K.; Akiyama, H.; Yano, K.-I. Nanosecond pulsed electric fields activate MAPK pathways in human cells. *Arch. Biochem. Biophys.* **2011**, *515*, 99–106. [CrossRef]
55. Morotomi-Yano, K.; Oyadomari, S.; Akiyama, H.; Yano, K.-I. Nanosecond pulsed electric fields act as a novel cellular stress that induces translational suppression accompanied by eIF2α phosphorylation and 4E-BP1 dephosphorylation. *Exp. Cell Res.* **2012**, *318*, 1733–1744. [CrossRef] [PubMed]
56. Yang, F.; Gu, N.; Chen, D.; Xi, X.; Zhang, D.; Li, Y.; Wu, J. Experimental study on cell self-sealing during sonoporation. *J. Control. Release* **2008**, *131*, 205–210. [CrossRef]
57. Lentacker, I.; De Cock, I.; Deckers, R.; De Smedt, S.; Moonen, C. Understanding ultrasound induced sonoporation: Definitions and underlying mechanisms. *Adv. Drug Deliv. Rev.* **2014**, *72*, 49–64. [CrossRef] [PubMed]
58. Wang, R.; Ganesan, S.; Zheng, X.F.S. Yin and yang of 4E-BP1 in cancer. *Cell Cycle* **2016**, *15*, 1401–1402. [CrossRef]

59. Qin, X.; Jiang, B.; Zhang, Y. 4E-BP1, a multifactor regulated multifunctional protein. *Cell Cycle* **2016**, *15*, 781–786. [CrossRef]
60. Preston, A.M.; Hendershot, L.M. Examination of a second node of translational control in the unfolded protein response. *J. Cell Sci.* **2013**, *126*, 4253–4261. [CrossRef]
61. Duluc, C.; Moatassim-Billah, S.; Chalabi-Dchar, M.; Perraud, A.; Samain, R.; Breibach, F.; Gayral, M.; Cordelier, P.; Delisle, M.-B.; Bousquet-Dubouch, M.-P.; et al. Pharmacological targeting of the protein synthesis mTOR/4E- BP 1 pathway in cancer-associated fibroblasts abrogates pancreatic tumour chemoresistance. *EMBO Mol. Med.* **2015**, *7*, 735–753. [CrossRef]
62. Roux, P.P.; Shahbazian, D.; Vu, H.; Holz, M.K.; Cohen, M.S.; Taunton, J.; Sonenberg, N.; Blenis, J. RAS/ERK Signaling Promotes Site-specific Ribosomal Protein S6 Phosphorylation via RSK and Stimulates Cap-dependent Translation. *J. Biol. Chem.* **2007**, *282*, 14056–14064. [CrossRef]
63. Snipstad, S.; Sulheim, E.; Davies, C.D.L.; Moonen, C.; Storm, G.; Kiessling, F.; Schmid, R.; Lammers, T. Sonopermeation to improve drug delivery to tumors: From fundamental understanding to clinical translation. *Expert Opin. Drug Deliv.* **2018**, *15*, 1249–1261. [CrossRef]

Publisher's Note: MDPI stays neutral with regard to jurisdictional claims in published maps and institutional affiliations.

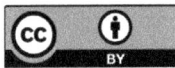

© 2020 by the authors. Licensee MDPI, Basel, Switzerland. This article is an open access article distributed under the terms and conditions of the Creative Commons Attribution (CC BY) license (http://creativecommons.org/licenses/by/4.0/).

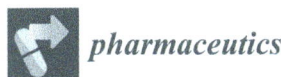

Review

Three-Dimensional Spheroids as In Vitro Preclinical Models for Cancer Research

Bárbara Pinto [1], Ana C. Henriques [1,2], Patrícia M. A. Silva [1] and Hassan Bousbaa [1,*]

[1] Cooperativa de Ensino Superior Politécnico e Universitário (CESPU), Instituto de Investigação e Formação Avançada em Ciências e Tecnologias da Saúde (IINFACTS), Instituto Universitário de Ciências da Saúde (IUCS), 4585-116 Gandra PRD, Portugal; barbara_fernandes_pinto@hotmail.com (B.P.); A24955@alunos.cespu.pt (A.C.H.); patricia.silva@cespu.pt (P.M.A.S.)
[2] Instituto Nacional de Engenharia Biomédica (INEB), Universidade do Porto, 4099-002 Porto, Portugal
* Correspondence: hassan.bousbaa@iucs.cespu.pt; Tel.: +351-224-157-186; Fax: +351-224-157-102

Received: 16 October 2020; Accepted: 4 December 2020; Published: 6 December 2020

Abstract: Most cancer biologists still rely on conventional two-dimensional (2D) monolayer culture techniques to test in vitro anti-tumor drugs prior to in vivo testing. However, the vast majority of promising preclinical drugs have no or weak efficacy in real patients with tumors, thereby delaying the discovery of successful therapeutics. This is because 2D culture lacks cell–cell contacts and natural tumor microenvironment, important in tumor signaling and drug response, thereby resulting in a reduced malignant phenotype compared to the real tumor. In this sense, three-dimensional (3D) cultures of cancer cells that better recapitulate in vivo cell environments emerged as scientifically accurate and low cost cancer models for preclinical screening and testing of new drug candidates before moving to expensive and time-consuming animal models. Here, we provide a comprehensive overview of 3D tumor systems and highlight the strategies for spheroid construction and evaluation tools of targeted therapies, focusing on their applicability in cancer research. Examples of the applicability of 3D culture for the evaluation of the therapeutic efficacy of nanomedicines are discussed.

Keywords: 3D cultures; tumor microenvironment; tumor spheroids; efficacy analysis; drug resistance; cancer therapy

---

1. Introduction

Significant investments are made in cancer research for drug discovery and development. Yet, the approval rate (≤5%) of drugs that reach the clinic remains very low [1,2]. Typically, anticancer compounds are tested in two dimensional (2D) cell culture models, that involve a panel of cancer cell lines, such as those used by the US National Cancer Institute [3]. Drugs that show promising cytotoxicity in 2D in vitro system progress to animal models of human cancers (mainly mice) for anti-tumor efficacy testing [4]. Unfortunately, most of the promising preclinical drugs have no or weak efficacy in real patients with tumors, resulting in a significant delay of anticancer drug development [5]. One of the main factors underlying this poor success is the inadequacy of the preclinical 2D cultures and animal models to recapitulate the human tumor microenvironment (TME). TME is a complex and heterogeneous structure made of cellular (e.g., transformed epithelial cells, fibroblasts, infiltrating lymphocytes, mesenchymal stem cells, endothelial cells) and non-cellular (e.g., extracellular matrix—ECM, growth factors, cytokines and chemokines) components, with a critical role in cancer development and progression [6,7]. The 2D culture systems lack the structural architecture and the microenvironment of the tumor, and display altered gene expression and activation of cell signaling pathways, compared to the in vivo tumor tissues (Table 1) [8–10]. Besides the associated higher cost and ethical issues, animal models also display significant limitations and poorly reflect the proprieties of human tumors. For instance, the stromal component of the xenograft is not of human origin, the rate of growth is higher in xenografts (doubling time of a few days) than in primary human tumors (doubling time of a few months), and, thus, they often tend to respond better to anticancer drugs [11].

Table 1. Differences between conventional 2D monolayer and 3D spheroid cultures.

Cell Culture System	Advantages	Disadvantages
2D cultures	<ul><li>Fast replication;</li><li>Low cost;</li><li>Easy to manipulate;</li><li>Establish long-term cultures.</li></ul>	<ul><li>Homogeneity in oxygen and nutrients perfusion;</li><li>Decreased cell–cell and cell–ECM interactions;</li><li>More susceptible to pharmacological action;</li><li>Poor cell differentiation;</li><li>Faster proliferation than in vivo tumors.</li><li>Modified genetic profile when compared to in vivo tissue.</li></ul>
3D cultures	<ul><li>Heterogeneity in oxygen and nutrients perfusion;</li><li>3 different layers (proliferation, quiescence and necrosis zones) resembling the in vivo tumors;</li><li>Increased cell–cell and cell–ECM interactions;</li><li>Mimic drug penetration in the tumor.</li><li>Recapitulate the genetic in vivo profile.</li></ul>	<ul><li>High cost;</li><li>Greater difficulty in carrying out methodological techniques.</li></ul>

Therefore, the development of preclinical models that better recapitulate patient tumor and microenvironment represents a promising challenge to improve the success rates in anticancer drug development. Since the discovery of the importance of the extracellular matrix (ECM) in cell behavior, it became clear that three-dimensional (3D) cell culture systems offer an excellent opportunity to recapitulate the real avascular tumor, by allowing cancer cells to be cultured, either alone or in co-culture with other cell types, in a spatial manner reminiscent of the structural architecture of the tumor that provides cell–cell and cell–ECM interactions, thereby mimicking the native tumor microenvironment (Table 1) [12–15]. Hopefully, besides circumventing the barriers and limitations imposed by 2D monolayer cultures, 3D cell culture models could reduce or, ideally, replace the use of animal models, thereby resolving the associated ethical and cost issues [16,17]. Here, common 3D cell culture methods are highlighted, the characterization tools for the evaluation of the targeted effect are reviewed, with focus on multicellular tumor spheroids (MCTS) and their applicability in cancer research.

2. Tumor Microenvironment as Pathophysiologic Barrier to Anticancer Therapy

The TME comprises the heterogeneous population of malignant cells, the ECM, and various tumor-associated cells such as cancer-associated fibroblasts (CAF), endothelial cells, adipocytes, and immune cells (Figure 1). Tumor-associated macrophages (TAMs) are monocyte-derived macrophages that can be categorized as inflammatory M1 macrophages, with roles in phagocytosis and cell killing, and immunosuppressive M2 macrophages, with roles in tissue repair [18]. The TME, mainly through hypoxia and secreted cytokines, promotes the M2 phenotype which favors, amongst others, tissue repair and tumor invasion and progression [19,20]. TAMs can constitute up to 50% of the tumor mass, and are associated with poor prognosis in many cancer types. CAFs are also a major component of the TME, characterized by a high interaction with tumor cells and the TME. In this context, CAFs contribute to tumor cell invasion, as well as to changes in tumor growth and immune microenvironment, through ECM remodeling and production of soluble factors [21,22].

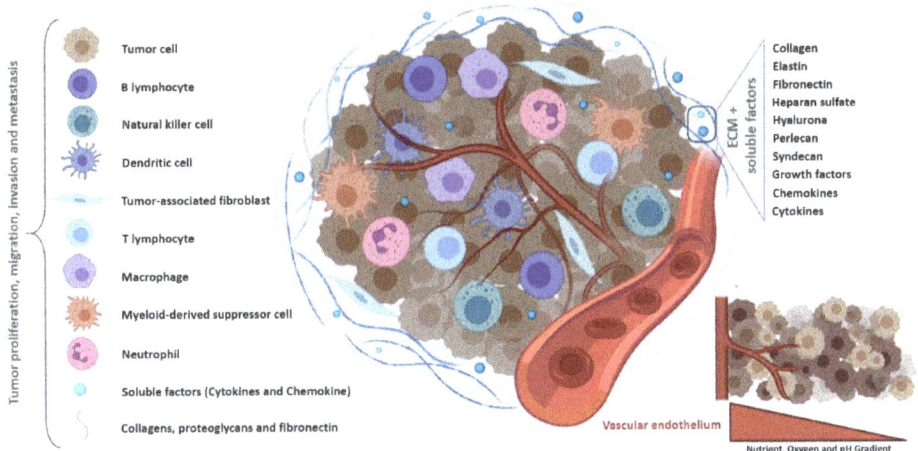

Figure 1. Schematic representation of the tumor microenvironment. The tumor ecosystem consists of a heterogeneous population formed by cancer and infiltrating immune cells, including tumor-associated fibroblasts, myeloid-derived suppressor cells and immune cells. The cross-talk between all these tumor microenvironment components play an essential role in tumor growth, development and metastasis, under hostile conditions. Soluble factors are constantly produced, triggering immunosuppressive responses and tumor survival. Created with BioRender.com.

The ECM provides structural support for cells in the extracellular space, and is composed of structural fibrous proteins (e.g., collagens and elastin), multiadhesive proteins (e.g., fibronectin and laminin), glycosaminoglycans (e.g., heparan sulfate, hyaluronan), proteoglycans (e.g., perlecan, syndecan), and sequestered growth factors, as well as secreted proteins [23–25]. The cross-talk between the different TME cells and components plays an essential role in tumor growth, progression and metastasis [26].

Many factors present in the TME, including transforming growth factor beta (TGF-β), cytokines (IL-10 and IL-1β), members of the VEGF, plateled-derived growth factor (PDGF), FGF, angiopoietin families, Bv8/PROK2, and hypoxia-inducible factor (HIF)-1α, provide molecular support to tumor growth and progression [27–30]. Additionally, cancer cells are experts in modifying their surrounding environments. For instance, cancer cells can co-opt fibroblasts to obtain growth factors, such as basic fibroblast growth factor (bFGF), necessary to sustain their growth and proliferation. additionally, tumor cells can interact with the surrounding endothelial cells, promoting the release of soluble factors, like vascular endothelial growth factor (VEGF), to trigger the angiogenic process. Tumor cells can also evade the immune-mediated cellular destruction through different strategies. For instance, loss of tumor antigen expression precludes their recognition by the immune system, production of immunosuppressive cytokines protects them from the cytotoxic lysis by immune cells, and development of immunosuppressive forces leads to local immunosuppression in the TME that shifts the phenotype and function of normal immune cells from an anti-tumor state to a pro-tumor state [31–36].

Currently, treatment options against cancer include surgery, chemotherapy, radiation therapy, hormonal therapy, and targeted therapy [37]. Basically, anticancer therapies aim to target tumor cells either directly, through DNA damage by cytotoxic drugs or local radiation causing apoptosis, or indirectly, through the destruction of TME so as to deprive cancer cells of the machinery that fuel their growth and progression. However, these therapies induce new biological tumor responses, mainly through immunological and angiogenic modulation, contributing to drug resistance, which remains a serious consequence of most anticancer treatments, impacting the patient's prognosis and quality of life [31,38].

The TME imposes many biological barriers that greatly hinder drug delivery to tumors [39,40]. These barriers include malformed vasculature, rigid extracellular matrix, hypoxia, acidic pH, abnormal enzyme level, altered metabolism pathway, and immunosuppressive environment. Uncontrolled cell growth and proliferation result in insufficient blood supply to cancer cells in the inner core and in the intermediate layer of the tumor mass, causing cellular hypoxia [39]. Hypoxia, one of the hallmarks of cancer, plays a fundamental role in tumor development and malignancy. This condition is able to modify the tumor endothelial cells morphology, reducing oxygen diffusion to cancer tissue [41]. While hypoxia is harmful to non-tumor cells, unfortunately, cancer cells readily switch from oxidative phosphorylation to aerobic glycolysis, a condition known as Warburg effect, orchestrated by the transcription factor HIF-1α through which cancer cells acquire many malignant properties [42,43]. Moreover, the tumor vessels exhibit a disordered structure, which leads to a decrease in the blood perfusion homogeneity [44]. This tumor vascular deficiency makes difficult drug distribution to all cancer cells, impacting therapy effectiveness [43]. TME pH also contributes to anticancer drug resistance. The increase in anaerobic metabolism leads to greater lactic acid production, reducing the extracellular pH, that ranges from 6.2 to 7.2 [45]. As pH levels decrease, metalloproteinases become activated, destroying cell interactions which facilitates tumor migration and invasion [46]. Acidic microenvironment causes the "ion trapping" phenomenon, process in which basic anticancer drugs are transformed into a cation substance, reducing their transmembrane permeability and, consequently, their effectiveness [47]. Immune cells such as macrophages, neutrophils, mast cells, myeloid-derived suppressor cells, and natural killer cells, secret many soluble factors that promote immunosuppression, angiogenesis, chronic inflammation, and drug resistance [43,48–50]. Additionally, the mechanisms associated with immune escape during tumor progression can promote resistance to anticancer drugs [31,43]. Tumor cells themselves can alter the organization and protein deposition of the ECM, forming a physical barrier that prevents drug penetration into tumor cells [51,52].

Therefore, new therapeutic strategies have been developed to target the tumor-promoting microenvironmental factors in a goal to block the interaction between tumor cells and the TME [53]. Such strategies include, for example, inhibition of the extracellular ligand-receptor interactions and downstream pathways, re-programming the immune response, and co-targeting of tumor cells and the microenvironment [43].

As outlined above, the tumors and their microenvironment provide multiple biological barriers against drug penetration, accumulation, and efficacy, leading to tumor resistance to therapy [54]. Thus, discovery and delivery testing of new anticancer drug candidates require preclinical models that are more physiological than conventional 2D cultures, capable of recapitulating these TME barriers. In this sense, the spheroids provide the appropriate model of the pathophysiologic parameters present in the real tumor, because they recapitulate the complex multicellular architecture, the barriers to mass transport, and extracellular matrix deposition, which explain their growing use as models for better prediction of drug effects and delivery in the last decades [55].

3. Common Characteristics of Spheroids and Tumors

Various cancer cells can spontaneously assemble into spheroids in culture environment that privileges cell–cell and cell–ECM interactions over cell–substrate interactions [14]. These predominant cell–cell and cell–ECM interactions result in the formation of a 3D structure that closely reproduces mimics the native spatial organization and environment of avascular tumors, where cells can proliferate, aggregate and differentiate (Figure 2) [56]. Common methods for spheroid generation are described in the next section. Spheroids have a diameter of 200 micrometers or more, generally with a spherical shape, and display three concentric zones of heterogeneous cell populations: an external zone of highly proliferating and migrating cells; a middle zone of quiescent cells, and an internal zone of necrotic cells [57,58]. These cell layers are so defined due to the nutrients and oxygen gradients that are established, as a result of limited diffusion, from the outside to the center of the spheroids. Thus, cells of the peripheral layer of the spheroids are exposed to sufficient oxygen and growth factors from the medium, which stimulate their proliferation. At the middle layer, limited diffusion of growth factors forces cell entry into quiescent state of the cell cycle. In large spheroids (>500 micrometers), oxygen deficiency (hypoxia) in the innermost zone induces altered gene expression, through stabilization of the transcription factor HIF-1α, and, consequently, triggers the Warburg effect, promoting aerobic glycolysis and lactic acid production, thereby lowering pH of the inner layer of spheroids [59]. Nutrient and oxygen deprivation, together with the accumulation of metabolic waste, triggers the necrotic death of cells at the innermost layer.

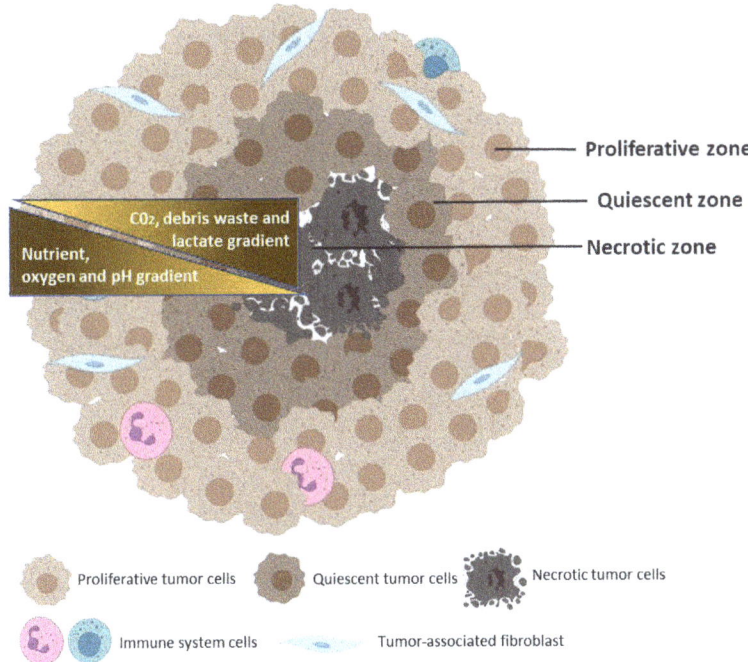

Figure 2. Typical structure of a multicellular tumor spheroid. The geometric rearrangement of the cells within the spheroid forms three concentric zones of heterogeneous cell populations: an external proliferating zone (Proliferative zone); a middle zone of quiescent cells (Quiescent zone), and an internal zone of necrotic cells (Necrotic zone). These cell layers are caused by the gradients of nutrients, oxygen, and pH (yellow), from the outside to the center of the spheroid, and by the gradients of CO_2, waste, and lactate, from the center to the outside. Created with BioRender.com.

Therefore, 3D culture systems recapitulate many characteristics of in vivo tumors, such as cell–cell and cell–ECM interactions, nutrient and oxygen gradients, and distinct layers of cell populations. Besides, the morphology and polarity of the cells, as well as gene expression and activation of cell signaling pathways, are also close to those of real tumors [8,9,60,61]. These features make spheroids a promising model for the study of cancer biology, cancer initiation, invasion and metastatic processes, as well as drug testing.

4. Methods for Spheroid Generation

Cells grown in culture environment of low binding or absence of adhesive surface can assemble into 3D spheroids, as these conditions favor cell–cell and cell–ECM interactions over cell–substrate interactions. Spheroids can be obtained after 1 to 7 days of culture, with various morphologies, depending on the cell line and the approach used. Examples of studies that performed spheroid generation techniques are shown in Table 2, providing information on cell lines, density and the time required to obtain the spheroids. According to the literature, spheroids of 300–500 µm of size are those that best mimic in vivo tumors in terms of hypoxia and proliferation gradients. Typically, spheroids are constructed from tumor cells, using scaffold-free or scaffold-based techniques [62].

4.1. Scaffold-Free Techniques

In scaffold-free techniques, different factors (e.g., low-adhesion substrates, gravity force and magnetic action) contribute to cellular aggregate formation and spheroid generation. During this process, the ECM is originated through continuous deposit of proteins produced by spheroid cells [63]. The most common scaffold-free techniques currently used are ultra-low attachment plates, hanging drop, magnetic levitation and magnetic 3D printing. The advantages and disadvantages of each method are summarized in Table 3.

4.1.1. Ultra-Low Attachment Plates

The surfaces of the plates are coated with a substrate to prevent cell adhesion, promoting cell aggregation and spheroid formation. Besides presenting low adhesion, the wells of these plates have a defined shape (round bottom, V-shaped or conical), allowing the positioning of a single spheroid [64,65]. Generally, the main substrates used to coat the plate are agar/agarose or poly(2-hydroxyethyl methacrylate), by adding 50 µL of solution in each well of 96-well plates, at concentrations of 15 mg/mL and 5 mg/mL, respectively [66–68]. With this technique, a large number of spheroids can be generated simultaneously on the same plate, facilitating experimental reproducibility, in addition to enable the monitoring of spheroid formation and growth. As disadvantages, some tumor cell lines do not form tight spheroids in ultra-low attachment plates [69].

4.1.2. Hanging Drop

In this method, approximately 25 µL of cell suspension is positioned inside of a petri dish lid, which contains phosphate-buffered saline (PBS) to avoid dehydration of the cellular solution. Then, the lid is inverted and due to surface tension, the droplets remain suspended. Owing to the force of gravity, the cells within the droplets spontaneously form cellular aggregates, giving rise to a single spheroid [70,71]. This method allows large production of spheroids and an easy control of their size. However, it is labor intensive due to its multistep process, and there is a risk of cell damage in case of media evaporation, requiring constant monitoring of the culture medium [71–74]. Moreover, the hanging drop method can originate spheroids with heterogeneous sizes and morphologies, impacting the spheroid standardization, which is essential for new drug screening. Recently, studies have developed different tools to minimize these limitations and facilitated the realization of this method [75–77]. For instance, the pressure-assisted network for droplet accumulation (PANDA) system consists of a pressure chip capable to create homogeneous and compact hanging drop array, enabling the fast and economical production of spheroids [75]. Another way to circumvent these barriers is through the use of 3D printed hanging-drop dripper array that allows in situ analysis of drug screening, tumor metastasis and tumor transendothelial migration, besides promoting heterotypic spheroid interaction [77].

4.1.3. Magnetic Levitation and Magnetic 3D Printing

Through a mixture of magnetic particles/nanoparticles, the cells are magnetized and incubated under magnetic forces to overcome the gravitational force, allowing their levitation and, consequently, formation of cellular aggregate [78]. In this method, after the cells absorb the magnetic particles, a magnet is positioned above (magnetic levitation) or below (magnetic 3D printing) the plate, promoting cells aggregation and spheroid generation [70]. Spheroids are usually formed in less than 16 h, being considered a fast-acting technique [72]. However, prior preparation of magnetic nanoparticles is necessary, and limited number of spheroids are generated [78].

4.2. Scaffold-Based Techniques

In scaffold-based techniques, external cell anchoring systems are used to mimic the ECM structure, allowing greater cell–cell and cell–matrix interaction. These systems can consist of porous microcarriers of natural, synthetic, and semisynthetic hydrogels made of cross-linked polymers. Porous scaffolds are widely used in the bioengineering sector, and have gained prominence in 3D cell culture implementation [63,72,79]. Due to their interconnected pores, these structures allow greater diffusion of nutrients, oxygen and metabolic debris, in addition to mimicking the ECM architecture, providing cellular support, attachment and proliferation [80–82]. 3D porous scaffolds also promote the formation of bigger spheroids, compared to non-porous scaffolds, and enhance tumor cell invasion and therapeutic resistance [83,84]. Although they are synthesized mainly by polymers such as poly(ε-caprolactone), porous microparticles can consist of different substances, including natural (e.g., chitosan, hyaluronic acid, alginate, collagen, gelatin, silk fibroin), and synthetic (e.g., poly(lactide-co-glycolide)) materials [85–90]. The porosity and pore size of the scaffold are essential for the establishment of effective 3D models, as they can affect the transport of oxygen, metabolites and nutrients, as well as cell adhesion and cell growth [91]. While porous 3D scaffold methods are useful to control the spheroid size, effective collecting and separation of spheroids from 3D scaffolds may be difficult [92]. Common scaffold-based methodologies include spinner flasks, micropatterned plates, matrix encapsulation, matrix on top, matrix embedded, microcarriers beads, and microfluidic devices.

4.2.1. Spinner Flasks

Continuous rotating agitation inhibits cell adhesion to the surface, leading to spheroid formation. The main means of rotation used are through spinner flasks and rotating flasks. In spinner flasks, a magnetic stirrer is positioned inside the flask, allowing homogeneous distribution of oxygen and nutrients. However, the cells are subjected to direct shearing force, which increases the risk of their damage. In the rotating flasks, the flask itself is rotated, allowing the dispersion of oxygen and nutrients, and the reduction of the shear forces on the cells [70]. As an advantage, this method allows large scale generation of spheroids. However, the continuous rotation prevents the visualization of the aggregates, can damage the cells, and is hard to monitor [71]. Yet, this method is considered as one of the most efficient systems for obtaining large amounts of spheroids under controlled nutritional conditions [72].

4.2.2. Micropatterned Plates

The plates are modified to create micrometer sized compartments with a low adhesion surface within each microspace, providing a micropattern or microwells which induce cells to grow as clusters. First, a layer of 3-trimethoxysilyl polymethacrylate is added to the glass plate, to ensure fixation of the hydrogel microwells to the plate, followed by a uniform layer of hydrogel. Soon after, using photolithography techniques, polydimethylsiloxane is added to the hydrogel for microwell formation [70]. The cell suspension is then seeded into hydrogel microwells, which can vary in size from 150–600 µm [93]. This method allows large scale production of spheroids. However, bubbles often form during the culture, and pipetting can damage micropatterned surfaces due to pipetting [64].

4.2.3. Matrix Encapsulation

Suspended cells are surrounded by hydrogel and placed in calcium free solution, forming cellular microcapsules. In these microcapsules, cells aggregate to form matrix encapsulated spheroids [70]. Generally, microcapsules have a size between 100 and 500 µm, are capable of generating monotypic or heterotypic spheroids, and allow cell–cell and cell–ECM interaction [94]. In these systems, the transport of nutrients and metabolic residues occurs by simple diffusion and, as the microcapsule increases, the nutrient transport becomes limited, which can cause cellular necrosis. Due to their viscoelastic capabilities, alginate hydrogels has been widely used to generate microcapsules [95]. An important advantage is that this method yields homogeneous sized spheroids.

4.2.4. Matrix on Top and Matrix Embedded

The matrix on top and matrix embedded methods are quite similar. In the matrix-on-top method, the cells are seeded and trapped on the top of the solid matrix, and spheroids are formed through cellular aggregation. In the matrix embedded method, cells suspended in the liquefied matrix are only incorporated into the matrix after the gelation process [70]. Several compounds have been used as a matrix, including agarose, matrigel, collagen, and synthetic polymers [96]. Matrix-on-top method facilitates post-culture processing and imaging of the generated spheroids.

4.2.5. Microcarrier Beads

This system has been used for more than 25 years for to generate 3D cell culture [97]. In this method, cells adhere to natural (e.g., collagen, cellulose) or synthetic (e.g., dextran, poly(D,L-lactide-co-glycolide)) matrix-coated beads, forming spheroidal structures [98,99]. The microcarrier beads provide a cell attachment surface, allowing the aggregation, especially of cells unable to aggregate spontaneously. This method is considered a fast, easy, and reproducible spheroid generation system, and allows the adhesion of different cell types to form heterogeneous spheroids. However, the presence of microcarrier beads in spheroids does not mimic the tumor physiological conditions in vivo [100].

4.2.6. Microfluidic Devices

The cells are placed in microchannels with a free perfusion system, allowing the distribution of oxygen and nutrients, and the elimination of metabolic waste. As an advantage, this system can mimic tumor microvasculature in vivo. However, this method requires specialized laboratories and equipment [101–103]. Due to its ability to guarantee gases permeability, polydimethylsiloxane (PDMS) is the most used material for making microfluidic devices [104]. In addition, PDMS are biocompatible, easy to make, and are low cost. However, under high pressure, PDMS microchannels can be deformed, causing changes in fluid speeds. Depending on the type of sealing, reversible or irreversible, the PDMS microfluidic devices can withstand pressure up to 0.3 or 2 bar, respectively. Moreover, when exposed to some fluids, PDMS microfluidic can swell, which impacts in device function [105–107]. Other microfluidic device polymers, such as thermoset polyester, polyurethane methacrylate and Norland Adhesive 81, also undergo structural changes when exposed to pressures above 10, 8 and 5 bar, respectively [108].

Table 2. Examples of tumors and respective cell lines, densities and time required for 3D cell culture formation by different spheroid generation methods.

Spheroid Techniques	Spheroid Generation Methods	Tumor/Cell Lines	Cell Seeding Densities	Period to Spheroid Formation/Observations	References
Scaffold-free techniques	1. Ultra-low attachment plates	• Head and neck squamous cell carcinoma lines (HNSCC): Cal27, Cal33, FaDu, UM-22B, BICR56, OSC-19, PCI-13, PCI52, Detroit-562, UM-SCC-1, and SCC-9.	• 625, 1250, 2500, 5×10^3, 1×10^4, or 2×10^4 cells/well.	• Although some HNSCC cell lines formed MCTSs within 24 h of seeding into 384-well ULA-plates, others required 2–3 days to self-assemble.	[109]
		• HNSCC cell lines: Cal33 and FaDu.	• 5×10^3 cells/well.	• Typically, the spheroids were formed 24 h after seeding.	[110]
		• Hepatocellular carcinoma cells: Huh-7; Hpatic stellate cells: LX-2.	• Monospheroids: 750 cells/well of Huh-7 or 2250 cells/well of LX-2; Mixed-cell spheroids: Huh-7 and LX-2 cells/well at a 1:3 ratio (750:2250).	• Spheroids were formed on day 1.	[111]
		• Human bone marrow mesenchymal stem cells (hBM-MSCs).	• 1.4×10^4, 3.5×10^4, 1.4×10^4, and 3.5×10^4 cells/well.	• Spheroids were observed 1 day after seeding; • 96-well plates were pre-coated with 20 mg/mL of poly(2-hydroxyethyl methacrylate).	[112]
	2. Hanging drop	• Human hepatoma cell line: HepG2.	• 1×10^4, 2×10^4, 4×10^4 and 5×10^4 cells/well.	• Spheroid formation was observed 1 day after seeding.	[113]
		• Human bone marrow mesenchymal stem cells (hBM-MSCs).	• 1×10^4, 2.5×10^4, 1×10^5, 2.5×10^5 cells/droplet.	• Spheroid formation was observed 1 day after seeding.	[112]

Table 2. *Cont.*

Spheroid Techniques	Spheroid Generation Methods	Tumor/Cell Lines	Cell Seeding Densities	Period to Spheroid Formation/Observations	References
Scaffold-based techniques		• Non-tumorigenic mammary cells: MCF10A; breast cancer cells: MDA-MB-231; and co-culture with MCF10A and mesenchymal stem/stromal cells (MSC).	• MCF10A (3000 cells/droplet); MDA-MB-231(2000 cells/droplet); co-culture with MCF10A and MSC (cells were seeded at 1:1 with 2000 total cells/droplet).	• Spheroid formation was observed 1 day after seeding.	[114]
		• Murine colon carcinoma: CT26.	• 5000 cells/droplet.	• Spheroid formation was observed 1 day after seeding.	[115]
		• Human breast cancer cell line: MCF-7.	• 1000 cells/well.	• Singular and concentrated 3D spheroids were observed 1 day after seeding; • Cells suspended in a diethylenetriaminepentaacetic acid gadolinium (III) dihydrogen salt hydrate (Gd-DTPA) medium.	[116]
	3. Magnetic levitation and Magnetic 3D printing	• Murine colon carcinoma: CT26 and human glioblastoma cells: U-87 MG.	• 1×10^6 cells/µL/mold.	• Spheroid formation was observed 1 day after seeding; • Magnetic spheroids of sizes of 0.4, 0.5, 1, and 1.6 mm were used.	[115]
		• Human pancreatic β-cell line (EndoC5H3) and human umbilical vein endothelial cells (HUVECs).	• 5000 cells/50 mL in corresponding cell culture media per well; • Cell ratio: 5000 cells to 5000 HUVECs.	• The exact beginning of spheroid formation was not described; spheroid formation was observed from day 5; β-cells and HUVECs were previously treated with NanoShuttle™-PL at a concentration of 40 µL/mL in media culture.	[117]
		• Mesenchymal stem cells (MSCs).	• 1×10^4 cells/well (before incubation with magnetic nanoparticles.	• Spheroid formation was observed 1 day after seeding.	[118]

Table 2. *Cont.*

Spheroid Techniques	Spheroid Generation Methods	Tumor/Cell Lines	Cell Seeding Densities	Period to Spheroid Formation/Observations	References
	4. Spinner flasks	• Human hepatoma cell line: SK-Hep-1.	• 1×10^6 cells were inoculated into a siliconized Cellspin flask containing 250 mL of growth medium.	• Cell aggregation was observed between 24–48 h after cell seeding. Spheroids were formed from 7–10 days, being well defined on day 10.	[119]
		• Human adenocarcinoma cells: HT29.	• 5×10^4 HT29 cells per 75 cm2 flask; • Aggregates were transferred to 250 mL spinner flasks containing 150 mL of culture medium.	• Cell aggregation was observed from day 3 and spheroids were observed in day 15.	[120]
	5. Micropatterned plates	• Sprague Dawley rats' hepatocytes and MSC.	• 4×10^5 cells/well.	• Spheroids formed gradually within 2 days.	[121]
		• Mouse colon carcinoma cells: CT26.	• 3×10^6 cells/mL.	• The exact beginning of spheroid formation was not described; spheroid formation was observed from day 5.	[122]
	6. Matrix encapsulation	• Human umbilical vein endothelial cells (HUVECs) and mesenchymal stem cells (MSCs).	• 6×10^5 cells/mL. (75% MSCs and 25% HUVECs).	• Spheroid formation was observed 1 day after seeding.	[123]
		• Neuroblastoma cells: SK-N-BE(2); lung cancer cells: H460; and glioblastoma cells: U87vIII.	• 4750 cells/ droplet.	• Spheroids began to form 1 day after seeding.	[124]
	7. Matrix-on top and Matrix embedded	• Human adenocarcinoma cell line derived from a metastatic site: MDA-MB 231 and murine Abelson leukemia transformed macrophage/monocyte line: RAW 264.7.	• 500 to 5000 of RAW 264.7 cells with 10,000 of MDA-MB 231 cells.	• Spheroids began to form 1 day after seeding.	[125]

Table 2. Cont.

Spheroid Techniques	Spheroid Generation Methods	Tumor/Cell Lines	Cell Seeding Densities	Period to Spheroid Formation/Observations	References
	8. Microcarriers beads	• Human hepatocarcinoma cell line: BEL7402.	• 1×10^4 cells/well.	• The exact beginning of spheroid formation was not described; on day 4 spheroids were already formed; • It was added 200 microcarrier beads/well (Cytodex-3); • The plate was coated with 10% poly(2-hydroxyethyl methacrylate).	[126]
		• Human melanoma cell line: BLM.	• 5×10^5 cells.	• Spheroid formation was described on the first day.	[127]
	9. Microfluidic devices	• Human cancer cell lines derived from ovarian solid tumor (TOV112D) or ascites (OV90).	• 12,000 cells/mL.	• The exact beginning of spheroid formation was not described; spheroid formation was observed from day 3; • Cell were seeded in single inlet multi-size spheroid synthesis (SIMSS) chips.	[128]
		• Human colorectal cancer cell line: HT-29, and human normal fibroblast cell line: CCD-18Co.	• 5×10^6/mL of HT-29 and 3×10^6/mL of CCD-18Co.	• Spheroid formation was observed 1 day after seeding; • Microfluidic chips were made using PDMS.	[129]

Table 3. Advantages and disadvantages of the main methods used for spheroid generation.

Spheroid Techniques	Spheroids Generation Methods	Advantages	Disadvantages	References
Scaffold-free techniques	1. Ultra-low attachment plates	• Large-scale spheroid production; • Inexpensive; • Easy handling.	• Difficulty in forming tight spheroids in some cell lines.	[64,65,71,72,130,131]
	2. Hanging drop	• Production of up to 384 spheroids in a single trial; • Control of cell composition and spheroid size; • No specialized equipment or reagents required.	• Difficulty in tracking spheroid formation; • It is not practical to add compounds and/or change the culture medium; • Risk of droplet dehydration; • Intense work/time for spheroid formation; • Difficulty in scale-up.	[70–74,114,132,133]
	3. Magnetic levitation (a) and Magnetic 3D printing (b)	• Easy development of heterotypic spheroids; • Fast spheroid formation.	• Require the preparation of magnetic particles; • Limited spheroid formation.	[70,72,78,134]

Table 3. *Cont.*

Spheroid Techniques	Spheroids Generation Methods	Advantages	Disadvantages	References
	4. Spinner (top) and rotating (bottom) flasks	• Large-scale spheroid production.	• Slow agitation speed generates cell dispersion; • High agitation speed generates shear force, damaging the cells; • Constant agitation prevents cell visualization; • Formation of spheroids with heterogeneous diameters; • Requires specialized equipment.	[70–72,135,136]
Scaffold-based techniques	5. Micropatterned plates	• Large-scale spheroid production; • Few well-to-well and plate-to-plate variation.	• Formation of spheroids with heterogeneous diameters; • Bubble formation during the culture; • Pipetting can damage micropattern surfaces.	[64,70,93,137,138]
	6. Matrix encapsulation	• Enables cell–cell and cell–ECM interaction.	• High risk of necrosis due to cell confinement.	[70,94,95,122]

Table 3. *Cont.*

Spheroid Techniques	Spheroids Generation Methods	Advantages	Disadvantages	References
	7. Matrix-on top and Matrix embedded	• No specialized equipment required; • Ease of obtaining spheroid images.	• Requires prior preparation and specialized matrix handling.	[70,96,124,139]
	8. Microcarrier beads	• Fast, easy and reproducible method; • Can form heterotypic spheroids.	• Does not resemble the physiological tumor conditions in vivo.	[97–100]
	9. Microfluidic devices	• Mimic tumor vasculature.	• Specialized equipment required; • PDMS devices can change the flow speed when under high pressure; • PDMS microfluidic can swell when exposed to some fluids; • Require trained users.	[101,102,104–106]

5. Tools to Evaluate Targeting Effect

Several techniques are available to characterize spheroids, either in viable, fixed, or dissociated state, before and after anticancer drug treatment. These techniques were described in details in a number of excellent review papers [63,140,141], and allow the characterization of the organization, size, shape, gene and protein expression, metabolic status, migration and invasion of anticancer drug-treated spheroids. In general, standard biological assays used for 2D culture can be applied to spheroids, with some drawbacks as outlined below (Table 4).

5.1. Optical Microscopy

Morphologic changes such as size and shape can be monitored over time by optical microscopy and analyzed by appropriate software [142,143]. For instance, with a standard phase-contrast microscope, the difference in the size or volume between treated and untreated spheroids at a defined endpoint, or even during treatment, can be used to evaluate the efficacy of an anticancer drug.

Fluorescence microscopy can provide information on ECM deposition in spheroids immunostained with antibodies against fibronectin, laminin, and collagen IV [144], while relevant information such as cytoskeletal arrangement, proliferation, and apoptosis in the spheroids can be obtained by Hoechst or DAPI, phalloidin, Ki-67, caspases, Annexin V, Propidium iodide, and TUNEL staining [63,145]. Confocal laser microscopy is required to obtain higher spatial resolution, needed to analyze spheroid architecture. However, this analysis is restricted to small spheroids due to limited light penetration and to light scattering in thick tissues [143].

To overcome these issues, spheroids can be processed for histological sectioning. Then, staining methods such as hematoxylin and eosin staining allow distinction of pyknotic nuclei and eosinophilic cytoplasm in spheroid sections. For proliferating and quiescent cell populations, the use of specific antibodies in immunohistological staining is required. However, spheroid fixation used in the histological procedure precludes the study of dynamic alterations in the spheroids over time. Additionally, sample fracture and morphology deformation can occur during spheroid sectioning. Due to the delicate nature and small size of spheroids, the fixation time may need to be reduced, comparatively to biopsies or organ fragments. Further spheroid processing has also presented some challenges. For example, the inclusion of several spheroids in a unique paraffin block may involve a more arduous and costly sectioning process, since the spheroids will localize in different section planes. The development of microwell-containing apparatuses facilitated this process, allowing the simultaneous analysis of multiple spheroids in a more organized and cheaper manner [146].

To overcome these drawbacks of spheroid fixation and sectioning, faster and noninvasive microscopy approaches have been developed in the last years to image the innermost layer of live and fixed spheroids, such as light sheet fluorescence microscopy (LSFM), single or selective plane illumination microscopy (SPIM), and multi-photon microscopy (MPM) [147–149]. These new microscopic approaches allow deep tissue imaging study without the need of physical sectioning, while allowing dynamic processes to be studied in live 3D cultures at high resolution, under reduced light exposure and phototoxicity.

5.2. Electron Microscopy

Electron microscopy techniques are widely used to characterize spheroids because they provide high resolution, at nanoscale levels. High-resolution images of the internal structures can be generated by transmission electron microscopy (TEM) while high-resolution images of the surface of spheroids can be achieved by scanning electron microscopy (SEM) [56].

The TEM technique provides information on cell–cell interaction in the spheroids, such as cell junctions, and ECM deposition, as well as information on treatment outcomes such as apoptosis, cell shrinkage and organelle swelling [150]. Importantly, TEM is mostly used to analyze the distribution of drugs or nanoparticles in the spheroid [151].

The SEM technique provides high-resolution images and is used to analyze, for instance, cellular protrusions, integrity of cell–cell interactions, integrity of cellular membrane after anticancer drug treatment [56,152,153].

Both TEM and SEM are very informative although specimen collapse and morphological alterations can be associated with the steps involved in the procedures [154].

5.3. Flow Cytometry

Quantitative measurements such as cell viability, proliferation kinetics, cell cycle, apoptosis, and uptake of anticancer drugs and nanomedicines in spheroids can be performed using flow cytometry. Mechanical or enzymatic disaggregation of spheroids by trypsin or less toxic enzyme cocktail (Accutase®) is needed to obtain single cell suspension that can be stained and manipulated similarly to 2D cultures, and analyzed by flow cytometry [155]. For instance, single cells can be stained with calcein and ethidium to evaluate live cells and dead cells, respectively [56]. Other fluorescent dyes are used to analyze proliferating or quiescent cells (e.g., Propidium iodide), entry intro S phase of the cell cycle (e.g., 5-bromo-2'-deoxyuridine (BrdU) detected by a fluorescently labeled secondary antibody), or the expression of specific cellular proteins with fluorescently labelled antibodies. Flow cytometry analysis does not enable evaluation of penetration of anticancer drugs due to spheroid disaggregation and cell dissociation. However, it was reported that Hoechst 33342 (a fluorescent DNA dye) forms a marked diffusion gradient into the inner space of spheroids, therefore enabling cells of the different layers to be sorted on the basis of Hoechst staining intensity [156,157]. One major limitation of flow cytometry analysis is the need of a large amount of spheroids due to loss of cells during the process of cell dissociation [140].

5.4. Colorimetric Methods

Cell viability in the spheroids can be evaluated without the need of cell dissociation. For this purpose, are used colorimetric, fluorometric and luminescent methods that include acid phosphatase assay, Alamar blue, MTT assay, and lactate dehydrogenase quantification [140,158,159]. Nowadays, specialized kits for cytotoxicity assessment in spheroids are made available from many manufacturers. For instance, commercially available cell viability assays such as CellTiter-Glo 3D with better penetration of the reagents into the spheroids are easy to implement, and enable more accurate cytotoxicity determination [142,160]

5.5. Molecular Biology Tools

Standard molecular biology assays such as Western blot and qRT-PCR are useful to evaluate differential protein and gene expression, respectively, between 2D and 3D systems and/or before and after drug treatment. These techniques involve the use of cell lysis during the procedures of cellular protein and RNA extraction from the spheroids [59,161].

Table 4. Methods currently used to characterize spheroids and to evaluate drug effect.

Method	Description	Staining Methods/Markers	Feature Evaluated	Advantages (↑) and Limitations (↓)	References
Phase contrast microscopy	Monitorization of morphology and general state of spheroids.	-	Size/volume and shape.	↑ Low cost and easy method to observe the general data on spheroids size and shape. ↑ Noninvasive. ↓ Does not provide enough quality in focus to obtain detailed data from complex 3D spheroid structures.	[140,142,162]
Fluorescence microscopy	Uses fluorescent dyes to analyze specific structures in the sample; Monitorization of stained/immunostained spheroids or spheroid sections.	DNA staining by Hoechst or DAPI. Fibronectin, laminin, and collagen IV staining. Phalloidin staining. Ki-67 staining. Caspase staining. Annexin V + propidium iodide (PI), and TUNEL staining methods. Calcein + ethidium homodimer-1 (EthD-1).	DNA, nucleus. ECM deposition. cytoskeletal arrangement. Cell proliferation. Cell death, apoptosis. Live/cell death assays.	↑ Allows easy monitoring of a wide range of features. ↓ For larger spheroids, processing for histological sectioning is required—spheroid fixation used in the histological procedure precludes the study of dynamic alterations in the spheroids over time.	[144,145,158,163–167]
Bright field microscopy	Light is transmitted through the sample, and denser areas attenuate light transmission, originating contrast.	e.g., hematoxylin and eosin staining.	Distinction of nuclei and cytoplasmic structures.	↑ Low-cost method that offers a general overview of the sample structure (of a section). ↓ Requires spheroid processing for histological sectioning.	[143,168–170]
Confocal laser microscopy	The use of a focused laser spot with the removal of the out-of-focus light allows to acquire higher spatial resolution images.	Same markers described for fluorescence microscopy.	Spheroid architecture. The features described for fluorescence microscopy can also be evaluated.	↑ High resolution data. ↑ 3D reconstruction. ↓ Restricted to small spheroids due to limited light penetration and to light scattering in thick tissues.	[143,171,172] [173–175]

Table 4. *Cont.*

Method	Description	Staining Methods/Markers	Feature Evaluated	Advantages (↑) and Limitations (↓)	References
Light sheet fluorescence microscopy (LSFM) and single or selective plane illumination microscopy (SPIM)	High resolution data from thick experiments through the use of planar illumination incident orthogonally to the direction of observation.			↑ High spatial resolution. ↑ 3D reconstruction. ↑ Noninvasive. ↑ Does not require physical sectioning. ↑ Reduced light exposure and phototoxicity. ↓ LSFM may imply high processing time and memory in order to produce high-resolution 3D images; scattering and absorption of light may limit the penetration into specimens, although some efforts have been recently made to improve those issues.	[147–149,175–180]
Multi-photon microscopy (MPM)	MPM pulsed long wavelength is used to excite fluorophores—two photon absorption-based fluorescence.	Same markers described for fluorescence microscopy.	The innermost layer of live and fixed spheroids.	↓ The upgrading of conventional microscopes to LSFM and/or SPIM technology may be complex and, in some cases, the optical sectioning capability may be limited. ↓ Some MPM limitations have been reported, such as weak endogenous signal strength, limited imaging materials, insufficient imaging depth.	[181–184]

205

Table 4. Cont.

Method		Description	Staining Methods/Markers	Feature Evaluated	Advantages (↑) and Limitations (↓)	References
Electron microscopy	Scanning electron microscopy (SEM)	The surface of the structures in the sample are scanned with a beam of electrons. The emitted signals provide high-resolution images of the surface of spheroids.	-	Cellular protrusions; Integrity of cell–cell interactions; Integrity of cellular membrane after anticancer drug treatment.	↑ High resolution. ↓ In some cases, specimen collapse and morphological alterations can be associated with the steps involved in the procedures.	[56,152–154,185–188]
	Transmission electron microscopy (TEM)	A beam of electrons hits the sample; part of the beam is transmitted through the specimen and used to generate high resolution images; information on cell–cell interactions is provided	-	Cell junctions and ECM deposition; Drug treatment outcomes such as apoptosis, cell shrinkage and organelle swelling; Distribution of drugs or nanoparticles in the spheroid.		
Flow cytometry		Analysis of physical and chemical properties of single cells. Mechanical or enzymatic disaggregation of spheroids is required	AnnexinV/PI	Cell death, apoptosis.	↑ Quantitative analysis. ↑ After disaggregation, samples can be manipulated similarly to 2D cultures. ↓ A large amount of spheroids are required due to loss of cells during the process of cell dissociation.	[189–191]
			PI/ribonuclease	Cell cycle analysis.		[56,192,193]
			5-bromo-2'-deoxyuridine (BrdU) + PI (or analog).	Cell cycle analysis, quiescent cells.		[194,195]
			Calcein + ethidium homodimer-1 (EthD-1) (PI analog).	Live/dead cell analysis, detection of quiescent cells.		[56]
			Hoechst 33342	DNA staining intensity dependent on the depth of cells in the spheroid.		[156,157,196]
			Fluorescent staining of specific cellular proteins.			[197,198]

Table 4. Cont.

Method		Description	Staining Methods/Markers	Feature Evaluated	Advantages (↑) and Limitations (↓)	References
Quantitative methods for cell viability analysis	MTT	Colorimetric Evaluation of the metabolic activity through tetrazolium salt reduction.			↑ Well-known methods so far implemented for 2D culture approaches. ↓ Limited efficacy in 3D spheroids and microtissues, due to difficulties of reagents to cross cell–cell junctions and/or 3D matrices.	[140,158,159,199–201]
	Lactate dehydrogenase quantification	Colorimetric Cytotoxicity evaluation through the quantification of lactate dehydrogenase (LDH) release.				
	Alamar blue	Fluorometric Evaluation of the metabolic activity through ATP measurement by resazurin reduction.			↑ Highly sensitive. ↑ Does not require spheroid dissociation. ↓ Complete removal of culture medium is required, which may not be practical and increases spheroid damage risk.	[201–203]
	Acid phosphatase assay (ACP)	Colorimetric Cytotoxicity evaluation through measurement of ACP activity.				
	CellTiter-Glo 3D	Luminescent Evaluation of the metabolic activity through ATP measurement, by luciferin oxidation.			↑ Better penetration of the reagents into the spheroids. ↑ Enables higher accuracy and reproducibility in large spheroids. ↑ Does not require removal of culture medium. ↓ ATP output may be affected by several factors and is not always proportional to cell number.	[142,204–207]
Molecular biology methods for quantification of gene expression	qRT-PCR	Quantification of gene expression at mRNA level.	-		↑ Accurate and well-known methods so far implemented for 2D culture models. ↑ After disaggregation, samples can be manipulated similarly to 2D cultures. ↓ Mechanical disruption and association with chemical buffers are required to extract proteins and RNA from the cells.	[59,161,208–211]
	Western blot	Quantification of gene expression at protein level.	-			

6. Application of 3D Cultures in Anti-Cancer Drug Discovery and Delivery

The capacity to reproduce the in vivo 3D tumor environment such as cellular heterogeneity, gene expression patterns, cell differentiation, generation of hypoxia, activation of cell signaling pathways, and cell–cell and cell–ECM adhesions, are amongst the many advantages that prompted the use of spheroids for in vitro evaluation of chemoresistance, migration and invasion, and other aspects of tumor biology (e.g., cancer stem cells/tumorigenicity, hypoxia and tumor metabolism). We will focus on chemoresistance and migration/invasion, and provide a brief overview on the use of spheroids to study drug delivery. Details of the other aspects were reviewed elsewhere [64,70,212,213].

6.1. Chemoresistance

Drug resistance is a major concern responsible for the failure of the current chemotherapeutics and their ability to fight cancer, especially in aggressive and highly metastatic tumors. It is now well established that cancer cells, grown in vitro as 3D spheroids, more accurately mimic the drug behavior in terms of sensibility and resistance than cells grown as 2D monolayers [214]. This difference is probably due to the TME and the spatial organization of the spheroids [215]. Increased cell–cell and cell–matrix adhesions may lead to changes in gene expression. Upregulation of cell-adhesion molecules, such as lumican, SNED1, DARP32, and miR-146a, was reported to increase chemotherapeutic resistance in pancreatic tumor spheroids as compared to 2D monolayers [59]. Fibronectin protected DU145 prostate cancer cell spheroids against ceramide and docetaxel-induced apoptosis through interaction with Insulin like growth factor-1 receptor [216]. A variety of apoptotic stimuli, including combinations of tumor necrosis factor-related apoptosis-inducing ligand (TRAIL), ribotoxic stressors, histone deacetylase, and proteasome inhibitors, were reported to be highly effective against mesothelioma cells when grown as monolayers than when grown as multicellular spheroids [214].

Increased resistance to chemotherapeutic drugs in spheroids is attributed to many factors associated with their constitution and organization, such as hypoxia, altered cellular energy metabolism, the acidic microenvironment, the cellular heterogeneity including the presence of cancer stem cells, and cell–cell and cell–ECM interactions [215,217–222]. The mechanisms by which these factors confer chemoresistance to spheroids were nicely reviewed in [223]. While most studies showed that cells in spheroids are more chemoresistant than cells in 2D monolayers, some studies reported that cells in MCTS are equally or even more sensitive to anticancer agents than their 2D monolayer counterparts. For example, the proteasome inhibitor PS-341 was shown to be equally effective in killing ovarian and prostate tumor cells grown in the form of multicellular spheroids, and tumor cells grown in monolayer cell culture [224].

A number of studies reported that spheroids are also more radioresistant than 2D monolayers. For instance, increased cell compaction increased the resistance of human colon adenocarcinoma spheroids to ionizing radiation [225]. Besides the aforementioned factors, radioresistance may be due to decreased radiation-induced DNA damage as a consequence of lack of oxygen in the spheroids, given that oxygen seems to be required to stabilize DNA damage upon radiation [226–228].

6.2. Migration and Invasion

The acquisition of motility and migratory ability is an important hallmark of malignant tumors. Common characteristics of solid tumors, such as hypoxia and soluble mediators-mediated interactions with stromal cells, drive tumor cell migration and invasion, through essential steps that involve, amongst others, actin cytoskeleton remodeling, changes in cell–cell and cell–ECM adhesion, and protein degradation of the surrounding ECM [229,230]. Therefore, the success of studying the multistep process of metastasis relies on a 3D microenvironment through which tumor cells can move and disseminate. In this sense, tumor spheroids are viewed as relevant in vitro models for studying invasion and migration processes [70,166,231,232]. For instance, 3D spheroids display adhesion and ECM molecule expression pattern similar to that of the tumor in vivo, and can also induce expression of proteins associated with metastasis [70,231,233]. Importantly, non-tumor cells are also present in the TME and continuously interact, through paracrine signaling, with cancer cells. For instance, fibroblasts were shown to promote contact-dependent cancer cell motility and invasion of 3D spheroids in co-culture with colorectal cancer cells, a finding validated in vivo [234]. Therefore, ideal migration/invasion assays should be performed in 3D co-cultures that also include non-tumor cells, such as macrophages, dendritic cells, endothelial cells, CAFs and immune cells, in order to better simulate the migration and invasion process found in tumor tissues. CAFs, through the release of cytokines and growth factors, together with the other stromal cells, promote the epithelial-mesenchymal transition in heterotypic 3D cell cultures, resulting in tumor development and metastasis [111,234–236]. At the same time, endothelial cells in 3D co-cultures tend to accumulate in the peripheral layer, facilitating the adhesion and infiltration of immune cells [28]. In fact, immune cells can secrete interleukin 6 and MMP-9, which cause inflammation, angiogenesis and ECM degradation, thereby promoting tumor invasion and metastasis [237].

Several assays are available to determine the invasion and migration potential of cells in spheroids [70,232]. In the transwell-based or Boyden chamber assays, the spheroids are seeded on the top of a filter coated with a thick layer of ECM-derived components, usually collagen I, and invasion, in response to a chemo-attractant such as growth factors, can be measured by determining the number of cells that move from the top chamber to the lower chamber [70,232,238]. Additionally, the ability of the cells to invade cellular barriers can be determined by adding a layer of fibroblasts or endothelial cells on top of the matrix [70]. This latter is particularly relevant to mimic the ability of cancer cells to cross the blood vessel barrier and to invade deeply the tissues. Alternatively, spheroids can be completely embedded into different matrices, usually between two layers of ECM gel, where cells leave the spheroids and invade the surrounding matrix [96,239]. Sophisticated techniques combined with computerized quantification are now available to reproducibly perform optimized experimental conditions and to calculate the invasive index of cells [70,239–241]. For instance, the extent and rate of tumor spheroid invasion, using the 3D spheroid invasion assay, was rapidly and reproducibly measured using imaging cytometer [238]. Spheroid invasion assays can also be used as a metric to measure drug efficacy [96]. For example, lower concentrations of the adjuvant gamma-linolenic acid caused an increase in glioma spheroid invasion, but increased the apoptotic index at higher concentrations [242]. In sum, spheroids have been widely utilized to study the role of mechanisms involved in cellular invasion, and represent a valuable tool for preclinical evaluation of therapeutic agents targeting invasion [96,166,232].

6.3. Spheroids and Nanomedicines

Systemic drug toxicity and poor efficacy remain a major concern in cancer therapy due to the lack of selective drug delivery to tumor tissues, stressing the need to improve tumor targeting [243]. Nanomedicines have thus emerged as promising approach to (actively) target tumor and improve drug delivery. These nanostructures are biocompatible, biodegradable, non-toxic, can be prepared on a large scale, can provide controlled drug release, and enhance tissue/cell-specific targeting, in addition to reducing side effects [244–248]. However, despite the promising preclinical outcome that was reported for a significant number of nanotherapeutics, only few nanodrugs reached the clinic and achieved the expected results in patients [243]. Many barriers influence the efficiency of nanomedicine delivery to the target tumor, that are not recapitulated by the 2D monolayer cultures.

Tissue penetration of nanoparticles (NPs) relies on their diffusion capacity through the ECM, which varies in density and size, and is also influenced by cell–cell interactions, necrotic core, hypoxia, and by the intravascular pressure irregularities due to vessel compressions applied by growing tumors [249–251]. In this sense, as outlined above, spheroids have gained in popularity over traditional 2D culture systems because their pathophysiological features are close to those of the native tumors, being an excellent model to evaluate nanodrugs and to better predict their clinical outcomes [101,197,212,252]. Consequently, spheroids have been used as valuable tool to study different physico-chemical proprieties of nanocarriers such as chemical composition, size, shape and surface properties, which are crucial for their penetration and antitumor efficacy [197,253,254].

A general observation from studies that used spheroids is that nanoparticles (NPs) penetration is inversely correlated to the particle size [159,254–256]. NPs with small size (<100 nm) penetrate deeply and faster in the spheroids and distribute homogeneously, as compared to larger NPs (>100 nm) which remain confined to the superficial layers [159,257–259]. However, NPs <50 nm were reported to interact with liver cells, and to be poorly retained in the tumor [260].

The surface charge of NPs also influences their penetration in the spheroids: negatively charged NPs penetrate deeply while their positive counterparts remain at the outer layers [56,199]. Yet, more effective drug delivery is warranted by NPs with positive surface charge due to electrostatic interactions with negatively charged cell membranes. To overcome this issue, it has been proposed the use of pH-responsive negatively charged NPs that can turn to positively charged ones once in contact with acidic conditions (e.g., tumor microenvironment), so that negative surface charge ensures deep penetration in the spheroids, while positive surface charge enables more effective drug delivery [199, 261].

Although little information exists on the influence of NP shape on penetration and accumulation in the spheroid, the existing literature indicates that nanorods seem to diffuse more rapidly in spheroids compared to nanospheres, and that short nanorods (400 nm in length) accumulate more rapidly and are better internalized than long nanorods (<2000 nm in length) [262–264].

Interestingly, NP penetration into spheroids has been enhanced by modification of the surface coating. For instance, ECM-degrading enzymes such as collagenases have been used to coat NPs of up to 100 nm in size, which demonstrated superior (4-fold increase) penetration over control NPs [258]. Drug efficacy is the most important endpoint of any formulation, and it depends greatly on the penetration and accumulation into the spheroids [254]. In general, nanocarrier formulations with high penetration and accumulation in the spheroids exhibited better antitumor activity [159].

Comparison between NP delivery and efficacy between 3D tumor spheroids and animal models revealed key similarities between the two systems. For instance, the photosensitizer verteporfin encapsulated into lipid nanocarriers strongly reduced tumor cell viability of ovarian spheroid cancer cells, and also inhibited tumor growth in an orthotopic murine ovarian cancer model, when compared to free drug [265]. Similar to in vivo tissues, HepG2 cells in 3D hydrogels were more resistant to biotin-conjugated pullulan acetate nanoparticles (Bio-PA NPs) treatments compared to the 2D system [266]. Moreover, Bio-PA NPs exhibited similar anti-tumor activity in 3D culture cells and in in vivo xenografted hepatic tumor model [266]. Studies also observed that iRGD-conjugated nanoparticles with doxorubicin were able to accumulate with more efficacy and penetrate deeply into tumor in both SH-SY5Y spheroids and H22 tumor-bearing mice, restraining tumor growth in both systems [267]. Overall, this highlights the predictive power of spheroids for in vivo therapeutic efficacy, and their potential as promising alternative to animal models for cancer study, hopefully resolving high cost and ethical issues associated with animal use.

7. Concluding Remarks and Perspectives

It is consensual that 3D tumor models enable evaluation of anticancer drugs and nanomedicines in a condition closer to the real tumor, owing to their key features such as spatial organization, cell–cell and cell–ECM, diffusive gradients, complex cell signaling, drug resistance and metabolic adaptation. As reviewed here, these features are missing in 2D culture systems and, consequently, 3D culture models in preclinical evaluation are expected to provide more accurate results of the therapeutic potential of anticancer drug candidates, thereby increasing the predictability of the in vivo efficacy. Identifying and eliminating those therapeutics that did not show any interesting efficacy in 3D cultures will reduce animal use and speed up the number of therapeutics that reach the clinic.

It is noteworthy that most of the published works used spheroids made of only cancer cells, and, thus, do not represent the complexity associated with the diversity of the cellular and non-cellular components present in the real tumor. Spheroids that incorporate cell types recapitulating the vasculature (e.g., endothelial cells), the immune system (e.g., leukocytes) and ECM production (e.g., fibroblasts) are, thus, highly recommended. This is important as it would make the geometry of drug penetration in the spheroids closely similar to that in vivo, therefore providing better prediction of drug effects and delivery mechanisms and, at the same time, reducing costly investments associated with the ultimate step of clinical investigations.

Standardized methodologies for generation and characterization of spheroids are urgently needed, this would avoid variability in size and homogeneity, as well as in biological effect evaluation. Although considerable progress has been made to adapt existing 2D culture analysis assays to the spheroid model, many challenges remain to be addressed. Enabling acquisition of high-resolution images from intact spheroids remains a major challenge, due to the size of spheroids and poor light scattering. On the other hand, histological procedures for spheroid sectioning require special care in handling, as specimen tend to collapse or fracture easily. Mass production, together with developing easy to handle spheroids that are time and cost effective, with reduced workflows of culture and analysis, is crucial in order to encourage their routine use in drug discovery research. We are, yet, still far from giving up using animal models for safety and efficacy studies of drugs. Meanwhile, and ideally, the use of spheroids in preclinical testing could reduce the number of compounds progressing to in vivo testing, thereby reducing the numbers of animals used.

In conclusion, the use of 3D models to assess tumor penetration, accumulation and antitumor activity of drug and nanomedicine candidates is becoming a reality, and should turn out a mandatory step between 2D and in vivo models in the near future, with a great impact on the transferability of new anticancer drugs from bench to bedside. Hopefully, the generation of tumor spheroids from the patient's own cells may enable personalized approaches to screening and selecting the appropriate drugs for the patients.

Author Contributions: Review topic and general structure, H.B.; data collection and writing the review draft, B.P. and H.B.; discussions, revising of text and generation of final version, B.P., A.C.H., P.M.A.S., and H.B.; preparation of the figures and tables, B.P., A.C.H., and P.M.A.S.; funding acquisition, H.B. All authors have read and agreed to the published version of the manuscript.

Funding: This work was funded by CESPU—Cooperativa de Ensino Superior Politécnico e Universitário under the project "IMPLDEBRIS-PL-3RL-IINFACTS-2019". Bárbara Fernandes Pinto is a PhD fellowship holder from CESPU (BD/CBAS/CESPU/01/2020). Ana C. Henriques acknowledges FCT—Fundação para a Ciência e a Tecnologia for financial support (grant SFRH/BD/116167/2016).

Acknowledgments: We thank the anonymous reviewers for their time, comments, and constructive criticism.

Conflicts of Interest: The authors declare no conflict of interest.

References

1. Hait, W.N. Anticancer drug development: The grand challenges. *Nat. Rev. Drug. Discov.* **2010**, *9*, 253–254. [CrossRef]
2. Hutchinson, L.; Kirk, R. High drug attrition rates—Where are we going wrong? *Nat. Rev. Clin. Oncol.* **2011**, *8*, 189–190. [CrossRef] [PubMed]
3. Rubinstein, L.V.; Shoemaker, R.H.; Paull, K.D.; Simon, R.M.; Tosini, S.; Skehan, P.; Scudiero, D.A.; Monks, A.; Boyd, M.R. Comparison of In Vitro Anticancer-Drug-Screening Data Generated With a Tetrazolium Assay Versus a Protein Assay Against a Diverse Panel of Human Tumor Cell Lines. *JNCI J. Natl. Cancer Inst.* **1990**, *82*, 1113–1117. [CrossRef] [PubMed]
4. Ocana, A.; Pandiella, A.; Siu, L.L.; Tannock, I.F. Preclinical development of molecular-targeted agents for cancer. *Nat. Rev. Clin. Oncol.* **2011**, *8*, 200–209. [CrossRef] [PubMed]
5. van der Worp, H.B.; Howells, D.W.; Sena, E.S.; Porritt, M.J.; Rewell, S.; O'Collins, V.; Macleod, M.R. Can animal models of disease reliably inform human studies? *PLoS Med.* **2010**, *7*, e1000245. [CrossRef] [PubMed]
6. Quail, D.F.; Joyce, J.A. Microenvironmental regulation of tumor progression and metastasis. *Nat. Med.* **2013**, *19*, 1423–1437. [CrossRef]

7. Belli, C.; Trapani, D.; Viale, G.; D'Amico, P.; Duso, B.A.; Della Vigna, P.; Orsi, F.; Curigliano, G. Targeting the microenvironment in solid tumors. *Cancer Treat. Rev.* **2018**, *65*, 22–32. [CrossRef]
8. Imamura, Y.; Mukohara, T.; Shimono, Y.; Funakoshi, Y.; Chayahara, N.; Toyoda, M.; Kiyota, N.; Takao, S.; Kono, S.; Nakatsura, T.; et al. Comparison of 2D- and 3D-culture models as drug-testing platforms in breast cancer. *Oncol. Rep.* **2015**, *33*, 1837–1843. [CrossRef]
9. Birgersdotter, A.; Sandberg, R.; Ernberg, I. Gene expression perturbation in vitro–a growing case for three-dimensional (3D) culture systems. *Semin. Cancer Biol.* **2005**, *15*, 405–412. [CrossRef]
10. Souza, A.G.; Silva, I.B.B.; Campos-Fernandez, E.; Barcelos, L.S.; Souza, J.B.; Marangoni, K.; Goulart, L.R.; Alonso-Goulart, V. Comparative Assay of 2D and 3D Cell Culture Models, Proliferation, Gene Expression and Anticancer Drug Response. *Curr. Pharm. Des.* **2018**, *24*, 1689–1694. [CrossRef]
11. Teicher, B.A. Tumor models for efficacy determination. *Mol. Cancer Ther.* **2006**, *5*, 2435–2443. [CrossRef] [PubMed]
12. Bissell, M.J. Architecture Is the Message, The role of extracellular matrix and 3-D structure in tissue-specific gene expression and breast cancer. *Pezcoller Found J.* **2007**, *16*, 2–17. [PubMed]
13. Ravi, M.; Paramesh, V.; Kaviya, S.R.; Anuradha, E.; Solomon, F.P. 3D cell culture systems: Advantages and applications. *J. Cell Physiol.* **2015**, *230*, 16–26. [CrossRef] [PubMed]
14. Białkowska, K.; Komorowski, P.; Bryszewska, M.; Miłowska, K. Spheroids as a Type of Three-Dimensional Cell Cultures-Examples of Methods of Preparation and the Most Important Application. *Int. J. Mol. Sci.* **2020**, *21*, 6225. [CrossRef] [PubMed]
15. Shehzad, A.; Ravinayagam, V.; AlRumaih, H.; Aljafary, M.; Almohazey, D.; Almofty, S.; Al-Rashid, N.A.; Al-Suhaimi, E.A. Application of Three-dimensional (3D) Tumor Cell Culture Systems and Mechanism of Drug Resistance. *Curr. Pharm. Des.* **2019**, *25*, 3599–3607. [CrossRef] [PubMed]
16. Park, J.I.; Lee, J.; Kwon, J.L.; Park, H.B.; Lee, S.Y.; Kim, J.Y.; Sung, J.; Kim, J.M.; Song, K.S.; Kim, K.H. Scaffold-Free Coculture Spheroids of Human Colonic Adenocarcinoma Cells and Normal Colonic Fibroblasts Promote Tumorigenicity in Nude Mice. *Transl. Oncol.* **2016**, *9*, 79–88. [CrossRef] [PubMed]
17. Szade, K.; Zukowska, M.; Szade, A.; Collet, G.; Kloska, D.; Kieda, C.; Jozkowicz, A.; Dulak, J. Spheroid-plug model as a tool to study tumor development, angiogenesis, and heterogeneity in vivo. *Tumour Biol. J. Int. Soc. Oncodev. Biol. Med.* **2016**, *37*, 2481–2496. [CrossRef]
18. Zhou, J.; Tang, Z.; Gao, S.; Li, C.; Feng, Y.; Zhou, X. Tumor-Associated Macrophages: Recent Insights and Therapies. *Front. Oncol.* **2020**, *10*, 188. [CrossRef]
19. Wei, C.; Yang, C.; Wang, S.; Shi, D.; Zhang, C.; Lin, X.; Liu, Q.; Dou, R.; Xiong, B. Crosstalk between cancer cells and tumor associated macrophages is required for mesenchymal circulating tumor cell-mediated colorectal cancer metastasis. *Mol. Cancer* **2019**, *18*, 64. [CrossRef]
20. Lin, Y.; Xu, J.; Lan, H. Tumor-associated macrophages in tumor metastasis: Biological roles and clinical therapeutic applications. *J. Hematol. Oncol.* **2019**, *12*, 76. [CrossRef]
21. Garufi, A.; Traversi, G.; Cirone, M.; D'Orazi, G. HIPK2 role in the tumor-host interaction, Impact on fibroblasts transdifferentiation CAF-like. *IUBMB Life* **2019**, *71*, 2055–2061. [CrossRef] [PubMed]
22. Sahai, E.; Astsaturov, I.; Cukierman, E.; DeNardo, D.G.; Egeblad, M.; Evans, R.M.; Fearon, D.; Greten, F.R.; Hingorani, S.R.; Hunter, T.; et al. A framework for advancing our understanding of cancer-associated fibroblasts. *Nat. Rev. Cancer* **2020**, *20*, 174–186. [CrossRef] [PubMed]
23. Wagner, J.; Rapsomaniki, M.A.; Chevrier, S.; Anzeneder, T.; Langwieder, C.; Dykgers, A.; Rees, M.; Ramaswamy, A.; Muenst, S.; Soysal, S.D.; et al. A Single-Cell Atlas of the Tumor and Immune Ecosystem of Human Breast Cancer. *Cell* **2019**, *177*, 1330–1345. [CrossRef]
24. Hinshaw, D.C.; Shevde, L.A. The Tumor Microenvironment Innately Modulates Cancer Progression. *Cancer Res.* **2019**, *79*, 4557–4566. [CrossRef] [PubMed]
25. Reina-Campos, M.; Moscat, J.; Diaz-Meco, M. Metabolism shapes the tumor microenvironment. *Curr. Opin. Cell Biol.* **2017**, *48*, 47–53. [CrossRef]
26. Gonzalez, H.; Hagerling, C.; Werb, Z. Roles of the immune system in cancer: From tumor initiation to metastatic progression. *Genes Dev.* **2018**, *32*, 1267–1284. [CrossRef]
27. Zhang, J.; Zhang, Q.; Lou, Y.; Fu, Q.; Chen, Q.; Wei, T.; Yang, J.; Tang, J.; Wang, J.; Chen, Y.; et al. Hypoxia-inducible factor-1α/interleukin-1β signaling enhances hepatoma epithelial-mesenchymal transition through macrophages in a hypoxic-inflammatory microenvironment. *Hepatology* **2018**, *67*, 1872–1889. [CrossRef]

28. Aung, A.; Kumar, V.; Theprungsirikul, J.; Davey, S.K.; Varghese, S. An Engineered Tumor-on-a-Chip Device with Breast Cancer-Immune Cell Interactions for Assessing T-cell Recruitment. *Cancer Res.* **2020**, *80*, 263–275. [CrossRef]
29. Kashyap, A.S.; Schmittnaegel, M.; Rigamonti, N.; Pais-Ferreira, D.; Mueller, P.; Buchi, M.; Ooi, C.H.; Kreuzaler, M.; Hirschmann, P.; Guichard, A.; et al. Optimized antiangiogenic reprogramming of the tumor microenvironment potentiates CD40 immunotherapy. *Proc. Natl. Acad. Sci. USA* **2020**, *117*, 541–551. [CrossRef]
30. Protopsaltis, N.J.; Liang, W.; Nudleman, E.; Ferrara, N. Interleukin-22 promotes tumor angiogenesis. *Angiogenesis* **2019**, *22*, 311–323. [CrossRef]
31. O'Donnell, J.S.; Teng, M.W.L.; Smyth, M.J. Cancer immunoediting and resistance to T cell-based immunotherapy. *Nat. Rev. Clin. Oncol.* **2019**, *16*, 151–167. [CrossRef] [PubMed]
32. Domschke, C.; Schneeweiss, A.; Stefanovic, S.; Wallwiener, M.; Heil, J.; Rom, J.; Sohn, C.; Beckhove, P.; Schuetz, F. Cellular Immune Responses and Immune Escape Mechanisms in Breast Cancer, Determinants of Immunotherapy. *Breast Care* **2016**, *11*, 102–107. [CrossRef] [PubMed]
33. Yuan, Y. Spatial Heterogeneity in the Tumor Microenvironment. *Cold Spring Harb. Perspect. Med.* **2016**, *6*, a026583. [CrossRef] [PubMed]
34. Janssen, L.M.E.; Ramsay, E.E.; Logsdon, C.D.; Overwijk, W.W. The immune system in cancer metastasis: Friend or foe? *J. Immunother. Cancer* **2017**, *5*, 79. [CrossRef]
35. Choi, H.; Moon, A. Crosstalk between cancer cells and endothelial cells: Implications for tumor progression and intervention. *Arch. Pharm. Res.* **2018**, *41*, 711–724. [CrossRef]
36. Houthuijzen, J.M.; Jonkers, J. Cancer-associated fibroblasts as key regulators of the breast cancer tumor microenvironment. *Cancer Metastasis Rev.* **2018**, *37*, 577–597. [CrossRef]
37. Wang, J.J.; Lei, K.F.; Han, F. Tumor microenvironment: Recent advances in various cancer treatments. *Eur. Rev. Med. Pharmacol. Sci.* **2018**, *22*, 3855–3864.
38. Shaked, Y. The pro-tumorigenic host response to cancer therapies. *Nat. Rev. Cancer* **2019**, *19*, 667–685. [CrossRef]
39. Jing, X.; Yang, F.; Shao, C.; Wei, K.; Xie, M.; Shen, H.; Shu, Y. Role of hypoxia in cancer therapy by regulating the tumor microenvironment. *Mol. Cancer* **2019**, *18*, 157. [CrossRef]
40. Zhong, S.; Jeong, J.H.; Chen ZChen, Z.; Luo, J.L. Targeting Tumor Microenvironment by Small-Molecule Inhibitors. *Transl. Oncol.* **2020**, *13*, 57–69. [CrossRef]
41. Luo, W.; Wang, Y. Hypoxia Mediates Tumor Malignancy and Therapy Resistance. *Adv. Exp. Med. Biol.* **2019**, *1136*, 1–18. [PubMed]
42. Gandhi, N.; Das, G.M. Metabolic Reprogramming in Breast Cancer and Its Therapeutic Implications. *Cells* **2019**, *8*, 89. [CrossRef] [PubMed]
43. Wu, T.; Dai, Y. Tumor microenvironment and therapeutic response. *Cancer Lett.* **2017**, *387*, 61–68. [CrossRef] [PubMed]
44. Thews, O.; Riemann, A. Tumor pH and metastasis: A malignant process beyond hypoxia. *Cancer Metastasis Rev.* **2019**, *38*, 113–129. [CrossRef]
45. Swenson, E.R. Hypoxia and Its Acid-Base Consequences, From Mountains to Malignancy. *Adv. Exp. Med. Biol.* **2016**, *903*, 301–323.
46. White, K.A.; Grillo-Hill, B.K.; Barber, D.L. Cancer cell behaviors mediated by dysregulated pH dynamics at a glance. *J. Cell Sci.* **2017**, *130*, 663–669. [CrossRef]
47. Paškevičiūtė, M.; Petrikaitė, V. Proton Pump Inhibitors Modulate Transport Of Doxorubicin And Its Liposomal Form Into 2D And 3D Breast Cancer Cell Cultures. *Cancer Manag. Res.* **2019**, *11*, 9761–9769. [CrossRef]
48. Pitt, J.M.; Marabelle, A.; Eggermont, A.; Soria, J.C.; Kroemer, G.; Zitvogel, L. Targeting the tumor microenvironment: Removing obstruction to anticancer immune responses and immunotherapy. *Ann. Oncol.* **2016**, *27*, 1482–1492. [CrossRef]
49. Jarosz-Biej, M.; Smolarczyk, R.; Cichoń, T.; Kułach, N. Tumor Microenvironment as A "Game Changer" in Cancer Radiotherapy. *Int. J. Mol. Sci.* **2019**, *20*, 3212. [CrossRef]
50. Riera-Domingo, C.; Audigé, A.; Granja, S.; Cheng, W.C.; Ho, P.C.; Baltazar, F.; Stockmann, C.; Mazzone, M. Immunity, Hypoxia, and Metabolism-the Ménage à Trois of Cancer, Implications for Immunotherapy. *Physiol. Rev.* **2020**, *100*, 1–102. [CrossRef]

51. Najafi, M.; Farhood, B.; Mortezaee, K. Extracellular matrix (ECM) stiffness and degradation as cancer drivers. *J. Cell Biochem.* **2019**, *120*, 2782–2790. [CrossRef] [PubMed]
52. Sangaletti, S.; Chiodoni, C.; Tripodo, C.; Colombo, M.P. The good and bad of targeting cancer-associated extracellular matrix. *Curr. Opin. Pharmacol.* **2017**, *35*, 75–82. [CrossRef] [PubMed]
53. Roma-Rodrigues, C.; Mendes, R.; Baptista, P.V.; Fernandes, A.R. Targeting Tumor Microenvironment for Cancer Therapy. *Int. J. Mol. Sci.* **2019**, *20*, 840. [CrossRef] [PubMed]
54. Hanahan, D.; Weinberg, R.A. Hallmarks of cancer: The next generation. *Cell* **2011**, *144*, 646–674. [CrossRef] [PubMed]
55. Kitaeva, K.V.; Rutland, C.S.; Rizvanov, A.A.; Solovyeva, V.V. Cell Culture Based in vitro Test Systems for Anticancer Drug Screening. *Front. Bioeng. Biotechnol.* **2020**, *8*, 322. [CrossRef] [PubMed]
56. Ma, H.L.; Jiang, Q.; Han, S.; Wu, Y.; Tomshine, J.C.; Wang, D.; Gan, Y.; Zou, G.; Liang, X.J. Multicellular tumor spheroids as an in vivo-like tumor model for three-dimensional imaging of chemotherapeutic and nano material cellular penetration. *Mol. Imaging* **2012**, *11*, 487–498. [CrossRef] [PubMed]
57. Baker, B.M.; Chen, C.S. Deconstructing the third dimension: How 3D culture microenvironments alter cellular cues. *J. Cell Sci.* **2012**, *125*, 3015–3024. [CrossRef]
58. Hirschhaeuser, F.; Menne, H.; Dittfeld, C.; West, J.; Mueller-Klieser, W.; Kunz-Schughart, L.A. Multicellular tumor spheroids: An underestimated tool is catching up again. *J. Biotechnol.* **2010**, *148*, 3–15. [CrossRef]
59. Longati, P.; Jia, X.; Eimer, J.; Wagman, A.; Witt, M.R.; Rehnmark, S.; Verbeke, C.; Toftgård, R.; Löhr, M.; Heuchel, R.L. 3D pancreatic carcinoma spheroids induce a matrix-rich, chemoresistant phenotype offering a better model for drug testing. *BMC Cancer* **2013**, *13*, 95. [CrossRef]
60. Yamada, K.M.; Cukierman, E. Modeling tissue morphogenesis and cancer in 3D. *Cell* **2007**, *130*, 601–610. [CrossRef]
61. Goldhammer, N.; Kim, J.; Timmermans-Wielenga, V.; Petersen, O.W. Characterization of organoid cultured human breast cancer. *Breast Cancer Res.* **2019**, *21*, 141. [CrossRef] [PubMed]
62. Baal, N.; Widmer-Teske, R.; McKinnon, T.; Preissner, K.T.; Zygmunt, M.T. In vitro spheroid model of placental vasculogenesis: Does it work? *Lab. Investig.* **2009**, *89*, 152–163. [CrossRef] [PubMed]
63. Costa, E.C.; Moreira, A.F.; de Melo-Diogo, D.; Gaspar, V.M.; Carvalho, M.P.; Correia, I.J. 3D tumor spheroids: An overview on the tools and techniques used for their analysis. *Biotechnol. Adv.* **2016**, *34*, 1427–1441. [CrossRef] [PubMed]
64. Fang, Y.; Eglen, R.M. Three-Dimensional Cell Cultures in Drug Discovery and Development. *SLAS Discov.* **2017**, *22*, 456–472.
65. Gao, W.; Wu, D.; Wang, Y.; Wang, Z.; Zou, C.; Dai, Y.; Ng, C.F.; Teoh, J.Y.C.; Chan, F.L. Development of a novel and economical agar-based non-adherent three-dimensional culture method for enrichment of cancer stem-like cells. *Stem Cell Res. Ther.* **2018**, *9*, 243. [CrossRef]
66. Xiang, X.; Phung, Y.; Feng, M.; Nagashima, K.; Zhang, J.; Broaddus, V.C.; Hassan, R.; FitzGerald, D.; Ho, M. The development and characterization of a human mesothelioma in vitro 3D model to investigate immunotoxin therapy. *PLoS ONE* **2011**, *6*, e14640. [CrossRef]
67. Sarisozen, C.; Abouzeid, A.H.; Torchilin, V.P. The effect of co-delivery of paclitaxel and curcumin by transferrin-targeted PEG-PE-based mixed micelles on resistant ovarian cancer in 3-D spheroids and in vivo tumors. *Eur. J. Pharm. Biopharm.* **2014**, *88*, 539–550. [CrossRef]
68. Sarisozen, C.; Dhokai, S.; Tsikudo, E.G.; Luther, E.; Rachman, I.M.; Torchilin, V.P. Nanomedicine based curcumin and doxorubicin combination treatment of glioblastoma with scFv-targeted micelles, In vitro evaluation on 2D and 3D tumor models. *Eur. J. Pharm. Biopharm.* **2016**, *108*, 54–67. [CrossRef]
69. Ekert, J.E.; Johnson, K.; Strake, B.; Pardinas, J.; Jarantow, S.; Perkinson, R.; Colter, D.C. Three-dimensional lung tumor microenvironment modulates therapeutic compound responsiveness in vitro–implication for drug development. *PLoS ONE* **2014**, *9*, e92248. [CrossRef]
70. Nath, S.; Devi, G.R. Three-dimensional culture systems in cancer research, Focus on tumor spheroid model. *Pharmacol. Ther.* **2016**, *163*, 94–108. [CrossRef]
71. Achilli, T.M.; Meyer, J.; Morgan, J.R. Advances in the formation, use and understanding of multi-cellular spheroids. *Expert Opin. Biol. Ther.* **2012**, *12*, 1347–1360. [CrossRef] [PubMed]
72. Verjans, E.T.; Doijen, J.; Luyten, W.; Landuyt, B.; Schoofs, L. Three-dimensional cell culture models for anticancer drug screening, Worth the effort? *J. Cell Physiol.* **2018**, *233*, 2993–3003. [CrossRef] [PubMed]

73. Froehlich, K.; Haeger, J.D.; Heger, J.; Pastuschek, J.; Photini, S.M.; Yan, Y.; Lupp, A.; Pfarrer, C.; Mrowka, R.; Schleußner, E.; et al. Generation of Multicellular Breast Cancer Tumor Spheroids, Comparison of Different Protocols. *J. Mammary Gland Biol. Neoplasia* **2016**, *21*, 89–98. [CrossRef] [PubMed]
74. Lee, D.; Pathak, S.; Jeong, J.-H. Design and manufacture of 3D cell culture plate for mass production of cell-spheroids. *Sci. Rep.* **2019**, *9*, 13976. [CrossRef] [PubMed]
75. Cho, C.Y.; Chiang, T.H.; Hsieh, L.H.; Yang, W.Y.; Hsu, H.H.; Yeh, C.K.; Huang, C.C.; Huang, J.H. Development of a Novel Hanging Drop Platform for Engineering Controllable 3D Microenvironments. *Front. Cell Dev. Biol.* **2020**, *8*, 327. [CrossRef] [PubMed]
76. Wu, H.-W.; Hsiao, Y.-H.; Chen, C.-C.; Yet, S.F.; Hsu, C.H. A PDMS-Based Microfluidic Hanging Drop Chip for Embryoid Body Formation. *Molecules* **2016**, *21*, 882. [CrossRef] [PubMed]
77. Zhao, L.; Xiu, J.; Liu, Y.; Zhang, T.; Pan, W.; Zheng, X.; Zhang, X. A 3D Printed Hanging Drop Dripper for Tumor Spheroids Analysis Without Recovery. *Sci. Rep.* **2019**, *9*, 1–14. [CrossRef] [PubMed]
78. Ryu, N.E.; Lee, S.H.; Park, H. Spheroid Culture System Methods and Applications for Mesenchymal Stem Cells. *Cells* **2019**, *8*, 1620. [CrossRef] [PubMed]
79. Rijal, G.; Li, W. A versatile 3D tissue matrix scaffold system for tumor modeling and drug screening. *Sci. Adv.* **2017**, *3*, e1700764. [CrossRef]
80. Kuriakose, A.E.; Hu, W.; Nguyen, K.T.; Menon, J.U. Scaffold-based lung tumor culture on porous PLGA microparticle substrates. *PLoS ONE* **2019**, *14*, e0217640. [CrossRef]
81. Zhang, M.; Boughton, P.; Rose, B.; Lee, C.S.; Hong, A.M. The use of porous scaffold as a tumor model. *Int. J. Biomater.* **2013**, *2013*, 396056. [CrossRef] [PubMed]
82. Xiao, Y.; Zhou, M.; Zhang, M.; Liu, W.; Zhou, Y.; Lang, M. Hepatocyte culture on 3D porous scaffolds of PCL/PMCL. *Colloids Surf. B Biointerfaces* **2019**, *173*, 185–193. [CrossRef] [PubMed]
83. Wang, X.; Dai, X.; Zhang, X.; Li, X.; Xu, T.; Lan, Q. Enrichment of glioma stem cell-like cells on 3D porous scaffolds composed of different extracellular matrix. *Biochem. Biophys. Res. Commun.* **2018**, *498*, 1052–1057. [CrossRef] [PubMed]
84. Vasanthan, K.S.; Subramaniam, A.; Krishnan, U.M.; Sethuraman, S. Influence of 3D porous galactose containing PVA/gelatin hydrogel scaffolds on three-dimensional spheroidal morphology of hepatocytes. *J. Mater. Sci. Mater. Med.* **2015**, *26*, 5345. [CrossRef]
85. Florczyk, S.J.; Wang, K.; Jana, S.; Wood, D.L.; Sytsma, S.K.; Sham, J.G.; Kievit, F.M.; Zhang, M. Porous chitosan-hyaluronic acid scaffolds as a mimic of glioblastoma microenvironment ECM. *Biomaterials* **2013**, *34*, 10143–10150. [CrossRef]
86. De, T.; Goyal, S.; Balachander, G.; Chatterjee, K.; Kumar, P.; Babu, K.G.; Rangarajan, A. A Novel Ex Vivo System Using 3D Polymer Scaffold to Culture Circulating Tumor Cells from Breast Cancer Patients Exhibits Dynamic E-M Phenotypes. *J. Clin. Med.* **2019**, *8*, 1473. [CrossRef]
87. Wang, K.; Kievit, F.M.; Florczyk, S.J.; Stephen, Z.R.; Zhang, M. 3D Porous Chitosan-Alginate Scaffolds as an In Vitro Model for Evaluating Nanoparticle-Mediated Tumor Targeting and Gene Delivery to Prostate Cancer. *Biomacromolecules* **2015**, *16*, 3362–3372. [CrossRef]
88. Bäcker, A.; Erhardt, O.; Wietbrock, L.; Schel, N.; Göppert, B.; Dirschka, M.; Abaffy, P.; Sollich, T.; Cecilia, A.; Gruhl, F.J. Silk scaffolds connected with different naturally occurring biomaterials for prostate cancer cell cultivation in 3D. *Biopolymers* **2017**, *107*, 70–79. [CrossRef]
89. Fischbach, C.; Chen, R.; Matsumoto, T.; Schmelzle, T.; Brugge, J.S.; Polverini, P.J.; Mooney, D.J. Engineering tumors with 3D scaffolds. *Nat. Methods* **2007**, *4*, 855–860. [CrossRef]
90. Zhang, J.; Wehrle, E.; Vetsch, J.R.; Paul, G.R.; Rubert, M.; Müller, R. Alginate dependent changes of physical properties in 3D bioprinted cell-laden porous scaffolds affect cell viability and cell morphology. *Biomed. Mater.* **2019**, *14*, 065009. [CrossRef]
91. Alghuwainem, A.; Alshareeda, A.T.; Alsowayan, B. Scaffold-Free 3-D Cell Sheet Technique Bridges the Gap between 2-D Cell Culture and Animal Models. *Int. J. Mol. Sci.* **2019**, *20*, 4926. [CrossRef] [PubMed]
92. Gong, X.; Lin, C.; Cheng, J.; Su, J.; Zhao, H.; Liu, T.; Wen, X.; Zhao, P. Generation of Multicellular Tumor Spheroids with Microwell-Based Agarose Scaffolds for Drug Testing. *PLoS ONE* **2015**, *10*, e0130348. [CrossRef] [PubMed]
93. Sant, S.; Johnston, P.A. The production of 3D tumor spheroids for cancer drug discovery. *Drug Discov. Today Technol.* **2017**, *23*, 27–36. [CrossRef] [PubMed]

94. Ferreira, L.P.; Gaspar, V.M.; Mano, J.F. Design of spherically structured 3D in vitro tumor models -Advances and prospects. *Acta Biomater.* **2018**, *75*, 11–34. [CrossRef] [PubMed]
95. Huang, X.; Zhang, X.; Wang, X.; Wang, C.; Tang, B. Microenvironment of alginate-based microcapsules for cell culture and tissue engineering. *J. Biosci. Bioeng.* **2012**, *114*, 1–8. [CrossRef]
96. Tevis, K.M.; Colson, Y.L.; Grinstaff, M.W. Embedded Spheroids as Models of the Cancer Microenvironment. *Adv. Biosyst.* **2017**, *1*, 1700083. [CrossRef] [PubMed]
97. Akins, R.E.; Schroedl, N.A.; Gonda, S.R.; Hartzell, C.R. Neonatal rat heart cells cultured in simulated microgravity. *In Vitro Cell Dev. Biol. Anim.* **1997**, *33*, 337–343. [CrossRef]
98. Antoni, D.; Burckel, H.; Josset, E.; Noel, G. Three-dimensional cell culture: A breakthrough in vivo. *Int. J. Mol. Sci.* **2015**, *16*, 5517–5527. [CrossRef]
99. Huang, L.; Abdalla, A.M.E.; Xiao, L.; Yang, G. Biopolymer-Based Microcarriers for Three-Dimensional Cell Culture and Engineered Tissue Formation. *Int. J. Mol. Sci.* **2020**, *21*, 1895. [CrossRef]
100. Liu, H.; Lu, T.; Kremers, G.-J.; Seynhaeve, A.L.; ten Hagen, T.L. A microcarrier-based spheroid 3D invasion assay to monitor dynamic cell movement in extracellular matrix. *Biol. Proced. Online* **2020**, *22*, 1–12. [CrossRef]
101. Mehta, G.; Hsiao, A.Y.; Ingram, M.; Luker, G.D.; Takayama, S. Opportunities and challenges for use of tumor spheroids as models to test drug delivery and efficacy. *J. Control. Release* **2012**, *164*, 192–204. [CrossRef] [PubMed]
102. Vadivelu, R.K.; Kamble, H.; Shiddiky, M.J.A.; Nguyen, N.-T. Microfluidic Technology for the Generation of Cell Spheroids and Their Applications. *Micromachines* **2017**, *8*, 94. [CrossRef]
103. Chen, C.; Townsend, A.D.; Hayter, E.; Birk, H.M.; Sell, S.A.; Martin, R.S. Insert-based microfluidics for 3D cell culture with analysis. *Anal. Bioanal. Chem.* **2018**, *410*, 3025–3035. [CrossRef] [PubMed]
104. Kuriu, S.; Kadonosono, T.; Kizaka-Kondoh, S.; Ishida, T. Slicing Spheroids in Microfluidic Devices for Morphological and Immunohistochemical Analysis. *Micromachines* **2020**, *11*, 480. [CrossRef] [PubMed]
105. Tanyeri, M.; Tay, S. Viable cell culture in PDMS-based microfluidic devices. *Methods Cell Biol.* **2018**, *148*, 3–33.
106. Hunter, L.; Gala de Pablo, J.; Stammers, A.C.; Thomson, N.H.; Evans, S.D.; Shim, J.U. On-chip pressure measurements and channel deformation after oil absorption. *SN Appl. Sci.* **2020**, *2*, 1–8. [CrossRef]
107. Kuncová-Kallio, J.; Kallio, P.J. PDMS and its suitability for analytical microfluidic devices. *Conf. Proc. IEEE Eng. Med. Biol. Soc.* **2006**, *2006*, 2486–2489.
108. Martin, A.; Teychené, S.; Camy, S.; Aubin, J. Fast and inexpensive method for the fabrication of transparent pressure-resistant microfluidic chips. *Microfluid. Nanofluidics* **2016**, *20*, 92. [CrossRef]
109. Kochanek, S.J.; Close, D.A.; Johnston, P.A. High Content Screening Characterization of Head and Neck Squamous Cell Carcinoma Multicellular Tumor Spheroid Cultures Generated in 384-Well Ultra-Low Attachment Plates to Screen for Better Cancer Drug Leads. *Assay Drug Dev. Technol.* **2019**, *17*, 17–36. [CrossRef]
110. Close, D.A.; Camarco, D.P.; Shan, F.; Kochanek, S.J.; Johnston, P.A. The Generation of Three-Dimensional Head and Neck Cancer Models for Drug Discovery in 384-Well Ultra-Low Attachment Microplates. *Methods Mol. Biol.* **2018**, *1683*, 355–369.
111. Khawar, I.A.; Park, J.K.; Jung, E.S.; Lee, M.A.; Chang, S.; Kuh, H.J. Three Dimensional Mixed-Cell Spheroids Mimic Stroma-Mediated Chemoresistance and Invasive Migration in hepatocellular carcinoma. *Neoplasia* **2018**, *20*, 800–812. [CrossRef] [PubMed]
112. Kim, M.; Yun, H.-W.; Choi, B.H.; Min, B.H. Three-Dimensional Spheroid Culture Increases Exosome Secretion from Mesenchymal Stem Cells. *Tissue Eng. Regen. Med.* **2018**, *15*, 427–436. [CrossRef]
113. Hurrell, T.; Ellero, A.A.; Masso, Z.F.; Cromarty, A.D. Characterization and reproducibility of HepG2 hanging drop spheroids toxicology in vitro. *Toxicol. In Vitro* **2018**, *50*, 86–94. [CrossRef] [PubMed]
114. Djomehri, S.I.; Burman, B.; Gonzalez, M.E.; Takayama, S.; Kleer, C.G. A reproducible scaffold-free 3D organoid model to study neoplastic progression in breast cancer. *J. Cell Commun. Signal.* **2019**, *13*, 129–143. [CrossRef] [PubMed]
115. Perez, J.E.; Nagle, I.; Wilhelm, C. Magnetic molding of tumor spheroids: Emerging model for cancer screening. *Biofabrication* **2020**. [CrossRef]
116. Mishriki, S.; Abdel Fattah, A.R.; Kammann, T.; Sahu, R.P.; Geng, F.; Puri, I.K. Rapid Magnetic 3D Printing of Cellular Structures with MCF-7 Cell Inks. *Research* **2019**, *2019*, 9854593. [CrossRef]

117. Urbanczyk, M.; Zbinden, A.; Layland, S.L.; Duffy, G.; Schenke-Layland, K. Controlled Heterotypic Pseudo-Islet Assembly of Human β-Cells and Human Umbilical Vein Endothelial Cells Using Magnetic Levitation. *Tissue Eng. Part A* **2020**, *26*, 387–399. [CrossRef] [PubMed]
118. Casson, J.; O'Kane, S.; Smith, C.-A.; Dalby, M.J.; Berry, C.C. Interleukin 6 Plays a Role in the Migration of Magnetically Levitated Mesenchymal Stem Cells Spheroids. *Appl. Sci.* **2018**, *8*, 412. [CrossRef]
119. Pawlik, T.M.; Souba, W.W.; Sweeney, T.J.; Bode, B.P. Amino acid uptake and regulation in multicellular hepatoma spheroids. *J. Surg. Res.* **2000**, *91*, 15–25. [CrossRef]
120. Yakavets, I.; Yankovsky, I.; Millard, M.; Lamy, L.; Lassalle, H.P.; Wiehe, A.; Zorin, V.; Bezdetnaya, L. The alteration of temoporfin distribution in multicellular tumor spheroids by β-cyclodextrins. *Int. J. Pharm.* **2017**, *529*, 568–575. [CrossRef]
121. Itaka, K.; Uchida, S.; Matsui, A.; Yanagihara, K.; Ikegami, M.; Endo, T.; Ishii, T.; Kataoka, K. Gene Transfection toward Spheroid Cells on Micropatterned Culture Plates for Genetically-modified Cell Transplantation. *J. Vis. Exp. JoVE* **2015**, e52384. [CrossRef] [PubMed]
122. Alessandri, K.; Sarangi, B.R.; Gurchenkov, V.V.; Sinha, B.; Kießling, T.R.; Fetler, L.; Rico, F.; Scheuring, S.; Lamaze, C.; Simon, A.; et al. Cellular capsules as a tool for multicellular spheroid production and for investigating the mechanics of tumor progression in vitro. *Proc Natl Acad Sci USA* **2013**, *110*, 14843–14848. [CrossRef] [PubMed]
123. Heo, D.N.; Hospodiuk, M.; Ozbolat, I.T. Synergistic interplay between human MSCs and HUVECs in 3D spheroids laden in collagen/fibrin hydrogels for bone tissue engineering. *Acta Biomater.* **2019**, *95*, 348–356. [CrossRef] [PubMed]
124. Utama, R.H.; Atapattu, L.; O'Mahony, A.P.; Fife, C.M.; Baek, J.; Allard, T.; O'Mahony, K.J.; Ribeiro, J.C.; Gaus, K.; Kavallaris, M.; et al. A 3D Bioprinter Specifically Designed for the High-Throughput Production of Matrix-Embedded Multicellular Spheroids. *iScience* **2020**, *23*. [CrossRef] [PubMed]
125. Tevis, K.M.; Cecchi, R.J.; Colson, Y.L.; Grinstaff, M.W. Mimicking the tumor microenvironment to regulate macrophage phenotype and assessing chemotherapeutic efficacy in embedded cancer cell/macrophage spheroid models. *Acta Biomater.* **2017**, *50*, 271–279. [CrossRef]
126. Jianmin, Z.; Hongfang, W.; Meifu, F. Resistance of multicellular aggregates to pharmorubicin observed in human hepatocarcinoma cells. *Braz. J. Med. Biol. Res.* **2002**, *35*, 255–260. [CrossRef]
127. Liu, H.; Seynhaeve, A.L.B.; Brouwer, R.W.W.; van IJcken, W.F.; Yang, L.; Wang, Y.; Chang, Z.; ten Hagen, T.L. CREPT Promotes Melanoma Progression Through Accelerated Proliferation and Enhanced Migration by RhoA-Mediated Actin Filaments and Focal Adhesion Formation. *Cancers* **2019**, *12*, 33. [CrossRef]
128. Marimuthu, M.; Rousset, N.; St-Georges-Robillard, A.; Lateef, M.A.; Ferland, M.; Mes-Masson, A.M.; Gervais, T. Multi-size spheroid formation using microfluidic funnels. *Lab Chip* **2018**, *18*, 304–314. [CrossRef]
129. Jeong, S.Y.; Lee, J.H.; Shin, Y.; Chung, S.; Kuh, H.J. Co-Culture of Tumor Spheroids and Fibroblasts in a Collagen Matrix-Incorporated Microfluidic Chip Mimics Reciprocal Activation in Solid Tumor Microenvironment. *PLoS ONE* **2016**, *11*, e0159013. [CrossRef]
130. Feng, H.; Ou, B.C.; Zhao, J.K.; Yin, S.; Lu, A.G.; Oechsle, E.; Thasler, W.E. Homogeneous pancreatic cancer spheroids mimic growth pattern of circulating tumor cell clusters and macrometastases: Displaying heterogeneity and crater-like structure on inner layer. *J. Cancer Res. Clin. Oncol.* **2017**, *143*, 1771–1786. [CrossRef]
131. Ivanov, D.P.; Parker, T.L.; Walker, D.A.; Alexander, C.; Ashford, M.B.; Gellert, P.R.; Garnett, M.C. Multiplexing spheroid volume, resazurin and acid phosphatase viability assays for high-throughput screening of tumour spheroids and stem cell neurospheres. *PLoS ONE* **2014**, *9*, e103817. [CrossRef] [PubMed]
132. Wang, S.; Wang, X.; Boone, J.; Wie, J.; Yip, K.P.; Zhang, J.; Wang, L.; Liu, R. Application of Hanging Drop Technique for Kidney Tissue Culture. *Kidney Blood Press. Res.* **2017**, *42*, 220–231. [CrossRef] [PubMed]
133. Acar, S.; Arslan, N.; Paketçi, A.; Okur, T.D.; Demir, K.; Böber, E.; Abacı, A. Presentation of central precocious puberty in two patients with Tay-Sachs disease. *Hormones* **2018**, *17*, 415–418. [CrossRef]
134. Jaganathan, H.; Gage, J.; Leonard, F.; Srinivasan, S.; Souza, G.R.; Dave, B.; Godin, B. Three-dimensional in vitro co-culture model of breast tumor using magnetic levitation. *Sci. Rep.* **2014**, *4*, 6468. [CrossRef] [PubMed]
135. Gonzalez-Fernandez, T.; Tenorio, A.J.; Leach, J.K. Three-Dimensional Printed Stamps for the Fabrication of Patterned Microwells and High-Throughput Production of Homogeneous Cell Spheroids. *3D Print Addit. Manuf.* **2020**, *7*, 139–147. [CrossRef] [PubMed]

136. Santos, J.M.; Camões, S.P.; Filipe, E.; Cipriano, M.; Barcia, R.N.; Filipe, M.; Teixeira, M.; Simões, S.; Gaspar, M.; Mosqueira, D. Three-dimensional spheroid cell culture of umbilical cord tissue-derived mesenchymal stromal cells leads to enhanced paracrine induction of wound healing. *Stem Cell Res. Ther.* **2015**, *6*, 90. [CrossRef] [PubMed]
137. Monjaret, F.; Fernandes, M.; Duchemin-Pelletier, E.; Argento, A.; Degot, S.; Young, J. Fully Automated One-Step Production of Functional 3D Tumor Spheroids for High-Content Screening. *J. Lab. Autom.* **2016**, *21*, 268–280. [CrossRef] [PubMed]
138. Otsuka, H.; Sasaki, K.; Okimura, S.; Nagamura, M.; Nakasone, Y. Micropatterned co-culture of hepatocyte spheroids layered on non-parenchymal cells to understand heterotypic cellular interactions. *Sci. Technol. Adv. Mater.* **2013**, *14*, 065003. [CrossRef] [PubMed]
139. Abe, Y.; Tada, A.; Isoyama, J.; Nagayama, S.; Yao, R.; Adachi, J.; Tomonaga, T. Improved phosphoproteomic analysis for phosphosignaling and active-kinome profiling in Matrigel-embedded spheroids and patient-derived organoids. *Sci. Rep.* **2018**, *8*, 1–12. [CrossRef]
140. Friedrich, J.; Seidel, C.; Ebner, R.; Kunz-Schughart, L.A. Spheroid-based drug screen: Considerations and practical approach. *Nat. Protoc.* **2009**, *4*, 309–324. [CrossRef]
141. Zanoni, M.; Pignatta, S.; Arienti, C.; Bonafè, M.; Tesei, A. Anticancer drug discovery using multicellular tumor spheroid models. *Expert Opin. Drug Discov.* **2019**, *14*, 289–301. [CrossRef] [PubMed]
142. Zanoni, M.; Piccinini, F.; Arienti, C.; Zamagni, A.; Santi, S.; Polico, R.; Bevilacqua, A.; Tesei, A. 3D tumor spheroid models for in vitro therapeutic screening: A systematic approach to enhance the biological relevance of data obtained. *Sci. Rep.* **2016**, *6*, 1–11. [CrossRef] [PubMed]
143. Piccinini, F.; Tesei, A.; Arienti, C.; Bevilacqua, A. Cancer multicellular spheroids: Volume assessment from a single 2D projection. *Comput. Methods Programs Biomed.* **2015**, *118*, 95–106. [CrossRef] [PubMed]
144. Correa de Sampaio, P.; Auslaender, D.; Krubasik, D.; Failla, A.V.; Skepper, J.N.; Murphy, G.; English, W.R. A heterogeneous in vitro three dimensional model of tumour-stroma interactions regulating sprouting angiogenesis. *PLoS ONE* **2012**, *7*, e30753. [CrossRef]
145. Ingeson-Carlsson, C.; Martinez-Monleon, A.; Nilsson, M. Differential effects of MAPK pathway inhibitors on migration and invasiveness of BRAF(V600E) mutant thyroid cancer cells in 2D and 3D culture. *Exp. Cell Res.* **2015**, *338*, 127–135. [CrossRef]
146. Moraes, G.S.; Wink, M.R.; Klamt, F.; Silva, A.O.; da Cruz Fernandes, M. Simplified low-cost methodology to establish, histologically process and analyze three-dimensional cancer cell spheroid arrays. *Eur. J. Cell Biol.* **2020**, *99*, 151095. [CrossRef]
147. Huisken, J.; Swoger, J.; Del Bene FWittbrodt, J.; Stelzer, E.H. Optical sectioning deep inside live embryos by selective plane illumination microscopy. *Science* **2004**, *305*, 1007–1009. [CrossRef]
148. Cella Zanacchi, F.; Lavagnino, Z.; Perrone Donnorso, M.; Del Bue, A.; Furia, L.; Faretta, M.; Diaspro, A. Live-cell 3D super-resolution imaging in thick biological samples. *Nat. Methods* **2011**, *8*, 1047–1049. [CrossRef]
149. Hwang, Y.J.; Kolettis, N.; Yang, M.; Gillard, E.R.; Sanchez, E.; Sun, C.H.; Tromberg, B.J.; Krasieva, T.B.; Lyubovitsky, J.G. Multiphoton imaging of actin filament formation and mitochondrial energetics of human ACBT gliomas. *Photochem. Photobiol.* **2011**, *87*, 408–417. [CrossRef]
150. Tesei, A.; Sarnelli, A.; Arienti, C.; Menghi, E.; Medri, L.; Gabucci, E.; Pignatta, S.; Falconi, M.; Silvestrini, R.; Zoli, W. In vitro irradiation system for radiobiological experiments. *Radiat. Oncol.* **2013**, *8*, 257. [CrossRef]
151. Huang, K.; Ma, H.; Liu, J.; Huo, S.; Kumar, A.; Wei, T.; Zhang, X.; Jin, S.; Gan, Y.; Wang, P.C. Size-dependent localization and penetration of ultrasmall gold nanoparticles in cancer cells, multicellular spheroids, and tumors in vivo. *ACS Nano* **2012**, *6*, 4483–4493. [CrossRef] [PubMed]
152. Costa, E.C.; Gaspar, V.M.; Coutinho, P.; Correia, I.J. Optimization of liquid overlay technique to formulate heterogenic 3D co-cultures models. *Biotechnol. Bioeng.* **2014**, *111*, 1672–1685. [CrossRef] [PubMed]
153. Yao, H.J.; Ju, R.J.; Wang, X.; Zhang, Y.; Li, R.J.; Yu, Y.; Zhang, L.; Lu, W.L. The antitumor efficacy of functional paclitaxel nanomicelles in treating resistant breast cancers by oral delivery. *Biomaterials* **2011**, *32*, 3285–3302. [CrossRef] [PubMed]
154. Uroukov, I.S.; Patton, D. Optimizing environmental scanning electron microscopy of spheroidal reaggregated neuronal cultures. *Microsc. Res. Tech.* **2008**, *71*, 792–801. [CrossRef] [PubMed]
155. Patra, B.; Peng, C.C.; Liao, W.H.; Lee, C.H.; Tung, Y.C. Drug testing and flow cytometry analysis on a large number of uniform sized tumor spheroids using a microfluidic device. *Sci. Rep.* **2016**, *6*. [CrossRef] [PubMed]

156. Beaumont, K.A.; Anfosso, A.; Ahmed, F.; Weninger, W.; Haass, N.K. Imaging- and Flow Cytometry-based Analysis of Cell Position and the Cell Cycle in 3D Melanoma Spheroids. *J. Vis. Exp.* **2015**, e53486. [CrossRef]
157. Durand, R.E. Use of Hoechst 33342 for cell selection from multicell systems. *J. Histochem. Cytochem.* **1982**, *30*, 117–122. [CrossRef]
158. Ho, W.Y.; Yeap, S.K.; Ho, C.L.; Rahim, R.A.; Alitheen, N.B. Development of multicellular tumor spheroid (MCTS) culture from breast cancer cell and a high throughput screening method using the MTT assay. *PLoS ONE* **2012**, *7*, e44640. [CrossRef]
159. Solomon, M.A.; Lemera, J.; D'Souza, G.G. Development of an in vitro tumor spheroid culture model amenable to high-throughput testing of potential anticancer nanotherapeutics. *J. Liposome Res.* **2016**, *26*, 246–260. [CrossRef]
160. Kessel, S.; Cribbes, S.; Bonasu, S.; Rice, W.; Qiu, J.; Chan, L.L.Y. Real-time viability and apoptosis kinetic detection method of 3D multicellular tumor spheroids using the Celigo Image Cytometer. *Cytom. A* **2017**, *91*, 883–892. [CrossRef]
161. Pignatta, S.; Orienti, I.; Falconi, M.; Teti, G.; Arienti, C.; Medri, L.; Zanoni, M.; Carloni, S.; Zoli, W.; Amadori, D. Albumin nanocapsules containing fenretinide: Pre-clinical evaluation of cytotoxic activity in experimental models of human non-small cell lung cancer. *Nanomedicine* **2015**, *11*, 263–273. [CrossRef] [PubMed]
162. Xin, H.; Sha, X.; Jiang, X.; Zhang, W.; Chen, L.; Fang, X. Anti-glioblastoma efficacy and safety of paclitaxel-loading Angiopep-conjugated dual targeting PEG-PCL nanoparticles. *Biomaterials* **2012**, *33*, 8167–8176. [CrossRef] [PubMed]
163. Robertson, F.; Ogasawara, M.A.; Ye, Z.; Chu, K.; Pickei, R.; Debeb, B.G.; Woodward, W.A.; Hittelman, W.N.; Cristofanilli, M.; Barsky, S.H. Imaging and analysis of 3D tumor spheroids enriched for a cancer stem cell phenotype. *J. Biomol. Screen* **2010**, *15*, 820–829. [CrossRef]
164. Schneckenburger, H.; Weber, P.; Wagner, M.; Schickinger, S.; Richter, V.; Bruns, T.; Strauss, W.; Wittig, R. Light exposure and cell viability in fluorescence microscopy. *J. Microsc.* **2011**, *245*, 311–318. [CrossRef] [PubMed]
165. Darrigues, E.; Nima, Z.A.; Nedosekin, D.A.; Watanabe, F.; Alghazali, K.M.; Zharov, V.P.; Biris, A.S. Tracking Gold Nanorods' Interaction with Large 3D Pancreatic-Stromal Tumor Spheroids by Multimodal Imaging, Fluorescence, Photoacoustic, and Photothermal Microscopies. *Sci. Rep.* **2020**, *10*, 1–14. [CrossRef]
166. Vinci, M.; Gowan, S.; Boxall, F.; Patterson, L.; Zimmermann, M.; Court, W.; Lomas, C.; Mendiola, M.; Hardisson, D.; Eccles, S.A.; et al. Advances in establishment and analysis of three-dimensional tumor spheroid-based functional assays for target validation and drug evaluation. *BMC Biol.* **2012**, *10*, 29. [CrossRef]
167. Yakavets, I.; Jenard, S.; Francois, A.; Maklygina, Y.; Loschenov, V.; Lassalle, H.-P.; Dolivet, G.; Bezdetnaya, L. Stroma-Rich Co-Culture Multicellular Tumor Spheroids as a Tool for Photoactive Drugs Screening. *J. Clin. Med.* **2019**, *8*, 1686. [CrossRef]
168. Shi, W.; Kwon, J.; Huang, Y.; Tan, J.; Uhl, C.G.; He, R.; Zhou, C.; Liu, Y. Facile Tumor Spheroids Formation in Large Quantity with Controllable Size and High Uniformity. *Sci. Rep.* **2018**, *8*, 6837. [CrossRef]
169. Ivanov, D.P.; Grabowska, A.M. Spheroid arrays for high-throughput single-cell analysis of spatial patterns and biomarker expression in 3D. *Sci. Rep.* **2017**, *7*, 1–12. [CrossRef]
170. Ansari, N.; Müller, S.; Stelzer, E.H.; Pampaloni, F. Quantitative 3D cell-based assay performed with cellular spheroids and fluorescence microscopy. *Methods Cell Biol.* **2013**, *113*, 295–309.
171. Leary, E.; Rhee, C.; Wilks, B.T.; Morgan, J.R. Quantitative Live-Cell Confocal Imaging of 3D Spheroids in a High-Throughput Format. *SLAS Technol.* **2018**, *23*, 231–242. [CrossRef] [PubMed]
172. Durymanov, M.; Kroll, C.; Permyakova, A.; O'Neill, E.; Sulaiman, R.; Person, M.; Reineke, J. Subcutaneous Inoculation of 3D Pancreatic Cancer Spheroids Results in Development of Reproducible Stroma-Rich Tumors. *Transl. Oncol.* **2019**, *12*, 180–189. [CrossRef] [PubMed]
173. Nürnberg, E.; Vitacolonna, M.; Klicks, J.; Von Molitor, E.; Cesetti, T.; Keller, F.; Bruch, R.; Ertongur-Fauth, T.; Riedel, K.; Scholz, P.; et al. Routine Optical Clearing of 3D-Cell Cultures, Simplicity Forward. *Front. Mol. Biosci.* **2020**, *7*, 20. [CrossRef]
174. Diaspro, A.; Federici, F.; Robello, M. Influence of refractive-index mismatch in high-resolution three-dimensional confocal microscopy. *Appl. Opt.* **2002**, *41*, 685–690. [CrossRef] [PubMed]
175. Lazzari, G.; Vinciguerra, D.; Balasso, A.; Nicolas, V.; Goudin, N.; Garfa-Traore, M.; Féher, A.; Dinnyés, A.; Nicolas, J.; Couvreur, P.; et al. Light sheet fluorescence microscopy versus confocal microscopy: In quest of a suitable tool to assess drug and nanomedicine penetration into multicellular tumor spheroids. *Eur. J. Pharm. Biopharm.* **2019**, *142*, 195–203. [CrossRef]

176. Buglak, N.E.; Lucitti, J.; Ariel, P.; Maiocchi, S.L.; Miller, F.J.; Bahnson, E.S.M. Light Sheet Fluorescence Microscopy as a New Method for Unbiased Three-Dimensional Analysis of Vascular Injury. *Cardiovasc. Res* **2020**. [CrossRef]
177. Smyrek, I.; Stelzer, E.H. Quantitative three-dimensional evaluation of immunofluorescence staining for large whole mount spheroids with light sheet microscopy. *Biomed. Opt. Express* **2017**, *8*, 484–499. [CrossRef]
178. Lazzari, G.; Nicolas, V.; Matsusaki, M.; Akashi, M.; Couvreur, P.; Mura, S. Multicellular spheroid based on a triple co-culture, A novel 3D model to mimic pancreatic tumor complexity. *Acta Biomater.* **2018**, *78*, 296–307. [CrossRef]
179. Stern, T.; Kaner, I.; Zer, N.L.; Shoval, H.; Dror, D.; Manevitch, Z.; Chai, L.; Brill-Karniely, Y.; Benny, O. Rigidity of polymer micelles affects interactions with tumor cells. *J. Control. Release* **2017**, *257*, 40–50. [CrossRef]
180. Wan, X.; Li, Z.; Ye, H.; Cui, Z. Three-dimensional perfused tumour spheroid model for anti-cancer drug screening. *Biotechnol. Lett.* **2016**, *38*, 1389–1395. [CrossRef]
181. Nylk, J.; McCluskey, K.; Preciado, M.A.; Mazilu, M.; Yang, Z.; Gunn-Moore, F.J.; Aggarwal, S.; Tello, J.A.; Ferrier, D.E.K.; Dholakia, K. Light-sheet microscopy with attenuation-compensated propagation-invariant beams. *Sci. Adv.* **2018**, *4*, eaar4817. [CrossRef] [PubMed]
182. Shemesh, Z.; Chaimovich, G.; Gino, L.; Ozana, N.; Nylk, J.; Dholakia, K.; Zalevsky, Z. Reducing data acquisition for light-sheet microscopy by extrapolation between imaged planes. *J. Biophotonics* **2020**, *13*, e202000035. [CrossRef] [PubMed]
183. Zhao, F.; Yang, Y.; Li, Y.; Jiang, H.; Xie, X.; Yu, T.; Wang, X.; Liu, Q.; Zhang, H.; Jia, H.; et al. Efficient and cost-effective 3D cellular imaging by sub-voxel-resolving light-sheet add-on microscopy. *J. Biophotonics* **2020**, *13*, e201960243. [CrossRef] [PubMed]
184. Lin, H.; Fan, T.; Sui, J.; Wang, G.; Chen, J.; Zhuo, S.; Zhang, H. Recent advances in multiphoton microscopy combined with nanomaterials in the field of disease evolution and clinical applications to liver cancer. *Nanoscale* **2019**, *11*, 19619–19635. [CrossRef]
185. Sato, R.; Yasukawa, T.; Kacza, J.; Eichler, W.; Nishiwaki, A.; Iandiev, I.; Ohbayashi, M.; Kato, A.; Yafai, Y.; Bringmann, A.; et al. Three-Dimensional Spheroidal Culture Visualization of Membranogenesis of Bruch's Membrane and Basolateral Functions of the Retinal Pigment Epithelium. *Investig. Ophthalmol. Vis. Sci.* **2013**, *54*, 1740–1749. [CrossRef]
186. Beauchamp, P.; Jackson, C.B.; Ozhathil, L.C.; Agarkova, I.; Galindo, C.L.; Sawyer, D.B.; Suter, T.M.; Zuppinger, C. 3D Co-culture of hiPSC-Derived Cardiomyocytes With Cardiac Fibroblasts Improves Tissue-Like Features of Cardiac Spheroids. *Front. Mol. Biosci.* **2020**, *7*, 14. [CrossRef]
187. Hortelão, A.C.; Carrascosa, R.; Murillo-Cremaes, N.; Patiño, T.; Sanchez, S. Targeting 3D Bladder Cancer Spheroids with Urease-Powered Nanomotors. *ACS Nano* **2019**, *13*, 429–439. [CrossRef]
188. Chelobanov, B.; Poletaeva, J.; Epanchintseva, A.; Tupitsyna, A.; Pyshnaya, I.; Ryabchikova, E. Ultrastructural Features of Gold Nanoparticles Interaction with HepG2 and HEK293 Cells in Monolayer and Spheroids. *Nanomaterials* **2020**, *10*, 2040. [CrossRef]
189. Salehi, F.; Behboudi, H.; Kavoosi, G.; Ardestani, S.K. Monitoring ZEO apoptotic potential in 2D and 3D cell cultures and associated spectroscopic evidence on mode of interaction with DNA. *Sci. Rep.* **2017**, *7*, 2553. [CrossRef]
190. Nigjeh, S.E.; Yeap, S.K.; Nordin, N.; Kamalideghan, B.; Ky, H.; Rosli, R. Citral induced apoptosis in MDA-MB-231 spheroid cells. *BMC Complement. Altern. Med.* **2018**, *18*, 56. [CrossRef]
191. Salehi, F.; Jamali, T.; Kavoosi, G.; Ardestani, S.K.; Vahdati, S.N. Stabilization of Zataria essential oil with pectin-based nanoemulsion for enhanced cytotoxicity in monolayer and spheroid drug-resistant breast cancer cell cultures and deciphering its binding mode with gDNA. *Int. J. Biol. Macromol.* **2020**, *164*, 3645–3655. [CrossRef] [PubMed]
192. Mirab, F.; Kang, Y.J.; Majd, S. Preparation and characterization of size-controlled glioma spheroids using agarose hydrogel microwells. *PLoS ONE* **2019**, *14*, e0211078. [CrossRef] [PubMed]
193. Svirshchevskaya, E.; Doronina, E.; Grechikhina, M.; Matushevskaya, E.; Kotsareva, O.; Fattakhova, G.; Sapozhnikov, A.; Felix, K. Characteristics of multicellular tumor spheroids formed by pancreatic cells expressing different adhesion molecules. *Life Sci.* **2019**, *219*, 343–352. [CrossRef] [PubMed]
194. Khaitan, D.; Chandna, S.; Arya, M.B.; Dwarakanath, B.S. Establishment and characterization of multicellular spheroids from a human glioma cell line; Implications for tumor therapy. *J. Transl. Med.* **2006**, *4*, 12. [CrossRef]

195. Liu, J.; Li, J.; Li, P.; Wang, Y.; Liang, Z.; Jiang, Y.; Li, J.; Feng, C.; Wang, R.; Chen, H.; et al. Loss of DLG5 promotes breast cancer malignancy by inhibiting the Hippo signaling pathway. *Sci. Rep.* **2017**, *7*, 42125. [CrossRef]
196. Wang, Q.; Bu, S.; Xin, D.; Li, B.; Wang, L.; Lai, D. Autophagy Is Indispensable for the Self-Renewal and Quiescence of Ovarian Cancer Spheroid Cells with Stem Cell-Like Properties. *Oxidative Med. Cell. Longev.* **2018**, *2018*, 7010472. [CrossRef]
197. Bauleth-Ramos, T.; Feijão, T.; Gonçalves, A.; Shahbazi, M.-A.; Liu, Z.; Barrias, C.; Oliveira, M.J.; Granja, P.; Santos, H.A.; Sarmento, B. Colorectal cancer triple co-culture spheroid model to assess the biocompatibility and anticancer properties of polymeric nanoparticles. *J. Control. Release* **2020**, *323*, 398–411. [CrossRef]
198. Guo, X.; Chen, Y.; Ji, W.; Chen, X.; Li, C.; Ge, R. Enrichment of cancer stem cells by agarose multi-well dishes and 3D spheroid culture. *Cell Tissue Res.* **2019**, *375*, 397–408. [CrossRef]
199. Lu, H.; Stenzel, M.H. Multicellular Tumor Spheroids (MCTS) as a 3D In Vitro Evaluation Tool of Nanoparticles. *Small* **2018**, *14*, e1702858. [CrossRef]
200. Askari, E.; Naghib, S.M.; Seyfoori, A.; Maleki, A.; Rahmanian, M. Ultrasonic-assisted synthesis and in vitro biological assessments of a novel herceptin-stabilized graphene using three dimensional cell spheroid. *Ultrason Sonochemistry* **2019**, *58*, 104615. [CrossRef]
201. Flampouri, E.; Imar, S.; Oconnell, K.; Singh, B. Spheroid-3D and Monolayer-2D Intestinal Electrochemical Biosensor for Toxicity/Viability Testing, Applications in Drug Screening, Food Safety, and Environmental Pollutant Analysis. *ACS Sens.* **2019**, *4*, 660–669. [CrossRef] [PubMed]
202. Friedrich, J.; Eder, W.; Castaneda, J.; Doss, M.; Huber, E.; Ebner, R.; Kunz-Schughart, L.A. A reliable tool to determine cell viability in complex 3-d culture: The acid phosphatase assay. *J. Biomol. Screen.* **2007**, *12*, 925–937. [CrossRef] [PubMed]
203. Rolver, M.G.; Elingaard-Larsen, L.O.; Pedersen, S.F. Assessing Cell Viability and Death in 3D Spheroid Cultures of Cancer Cells. *J. Vis. Exp.* **2019**, e59714. [CrossRef]
204. Kijanska, M.; Kelm, J. In vitro 3D Spheroids and Microtissues, ATP-based Cell Viability and Toxicity Assays. In *Assay Guidance Manual*; Markossian, S., Sittampalam, G.S., Grossman, A., Brimacombe, K., Arkin, M., Auld, D., Austin, C.P., Baell, J., Caaveiro, J.M.M., Chung, T.D.Y., et al., Eds.; Eli Lilly & Company and the National Center for Advancing Translational Sciences: Bethesda, MD, USA, 2004.
205. Aughton, K.; Shahidipour, H.; Djirackor, L.; Coupland, S.E.; Kalirai, H. Characterization of Uveal Melanoma Cell Lines and Primary Tumor Samples in 3D Culture. *Transl. Vis. Sci. Technol.* **2020**, *9*, 39. [CrossRef]
206. Huang, Z.; Yu, P.; Tang, J. Characterization of Triple-Negative Breast Cancer MDA-MB-231 Cell Spheroid Model. *OncoTargets Ther.* **2020**, *13*, 5395–5405. [CrossRef]
207. Posimo, J.M.; Unnithan, A.S.; Gleixner, A.M.; Choi, H.J.; Jiang, Y.; Pulugulla, S.H.; Leak, R.K. Viability assays for cells in culture. *J. Vis. Exp.* **2014**, e50645. [CrossRef] [PubMed]
208. Norberg, K.J.; Liu, X.; Moro, C.F.; Strell, C.; Nania, S.; Blümel, M.; Balboni, A.; Bozóky, B.; Heuchel, R.L.; Löhr, J.M. A novel pancreatic tumour and stellate cell 3D co-culture spheroid model. *BMC Cancer* **2020**, *20*, 1–13. [CrossRef]
209. Sano, K.; Usui, M.; Moritani, Y.; Nakazawa, K.; Hanatani, T.; Kondo, H.; Nakatomi, M.; Onizuka, S.; Iwata, T.; Sato, T.; et al. Co-cultured spheroids of human periodontal ligament mesenchymal stem cells and vascular endothelial cells enhance periodontal tissue regeneration. *Regen. Ther.* **2020**, *14*, 59–71. [CrossRef]
210. Mori, Y.; Yamawaki, K.; Ishiguro, T.; Yoshihara, K.; Ueda, H.; Sato, A.; Ohata, H.; Yoshida, Y.; Minamino, T.; Okamoto, K.; et al. ALDH-Dependent Glycolytic Activation Mediates Stemness and Paclitaxel Resistance in Patient-Derived Spheroid Models of Uterine Endometrial Cancer. *Stem Cell Rep.* **2019**, *13*, 730–746. [CrossRef]
211. Joshi, J.; Mahajan, G.; Kothapalli, C.R. Three-dimensional collagenous niche and azacytidine selectively promote time-dependent cardiomyogenesis from human bone marrow-derived MSC spheroids. *Biotechnol. Bioeng.* **2018**, *115*, 2013–2026. [CrossRef]
212. Khaitan, D.; Dwarakanath, B.S. Multicellular spheroids as an in vitro model in experimental oncology: Applications in translational medicine. *Expert Opin. Drug Discov.* **2006**, *1*, 663–675. [CrossRef] [PubMed]
213. Sacks, D.; Baxter, B.; Campbell, B.C.; Carpenter, J.S.; Cognard, C.; Dippel, D.; Eesa, M.; Fischer, U.; Hausegger, K.; Hirsch, J.A. Multisociety Consensus Quality Improvement Revised Consensus Statement for Endovascular Therapy of Acute Ischemic Stroke. *Int. J. Stroke* **2018**, *13*, 612–632. [CrossRef] [PubMed]

214. Barbone, D.; Yang, T.M.; Morgan, J.; Gaudino, G.; Broaddus, V.C. Mammalian target of rapamycin contributes to the acquired apoptotic resistance of human mesothelioma multicellular spheroids. *J. Biol. Chem.* **2008**, *283*, 13021–13030. [CrossRef] [PubMed]
215. Huanwen, W.; Zhiyong, L.; Xiaohua, S.; Xinyu, R.; Kai, W.; Tonghua, L. Intrinsic chemoresistance to gemcitabine is associated with constitutive and laminin-induced phosphorylation of FAK in pancreatic cancer cell lines. *Mol. Cancer* **2009**, *8*, 125. [CrossRef] [PubMed]
216. Thomas, F.; Holly, J.M.; Persad, R.; Bahl, A.; Perks, C.M. Fibronectin confers survival against chemotherapeutic agents but not against radiotherapy in DU145 prostate cancer cells: Involvement of the insulin like growth factor-1 receptor. *Prostate* **2010**, *70*, 856–865. [CrossRef]
217. Weigelt, B.; Lo, A.T.; Park, C.C.; Gray, J.W.; Bissell, M.J. HER2 signaling pathway activation and response of breast cancer cells to HER2-targeting agents is dependent strongly on the 3D microenvironment. *Breast Cancer Res. Treat.* **2010**, *122*, 35–43. [CrossRef]
218. Liao, J.; Qian, F.; Tchabo, N.; Mhawech-Fauceglia, P.; Beck, A.; Qian, Z.; Wang, X.; Huss, W.J.; Lele, S.B.; Morrison, C.D.; et al. Ovarian cancer spheroid cells with stem cell-like properties contribute to tumor generation, metastasis and chemotherapy resistance through hypoxia-resistant metabolism. *PLoS ONE* **2014**, *9*, e84941. [CrossRef]
219. Wartenberg, M.; Hoffmann, E.; Schwindt, H.; Grünheck, F.; Petros, J.; Arnold, J.R.S.; Hescheler, J.; Sauer, H. Reactive oxygen species-linked regulation of the multidrug resistance transporter P-glycoprotein in Nox-1 overexpressing prostate tumor spheroids. *FEBS Lett.* **2005**, *579*, 4541–4549. [CrossRef]
220. Hoffmann, O.; Ilmberger, C.; Magosch, S.; Joka, M.; Jauch, K.-W.; Mayer, B. Impact of the spheroid model complexity on drug response. *J. Biotechnol.* **2015**, *205*, 14–23. [CrossRef]
221. Sethi, T.; Rintoul, R.C.; Moore, S.M.; MacKinnon, A.C.; Salter, D.; Choo, C.; Chilvers, E.R.; Dransfield, I.; Donnelly, S.C.; Strieter, R.M.; et al. Extracellular matrix proteins protect small cell lung cancer cells against apoptosis: A mechanism for small cell lung cancer growth and drug resistance in vivo. *Nat. Med.* **1999**, *5*, 662–668. [CrossRef]
222. Aoudjit, F.; Vuori, K. Integrin signaling inhibits paclitaxel-induced apoptosis in breast cancer cells. *Oncogene* **2001**, *20*, 4995–5004. [CrossRef] [PubMed]
223. Nunes, A.S.; Barros, A.S.; Costa, E.C.; Moreira, A.F.; Correia, I.J. 3D tumor spheroids as in vitro models to mimic in vivo human solid tumors resistance to therapeutic drugs. *Biotechnol. Bioeng.* **2019**, *116*, 206–226. [CrossRef] [PubMed]
224. Frankel, A.; Man, S.; Elliott, P.; Adams, J.; Kerbel, R.S. Lack of multicellular drug resistance observed in human ovarian and prostate carcinoma treated with the proteasome inhibitor PS-341. *Clin. Cancer Res.* **2000**, *6*, 3719–3728. [PubMed]
225. Ferrante, A.; Rainaldi, G.; Indovina, P.; Indovina, P.L.; Santini, M.T. Increased cell compaction can augment the resistance of HT-29 human colon adenocarcinoma spheroids to ionizing radiation. *Int. J. Oncol.* **2006**, *28*, 111–118. [CrossRef]
226. Olive, P.L.; Durand, R.E. Drug and radiation resistance in spheroids: Cell contact and kinetics. *Cancer Metastasis Rev.* **1994**, *13*, 121–138. [CrossRef]
227. Robert Grimes, D.; Partridge, M. A mechanistic investigation of the oxygen fixation hypothesis and oxygen enhancement ratio. *Biomed. Phys. Eng. Express* **2015**, *1*, 045209. [CrossRef]
228. Horan, A.D.; Giandomenico, A.R.; Koch, C.J. Effect of oxygen on radiation-induced DNA damage in isolated nuclei. *Radiat. Res.* **1999**, *152*, 144–153. [CrossRef]
229. Lefranc, F.; Brotchi, J.; Kiss, R. Possible future issues in the treatment of glioblastomas: Special emphasis on cell migration and the resistance of migrating glioblastoma cells to apoptosis. *J. Clin. Oncol.* **2005**, *23*, 2411–2422. [CrossRef]
230. Erler, J.T.; Weaver, V.M. Three-dimensional context regulation of metastasis. *Clin. Exp. Metastasis* **2009**, *26*, 35–49. [CrossRef]
231. Jessup, J.M.; Brown, D.; Fitzgerald, W.; Ford, R.D.; Nachman, A.; Goodwin, T.J.; Spaulding, G. Induction of carcinoembryonic antigen expression in a three-dimensional culture system. *In Vitro Cell Dev. Biol. Anim.* **1997**, *33*, 352–357. [CrossRef]
232. Vinci, M.; Box, C.; Zimmermann, M.; Eccles, S.A. Tumor spheroid-based migration assays for evaluation of therapeutic agents. *Methods Mol. Biol.* **2013**, *986*, 253–266. [PubMed]

233. Weiswald, L.B.; Bellet, D.; Dangles-Marie, V. Spherical cancer models in tumor biology. *Neoplasia* **2015**, *17*, 1–15. [CrossRef] [PubMed]
234. Cattin, S.; Ramont, L.; Rüegg, C. Characterization and In Vivo Validation of a Three-Dimensional Multi-Cellular Culture Model to Study Heterotypic Interactions in Colorectal Cancer Cell Growth, Invasion and Metastasis. *Front. Bioeng. Biotechnol.* **2018**, *6*, 97. [CrossRef] [PubMed]
235. Almahmoudi, R.; Salem, A.; Murshid, S.; Dourado, M.R.; Apu, E.H.; Salo, T.; Al-Samadi, A. Interleukin-17F Has Anti-Tumor Effects in Oral Tongue Cancer. *Cancers* **2019**, *11*, 650. [CrossRef]
236. Gao, Q.; Yang, Z.; Xu, S.; Li, X.; Yang, X.; Jin, P.; Liu, Y.; Zhou, X.; Zhang, T.; Gong, C.; et al. Heterotypic CAF-tumor spheroids promote early peritoneal metastatis of ovarian cancer. *J. Exp. Med.* **2019**, *216*, 688–703. [CrossRef]
237. Yamamoto, S.; Hotta, M.M.; Okochi, M.; Honda, H. Effect of vascular formed endothelial cell network on the invasive capacity of melanoma using the in vitro 3D co-culture patterning model. *PLoS ONE* **2014**, *9*, e103502. [CrossRef]
238. Vinci, M.; Box, C.; Eccles, S.A. Three-dimensional (3D) tumor spheroid invasion assay. *J. Vis. Exp.* **2015**, e52686. [CrossRef]
239. Berens, E.B.; Holy, J.M.; Riegel, A.T.; Wellstein, A. A Cancer Cell Spheroid Assay to Assess Invasion in a 3D Setting. *J. Vis. Exp.* **2015**, e53409. [CrossRef]
240. De Wever, O.; Hendrix, A.; De Boeck, A.; Eertmans, F.; Westbroek, W.; Braems, G.; Bracke, M.E. Single cell and spheroid collagen type I invasion assay. *Methods Mol. Biol.* **2014**, *1070*, 13–35.
241. Febles, N.K.; Ferrie, A.M.; Fang, Y. Label-free single cell kinetics of the invasion of spheroidal colon cancer cells through 3D Matrigel. *Anal. Chem.* **2014**, *86*, 8842–8849. [CrossRef]
242. Bell, H.S.; Wharton, S.B.; Leaver, H.A.; Whittle, I.R. Effects of N-6 essential fatty acids on glioma invasion and growth: Experimental studies with glioma spheroids in collagen gels. *J. Neurosurg.* **1999**, *91*, 989–996. [CrossRef] [PubMed]
243. Marchal, S.; El Hor, A.; Millard, M.; Gillon, V.; Bezdetnaya, L. Anticancer Drug Delivery, An Update on Clinically Applied Nanotherapeutics. *Drugs* **2015**, *75*, 1601–1611. [CrossRef] [PubMed]
244. Aldawsari, H.M.; Singh, S. Rapid Microwave-Assisted Cisplatin-Loaded Solid Lipid Nanoparticles, Synthesis, Characterization and Anticancer Study. *Nanomaterials* **2020**, *10*, 510. [CrossRef] [PubMed]
245. Wang, H.; Li, L.; Ye, J.; Wang, R.; Wang, R.; Hu, J.; Wang, Y.; Dong, W.; Xia, X.; Yang, Y.; et al. Improving the Oral Bioavailability of an Anti-Glioma Prodrug CAT3 Using Novel Solid Lipid Nanoparticles Containing Oleic Acid-CAT3 Conjugates. *Pharmaceutics* **2020**, *12*, 126. [CrossRef]
246. Zielińska, A.; Ferreira, N.R.; Durazzo, A.; Lucarini, M.; Cicero, N.; Mamouni, S.E.; Silva, A.M.; Nowak, I.; Santini, A.; Souto, E.B. Development and Optimization of Alpha-Pinene-Loaded Solid Lipid Nanoparticles (SLN) Using Experimental Factorial Design and Dispersion Analysis. *Molecules* **2019**, *24*, 2683. [CrossRef]
247. Lukowski, J.K.; Hummon, A.B. Quantitative evaluation of liposomal doxorubicin and its metabolites in spheroids. *Anal. Bioanal. Chem.* **2019**, *411*, 7087–7094. [CrossRef]
248. Yang, S.; Gao, H. Nanoparticles for modulating tumor microenvironment to improve drug delivery and tumor therapy. *Pharmacol. Res.* **2017**, *126*, 97–108. [CrossRef]
249. Davies Cde, L.; Berk, D.A.; Pluen, A.; Jain, R.K. Comparison of IgG diffusion and extracellular matrix composition in rhabdomyosarcomas grown in mice versus in vitro as spheroids reveals the role of host stromal cells. *Br. J. Cancer* **2002**, *86*, 1639–1644. [CrossRef]
250. Hobbs, S.K.; Monsky, W.L.; Yuan, F.; Roberts, W.G.; Griffith, L.; Torchilin, V.P.; Jain, R.K. Regulation of transport pathways in tumor vessels: Role of tumor type and microenvironment. *Proc Natl Acad Sci USA* **1998**, *95*, 4607–4612. [CrossRef]
251. Prabhakar, U.; Maeda, H.; Jain, R.K.; Sevick-Muraca, E.M.; Zamboni, W.; Farokhzad, O.C.; Barry, S.T.; Gabizon, A.; Grodzinski, P.; Blakey, D.C. Challenges and key considerations of the enhanced permeability and retention effect for nanomedicine drug delivery in oncology. *Cancer Res.* **2013**, *73*, 2412–2417. [CrossRef]
252. Patel, N.R.; Aryasomayajula, B.; Abouzeid, A.H.; Torchilin, V.P. Cancer cell spheroids for screening of chemotherapeutics and drug-delivery systems. *Ther. Deliv.* **2015**, *6*, 509–520. [CrossRef] [PubMed]
253. Jin, H.; Gui, R.; Sun, J.; Wang, Y. RETRACTED, Facilely self-assembled magnetic nanoparticles/aptamer/carbon dots nanocomposites for highly sensitive up-conversion fluorescence turn-on detection of tetrodotoxin. *Talanta* **2018**, *176*, 277–283. [CrossRef] [PubMed]

254. Millard, M.; Yakavets, I.; Zorin, V.; Kulmukhamedova, A.; Marchal, S.; Bezdetnaya, L. Drug delivery to solid tumors: The predictive value of the multicellular tumor spheroid model for nanomedicine screening. *Int. J. Nanomed.* **2017**, *12*, 7993–8007. [CrossRef] [PubMed]
255. Bugno, J.; Hsu, H.-J.; Pearson, R.M.; Noh, H.; Hong, S. Size and Surface Charge of Engineered Poly(amidoamine) Dendrimers Modulate Tumor Accumulation and Penetration, A Model Study Using Multicellular Tumor Spheroids. *Mol. Pharm.* **2016**, *13*, 2155–2163. [CrossRef]
256. Ni, D.; Ding, H.; Liu, S.; Yue, H.; Bao, Y.; Wang, Z.; Su, Z.; Wei, W.; Ma, G. Superior intratumoral penetration of paclitaxel nanodots strengthens tumor restriction and metastasis prevention. *Small* **2015**, *11*, 2518–2526. [CrossRef]
257. Agarwal, R.; Jurney, P.; Raythatha, M.; Singh, V.; Sreenivasan, S.V.; Shi, L.; Roy, K. Effect of shape, size, and aspect ratio on nanoparticle penetration and distribution inside solid tissues using 3D spheroid models. *Adv. Healthc. Mater.* **2015**, *4*, 2269–2280. [CrossRef]
258. Goodman, T.T.; Olive, P.L.; Pun, S.H. Increased nanoparticle penetration in collagenase-treated multicellular spheroids. *Int. J. Nanomed.* **2007**, *2*, 265–274.
259. Hinger, D.; Navarro, F.P.; Käch, A.; Thomann, J.-S.; Mittler, F.; Couffin, A.-C.; Maake, C. Photoinduced effects of m-tetrahydroxyphenylchlorin loaded lipid nanoemulsions on multicellular tumor spheroids. *J. Nanobiotechnology* **2016**, *14*, 68. [CrossRef]
260. Ernsting, M.J.; Murakami, M.; Roy, A.; Li, S.D. Factors controlling the pharmacokinetics, biodistribution and intratumoral penetration of nanoparticles. *J Control. Release* **2013**, *172*, 782–794. [CrossRef]
261. Kim, B.; Han, G.; Toley, B.J.; Kim, C.; Rotello, V.M.; Forbes, N.S. Tuning payload delivery in tumour cylindroids using gold nanoparticles. *Nat. Nanotechnol.* **2010**, *5*, 465–472. [CrossRef]
262. Chauhan, V.P.; Popović, Z.; Chen, O.; Cui, J.; Fukumura, D.; Bawendi, M.G.; Jain, R.K. Fluorescent nanorods and nanospheres for real-time in vivo probing of nanoparticle shape-dependent tumor penetration. *Angew. Chem. Int. Ed. Engl.* **2011**, *50*, 11417–11420. [CrossRef] [PubMed]
263. Wang, Y.; Kibbe, M.R.; Ameer, G.A. Photo-crosslinked Biodegradable Elastomers for Controlled Nitric Oxide Delivery. *Biomater. Sci.* **2013**, *1*, 625–632. [CrossRef] [PubMed]
264. Zhao, J.; Lu, H.; Xiao, P.; Stenzel, M.H. Cellular Uptake and Movement in 2D and 3D Multicellular Breast Cancer Models of Fructose-Based Cylindrical Micelles That Is Dependent on the Rod Length. *ACS Appl. Mater. Interfaces* **2016**, *8*, 16622–16630. [CrossRef] [PubMed]
265. Michy, T.; Massias, T.; Bernard, C.; VanWonterghem, L.; Henry, M.; Guidetti, M.; Royal, G.; Coll, J.-L.; Texier, I.; Josserand, V.; et al. Verteporfin-Loaded Lipid Nanoparticles Improve Ovarian Cancer Photodynamic Therapy In Vitro and In Vivo. *Cancers* **2019**, *11*, 1760. [CrossRef] [PubMed]
266. Chen, H.; Wei, X.; Chen, H.; Wei, H.; Wang, Y.; Nan, W.; Zhang, Q.; Wen, X. The study of establishment of an in vivo tumor model by three-dimensional cells culture systems methods and evaluation of antitumor effect of biotin-conjugated pullulan acetate nanoparticles. *Artif. Cells Nanomed. Biotechnol.* **2019**, *47*, 123–131. [CrossRef]
267. Wang, X.; Zhen, X.; Wang, J.; Zhang, J.; Wu, W.; Jiang, X. Doxorubicin delivery to 3D multicellular spheroids and tumors based on boronic acid-rich chitosan nanoparticles. *Biomaterials* **2013**, *34*, 4667–4679. [CrossRef]

Publisher's Note: MDPI stays neutral with regard to jurisdictional claims in published maps and institutional affiliations.

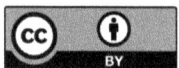

© 2020 by the authors. Licensee MDPI, Basel, Switzerland. This article is an open access article distributed under the terms and conditions of the Creative Commons Attribution (CC BY) license (http://creativecommons.org/licenses/by/4.0/).

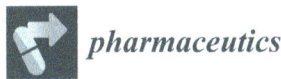

Review

Extracellular Vesicles as Drug Delivery Systems in Cancer

Laia Hernandez-Oller [1], Joaquin Seras-Franzoso [1], Fernanda Andrade [1,2], Diana Rafael [1,2], Ibane Abasolo [1,2], Petra Gener [1,2,*] and Simo Schwartz Jr. [1,2,*]

[1] Drug Delivery and Targeting Group, Molecular Biology and Biochemistry Research Centre for Nanomedicine (CIBBIM-Nanomedicine), Vall d'Hebron Institut de Recerca, Universitat Autònoma de Barcelona, 08035 Barcelona, Spain; laia.hernandez@alumni.vhir.org (L.H.-O.); joaquin.seras@vhir.org (J.S.-F.); fernanda.silva@vhir.org (F.A.); diana.fernandes_de_so@vhir.org (D.R.); ibane.abasolo@vhir.org (I.A.)

[2] Networking Research Centre for Bioengineering, Biomaterials, and Nanomedicine (CIBER-BBN), Instituto de Salud Carlos III, 50004 Zaragoza, Spain

* Correspondence: petra.gener@vhir.org (P.G.); simo.schwartz@vhir.org (S.S.J.); Tel.: +34-93489-4055 (P.G. & S.S.J.)

Received: 30 September 2020; Accepted: 23 November 2020; Published: 26 November 2020

Abstract: Within tumors, Cancer Stem Cell (CSC) subpopulation has an important role in maintaining growth and dissemination while preserving high resistance against current treatments. It has been shown that, when CSCs are eliminated, the surrounding Differentiated Cancer Cells (DCCs) may reverse their phenotype and gain CSC-like features to preserve tumor progression and ensure tumor survival. This strongly suggests the existence of paracrine communication within tumor cells. It is evidenced that the molecular crosstalk is at least partly mediated by Extracellular Vesicles (EVs), which are cell-derived membranous nanoparticles that contain and transport complex molecules that can affect and modify the biological behavior of distal cells and their molecular background. This ability of directional transport of small molecules prospects EVs as natural Drug Delivery Systems (DDS). EVs present inherent homing abilities and are less immunogenic than synthetic nanoparticles, in general. Currently, strong efforts are focused into the development and improvement of EV-based DDS. Even though EV-DDS have already reached early phases in clinical trials, their clinical application is still far from commercialization since protocols for EVs loading, modification and isolation need to be standardized for large-scale production. Here, we summarized recent knowledge regarding the use of EVs as natural DDS against CSCs and cancer resistance.

Keywords: cancer stem cells; extracellular vesicles; drug delivery systems

---

1. Introduction

Despite achieving great advances in oncology in the past few years, in terms of treatment and patient survival, cancer still represents the second cause of death worldwide. In particular, treatment resistance and metastasis in vital organs account for 90% of cancer related deaths [1]. New treatments and therapeutic approaches are needed to successfully fight tumor resistance, cancer progression and metastasis to improve clinical outcomes.

A tumor is a highly complex and heterogenic dynamic entity that evolves over time, adapting and therefore surviving to adverse conditions [2]. As the disease progresses, it becomes more difficult to treat, since it spreads to distant organs and/or acquires resistance to the treatment [3–5].

Within the tumor, a heterogeneous mix of different environments and cell types, such as CSCs (Cancer Stem Cells), DCCs (Differentiated Cancer Cells), CAFs (Cancer Associated Fibroblasts), mesenchymal cells, tumor-infiltrated immune cells, endothelial cells and stromal cells can be found. All of them are located within the extracellular matrix and together contribute to disease progression [6–10]. The constant exchange of information among these cells is essential to guarantee survival and progression of the tumor and to orchestrate the coordination and collaboration of different cells.

In this review, we assess the versatility of TME (Tumor Micro Environment) and the main player of communication within TME, the Extracellular Vesicles (EVs) and its use as a drug delivery system (DDS) for cancer treatment. We cover mostly in vitro studies taking into account the main cells currently used as EV sources. However, in vivo studies and a few ongoing (phase I or II) clinical studies are also described. We advocate for EVs, either natural or engineered, by comparison with liposomes or synthetic drug delivery particles. Indeed, we are well aware of the many challenges, which remain to be solved in order to translate the worldwide increasing current knowledge about EVs from the bench to the clinical care of cancer patients.

Cancer Stem Cells, Cancer Resistance and Cell Communication

CSCs substantially contribute to tumor growth and progression. They are an undifferentiated subset of cells within the tumor with stem-like properties, high proliferation rate, ability to differentiate and self-renewal potential [2,11–14]. CSCs are believed to sustain uncontrolled tumor growth and to be responsible for cancer progression, recurrence, metastatic spread, invasiveness, multidrug resistance and treatment failure [4,6,7,15–18]. Therefore, after treatment, the tumor percentage of CSC subpopulation frequently rises when compared to other tumor cells types [4–6,19]. It has been shown that only a few CSCs are needed for tumor regeneration in vivo, and they can enter to an undetectable quiescence state when the conditions of the TME are not favorable and proliferate afterwards [2,4,17].

Until the 1990s, the initiation and progression of a tumor was explained by the clonal cancer model, in which cancer was thought to be driven by accumulated somatic mutations that confer uncontrolled growth, a more aggressive behavior and higher fitness to a malignant transformed cell [17,20].

However, it was later shown that not all the cells within the tumor presented the same tumorigenic potential. With this knowledge, a hierarchical model (also referred to as the CSC model) (Figure 1A) has been described. Accordingly, only a small and distinct subpopulation of CSCs is alleged to have the capacity to generate and maintain the tumor [4,5]. In this model, cancer cells are created from a precursor cell, which undergoes either symmetric (generating two CSCs or two DCCs) or asymmetric (generating a CSCs and a DCCs) divisions [10]. Here, DCCs do not present the ability to self-renew indefinitely and can only generate cells of their same type. On the other hand, CSCs can generate multiple and heterogeneous tumor subpopulations that differentiate into diverse lineages [17,21]. In terms of cancer treatment, according to the hierarchical model, the complete eradication of the CSCs population should be enough to eradicate the tumor and prevent the relapse of the disease [6,13]. Therefore, strong efforts have been invested over the past decade, in the identification of CSCs within the tumor in order to target treatments against them [10].

Nevertheless, this hierarchical model cannot explain the dynamic behavior seen in the CSC subpopulation, as the concepts of DCC and CSC were not conceived within the same cell [16]. Therefore, a new stochastic model has been recently postulated (Figure 1B) [16,22,23]. According to this model, a tumor is composed by different cell populations that maintain a stable communication among them. Through this communication, they can "sense" if one specific subpopulation of the tumor cells is redundant, absent or has been depleted. In this model, the amount of CSCs seems to remain constant, to maintain the mentioned equilibrium within the TME [4,6,17]. According to a stochastic model, any cell of the tumor can initiate the progression of the disease due to the existing phenotypic plasticity, and, further, any cancer cell can recover the stem-cell-like phenotype by dedifferentiation [6,13,24].

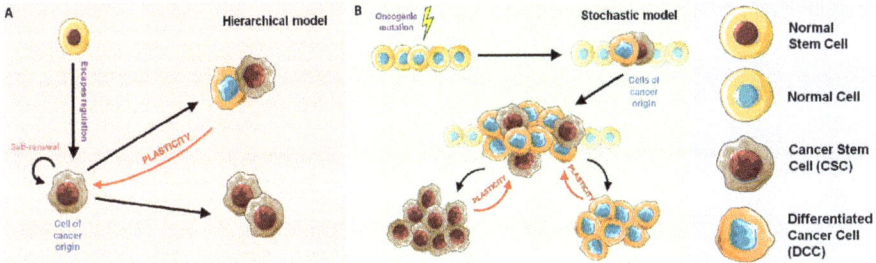

Figure 1. Tumor cell models. (**A**) Hierarchical model of division: a cancer stem cell (CSC) is originated from a normal stem cell that escapes from cell cycle regulation. This CSC has self-renewal capacity and acts as the cell of origin of the tumor and can generate different types of tumor cells. Because of plasticity, those differentiated cells can reverse their phenotype into CSCs. (**B**) Stochastic model of division: The cells of origin of the tumor can be any type of cell that experiences oncogenic mutations. Some mutations can lead to stem-like phenotypes and thus the cells become CSCs. This phenomenon (plasticity) unites the hierarchical model with the stochastic model.

Although the hierarchical model and the stochastic model have different considerations regarding the importance of CSCs in tumor initiation and progression, they are not mutually exclusive because of cellular plasticity (Figure 1) [6]. Essentially, the tumor is formed in a hierarchical manner, that is unstable since constant stochastic actions allow for the introduction of newly hierarchically organized cell populations [6,25,26].

In this context, cancer cells interact with other cells from the TME through direct cell–cell contact and/or using paracrine signaling, particularly for distant cells. Both cellular and non-cellular components of the niche have a role in maintaining stable the stemness potential of the tumor and further regulate CSC plasticity and EMT (epithelial to mesenchymal transition) [6,17,27,28].

Besides, different stress situations can also have critical involvement in the initiation and progression of the tumor. Previous studies have reported the important influence of hypoxia, intratumoral pH and other stress conditions, such as chemotherapeutic treatments, in the CSC niche. These stimuli can promote angiogenesis and the activation of stemness genes and therefore can initiate the dedifferentiation of DCCs [17,29]. Moreover, CSCs present adaptations to survive under hypoxia or acid environments [7]. These examples support the existence of a controlled balance between both cellular populations within the TME and suggest that any alteration in their stable state can have a potential influence in the clinical outcome of a patient [17].

Elucidating the molecular mechanisms that govern cellular plasticity may be essential to overcome the challenge that current therapies face when fighting against cancer. Effective targeting therapies need to be developed to eliminate the roots of continuously evolving tumor cell populations and to avoid the regeneration of CSCs [17,25].

2. Extracellular Vesicles in Cellular Communication

As mentioned before, CSC are not a static cell subpopulation of tumor cells, but a population with a highly dynamic phenotype [12]. However, the mechanisms behind these phenomena are still unclear. Recent evidence suggests that the molecular crosstalk between CSCs and DCCs within the TME has a determining role in this process [12]. Moreover, as the reversion process seems to be an important factor for the tumor to gain therapeutic resistance, this crosstalk may represent a crucial mechanism to promote tumor survival. Extracellular vesicles (EVs), mostly exosomes, derived from CSCs are probably one of the most important elements of this crosstalk (Figure 2a) [12,30].

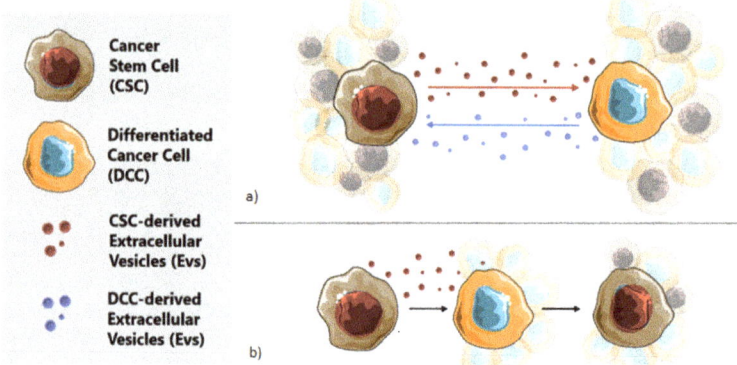

Figure 2. Cellular crosstalk with Extracellular vesicles (EVs). (**a**) EV-mediated molecular crosstalk between cancer stem cells (CSCs) and differentiated cancer cells (DCCs) allows for maintaining stable subpopulations. (**b**) Thanks to this cellular communication, DCCs can reverse to the CSCs phenotype when the CSC population decreases and vice versa.

EVs are naturally cell-derived membranous nanoparticles that contain and transport a wide range of complex molecules such as proteins, nucleic acids, sugars and lipids to specific targeted cells, which can affect and modify their behavior [31–35]. They form an endogenous natural transport system throughout which biomolecules can be exchanged among neighboring recipient cells or even to distant organs [1]. They carry a similar set of molecules as the original cell, reflecting thus its biological status, which changes in pathological conditions such as cancer [34,36]. Almost all cell types have been reported to release these vesicles, including human cells [33]. EVs are commonly classified conferring to their biosynthesis mechanism and size in three subtypes: exosomes, microvesicles and apoptotic bodies [37].

As introduced previously, EVs have been found to participate in the pathogenesis of cancer cell-to-cell communication, as they can transport biomolecules that promote tumor growth, cancer progression, treatment resistance and facilitate metastasis [1,34,38–40]. EVs participate in the creation of the pre-metastatic niche and can also influence therapeutic efficacy, as they may grant chemo-protective properties for tumor cells [41,42]. Among EVs, exosomes present inherent roles in cell-to-cell communication because of their small size (30–100 nm in diameter [12]) and the expression on their lipid bilayer membrane of cell-specific markers [43]. Exosomes are considered to be information carriers between CSC and other cells within the TME, which are essential for the survival of the tumor [12,40,44]. Of interest, it has been shown that cancer cells secrete significantly more exosomes than other cells [45]. Those secreted from cancer cells can regulate the cellular metabolism of the recipient cells, reprograming them to promote or enhance functions such as EMT, apoptosis, proliferation, angiogenesis, immune response suppression, stemness and cellular migration, as they may carry and transfer stemness-related molecules, oncogenic factors and capacity of multidrug resistance to antitumoral treatment [1,12,40,46–49].

Many studies have shown that cancer cell-derived exosomes can also affect and change the surrounding microenvironment by reprogramming the stromal cells to create a favorable niche for tumor progression [10,38,40,41]. At the same time, CSCs can modulate all components of the tumoral niche, facilitating CSCs growth and dissemination [10]. This tumoral niche components can simultaneously regulate the required equilibrium of CSCs and the process of cellular plasticity and are required for the maintenance of the CSC population (Figure 2b) [10,12,17,27].

3. Extracellular Vesicles as Natural Drug Delivery Systems

An ideal anticancer therapy should therefore target both CSCs and DCCs, and also the signals that promote the reversion to the CSC phenotype, to avoid progression and future relapses of the disease.

In this context, specific drug delivery may promote efficiency of anti-cancer therapy. The use of synthetic nanoparticles as drug delivery systems has been in the limelight for the past years [50,51]. Nanomedicine uses nanoscale materials, ranging from 1 to 1000 nm of size, as a consequence of their unique medical benefits regarding their structure and functionality [50]. However, rather few results have been reported in cancer drug delivery and only few prototypes have reached clinical trials; thus, very few of these treatment strategies have successfully transited from bench to bedside [26,52,53]. The main challenges of nanocarriers are still inadequate PK/PD (pharmacokinetic/pharmacodynamic) features, toxicity and immunogenicity, and unspecific targeting capacity. In addition, conventional DDS present significant difficulties in overcoming natural barriers and reaching their expected targets. Therefore, a new focus and a new paradigm of this prospective scientific field is urgently needed [33].

In this context, EVs are attractive, promising candidates to optimize drug delivery for clinical uses. These novel carriers present inherent targeting abilities and less immunogenicity than synthetic nanoparticles and seem to be able to successfully deliver drugs to the tumor site. Nevertheless, our current knowledge on the functions of the molecules exposed at the external surface or incorporated in the lumen of the EVs is still very limited, which hampers the exploitation of specific therapeutic and diagnostic uses and their translation into clinical applications. It is necessary to gain insight in the fundamental processes of EVs biology, to understand the basic mechanisms by which these vehicles can load their specific cargos and target specific cell types, as well as orchestrating their different functional roles as intercellular messengers.

Exosomes, which are considered to develop a principal role in cell-to-cell communication in cancer and in the maintenance of the dynamic equilibrium of CSCs, are being investigated for their potential use against cancer [10,12].

EVs are proposed as natural carriers with manipulated cargo to fight multidrug resistance and metastatic dissemination. EVs may well have advantages compared to the currently available DDS, as they seem to be stable in circulation, they can inherently overcome biological barriers (even the blood-brain barrier), and present intrinsic cell-specific targeting properties [1,12,33,54]. Additionally, EVs can avoid phagocytosis, present significantly low autologous immunogenicity and may use endogenous mechanisms for cargo uptake, trafficking and delivery [1,33,54,55]. The structure of the EVs resembles liposomes but with a more complex lipid layer composition. This complexity in the composition of their membrane helps to deliver the carried material directly into the targeted cell [10]. Moreover, EVs surface markers can be modified or replaced to enhance tumor-targeting specificity, and reduce the systemic toxicity [12,34]. For example, EVs could be coated with CSC marker antibodies to direct the vesicle to this specific cell population within the tumor, which is responsible for tumor progression [12]. They could also be used to present tumor CSC-specific antigens to T cells and consequently help the immune system to fight the disease more efficiently. Up today, chemotherapeutic drugs delivered by exosomes have been shown to have much more stability and effectiveness without toxicity, compared to conventional therapies [12].

Besides, the presence in EVs of different cell-type specific molecular signatures as biomarkers has placed them at the forefront of diagnostics in a wide variety of diseases. Currently, there is a huge interest in applying EVs or synthetic EVs as drug delivery systems. However, not all components in the natural EVs are essential for their function and delivery properties [10]. Therefore, understanding which are the crucial components of natural EVs responsible for specific biological functionalities, such as efficient homing to target cells and efficacious intracellular delivery of their cargo, is still a focus of current studies.

Among all properties that make EVs prospective candidates for drug delivery, probably their most interesting quality is their capacity to transmit nucleic acids and proteins to other cells, and the possibility to directly release their cargo into the cytoplasm of the recipient cells [10,33]. For instance, siRNA and microRNA could be delivered to specific organs or tissues with the aim to target CSC signaling pathways or for gene therapy [12]. Besides, it is important to comprehend the role of EVs in cancer progression and metastatic growth in order to use this knowledge against the disease [43].

3.1. Sources of EV-Based Drug Delivery

During the production process of EVs for cancer treatment, it is important to ensure optimal consideration of certain variables known to influence EV properties: cell type, cell collection process and/or expansion methods, the triggering mechanism for the release of EVs and the isolation and storage methods. All these steps can affect EVs population size, membrane markers (especially important for targeting), purity and content [43]. Applications for EVs as drug delivery vehicles includes allogenic and autologous treatments [34,56]. Moreover, the cell source of these EVs is important to avoid immune rejection responses and to allow specific applications. Until now, the most used cell sources of EVs for drug delivery have been immune cells, mesenchymal stem cells (MSCs), cancer cells, and commonly used commercial cell lines.

3.1.1. Immune Cell-Derived EVs

Immune cell-derived EVs are especially promising for cancer therapy, as they seem to share a common action mechanism with the cellular function of their secreting cells, and therefore protect against different diseases and foreign antigens. For instance, natural killer cells when fighting cancer cells, secrete EVs containing different cytotoxic proteins, which are targeted to kill those specific cells and stimulate the action of the immune system [34,57,58]. Therefore, genetic engineered EVs derived from the immune system cells, may represent an advantage for cancer treatment. This has already been seen in vitro and in vivo models [59–61]. In a recent study, EVs derived from macrophages and loaded through sonication with Paclitaxel (PTX) prevented metastasis in a lung cancer mouse model. Moreover, when these EVs were modified to reduce their immunogenicity by adding an aminoethylanisamide-polyethylene glycol vector, the EVs enhanced their circulation time and were directly targeted to lung metastases [59–61].

3.1.2. MSC-Derived EVs

MSC-derived EVs come from a cell source thought to possess limited immunogenicity and consequently, are suitable for allogenic transplantation. This happens when the expression of co-stimulatory molecules, such as class I major histocompatibility complex molecules, is very low. This quality would be a major goal to avoid immune rejection of the treatment. Moreover, EVs from MSCs present inflammatory tropism and one of their natural functions is to exert therapeutic effects, which comes along with the desired purpose of the natural drug delivery systems [34,53,57]. However, until now, MSCs have had limited use in therapy because of their potential oncogenicity. Nevertheless, several studies have been carried out, using MSCs as a source of EVs for different treatments. As, for example, tumor proliferation has been inhibited by PTX-loaded EVs, which had been released from PTX-treated MSCs in vitro [58,62]. Moreover, MSCs-EVs have reached clinical trials in regenerative medicine for tissue repair after myocardial infarction [63]. In this pathology, the affected cardiomyocytes are usually replaced by a non-elastic collagen scar, which impairs the heart function. However, MSC-derived EVs have been demonstrated to improve recovery after myocardial infarction by promoting neoangiogenesis [63].

3.1.3. Cancer Cell-Derived EVs

Cancer cell-derived EVs are produced in large quantities with special homing abilities due to the TME influence [34,57]. EVs produced in cancer cells express tumor-specific antigens on their membrane, which could help in the generation of the anti-tumor immune response, which has been recently confirmed using a mouse model [34,58]. Moreover, it has been seen that EVs from cancer cells loaded with chemotherapeutic agents can reduce resistance of CSCs to the applied treatment [12,34]. For example, a mouse lung cancer model study showed promising results, as when chemotherapy-loaded EVs were injected, the tumor load was reduced and therefore the survival was prolonged when compared to free chemotherapy treatment [34]. On the other hand, a clinical study has used cisplatin-loaded EVs from A549 human lung cancer cells in three end-stage lung cancer patients, resistant to cisplatin. The results showed that the global quantity of tumor cells and the incidence of CSCs was reduced drastically, while treatment with free cisplatin did not show any beneficial effects for the patients [34,64].

However, it is very important to take into consideration the possibility that this type of EV could also cause tumor growth and metastasis, since such EVs may help tumors to adapt and survive, particularly by the activation of pathological pathways and exerting immune-suppressive effects. Consequent studies were performed to assess how to block this immune-suppressive response, and it was found that, when those EVs were mixed with the adequate immune stimulatory adjuvants, the immune-inhibitory effect could be suppressed, and, therefore, an antitumoral response was promoted [58].

3.1.4. Commonly Used Cellular Lines-Derived Evs

Other common cellular lines, used on a regular basis in the laboratory, can also be a source of EVs for drug delivery. These cell lines (such as human embryonic kidney 293 cell line (HEK293T), Chinese hamster ovary cell line (CHO) or the cervical cancer immortal (HeLa) cell line) are easy to be genetically manipulated and have been commonly used for protein modification and overexpression. For example, the cellular line HEK293T, is one of the most used cellular lines for research on EV-mediated drug delivery and shows potential for industrial applications. Although EVs derived from HEK293T cells can be enriched with some molecules from cancer-related pathways, HEK293T-derived EVs display high transfection efficiency and are easy to load with small therapeutic RNA molecules [65].

3.2. *Modification and Loading of EVs*

Different methods have been proven useful to upload therapeutic molecules into EVs. These therapeutic agents can either be chemotherapeutic agents or nucleic acids (RNA-based therapies) [34]. At the moment, there are two ways to create EVs containing a desired drug or molecule. It is possible to either load the drugs/molecules first into parental cells and then generate the release of EVs, which will already contain the given molecules, or incorporate the drugs/molecules into previously isolated EVs [1,43].

3.2.1. Modification of Parental Cells

The engineering of parental cells, with the aim to transmit a determinate molecule to the EVs these cells secrete, can be performed through different methods. Subsequently, altered cells are cultured and secrete modified EVs containing the molecules of interest [66]. Of note, modifying the cells that will later produce the EVs may allow for designing exosomes to target specific tissues [10]. Moreover, using this methodology for cargo upload preserves the intact integrity of EVs membrane, which is usually damaged when other post-isolation loading techniques are employed [34]. Two of the perhaps most used approaches to engineer parental cells are the loading of these cells with exogenous cargo and the transfection of parental cells with DNA (Figure 3a) [1,56].

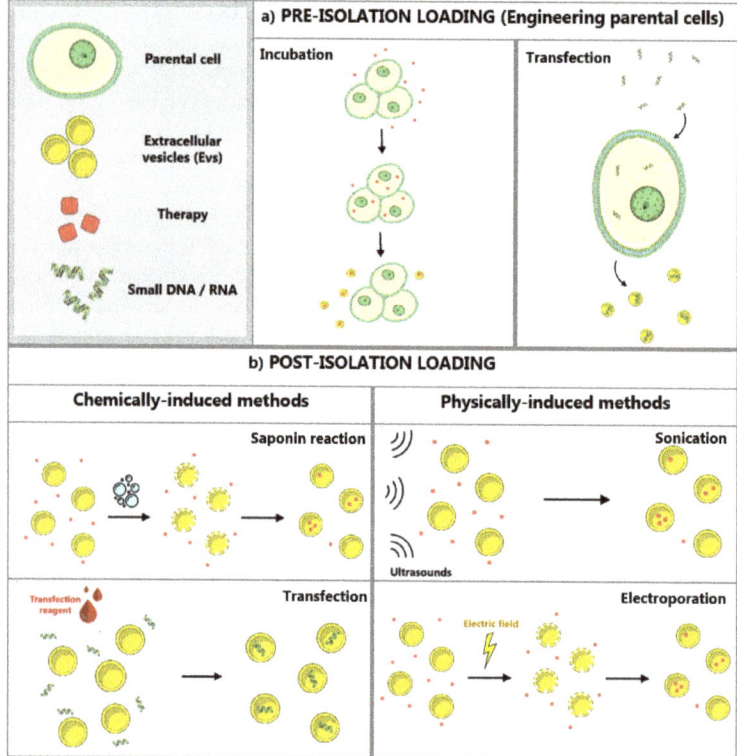

Figure 3. Extracellular vesicles (EVs) loading methods. (a) EVs can be loaded before isolation by engineering their parental cells. This procedure can be achieved by incubation of the parental cells with the desired cargo or by transfection of the cells. EVs secreted by those cells will already contain the cargo. (b) EVs can be loaded with a desired cargo after being isolated from the sample. This procedure can be chemically induced (through transfection or saponin reaction) or physically induced (through sonication or electroporation).

On one hand, the therapeutic of interest could be simply loaded in the parental cells from which exosomes will be isolated, through incubation of the cells with the drug [67]. For example, when a high dosage of PTX was cultured together with MSCs cell line SR4987 during 24 h, it was internalized by the cells and later released inside most EVs. Those EVs showed significant anticancer effect in vitro and in vivo when compared to a control group [62,68]. However, this method can cause cytotoxicity to the parental cell due to the drug loading and low efficacy of this drug loading within exosomes [1].

On the other hand, the DNA of interest could be transfected, and consequently alter and control the phenotype and cargo of the EVs derived from genetically modified cells [1]. Of note, not all cell lines are suitable for exogneneos expression, and the loading of EVs is difficult to control. In the study performed by O'Brien et al., the invasive triple negative breast cancer cell line (Hs578T) was engineered to overexpress miR-134. As a consequence, the EVs released by these cells contained the desired miRNA. Those were isolated and used with the aim to decrease the expression of Hsp90 in the cancer cell line. When the miR-134 entered via EVs to the targeted cells, cell migration has been reduced and the efficacy of the anti-Hsp90 treatments increased [1,69].

3.2.2. Direct Loading of EVs

There is also the possibility to load functional therapeutic molecules, such as biomolecules, synthetic compounds or drugs, directly to previously isolated EVs (Figure 3b) [67,68]. Since the lipid bilayer represents in these cases a restriction for the loading, the different techniques must accomplish the final goal of bypassing the EV membrane without causing excessive damage [1]. They are usually referred to as active loading strategies, which can be chemically induced (with chemical agents such as transfection reagents or saponin) or physically induced (involving the disruption of the membrane with methodologies such as electroporation or sonication) [33,34]. Loaded EVs may be structurally modified and engineered to improve cancer therapy after loading, to enhance its homing abilities [70].

Depending on the nature of the cargo, different loading methods may be chosen, and, occasionally, the simple mixing of EVs with a free drug is enough [1,54]. For example, with some hydrophobic drugs (such as PTX), it is only required to mix the cargo with EVs to accomplish the loading and encapsulation in the vesicles. This allows for increasing drug solubility and stability. Some clinical trials have already used this methodology to deliver specific cargo to the tumor, for instance, curcumin-loaded EVs [58]. Free curcumin (an anti-inflammatory agent used for treating cancer) has been mixed with previously purified exosomes from a mouse tumor cell line (EL-4). The curcumin particles were successfully internalized by the exosomes, and those exosomes exerted positive effects when delivered to inflammatory cells, increasing the efficacy of the curcumin particles [68].

3.3. Evs Isolation Techniques

Once the best cellular line for a specific experiment has been chosen and, if required, parental cells have been engineered and loaded with the desired cargo, EVs (containing the drug or not yet modified) need to be isolated. Several EV isolation techniques can be used for this purpose. An optimal method is expected to demonstrate the high purity, high efficiency and high recovery yield of exosomes, as well as scalability and reproducibility [1,33].

Until date, several methods for EVs/exosome isolation have been described (Table 1).

Table 1. Extracellular vesicle (EV) isolation techniques.

Isolation Method	Procedure	Advantages	Disadvantages
Differential Ultracentrifugation (UC)	The different molecules in a fluid sample are separated by centrifugation at high g-forces. Can be combined with sucrose density gradients or SEC for higher purity.	As the gold standard for EVs isolation, it is a cheap and scalable technique.	Low-yield technique with a time-consuming protocol, difficult to automatize. Moreover, specialized instruments and training are needed. EVs may collapse and the resulting sample is usually contaminated.
Size-Based Filtration, Chromatography and Fractionation	Technique based on a column filled with different sized pores. Smaller size molecules will have to go through many pores while larger molecules will be faster eluted.	Fast (normally a single step) and automatable method with high purity and integrity of the resulting sample.	The type of membrane used can have a large impact on the quality of the isolated EVs.
Immunoaffinity	Selective antibody-mediated arrest of EVs with specific surface antigens.	Allows a more selective isolation of EVs.	Protocols for immunoaffinity procedure are set on a very small scale and the costs for large volume samples isolation are high. Also, it is hard to recover fully intact EVs.
Polymer precipitation	The sample containing the EVs is precipitated with a solution of PEG and concentrated by centrifugation	Easy, scalable technique that does not require long runs or specific equipment.	The purity of the sample obtained should be improved. It is frequent to have samples contaminated with other particles and proteins.
Microfluidic separation	This method uses different techniques like immunoaffinity or filtrations to isolate EVs.	Fast technique with high sensitivity and efficiency.	This method presents a low sample volume restriction and needs expensive devices.

3.3.1. Differential Ultracentrifugation and Density Gradient Centrifugation

Differential ultracentrifugation (UC) is the current gold standard and most commonly used method for EV purification, as it is a cheap scalable technique and can be used in most circumstances. However, this method still presents some drawbacks. It is a low-yield, time-consuming method, difficult to automatize and with a high risk of EVs collapse or aggregation. Moreover, this process requires access to specialized instruments and training [33,41,71]. This isolation technique is based on sequential centrifugation for the sedimentation of EVs at high g-forces. It starts with low-speed spins to remove cells and large cellular debris. Later high-speed UC is used to pellet EVs. However, the resulting sample is usually contaminated with various types of EVs and protein aggregates. It is possible to further separate the different vesicle types by later sucrose density gradients to significantly improve the purity of the sample [1,33,40,43,72].

3.3.2. Size-Based Filtration, Chromatography and Fractionation

Size-based filtration methods (i.e., tangential filtration, flow-field franctionation) together with chromatography-based separation are emergent large-scale EV isolation techniques, that are fast and automatable [33]. Nevertheless, the major weakness of this methodology is that the type of membrane used can have large impact on the quality of the isolated EVs [40]. With this methodology, EVs can be separated from the rest of the sample via sequential filtration using different filters with the desired pore size or molecular weight limit [1,72]. Heinemann et al. designed a three-step protocol with the aim to isolate EVs using only a filtration technique [33,73]. Initially, cell debris is being removed using a 0.1 μm pore size polyethersulfone (PES) membrane. Then, proteins and a large volume of the sample are reduced using a 500 kDa molecular weight cut-off modified Polyethersulfone (PES) filter. The last step of the protocol consisted in the final EVs isolation with a 0.1 um Track Etch filter [33].

In addition, a chromatography method of special relevance for EVs isolation is size-exclusion chromatography (SEC). It is a promising technique as it allows for the separation of nanoscale particles depending on their hydrodynamic size [72]. It consists of a column filled with different-sized pores. Smaller-sized molecules will have to go through many pores, while larger molecules will be eluted faster [1]. SEC seems to present the high purity and integrity of the sample and advantages in different types of fluid, such as plasma or serum [40]. It is possible to combine SEC with UC for a better result [1,33,74].

Asymmetric Flow Field-Flow Fractionation is another used technique for EVs isolation based on their size. More commonly used for the separation of other types of nanoparticles, this methodology consists of the application of a laminar flow on the sample and a crossflow separation field which pushes the particulate molecules to an accumulation wall. Smaller particles will be reflected to the center of the chamber faster and eluted before larger ones. This technique has been reported to successfully isolate EVs sorted from a mouse melanoma cell line [1].

3.3.3. Immunoaffinity

Immunoaffinity, is a method based on selective antibody-mediated arrest of EVs with specific surface proteins. Thanks to the specificity of antibodies receptors, this technique allows for a more selective isolation of exosomes. Specific antibodies are fixed on a surface of exosomes. Several washes are performed, consequently exosomes detached and are collected [1]. This technique allows one to obtain a higher purity of the sample, and the separation from the different subtypes of EVs could be performed [33,75]. It is used to isolate subpopulations of EVs derived from cell sources, such as cancer cells. For example, a method to specifically isolate exosomes derived from antigen-presenting cells used antibody-coated magnetic beads to capture a precise subtype of exosomes through the major histocompatibility complex class II [33]. However, protocols for immunoaffinity procedure are set on a very small scale and the costs for large volume samples isolation are highly expensive, which are important drawbacks for the clinical translation [33,40]. Moreover, it is hard to recover fully intact EVs [76].

3.3.4. Polymer Precipitation

Another technique for EV isolation is a method based on polymer precipitation, commonly used to precipitate other molecules such as viruses. In this method, the sample containing the EVs is precipitated with a solution of polyethylene glycol (PEG). Then, with a centrifugation, it is possible to obtain a pellet containing EVs [1]. This approach for EVs isolation is easy, scalable and does not require long runs or specific equipment. Actually, different commercial EV isolation kits, such as Exosome Isolation (Thermo Fisher Scientific) or ExoQuick (System Biosciences), are used to simplify the EVs isolation process [40]. However, the purity of the sample obtained this way is not currently suitable for clinical application [40,77].

3.3.5. Microfluidic Separation

Finally, microfluidics is a separation method widely used for other nanoparticles. This method is fast and presents high sensitivity as it can be combined with other techniques such as immunoaffinity methodologies, using surface protein markers to enrich the sample of exosomes without contamination [1,41,72]. This technique allows one to obtain relatively pure samples of EVs. For instance, CD41-positive platelet-derived EVs were isolated from plasma through a quick process using an anti-CD41 antibody-coated surface [33]. However, a strong limitation of this method is the low sample volume restriction [1,72].

3.4. EVs for Drug Delivery in the Clinics

The race to find the best type of EVs, isolation method and source for these potential drug delivery systems has already started. Currently, some clinical trials have by now demonstrated the promising application of EVs in the clinics (Table 2). Yet, these methodologies are at the early stages of investigation and clinical application [33]. It is, however, possible to find a few listed clinical trials already using EVs of different sources as drug delivery systems to treat cancer (Table 2) (http://clinicaltrials.gov [78]). Here, we highlight a study in phase I carried out in the USA (NCT03608631), expected to present results by March 2022, which aims to use mesenchymal stromal cell-derived EVs loaded with KrasG12D siRNA to fight against a specific type of pancreatic cancer. Another clinical trial in France (phase II), completed in 2018 (NCT01159288), assessed the potential of vaccinations with tumor antigen-loaded dendritic cell-derived exosomes against lung cancer, with the aim to activate the innate and adaptive immunity of the patients. Phase I of this study already showed safety of the treatment and feasibility [79]. However, the final results of its phase II have not yet been revealed.

Table 2. Clinical trials with EVs as drug delivery systems.

Type of Cancer	EV Source	Isolation Method	Loading Method	Therapeutic Cargo	Phase	Ref.
Malignant pleural effusion	Tumor cells	Not mentioned	Not mentioned	Chemotherapy	Phase II	NCT01854866
Non-small cell lung cancer	Dendritic cells	Ultrafiltration/UC	Not mentioned	Peptides	Phase II	NCT01159288
Pancreatic cancer	Mesenchymal stromal cells	Not mentioned	Not mentioned	KrasG12D siRNA	Phase I	NCT03608631
Melanoma (stage III/IV)	Autologous monocyte-derived dendritic cells	Ultrafiltration/UC	Incubation with parental cells	MAGE3	Phase I	[78]
Lung cancer (stage IV)	Human lung carcinoma cell line A549	Differential gradient centrifugation	Passive incubation	Cisplatin	Phase I	[64]
Colon cancer	Plant nanovesicles	Not mentioned	Not mentioned	Curcumin	Phase I	NCT01294072

To exemplify the use of non-human EVs sources for drug delivery, there is a phase I clinical study being carried out in the USA (NCT01294072), with the purpose of using plant-derived exosomes for the delivery of curcumin to targeted colon tumors, as previous clinical trials showed low efficiency and limited bioavailability of oral consumed curcumin, even in high doses [79]. This phase I study is scheduled to end by December 2022.

3.5. Artificial Extracellular Vesicles as Ideal Drug Delivery Systems

Each cellular type, loading method or isolation technique has certain potential for the production and obtention of efficient EVs for drug delivery. However, these qualities may not be enough on their own to generate an ideal EV-based DDS. Moreover, clinical use of this drug carriers is at the moment limited due to the low yield production of EVs by the different cell sources [80,81]. Yet, this knowledge could be used to synthesize artificial EVs specifically designed for drug delivery against a specific type of cancer. Several methodologies have already been described for the generation of artificial EVs, although more research and consensus among scientists in terms of biomaterials is needed [82].

Within the concept of artificial EVs as novel delivery systems, these can be separated into semi-synthetic EVs (which have been only modified before or after isolation) or fully synthetic EVs/EV mimetics (cell culture generated or artificial structures that mimic native EVs) [80,82]. These EV mimetic vehicles are usually produced on a large-scale by extrusion of specific cells (using micrometer-sized membranes) or built up from synthetic lipid materials forming liposomes [80,81]. Synthetic liposomes have been considered to be a viable vehicles for cancer therapy for a long time, as most cancers present a high number of light density lipoprotein receptors [83]. Therefore, liposomes or lipid-based nanoparticles have centered many efforts in the past few years. They were demonstrated to effectively load different drugs such as RNAs or chemotherapeutic agents. However, they were prone to present immunogenicity and toxicity as well as low ability to reach specific organs or tissues, which is a major drawback for human treatments [83]. The benefits of engineered vesicles that carry both the simplicity of liposomes, which can be easily modified, as well as specific EV membrane proteins, grant these artificial EVs the ideal characteristics for drug delivery [80,84].

Furthermore, artificial EVs can be engineered to present on their cell membrane surface other targeting ligands to improve their biodistribution and targeting capabilities. This method has been used as an example to create EVs expressing a fusion protein for the treatment of chronic myelogenous leukemia, a disease in which some patients develop drug resistance against common treatments (i.e., tyrosine kinase inhibitors) or have strong side effects because of inefficient site-specific accumulation of the drug [34,85]. In this case, HEK293T cells were used as the source of EVs, being first transfected with a plasmid containing the exosomal protein Lamp2b fused with interleukin 3 (IL-3). The IL-3 receptor is overexpressed in blasts from patients suffering chronic myelogenous leukemia; therefore, this molecule could be used for targeting purposes against this type of cancer. Moreover, EVs were loaded with Imantib, a first line leukemia treatment. In cell culture and mouse models, the efficacy of such EVs as drug delivery vehicles has been confirmed since the cytotoxicity of Imantib, when compared to EVs without the lamp2b-IL-3 fusion protein, was significantly reduced, while the survival rate augmented [85]. These results show that using targeting ligands can improve drug delivery to specific sites and this significantly improves the treatment.

Likewise, elements to avoid the activation of the immune system against the EVs could be incorporated into the vesicles to enhance their immune evasion properties. The most common approach in this context is the use of PEG (also used in polymer precipitation isolation technique), a molecule that forms a hydration layer around the vesicles which reduces their recognition by immune cells and therefore enhances the circulation time of the particles [34]. This was confirmed by a study where mice were injected with EVs from human epidermoid carcinoma cells fused with PEG. These vesicles could be found in blood after one hour, while non-PEGylated EVs had been completely cleared from circulation within ten minutes [34,86].

In addition, stimuli-responsive elements could be used to improve functionality and spatial action by adding, for example, peptides that are sensitive to the acid TME, such as pH-sensitive functional groups, generating the extracellular release of the drug only when the EVs are exposed to the acidic tumor environment [34]. As an example, EVs were modified with 3-(diethylamino) propylamine (DEAP), which causes the collapse of the EV membrane when the pH is below 7.0 [34,87]. Another pH-sensitive membrane functionalization approach which enhances EV uptake and cytosolic release is cationic lipid and pH-sensitive peptide (GALA) conjugation [10]. In both cases, the disruption of the membrane from EVs containing a drug allow the release of the drug to a targeted site [34]. However, additional types of stimuli-induced responses could also be useful to fight cancer and overcome the current failures (Figure 4).

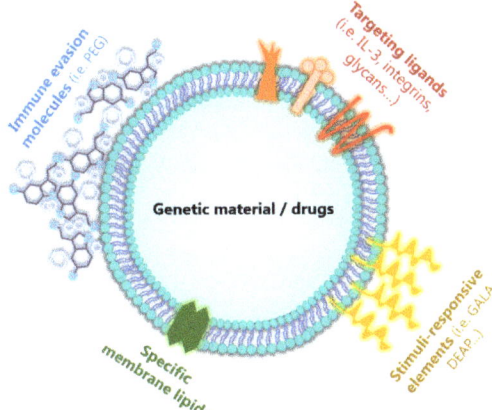

Figure 4. Structure of an ideal extracellular vesicle (EV) for drug delivery. EVs can be artificially synthetized or engineered to gain potential as ideal Drug Delivery Systems (DDS). While maintaining their natural membrane or synthetizing a simple liposome, immunosuppressive molecules (such as polyethylene glycol (PEG)) could be added to the membrane to avoid the action of the immune system of the patient. Moreover, different targeted ligands (like IL-3, integrins or glycans) could be used to direct the vesicles with the therapy to specific cells or tissues delivery. Moreover, stimuli-responsive elements (for instance pH-sensitive peptide (GALA) or 3-(diethylamino) propylamine (DEAP)) help to deliver their cargo with more specificity. Within the inner core, EVs may contain genetic material (like siRNA for therapy) of drugs against cancer or other diseases.

4. Discussion

Efforts to develop new treatments based on nanomedicine applications have exponentially grown for the past decades with the final aim of improving the delivery of different treatments by using nanocarriers to a wide range of diseases, including cancer. This kind of therapy presents advantages when compared to conventional cancer therapy (i.e., Chemotherapy), in terms of improved solubility, enhanced circulation time, targeted delivery and reduction of adverse side effects. Yet, only a few synthetic DDS have reached the market so far, as only few of them have been completely safe and significantly improved patient outcomes [88,89]. One of the major drawbacks of synthetic nanoparticles is the insufficient accumulation of drug in the desired organ or tissue [88,90]. Indeed, despite many preclinical studies, only one synthetic nanoparticle with active targeting capacity is on the market today [91].

Many studies and reviews have discussed the possibility to modify EVs to target various diseases [1,34,38,54,56,66,67]. This interest arises from the specific role of EVs in cellular communication and their capacity to alter the recipient cell phenotype by transferring their inner content [33].

Possibly, the utmost benefit of EVs is their lack of immunogenicity [43]. Contrarily, synthetic nanoparticles such as liposomes may cause hypersensitivity reactions and immune rejection [65]. On the other hand, EVs present intrinsic targeting capabilities through ligands and receptors expressed on their membranes, which is a very important feature in order to achieve a targeted drug delivery system and might offer serious advantages in reduction of side effects and enhanced efficacy over other synthetic nanoparticles [43]. Synthetic nanoparticles have the tendency to become very fast opsonized with proteins in the blood stream, while the targeting features of EVs confer an important influence on bio-distribution of the drug, enhancing circulation time and cellular interactions with intrinsic homing abilities [55,58,92]. The complex composition of their surface membrane enables high specificity and selectivity for their targets [55]. Besides, nucleic acids (i.e., small RNA) might especially benefit from being delivered by EVs [58]. Although the benefits in using natural nanoparticles for drug delivery in cancer seem obvious, the mechanisms by which EVs are transported through the body and to their target cells or tissue are not yet fully understood. EV-based DDS need to be further studied and validated [34,93]. An additional problem of EVs-based DDS is the lack of high-throughput methods of isolation and efficient drug loading for clinical applications. Currently, most studies have been made under a small-scale EVs production protocol [33]. Yet, large-scale synthesis would be required for their clinical translation. Furthermore, it is also important to take into account the feasibility of manufacturing EV-based DDS under good manufacturing practices (GMP) [10]. On the other hand, synthetic DDS can be produced as a large-scale homogeneous population, with standardized protocols [34].

For EVs application as DDS, it is very important to consider the different features of the EVs. Some EVs, depending on their cell of origin, can stimulate immune and anti-tumor responses [58]. This illustrates that the choice of an appropriate cell type or cell state are essential questions for the production of efficient EV-based DDS in a given disease or therapeutic application [59,65]. As mentioned above, the most used sources for EVs are immune cells, MSCs, cancer cells or common cell lines. Immune cells used as an EVs source in clinical trials demonstrated that non-modified EVs are usually not enough to induce potent beneficial effects in vivo [59]. On the other hand, MSC-derived EVs do not affect the immune system [59]. Still, this kind of EV proved to reach targeted organs after infusion bypassing the lung microvasculature [94,95]. Confirmed differences exist in biological effects of MSC-derived EVs from different sources (bone marrow, adipose tissue or endothelium) [94]. Although this cell source seems to be the most extended in use, its application in clinical trials is still limited, as some critical parameters, such as culture conditions or protocols for production, storage or administration, are not standardized [94–96]. On the other hand, the use of cancer cell lines as a source of EVs may simplify their isolation. However, the yet unknown content shared through cancer cells with EVs may represent an important safety risk [58]. Finally, EVs obtained from common cellular lines may be easier to produce in large quantities, although with fewer biological benefits. Other studies point to using EVs of vegetable origin (from freshly prepared juice of edible plants) as a source for drug delivery. For example, EVs derived from grapefruit juice proved to successfully deliver interfering RNA, proteins or chemotherapeutic agents in animal models [58]. Moreover, other non-human sources of EVs are being tested, like EVs derived from animal milk, which proved to successfully function as drug carriers. Attention should be paid to this particular source of EVs as it might allow the production of low-budgeted and up- scaled EVs [58,97].

Further, the need to find efficient isolation methods for EVs is one of the major limitations to use EVs for drug delivery [40,63]. Conventional isolation techniques usually present low purity of the sample and limited recovery yields [34]. Moreover, standardized protocols for the purification and isolation processes are also needed. These protocols should be scalable to translate the techniques into large-scale EVs production under GMP [33,43]. Yet, it is important to bear in mind that the combination of two or more methods may improve the isolation of EVs and the scalability of the process [1]. Likewise, with the current isolation methods, it was formerly impossible to completely isolate pure exosome samples [59]. Until date, the most used EVs isolation techniques have been UC combined with density gradient centrifugation, polymer precipitation or SEC for further purification and possible large-scale production of EVs [40,58,63,74]. Lately, novel technologies to isolate EVs are being developed. Microfluidic platforms are an example of such technologies; they have great potential but still need to be optimized in order to standardize the protocols and storage conditions, to maintain the functionality of EVs and make large-scale isolation feasible [58,63,72].

As synthetic nanoparticles have so far failed in their translation to the clinics, and the development of EVs for drug delivery is still facing some major challenging issues for large-scale production, artificial extracellular vesicles may represent an ideal DDS connecting the best of both systems [98]. These carriers mimic the structure of EVs, although conserving the simple structure and characteristics of synthetic DDS [80]. Additionally, large-scale production would be easily achieved in a short time period, and vesicle loading would become a simpler process [80,81,99]. Some in-between alternatives for synthetic nanoparticles and EVs have already been investigated, such as cell-membrane-coated nanoparticles. They use natural membranes and therefore benefit from their biological characteristics as EVs [34]. Cell-membrane-coated nanoparticles thus carry both properties of synthetic nanoparticles and cellular membranes. As a drawback, the extraction of this cell membrane is a complicated and time-consuming process [34,100].

5. Conclusions

Altogether, EVs are prospective for cancer treatment; however, their functionality and physiological role are still under investigation [40,63]. Moreover, stronger preclinical models (immunocompetent mice, humanized patient derived xenograft (PDX) models) to predict the human response to the treatment are needed for early phase clinical trials [58]. Additionally, a better understanding of EV biological function is needed, and several issues related to the purification, loading, targeting and scaling-up of EVs as DDS must be carefully considered to successfully transit these particles from bench to bedside [40,63,94].

Author Contributions: L.H.-O. drafted the work, P.G., S.S.J. revised the manuscript critically for important intellectual content and approved the final version, J.S.-F., F.A., D.R., I.A. made substantial contributions to conception and design of the review. All authors have read and agreed to the published version of the manuscript.

Funding: This work was partially supported by grant PI17/02242 and PI20/01474 from Fondo de Investigaciones Sanitarias (FIS) of Instituto Carlos III (ISCIII), co-financed by the European Regional Development Fund (FEDER) and the EvoNano project, and was funded by the European Union's Horizon 2020 FET Open programme under grant agreement No. 800983.

Conflicts of Interest: The authors declare no conflict of interest.

References

1. Zhang, Z.; Dombroski, J.A.; King, M.R. Engineering of Exosomes to Target Cancer Metastasis. *Cell. Mol. Bioeng.* **2020**, *13*, 1–16. [CrossRef] [PubMed]
2. Gener, P.; Seras-Franzoso, J.; Callejo, P.G.; Andrade, F.; Rafael, D.; Martínez, F.; Montero, S.; Arango, D.; Sayós, J.; Abasolo, I.; et al. Dynamism, Sensitivity, and Consequences of Mesenchymal and Stem-Like Phenotype of Cancer Cells. *Stem Cells Int.* **2018**, *2018*, 1–12. [CrossRef] [PubMed]
3. Gener, P.; Gouveia, L.; Sabat, G.R.; Rafael, D.; Fort, N.B.; Arranja, A.; Fernández, Y.; Prieto, R.M.; Ortega, J.S.; Arango, D.; et al. Fluorescent CSC models evidence that targeted nanomedicines improve treatment sensitivity of breast and colon cancer stem cells. *Nanomed. Nanotechnol. Biol. Med.* **2015**, *11*, 1883–1892. [CrossRef] [PubMed]
4. Gener, P.; Rafael, D.; Fernandez, Y.; Ortega, J.S.; Arango, D.; Abasolo, I.; Videira, M.; Schwartz, S.; Schwartz, S. Cancer stem cells and personalized cancer nanomedicine. *Nanomedicine* **2016**, *11*, 307–320. [CrossRef] [PubMed]
5. Nassar, D.; Blanpain, C. Cancer Stem Cells: Basic Concepts and Therapeutic Implications. *Annu. Rev. Pathol. Mech. Dis.* **2016**, *11*, 47–76. [CrossRef] [PubMed]
6. Plaks, V.; Kong, N.; Werb, Z. The Cancer Stem Cell Niche: How Essential Is the Niche in Regulating Stemness of Tumor Cells? *Cell Stem Cell* **2015**, *16*, 225–238. [CrossRef]

7. Eun, K.; Ham, S.W.; Kim, H. Cancer stem cell heterogeneity: Origin and new perspectives on CSC targeting. *BMB Rep.* **2017**, *50*, 117–125. [CrossRef] [PubMed]
8. Wang, M.; Zhao, J.; Zhang, L.; Wei, F.; Lian, Y.; Wu, Y.; Gong, Z.; Zhang, S.; Zhou, J.; Cao, K.; et al. Role of tumor microenvironment in tumorigenesis. *J. Cancer* **2017**, *8*, 761–773. [CrossRef] [PubMed]
9. Hanahan, D.; Weinberg, R.A. Hallmarks of Cancer: The Next Generation. *Cell* **2011**, *144*, 646–674. [CrossRef] [PubMed]
10. Gener, P.; Callejo, P.G.; Seras-Franzoso, J.; Andrade, F.; Rafael, D.; Abasolo, I.; Schwartz, S. The potential of nanomedicine to alter cancer stem cell dynamics: The impact of extracellular vesicles. *Nanomedicine* **2020**, 1–24. [CrossRef] [PubMed]
11. Gener, P.; Rafael, D.; Seras-Franzoso, J.; Perez, A.; Pindado, L.A.; Casas, G.; Arango, D.; Fernández, Y.; Díaz-Riascos, Z.V.; Abasolo, I.; et al. Pivotal Role of AKT2 during Dynamic Phenotypic Change of Breast Cancer Stem Cells. *Cancers* **2019**, *11*, 1058. [CrossRef] [PubMed]
12. Sun, Z.; Wang, L.; Dong, L.; Wang, X. Emerging role of exosome signalling in maintaining cancer stem cell dynamic equilibrium. *J. Cell. Mol. Med.* **2018**, *22*, 3719–3728. [CrossRef] [PubMed]
13. Olmeda, F.; Ben Amar, M. Clonal pattern dynamics in tumor: The concept of cancer stem cells. *Sci. Rep.* **2019**, *9*, 15607. [CrossRef] [PubMed]
14. Soteriou, D.; Fuchs, Y. A matter of life and death: Stem cell survival in tissue regeneration and tumour formation. *Nat. Rev. Cancer* **2018**, *18*, 187–201. [CrossRef] [PubMed]
15. Jung, Y.; Kim, W. Cancer stem cell targeting: Are we there yet? *Arch. Pharmacal Res.* **2015**, *38*, 414–422. [CrossRef]
16. Kreso, A.; Dick, J.E. Evolution of the Cancer Stem Cell Model. *Cell Stem Cell* **2014**, *14*, 275–291. [CrossRef]
17. Lee, G.; R Hall III, R.; Ahmed, A.U. Cancer Stem Cells: Cellular Plasticity, Niche, and its Clinical Relevance. *J. Stem Cell Res. Ther.* **2016**, *176*, 139–148. [CrossRef]
18. Chen, J.; Li, Y.; Yu, T.-S.; McKay, R.M.; Burns, D.K.; Kernie, S.G.; Parada, L.F. A restricted cell population propagates glioblastoma growth after chemotherapy. *Nat. Cell Biol.* **2012**, *488*, 522–526. [CrossRef]
19. Lagadec, C.; Vlashi, E.; Della Donna, L.; Meng, Y.; Dekmezian, C.; Kim, K.; Pajonk, F. Survival and self-renewing capacity of breast cancer initiating cells during fractionated radiation treatment. *Breast Cancer Res.* **2010**, *12*, R13. [CrossRef]
20. Lengauer, C.; Kinzler, K.W.; Vogelstein, B. Genetic instabilities in human cancers. *Nat. Cell Biol.* **1998**, *396*, 643–649. [CrossRef]
21. Meacham, C.E.; Morrison, S.J. Tumour heterogeneity and cancer cell plasticity. *Nat. Cell Biol.* **2013**, *501*, 328–337. [CrossRef] [PubMed]
22. Gupta, P.B.; Fillmore, C.M.; Jiang, G.; Shapira, S.D.; Tao, K.; Kuperwasser, C.; Lander, E.S. Stochastic State Transitions Give Rise to Phenotypic Equilibrium in Populations of Cancer Cells. *Cell* **2011**, *146*, 633–644. [CrossRef] [PubMed]
23. Shackleton, M.; Quintana, E.; Fearon, E.R.; Morrison, S.J. Heterogeneity in Cancer: Cancer Stem Cells versus Clonal Evolution. *Cell* **2009**, *138*, 822–829. [CrossRef] [PubMed]
24. Cabrera, M.C. Cancer stem cell plasticity and tumor hierarchy. *World J. Stem Cells* **2015**, *7*, 27–36. [CrossRef]
25. Chaffer, C.L.; Weinberg, R.A. How does multistep tumorigenesis really proceed? *Cancer Discov.* **2015**, *5*, 22–24. [CrossRef]
26. Puré, E.; Lo, A. Can Targeting Stroma Pave the Way to Enhanced Antitumor Immunity and Immunotherapy of Solid Tumors? *Cancer Immunol. Res.* **2016**, *4*, 269–278. [CrossRef]
27. Varas-Godoy, M.; E Rice, G.; Illanes, S.E. The Crosstalk between Ovarian Cancer Stem Cell Niche and the Tumor Microenvironment. *Stem Cells Int.* **2017**, *2017*, 1–8. [CrossRef]
28. Oh, M.; Nör, J.E. The Perivascular Niche and Self-Renewal of Stem Cells. *Front. Physiol.* **2015**, *6*, 367. [CrossRef]
29. Campos-Sánchez, E.; Cobaleda, C. Tumoral reprogramming: Plasticity takes a walk on the wild side. *Biochim. Biophys. Acta BBA Bioenergy* **2015**, *1849*, 436–447. [CrossRef]
30. Maia, J.; Caja, S.; Moraes, M.C.S.; Couto, N.; Costa-Silva, B. Exosome-Based Cell-Cell Communication in the Tumor Microenvironment. *Front. Cell Dev. Biol.* **2018**, *6*, 18. [CrossRef]
31. Yáñez-Mó, M.; Siljander, P.R.M.; Andreu, Z.; Bedina Zavec, A.; Borràs, F.E.; Buzas, E.I.; Buzas, K.; Casal, E.; Cappello, F.; Carvalho, J.; et al. Biological properties of extracellular vesicles and their physiological functions. *J. Extracell. Vesicles* **2015**, *4*, 27066. [CrossRef] [PubMed]

32. Ramteke, A.; Ting, H.; Agarwal, C.; Mateen, S.; Somasagara, R.; Hussain, A.; Graner, M.; Frederick, B.; Agarwal, R.; Deep, G. Exosomes secreted under hypoxia enhance invasiveness and stemness of prostate cancer cells by targeting adherens junction molecules. *Mol. Carcinog.* **2015**, *54*, 554–565. [CrossRef]
33. Vader, P.; Mol, E.A.; Pasterkamp, G.; Schiffelers, R. Extracellular vesicles for drug delivery. *Adv. Drug Deliv. Rev.* **2016**, *106*, 148–156. [CrossRef] [PubMed]
34. Walker, S.; Busatto, S.; Pham, A.; Tian, M.; Suh, A.; Carson, K.; Quintero, A.; Lafrence, M.; Malik, H.; Santana, M.X.; et al. Extracellular vesicle-based drug delivery systems for cancer treatment. *Theranostics* **2019**, *9*, 8001–8017. [CrossRef] [PubMed]
35. Zhang, H.-G.; Grizzle, W.E. Exosomes. *Am. J. Pathol.* **2014**, *184*, 28–41. [CrossRef] [PubMed]
36. Rilla, K.; Siiskonen, H.; Tammi, M.; Tammi, R. Hyaluronan-Coated Extracellular Vesicles—A Novel Link Between Hyaluronan and Cancer. *Adv. Cancer Res.* **2014**, *123*, 121–148. [CrossRef]
37. Verdera, H.C.; Gitz-Francois, J.J.; Schiffelers, R.M.; Vader, P. Cellular uptake of extracellular vesicles is mediated by clathrin-independent endocytosis and macropinocytosis. *J. Control. Release* **2017**, *266*, 100–108. [CrossRef]
38. Wu, M.; Wang, G.; Hu, W.; Yao, Y.; Yu, X.-F. Emerging roles and therapeutic value of exosomes in cancer metastasis. *Mol. Cancer* **2019**, *18*, 1–11. [CrossRef]
39. Becker, A.; Thakur, B.K.; Weiss, J.M.; Kim, H.S.; Peinado, H.; Lyden, D. Extracellular Vesicles in Cancer: Cell-to-Cell Mediators of Metastasis. *Cancer Cell* **2016**, *30*, 836–848. [CrossRef]
40. Wu, K.; Xing, F.; Wu, S.-Y.; Watabe, K. Extracellular vesicles as emerging targets in cancer: recent development from bench to bedside. *Biochim. Biophys. Acta* **2017**, *1868*, 1–59. [CrossRef]
41. Srivastava, A.; Amreddy, N.; Pareek, V.; Chinnappan, M.; Ahmed, R.; Mehta, M.; Razaq, M.; Munshi, A.; Ramesh, R. Progress in extracellular vesicle biology and their application in cancer medicine. *Wiley Interdiscip. Rev. Nanomed. Nanobiotechnol.* **2020**, *12*, e1621. [CrossRef] [PubMed]
42. Fu, X.; Liu, M.; Qu, S.; Ma, J.; Zhang, Y.; Shi, T.; Wen, H.; Shengyang, Q.; Wang, S.; Wang, J.; et al. Exosomal microRNA-32-5p induces multidrug resistance in hepatocellular carcinoma via the PI3K/Akt pathway. *J. Exp. Clin. Cancer Res.* **2018**, *37*, 52. [CrossRef] [PubMed]
43. Burnouf, T.; Agrahari, V.; Agrahari, V. Extracellular Vesicles as Nanomedicine: Hopes and Hurdles in Clinical Translation. *Int. J. Nanomed.* **2019**, *14*, 8847–8859. [CrossRef] [PubMed]
44. Kumar, D.; Gupta, D.; Shankar, S.; Srivastava, R.K. Biomolecular characterization of exosomes released from cancer stem cells: Possible implications for biomarker and treatment of cancer. *Oncotarget* **2015**, *6*, 3280–3291. [CrossRef] [PubMed]
45. Tickner, J.A.; Urquhart, A.J.; Stephenson, S.-A.; Richard, D.J.; O'Byrne, K.J. Functions and Therapeutic Roles of Exosomes in Cancer. *Front. Oncol.* **2014**, *4*, 127. [CrossRef]
46. Maacha, S.; Bhat, A.A.; Jimenez, L.; Raza, A.; Haris, M.; Uddin, S.; Grivel, J.-C. Extracellular vesicles-mediated intercellular communication: Roles in the tumor microenvironment and anti-cancer drug resistance. *Mol. Cancer* **2019**, *18*, 1–16. [CrossRef]
47. Feng, W.; Dean, D.C.; Hornicek, F.J.; Shi, H.; Duan, Z. Exosomes promote pre-metastatic niche formation in ovarian cancer. *Mol. Cancer* **2019**, *18*, 1–11. [CrossRef]
48. Guo, Y.; Ji, X.; Liu, J.; Fan, D.; Zhou, Q.; Chen, C.; Wang, W.; Wang, G.; Wang, H.; Yuan, W.; et al. Effects of exosomes on pre-metastatic niche formation in tumors. *Mol. Cancer* **2019**, *18*, 39. [CrossRef]
49. Fanini, F.; Fabbri, M. Cancer-derived exosomic microRNAs shape the immune system within the tumor microenvironment: State of the art. *Semin. Cell Dev. Biol.* **2017**, *67*, 23–28. [CrossRef]
50. Wagner, V.; Dullaart, A.; Bock, A.-K.; Zweck, A. The emerging nanomedicine landscape. *Nat. Biotechnol.* **2006**, *24*, 1211–1217. [CrossRef]
51. Freitas, R.A. What is nanomedicine? *Nanomed. Nanotechnol. Biol. Med.* **2005**, *1*, 2–9. [CrossRef] [PubMed]
52. Youn, Y.S.; Bae, Y.H. Perspectives on the past, present, and future of cancer nanomedicine. *Adv. Drug Deliv. Rev.* **2018**, *130*, 3–11. [CrossRef] [PubMed]
53. Borrelli, D.A.; Yankson, K.; Shukla, N.; Vilanilam, G.; Ticer, T.; Wolfram, J. Extracellular vesicle therapeutics for liver disease. *J. Control. Release* **2018**, *273*, 86–98. [CrossRef]
54. Bunggulawa, E.J.; Wang, W.; Yin, T.; Wang, N.; Durkan, C.; Wang, Y.; Wang, G. Recent advancements in the use of exosomes as drug delivery systems. *J. Nanobiotechnol.* **2018**, *16*, 1–13. [CrossRef] [PubMed]

55. De Jong, O.G.; Kooijmans, S.A.A.; Murphy, D.E.; Jiang, L.; Evers, M.J.W.; Sluijter, J.P.G.; Vader, P.; Schiffelers, R.M. Drug Delivery with Extracellular Vesicles: From Imagination to Innovation. *Acc. Chem. Res.* **2019**, *52*, 1761–1770. [CrossRef] [PubMed]
56. Batrakova, E.V.; Kim, M.S. Using exosomes, naturally-equipped nanocarriers, for drug delivery. *J. Control. Release* **2015**, *219*, 396–405. [CrossRef] [PubMed]
57. Chulpanova, D.S.; Kitaeva, K.V.; James, V.; Rizvanov, A.A.; Solovyeva, V.V. Therapeutic Prospects of Extracellular Vesicles in Cancer Treatment. *Front. Immunol.* **2018**, *9*, 1534. [CrossRef]
58. Lener, T.; Gimona, M.; Aigner, L.; Börger, V.; Buzas, E.; Camussi, G.; Chaput, N.; Chatterjee, D.; Court, F.A.; del Portillo, H.A.; et al. Applying extracellular vesicles based therapeutics in clinical trials—An ISEV position paper. *J. Extracell. Vesicles* **2015**, *4*, 1–31. [CrossRef]
59. Veerman, R.E.; Akpinar, G.G.; Eldh, M.; Gabrielsson, S. Immune Cell-Derived Extracellular Vesicles-Functions and Therapeutic Applications. *Trends Mol. Med.* **2019**, *25*, 382–394. [CrossRef]
60. Kim, M.S.; Haney, M.J.; Zhao, Y.; Mahajan, V.; Deygen, I.; Klyachko, N.L.; Inskoe, E.; Piroyan, A.; Sokolsky, M.; Okolie, O.; et al. Development of Exosome-encapsulated Paclitaxel to Overcome MDR in Cancer cells. *Nanomedicine* **2016**, *12*, 655–664. [CrossRef]
61. Kim, M.S.; Haney, M.J.; Zhao, Y.; Yuan, D.; Deygen, I.; Klyachko, N.L.; Kabanov, A.V.; Batrakova, E.V. Engineering macrophage-derived exosomes for targeted paclitaxel delivery to pulmonary metastases: In vitro and in vivo evaluations. *Nanomed. Nanotechnol. Biol. Med.* **2018**, *14*, 195–204. [CrossRef] [PubMed]
62. Pascucci, L.; Coccè, V.; Bonomi, A.; Ami, D.; Ceccarelli, P.; Ciusani, E.; Viganò, L.; Locatelli, A.; Sisto, F.; Doglia, S.M.; et al. Paclitaxel is incorporated by mesenchymal stromal cells and released in exosomes that inhibit in vitro tumor growth: A new approach for drug delivery. *J. Control. Release* **2014**, *192*, 262–270. [CrossRef] [PubMed]
63. Fuster-Matanzo, A.; Gessler, F.; Leonardi, T.; Iraci, N.; Pluchino, S. Acellular approaches for regenerative medicine: On the verge of clinical trials with extracellular membrane vesicles? *Stem Cell Res. Ther.* **2015**, *6*, 1–10. [CrossRef] [PubMed]
64. Ma, J.; Zhang, Y.; Tang, K.; Zhang, H.; Yin, X.; Li, Y.; Xu, P.; Sun, Y.; Ma, R.; Ji, T.; et al. Reversing drug resistance of soft tumor-repopulating cells by tumor cell-derived chemotherapeutic microparticles. *Cell Res.* **2016**, *26*, 713–727. [CrossRef]
65. Li, J.; Chen, X.; Yi, J.; Liu, Y.; Li, D.; Wang, J.; Hou, D.; Jiang, X.; Zhang, J.; Wang, J.; et al. Identification and Characterization of 293T Cell-Derived Exosomes by Profiling the Protein, mRNA and MicroRNA Components. *PLoS ONE* **2016**, *11*, e0163043. [CrossRef]
66. You, B.; Xu, W.; Zhang, B. Engineering exosomes: A new direction for anticancer treatment. *Am. J. Cancer Res.* **2018**, *8*, 1332–1342.
67. Luan, X.; Sansanaphongpricha, K.; Myers, I.; Chen, H.; Yuan, H.; Sun, D. Engineering exosomes as refined biological nanoplatforms for drug delivery. *Acta Pharmacol. Sin.* **2017**, *38*, 754–763. [CrossRef]
68. Rahbarghazi, R.; Jabbari, N.; Sani, N.A.; Asghari, R.; Salimi, L.; Kalashani, S.A.; Feghhi, M.; Etemadi, T.; Akbariazar, E.; Mahmoudi, M.; et al. Tumor-derived extracellular vesicles: Reliable tools for Cancer diagnosis and clinical applications. *Cell Commun. Signal.* **2019**, *17*, 1–17. [CrossRef]
69. O'Brien, K.; Lowry, M.C.; Corcoran, C.; Martinez, V.G.; Daly, M.; Rani, S.; Gallagher, W.M.; Radomski, M.W.; MacLeod, R.A.; O'Driscoll, L. miR-134 in extracellular vesicles reduces triple-negative breast cancer aggression and increases drug sensitivity. *Oncotarget* **2015**, *6*, 32774–32789. [CrossRef]
70. Syn, N.L.; Wang, L.; Chow, E.K.-H.; Lim, C.T.; Goh, B.-C. Exosomes in Cancer Nanomedicine and Immunotherapy: Prospects and Challenges. *Trends Biotechnol.* **2017**, *35*, 665–676. [CrossRef]
71. Taylor, D.D.; Shah, S. Methods of isolating extracellular vesicles impact down-stream analyses of their cargoes. *Methods* **2015**, *87*, 3–10. [CrossRef] [PubMed]
72. Konoshenko, M.Y.; Lekchnov, E.A.; Vlassov, A.V.; Laktionov, P.P. Isolation of Extracellular Vesicles: General Methodologies and Latest Trends. *BioMed Res. Int.* **2018**, *2018*, 1–27. [CrossRef] [PubMed]
73. Heinemann, M.L.; Ilmer, M.; Silva, L.P.; Hawke, D.H.; Recio, A.; Vorontsova, M.A.; Alt, E.; Vykoukal, J. Benchtop isolation and characterization of functional exosomes by sequential filtration. *J. Chromatogr. A* **2014**, *1371*, 125–135. [CrossRef] [PubMed]

74. Nordin, J.Z.; Lee, Y.; Vader, P.; Mäger, I.; Johansson, H.J.; Heusermann, W.; Wiklander, O.P.; Hällbrink, M.; Seow, Y.; Bultema, J.J.; et al. Ultrafiltration with size-exclusion liquid chromatography for high yield isolation of extracellular vesicles preserving intact biophysical and functional properties. *Nanomed. Nanotechnol. Biol. Med.* **2015**, *11*, 879–883. [CrossRef] [PubMed]
75. Yu, L.-L.; Zhu, J.; Liu, J.-X.; Jiang, F.; Ni, W.-K.; Qu, L.-S.; Ni, R.-Z.; Lu, C.-H.; Xiao, M. A Comparison of Traditional and Novel Methods for the Separation of Exosomes from Human Samples. *BioMed Res. Int.* **2018**, *2018*, 1–9. [CrossRef] [PubMed]
76. Nakai, W.; Yoshida, T.; Diez, D.; Miyatake, Y.; Nishibu, T.; Imawaka, N.; Naruse, K.; Sadamura, Y.; Hanayama, R. A novel affinity-based method for the isolation of highly purified extracellular vesicles. *Sci. Rep.* **2016**, *6*, 33935. [CrossRef]
77. Martins, T.S.; Catita, J.; Rosa, I.M.; Silva, O.A.B.D.C.E.; Henriques, A.G. Exosome isolation from distinct biofluids using precipitation and column-based approaches. *PLoS ONE* **2018**, *13*, e0198820. [CrossRef]
78. Escudier, B.; Dorval, T.; Chaput, N.; André, F.; Caby, M.-P.; Novault, S.; Flament, C.; Leboulaire, C.; Borg, C.; Amigorena, S.; et al. Vaccination of metastatic melanoma patients with autologous dendritic cell (DC) derived-exosomes: Results of the first phase I clinical trial. *J. Transl. Med.* **2005**, *3*, 10. [CrossRef]
79. Haoyao, S.; Burrola, S.; Wu, J.; Ding, W.Q. Extracellular Vesicles in the Development of Cancer Therapeutics. *Int. J. Mol. Sci.* **2020**, *21*, 6097. [CrossRef]
80. Gangadaran, P.; Ahn, B.-C. Extracellular Vesicle- and Extracellular Vesicle Mimetics-Based Drug Delivery Systems: New Perspectives, Challenges, and Clinical Developments. *Pharmaceutics* **2020**, *12*, 442. [CrossRef]
81. Gangadaran, P.; Hong, C.M.; Oh, J.M.; Rajendran, R.L.; Kalimuthu, S.; Son, S.H.; Gopal, A.; Zhu, L.; Baek, S.H.; Jeong, S.Y.; et al. In vivo Non-invasive Imaging of Radio-Labeled Exosome-Mimetics Derived from Red Blood Cells in Mice. *Front. Pharmacol.* **2018**, *9*, 817. [CrossRef] [PubMed]
82. García-Manrique, P.; Matos, M.; Gutiérrez, G.; Pazos, C.; Blanco-López, M.C. Therapeutic biomaterials based on extracellular vesicles: Classification of bio-engineering and mimetic preparation routes. *J. Extracell. Vesicles* **2018**, *7*, 1422676. [CrossRef] [PubMed]
83. Fais, S.; O'Driscoll, L.; Borras, F.E.; Buzas, E.; Camussi, G.; Cappello, F.; Carvalho, J.; Da Silva, A.C.; Del Portillo, H.; El Andaloussi, S.; et al. Evidence-Based Clinical Use of Nanoscale Extracellular Vesicles in Nanomedicine. *ACS Nano* **2016**, *10*, 3886–3899. [CrossRef] [PubMed]
84. Gangadaran, P.; Hong, C.M.; Ahn, B.-C. An Update on in Vivo Imaging of Extracellular Vesicles as Drug Delivery Vehicles. *Front. Pharmacol.* **2018**, *9*, 169. [CrossRef] [PubMed]
85. Bellavia, D.; Raimondo, S.; Calabrese, G.; Forte, S.; Cristaldi, M.; Patinella, A.; Memeo, L.; Manno, M.; Raccosta, S.; Diana, P.; et al. Interleukin 3- receptor targeted exosomes inhibit in vitro and in vivo Chronic Myelogenous Leukemia cell growth. *Theranostics* **2017**, *7*, 1333–1345. [CrossRef]
86. Kooijmans, S.; Fliervoet, L.; Van Der Meel, R.; Fens, M.H.A.M.; Heijnen, H.; Henegouwen, P.V.B.E.; Vader, P.C.V.V.; Schiffelers, R.M. PEGylated and targeted extracellular vesicles display enhanced cell specificity and circulation time. *J. Control. Release* **2016**, *224*, 77–85. [CrossRef]
87. Lee, H.; Park, H.; Noh, G.J.; Lee, E.S. pH-responsive hyaluronate-anchored extracellular vesicles to promote tumor-targeted drug delivery. *Carbohydr. Polym.* **2018**, *202*, 323–333. [CrossRef]
88. Han, X.; Xu, Y.; Geranpayehvaghei, M.; Anderson, G.J.; Li, Y.; Nie, G. Emerging nanomedicines for anti-stromal therapy against desmoplastic tumors. *Biomaterials* **2020**, *232*, 119745. [CrossRef]
89. Shi, J.; Kantoff, P.W.; Wooster, R.; Farokhzad, O.C. Cancer nanomedicine: Progress, challenges and opportunities. *Nat. Rev. Cancer* **2017**, *17*, 20–37. [CrossRef]
90. Ji, T.; Lang, J.; Wang, J.; Cai, R.; Zhang, Y.; Qi, F.; Zhang, L.; Zhao, X.; Wu, W.; Hao, J.; et al. Designing Liposomes to Suppress Extracellular Matrix Expression To Enhance Drug Penetration and Pancreatic Tumor Therapy. *ACS Nano* **2017**, *11*, 8668–8678. [CrossRef]
91. Ventola, C.L. Progress in Nanomedicine: Approved and Investigational Nanodrugs. *Pharm. Ther.* **2017**, *42*, 742–755.
92. Wiklander, O.P.B.; Nordin, J.Z.; O'Loughlin, A.; Gustafsson, Y.; Corso, G.; Mäger, I.; Vader, P.; Lee, Y.; Sork, H.; Seow, Y.; et al. Extracellular vesicle in vivo biodistribution is determined by cell source, route of administration and targeting. *J. Extracell. Vesicles* **2015**, *4*, 26316. [CrossRef] [PubMed]
93. Johnsen, K.B.; Gudbergsson, J.M.; Duroux, M.; Moos, T.; Andresen, T.L.; Simonsen, J.B. On the use of liposome controls in studies investigating the clinical potential of extracellular vesicle-based drug delivery systems-A commentary. *J. Control. Release* **2018**, *269*, 10–14. [CrossRef] [PubMed]

94. Mendt, M.; Rezvani, K.; Shpall, E. Mesenchymal stem cell-derived exosomes for clinical use. *Bone Marrow Transplant.* **2019**, *54*, 789–792. [CrossRef]
95. Börger, V.; Bremer, M.; Ferrer-Tur, R.; Gockeln, L.; Stambouli, O.; Becic, A.; Giebel, B. Mesenchymal Stem/Stromal Cell-Derived Extracellular Vesicles and Their Potential as Novel Immunomodulatory Therapeutic Agents. *Int. J. Mol. Sci.* **2017**, *18*, 1450. [CrossRef]
96. Squillaro, T.; Peluso, G.; Galderisi, U. Clinical Trials with Mesenchymal Stem Cells: An Update. *Cell Transplant.* **2016**, *25*, 829–848. [CrossRef] [PubMed]
97. Munagala, R.; Aqil, F.; Jeyabalan, J.; Gupta, R.C. Bovine milk-derived exosomes for drug delivery. *Cancer Letters.* **2016**, *371*, 48–61. [CrossRef]
98. Zhang, K.-L.; Wang, Y.-J.; Sun, J.; Zhou, J.; Xing, C.; Huang, G.; Li, J.; Yang, H.-H. Artificial chimeric exosomes for anti-phagocytosis and targeted cancer therapy. *Chem. Sci.* **2019**, *10*, 1555–1561. [CrossRef]
99. Kalimuthu, S.; Gangadaran, P.; Rajendran, R.L.; Zhu, L.; Oh, J.M.; Lee, H.W.; Gopal, A.; Baek, S.H.; Jeong, S.Y.; Lee, S.-W.; et al. A New Approach for Loading Anticancer Drugs into Mesenchymal Stem Cell-Derived Exosome Mimetics for Cancer Therapy. *Front. Pharmacol.* **2018**, *9*, 1116. [CrossRef]
100. Wu, M.; Le, W.; Mei, T.; Wang, Y.; Chen, B.; Liu, Z.; Xue, C. Cell membrane camouflaged nanoparticles: A new biomimetic platform for cancer photothermal therapy. *Int. J. Nanomed.* **2019**, *14*, 4431–4448. [CrossRef]

Publisher's Note: MDPI stays neutral with regard to jurisdictional claims in published maps and institutional affiliations.

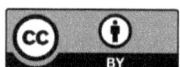

© 2020 by the authors. Licensee MDPI, Basel, Switzerland. This article is an open access article distributed under the terms and conditions of the Creative Commons Attribution (CC BY) license (http://creativecommons.org/licenses/by/4.0/).

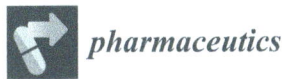

Article

Tumor-Homing pH-Sensitive Extracellular Vesicles for Targeting Heterogeneous Tumors

Jaeduk Park [1], Hyuk Lee [1], Yu Seok Youn [2], Kyung Taek Oh [3] and Eun Seong Lee [1,4,*]

1. Department of Biotechnology, The Catholic University of Korea, 43 Jibong-ro, Bucheon-si, Gyeonggi-do 14662, Korea; jduck0309@naver.com (J.P.); ahld1421@naver.com (H.L.)
2. School of Pharmacy, Sungkyunkwan University, 2066 Seobu-ro, Jangan-gu, Suwon, Gyeonggi-do 16419, Korea; ysyoun@skku.edu
3. College of Pharmacy, Chung-Ang University, 221 Heukseok dong, Dongjak-gu, Seoul 06974, Korea; kyungoh@cau.ac.kr
4. Department of Biomedical Chemical Engineering, The Catholic University of Korea, 43 Jibong-ro, Bucheon-si, Gyeonggi-do 14662, Korea
* Correspondence: eslee@catholic.ac.kr; Tel.: +82-02-2164-4921

Received: 31 March 2020; Accepted: 15 April 2020; Published: 17 April 2020

Abstract: In this study, we fabricated tumor-homing pH-sensitive extracellular vesicles for efficient tumor treatment. These vesicles were prepared using extracellular vesicles (EVs; BTEVs extracted from BT-474 tumor cells or SKEVs extracted from SK-N-MC tumor cells), hyaluronic acid grafted with 3-(diethylamino)propylamine (HDEA), and doxorubicin (DOX, as a model antitumor drug). Consequently, HDEA/DOX anchored EVs (HDEA@EVs) can interact with origin tumor cells owing to EVs' homing ability to origin cells. Therefore, EV blends of HDEA@BTEVs and HDEA@SKEVs demonstrate highly increased cellular uptake in both BT-474 and SK-N-MC cells: HDEA@BTEVs for BT-474 tumor cells and HDEA@SKEVs for SK-N-MC tumor cells. Furthermore, the hydrophobic HDEA present in HDEA@EVs at pH 7.4 can switch to hydrophilic HDEA at pH 6.5 as a result of acidic pH-induced protonation of 3-(diethylamino)propylamine (DEAP) moieties, resulting in an acidic pH-activated EVs' disruption, accelerated release of encapsulated DOX molecules, and highly increased cell cytotoxicity. However, EV blends containing pH-insensitive HA grafted with deoxycholic acid (HDOC) (HDOC@BTEVs and HDOC@SKEVs) showed less cell cytotoxicity for both BT-474 and SK-N-MC tumor cells, because they did not act on EVs' disruption and the resulting DOX release. Consequently, the use of these tumor-homing pH-sensitive EV blends may result in effective targeted therapies for various tumor cells.

Keywords: tumor-homing extracellular vesicles; pH-sensitive extracellular vesicles; doxorubicin; tumor therapy

1. Introduction

Extracellular vesicles (EVs) are nanosized cellular vesicles released from various types of tumor cells [1–5]. To achieve quick and extensive intercellular communication between tumor cells, EVs are secreted out of the cells so that they can enter the recipient cells [4–7]. These EVs perform various biological functions, such as the disposal of cellular waste products, release of foreign invaders, control of gene expression, and activation of the immune system [8–10].

In addition, EVs intrinsically express various membrane proteins, cell adhesion molecules, and tumor specific ligands, thereby enabling the homing of EVs to origin cells [4,11–16]. These properties of EVs enable tumor-homing ability and render them potential candidates as tumor-recognizing drug carriers. In particular, recent studies suggest that these EVs have the ability to interact with their released parental cells, and this property has been used to target tumor cells [4,11–16]. This means that these EVs are suitable as tumor-targeting and tumor-penetrating drug carriers, as they can be selectively homed to their parent tumor cells [4,13–22]. Furthermore, the immunogenicity of these EVs is relatively low; therefore, they exhibit excellent body safety for biomedical applications [4,10,19,20].

In this study, we fabricated tumor-homing pH-sensitive EVs. These EVs were prepared using EVs (BTEVs extracted from BT-474 tumor cells or SKEVs extracted from SK-N-MC tumor cells), hyaluronic acid grafted with 3-(diethylamino)propylamine (HDEA), and doxorubicin (DOX) [3]. In particular, we prepared EV blends using HDEA/DOX anchored EVs (HDEA@BTEVs and HDEA@SKEVs) to target different tumor cells. The EV blends are expected to yield efficient cellular uptake for parent BT-474 and SK-N-MC tumor cells. Therefore, we hypothesize that these different EVs can target their origin tumor cells, owing to their homing ability to origin cells, allowing their efficient accumulation into heterogeneous tumor cells. Furthermore, 3-(diethylamino)propylamine (DEAP) moieties present in HDEA can be protonated at endosomal pH and induce the destabilization of EVs, owing to DEAP-mediated vesicle destabilization, followed by the release of encapsulated DOX [3,23–31]. In this study, we investigated the tumor targeting ability, pH-sensitive properties, and antitumor efficacy of EV blends against BT-474 and SK-N-MC tumor cells.

2. Materials and Methods

2.1. Materials

Hyaluronic acid (HA, Mw = 4.8 kDa), 3-(diethylamino)propylamine (DEAP), N-hydroxysuccinimide (NHS), N,N'-dicyclohexylcarbodiimide (DCC), triethylamine (TEA), deoxycholic acid (DOCA), 4-dimethylaminopyridine (DMAP), pyridine, dimethyl sulfoxide (DMSO), sodium tetraborate, adipic acid dihydrazide (ADH), doxorubicin hydrochloride (DOX), paraformaldehyde, heparin, and Triton X-100, 4′,6-diamidino-2-phenylindole dihydrochloride (DAPI) were purchased from Sigma-Aldrich (St. Louis, MO, USA). Chlorin e6 (Ce6) was purchased from Frontier Scientific Inc (Logan, UT, USA). RPMI-1640 medium, DMEM medium, fetal bovine serum (FBS), phosphate buffered saline (PBS), ethylene diamine tetra-acetic acid (EDTA), penicillin, trypsin, and streptomycin were purchased from Welgene Inc (Seoul, Korea). EV-depleted FBS was purchased from System Biosciences Inc. (Palo Alto, CA, USA). Cell Counting Kit-8 (CCK-8) was purchased from Dojindo Molecular Technologies Inc. (Santa Clara, CA, USA). Wheat Germ Agglutinin Alexa Fluor® 488 Conjugate (WGA-Alexa Fluor® 488), fluorescein isothiocyanate (FITC) were purchased from Life Technologies (Carlsbad, CA, USA).

2.2. Synthesis of HA-g-DEAP

The detailed synthesis method of HA grafted with DEAP (HA-g-DEAP: HDEA) was described in our previous report [3,29–31]. Briefly, HA (200 mg) was reacted with DEAP (55 mg) in DMSO (10 mL) containing DCC (110 mg), NHS (60 mg), and TEA (500 µL) at 25 °C for 3 days, to produce HDEA (Figure S1). HA grafted with DOCA (HA-g-DOCA: HDOC) was prepared as a pH-insensitive control group against pH-sensitive HDEA. The detailed synthesis method of HDOC was described in our previous report [3,29–31]. Briefly, HA (200 mg) was reacted with DOCA (650 mg) in DMSO (10 mL) containing DCC (340 mg), DMAP (20 mg), and pyridine (500 µL) at 25 °C for 3 days, to produce HDOC (Figure S2). In addition, HDEA (100 mg) or HDOC (100 mg) were reacted with Ce6 (15 mg) in DMSO (10 mL) containing DCC (10 mg), ADH (9 mg), NHS (6 mg), and TEA (200 µL) at 25 °C for 2 days, to produce Ce6-labeled HDEA or Ce6–labeled HDOC [3,30,31]. The non-reacted chemicals were removed via dialysis against fresh DMSO for 3 days, and then deionized water for 3 days using a pre-swollen dialysis membrane (Spectra/Por®6 MWCO 2 kDa, Spectrum Laboratories Inc, Rancho Dominguez, CA, USA). The dialyzed solution was freeze-dried; subsequently, the final product was obtained [3,29–31].

2.3. Harvest of EVs

To harvest EVs, human breast carcinoma BT-474 cells and human neuroblastoma SK-N-MC cells were selected as the EV secreting cell lines and purchased from the Korean Cell Line Bank (Seoul, Korea). BT-474 cells were cultured in an RPMI-1640 medium containing 1% penicillin-streptomycin and 10% EV-depleted FBS in a 5% CO_2 atmosphere at 37 °C. SK-N-MC cells were cultured in the DMEM medium containing 1% penicillin-streptomycin and 10% EV-depleted FBS in a 5% CO_2 atmosphere at 37 °C. The cell culture medium was centrifuged at 2000 g for 20 min at 4 °C and additionally centrifuged at 10,000 g for 30 min to eliminate large cell debris and dead cells. Subsequently, the supernatant was again ultracentrifuged at 100,000 g at 4 °C for 70 min to separate EVs pellets. The obtained pellets were washed using fresh PBS (150 mM, pH 7.4) and then ultracentrifuged at 100,000 g at 4 °C for 70 min. These purified EVs were stored at −80 °C, after being suspended in fresh PBS (150 mM, pH 7.4) [3,30,32–34]. In addition, the suspended EVs concentration was analyzed using Nanosight (LM10, Malvern Instruments, Malvern, UK) with NTA 2.3 software [3,35].

2.4. Preparation of EV Samples

Sonication was performed to incorporate HDEA (or HDOC) and DOX to EVs [3,30,36]. HDEA (300 µg, or Ce6-labeled HDEA) or HDOC (200 µg, or Ce6-labeled HDOC) dissolved in DMSO (0.1 mL) containing DOX (400 µg) were mixed with EVs (200 µg) suspended in PBS (10 mL, 150 mM, pH 7.4) at 25 °C, and the solution was sonicated using a tip sonicator, vcx-130 with cv-18 (Sonics, Newtown, CT, USA) with a 30% amplitude for 30 s. This sonication process was repeated 6 times at 3 min intervals. The obtained solution was incubated at 37 °C for 60 min to recover the EVs. The filtration method using 0.22 µm membranes was performed to remove HDEA (or HDOC) or DOX aggregates. Ultracentrifugation at 100,000 g at 4 °C for 70 min was performed to remove free HDEA (or HDOC) and DOX to yield HDEA@EVs or HDOC@EVs [3,30,36]. In addition, DOX@EVs with DOX and without HDEA and HDOC were prepared following the same procedure as described above.

2.5. Measurement of Loading Contents

The concentration of HDEA or HDOC (with fluorescent Ce6 dye) in the EVs was measured using a fluorescence spectrofluorometer (RF-5301PC, Shimadzu, Kyoto, Japan) at λ_{ex} of 450 nm and λ_{em} of 670 nm using a DMSO/PBS solution (90/10 vol.%) [3,30,31]. The HDEA or HDOC loading content (%) was calculated as the weight percentage of HDEA or HDOC in the EVs. The concentration of DOX entrapped in the EVs was measured using a fluorescence spectrofluorometer at λ_{ex} of 470 nm and λ_{em} of 592 nm using a DMSO/PBS solution (90/10 vol.%). The DOX loading content (%) was calculated as the weight percentage of DOX in the EVs [3,30,31].

2.6. Characterization of EV Samples

The particle size and zeta potential of the EV samples at pH 7.4 or 6.5 were measured using a Zetasizer 3000 instrument (Malvern Instruments, Malvern, UK) [3,30,37–40]. The morphologies of the EV samples at pH 7.4 or 6.5 were analyzed using a transmission electron microscope (Talos L120C, FEI, Hillsboro, OR, USA) [3,31,37,38].

2.7. In Vitro DOX Release Test

The EV samples (equivalent to DOX of 100 µg/mL) in PBS (3 mL, 150 mM, pH 7.4) were added to a dialysis membrane (Spectra/Por® MWCO 10 K) and immersed in fresh PBS (15 mL, 150 mM, pH 7.4 or 6.5) [3,30,31,40]. A DOX release test was conducted using a mechanical shaker (100 rpm) at 37 °C [3,30,31,40]. The external PBS of the dialysis membrane was extracted and replaced with fresh PBS at the specified time point. The amount of DOX released from the EV samples was measured using a fluorescence spectrofluorometer at λ_{ex} of 470 nm and λ_{em} of 592 [3,27].

2.8. Hemolysis Test

To determine the endosomolytic activity of the EV samples, a hemolysis test was conducted using red blood cells (RBCs) collected from BALB/c mice (7-week-old female) [31,41,42]. The RBC solutions (10^6 cells/mL) at pH 7.4 or 6.5 were incubated with the EV samples (equivalent to EVs of 30 µg/mL, without DOX) at 37 °C for 1 h. The RBC solutions were centrifuged at 1500 g for 10 min at 4 °C and the supernatant was collected. The light absorbance (LA) value of the supernatant was measured using a spectrophotometer at a wavelength of 541 nm. A 0% (as a negative control) LA was acquired from a PBS-treated intact RBC solution and the 100% (as a positive control) of LA value was obtained from completely lysed RBC solution using 2 wt.% Triton X-100. The hemolysis (%) of each EV sample was determined as the LA of the RBC solution treated with each sample relative to the control LA value [31,41,42].

2.9. Cell Culture

Human breast carcinoma BT-474 cells, human neuroblastoma SK-N-MC cells, and human liver carcinoma Huh7 cells were purchased from the Korean Cell Line Bank. When the cells were grown as a monolayer (1×10^6 cells/mL), they were harvested by trypsinization using a 0.25% (wt./vol.) trypsin/0.03% (wt./vol.) EDTA solution. Subsequently, the cells suspended in the RPMI-1640 or DMEM medium were seeded in well plates before cell test [37–40].

2.10. In Vitro Cellular UPTAKE test

BT-474, SK-N-MC, or Huh7 tumor cells were incubated with EV samples (equivalent to DOX of 5 µg/mL) or free DOX (5 µg/mL) for 4 h. After washing the cells using fresh PBS (150 mM, pH 7.4), the fluorescence intensity of the cells was determined using a FACSCaliburTM flow cytometer (FACS Canto II, Becton Dickinson, Franklin lakes, NJ, USA) [3,31,37–39]. In addition, to visualize the cellular uptake of the EV samples, BT-474 or SK-N-MC tumor cells were incubated with the EV samples for 4 h and then fixed using 3.7% formaldehyde in PBS. The fixed cells were monitored using a Nikon microscope equipped with a VNIR hyperspectral camera system (Cytoviva high-resolution adapter, Cytoviva, Auburn, AL, USA) [43–45]. For confocal microscopy analysis, the treated cells were stained with WGA-Alexa Fluor® 488 and DAPI. The stained cells were then fixed using 3.7% formaldehyde in PBS and analyzed using a confocal laser scanning microscope (LSM710, Carl Zeiss, Oberkochen, Germany) [3,30,31].

2.11. In Vitro Cytotoxicity Test

To determine the cytotoxicity, BT-474, SK-N-MC, or Huh7 tumor cells were incubated with the EV samples (equivalent to DOX of 5 µg/mL) or free DOX (5 µg/mL) at pH 7.4 for 4 h. After washing the cells using fresh PBS (150 mM, pH 7.4), the treated cells were further incubated with fresh RPMI-1640 or DMEM medium at 37 °C for 24 h. CCK-8 assay was used to determine the cell viability [3,31,38–40]. In addition, the viability of the cells incubated with drug-free EVs for 24 h was measured using the CCK-8 assay to determine the original toxicity of the EVs and polymers [3,31,38–40].

2.12. In Vitro Cellular Uptake Test of EV Blends

BTEVs (with fluorescent Ce6 dye incorporation) and SKEVs (with fluorescent FITC dye incorporation) were used to visualize the cellular uptake of the EV blends. Here, Ce6 dye or FITC dye was incorporated into the EVs through sonication [3,30,36]. Briefly, Ce6 dye (200 µg) or FITC dye (200 µg) dissolved in DMSO (0.1 mL) were mixed with EVs (200 µg) suspended in PBS (10 mL, 150 mM, pH 7.4) at 25 °C; subsequently, the solution was sonicated using a tip sonicator, vcx-130 with cv-18 (Sonics, Newtown, CT, USA) with 30% amplitude for 30 s. The obtained solution was incubated at 37 °C for 60 min to recover the EVs. The filtration method using 0.22 µm membrane was performed to remove Ce6 or FITC aggregates. Ultracentrifugation at 100,000 g at 4 °C for 70 min was performed to remove free Ce6 or FITC. The measured weight of the Ce6 or FITC dye incorporated in the EVs was 1–2 wt.%, as evaluated using a fluorescence spectrofluorometer. The obtained EV blends [HDEA@BTEVs/HDEA@SKEVs (50/50 wt.%)] (equivalent to EVs of 30 µg/mL, without DOX) were added to the tumor cells seeded on coverslips in a culture plate at 37 °C for 4 h. After washing the cells using fresh PBS (150 mM, pH 7.4), the treated cells were fixed using 3.7% formaldehyde in PBS. The fixed cells were analyzed using a confocal laser scanning microscope (LSM710, Carl Zeiss, Oberkochen, Germany) [3,30,31].

2.13. In Vitro Cytotoxicity Test of EV Blends

The mixed tumor cells (BT-474/SK-N-MC = 50:50 ratio of the number of cells) were prepared before the cell test and incubated with EV blends [HDEA@BTEVs/HDEA@SKEVs (50/50 wt.%)] (equivalent to DOX of 5 µg/mL), HDEA@BTEVs (equivalent to DOX of 5 µg/mL), or HDEA@SKEVs (equivalent to DOX of 5 µg/mL) for 4 h at 37 °C. After washing the cells using fresh PBS (150 mM, pH 7.4), the treated cells were additionally cultured with fresh RPMI-1640/DMEM mixed medium (50/50 vol.%) at 37 °C for 24 h. The CCK-8 assay was used to determine the cell viability [3,31,38–40].

2.14. Statistics

All the experimental results were analyzed using Student's t-test or ANOVA at a significance level of $p < 0.01$ (**) [37].

3. Results and Discussion

3.1. Characterization of EV Samples

To fabricate pH-sensitive EV blends for targeting heterogeneous tumor cells, we first harvested EVs (BTEVs from BT-474 tumor cells and SKEVs from SK-N-MC tumor cells). The harvested BTEVs and SKEVs were almost spherical, as shown in the TEM image (Figure S3a). Subsequently, these EVs (BTEVs and SKEVs) were identified to exhibit specific protein expressions (Figure S3b). In particular, TSG 101, a conventional marker for EVs, was highly expressed in all EVs [46–48]. The estrogen receptor alpha (ER-α) was significantly detected in the SKEVs, whereas the tau protein (Tau) was only detected in the BTEVs (Figure S3b) [49–52]. Next, we incorporated pH-sensitive polymers (HDEA) and an antitumor model drug (DOX) to the EVs through sonication, as described in the experimental methods section. Finally, we obtained HDEA-anchored BTEVs (HDEA@BTEVs) or HDEA-anchored SKEVs (HDEA@SKEVs). HDOC@BTEVs and HDOC@SKEVs were prepared as pH-insensitive EVs to evaluate the pH-sensitive properties of HDEA@BTEVs and HDEA@SKEVs, respectively. The loading content of HDEA or HDOC in the EV samples was 29–31 wt.%, and the loading content of DOX in the EV samples was 12–16 wt.% (data not shown). Next, we prepared EV blends by physically mixing HDEA@BTEVs and HDEA@SKEVs (a weight ratio of 50/50) in PBS (pH 7.4).

As shown in Figure 1a, we expect the EV blends to home to their parent cells owing to the EVs' homing ability [4,11–17]. Here, the DEAP moieties in the EVs can be protonated at the endosomal pH 6.5, inducing EV destabilization and accelerating the release of encapsulated DOX [3,23–31].

Figure 1b,c shows that the average particle sizes of intact EVs and the EV samples ranged from 105 to 120 nm at pH 7.4. However, the particle size of the HDEA@BTEVs and HDEA@SKEVs increased from 105 nm at pH 7.4 to 200 nm at endosomal pH 6.5 (Figure 1b,c), likely owing to the destabilized membrane of EVs due to the protonated DEAP [3,30,31]. By contrast, intact BTEVs, intact SKEVs, HDOC@BTEVs, and HDOC@SKEVs indicated no significant difference in particle size when the pH of the solution was reduced to pH 6.5; this could be due to the absence of pH-sensitive polymers (HDEA). In addition, as the pH of the solution decreased from 7.4 to 6.5, the zeta potentials of the HDEA@BTEVs and HDEA@SKEVs increased from −18.3 and −18.6 mV to −8.6 mV and −9.2 mV, respectively (Figure 1d,e). It was assumed that the protonated DEAP at pH 6.5 elevated the zeta potential of the HDEA@BTEVs and HDEA@SKEVs [3,30,31]. However, the zeta potential of intact

BTEVs, intact SKEVs, HDOC@BTEVs, and HDOC@SKEVs indicated no significant difference at pH 7.4 and 6.5. Furthermore, the morphological images obtained from TEM reveal that almost spherical HDEA@BTEVs and HDEA@SKEVs at pH 7.4 were destabilized at pH 6.5, and that their structures were partially cracked (Figure 1f). However, the HDOC@BTEVs and HDOC@SKEVs did not show any noticeable changes between pH 7.4 and 6.5. These results demonstrated that pH-sensitive DEAP in the HDEA@BTEVs and HDEA@SKEVs mediated the destabilization of the EVs structure, owing to the protonation of HDEA [3,30,31] at endosomal pH 6.5.

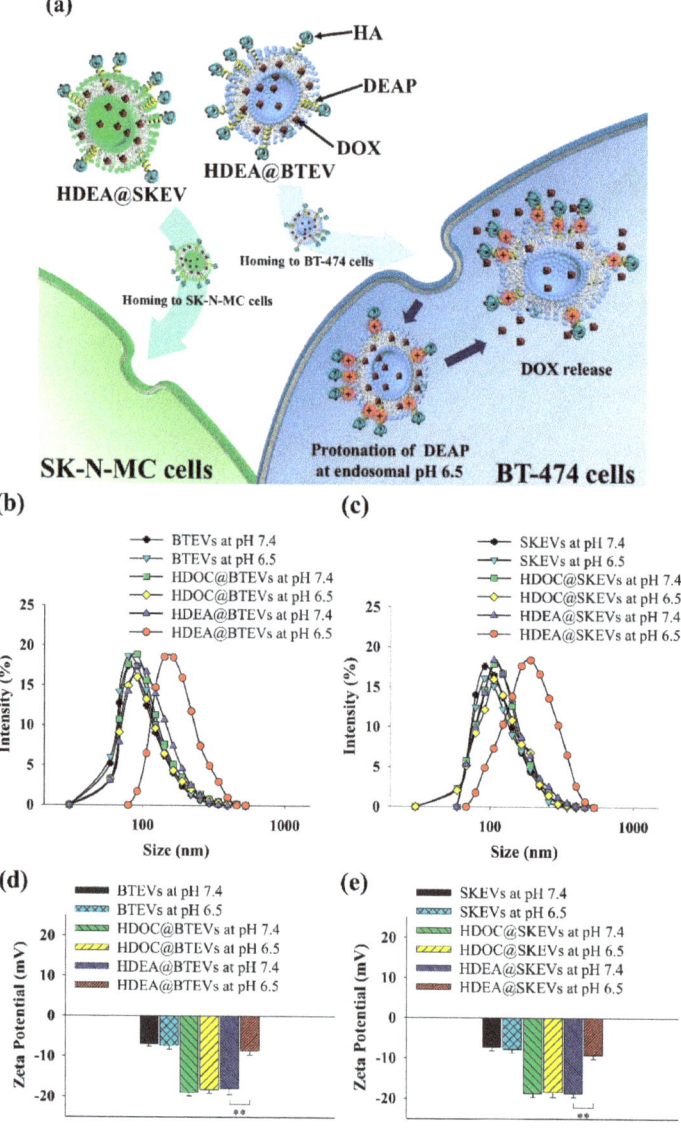

Figure 1. Cont.

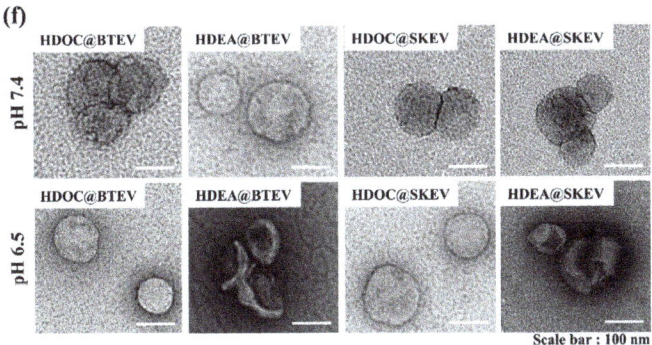

Figure 1. (a) Schematic illustration of tumor-homing pH-sensitive extracellular vesicles (EVs). Particle size distribution of (b) BTEVs and (c) SKEVs at pH 7.4 or 6.5. Zeta potential changes of (d) BTEVs and (e) SKEVs at pH 7.4 or 6.5 ($n = 3$, as multiple experiments, ** $p < 0.01$ compared to EVs at pH 7.4). (f) TEM images of EVs at pH 7.4 or 6.5.

3.2. pH-Triggered DOX Release

The DOX release profile of the EV samples was monitored at pH 7.4 or 6.5 (Figure 2). At pH 7.4, all the EV samples released DOX gradually, and no significant differences were observed in the DOX release rates. However, at pH 6.5, the HDEA@BTEVs and HDEA@SKEVs exhibited a significant increase in the DOX release rates. Specifically, in 48 h, they released approximately 80–85 wt.% of the encapsulated DOX. In addition, regardless of pH change, the DOX@BTEVs, HDOC@BTEVs, DOX@SKEVs, and HDOC@SKEVs showed a passive DOX release of 40–45 wt.%. These results indicate that the HDEA@BTEVs and HDEA@SKEVs recognized a slight pH change, resulting in an accelerated DOX release at pH 6.5.

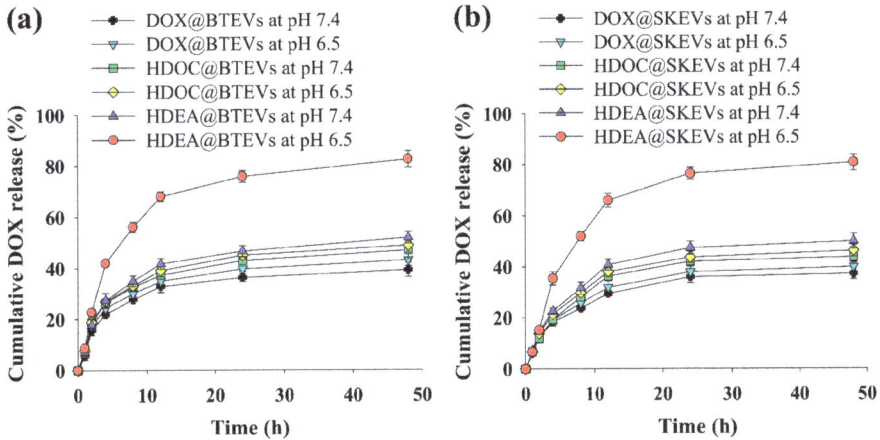

Figure 2. Cumulative doxorubicin hydrochloride (DOX) release from (a) BTEVs and (b) SKEVs at pH 7.4 or 6.5 in 48 h ($n = 3$, as multiple experiments).

3.3. Endosomolytic Activity Test

To evaluate the endosomolytic activity of EV samples, we performed a hemolysis test using RBCs with an endosomal-like membrane (Figure 3). At pH 7.4, intact EVs and all the EV samples exhibited negligible hemolytic activity. However, in response to endosomal pH 6.5, the hemolytic activities of the HDEA@BTEVs and HDEA@SKEVs increased significantly, likely owing to the proton sponge effect [3,30,31] of the protonated DEAP. By contrast, intact BTEVs, HDOC@BTEVs, intact SKEVs, and HDOC@SKEVs indicated no significant difference in hemolytic activity at pH 6.5. These results indicate that the endosomolytic activity of the HDEA@BTEVs and HDEA@SKEVs facilitated the cytosolic release of drugs in the tumor cells.

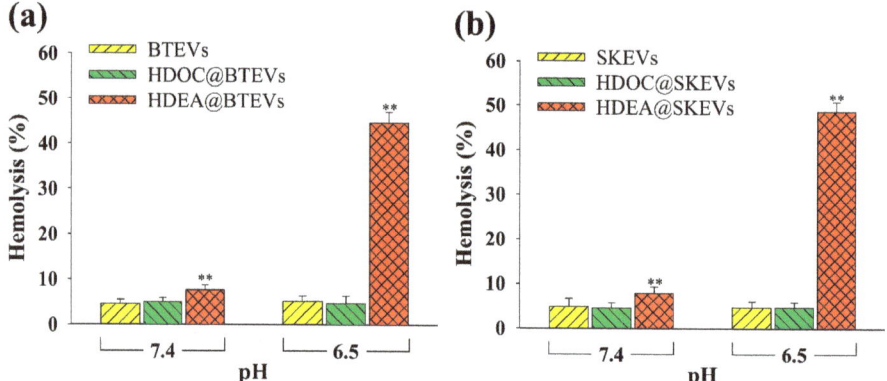

Figure 3. Hemolysis activities of (**a**) BTEVs and (**b**) SKEVs (n = 3, as multiple experiments, ** p < 0.01 compared with the control EVs).

3.4. In Vitro Cellular Uptake and Cytotoxicity of EV Blends

We verified the cellular uptake behaviors of EV samples for tumor cells (BT-474, SK-N-MC, and Huh7 cells) using a FACSCaliburTM flow cytometer [3,31,37–39]. Figure 4 shows the quantitative results of the cellular uptake of EV samples in tumor cells (BT-474, SK-N-MC, and Huh7). The average fluorescence intensity of BTEVs samples (HDEA@BTEVs, HDOC@BTEVs, and DOX@BTEVs) in BT-474 tumor cells was ~1.4 × 10^3; however, those of the SKEV samples (HDEA@SKEVs, HDOC@SKEVs, and DOX@SKEVs) and free DOX were ~1.2 × 10^2 and ~45 (Figure 4a), respectively. Consequently, the uptake of the BTEV samples by the BT-474 tumor cells increased significantly, compared with that of the SKEV samples and free DOX. Meanwhile, as shown in Figure 4b, the uptake of the SKEV samples by the SK-N-MC tumor cells increased, compared with that of the BTEV samples and free DOX. The average fluorescence intensity of the SKEV samples in SK-N-MC tumor cells was ~1.6 × 10^3; however, those of the BTEV samples and free DOX were ~1.5× 10^2 and ~57, respectively. However, the uptake of all the EV samples in the Huh7 tumor cells was extremely low and did not exhibit a noticeable difference between all samples (Figure 4c). In addition, the average fluorescence intensity of all EV samples in the Huh7 tumor cells was ~1.1 × 10^2. Overall, these results indicate that EVs with homing ability were efficiently endocytosed to their parent tumor cells [4,11–17].

To further evaluate the internalization of EVs to their parent tumor cells, we also performed in vitro cell imaging studies using a VNIR hyperspectral camera system and a confocal laser scanning microscope [3,30,31,43–45]. The hyperspectral images shows that the DOX (present in EV samples) signal of BT-474 tumor cells treated using BTEV samples (HDEA@BTEVs and HDOC@BTEVs) was higher than that of BT-474 tumor cells treated with SKEV samples (HDEA@SKEVs and HDOC@SKEVs) (Figure 5a), whereas the DOX signal of SK-N-MC tumor cells treated using SKEV samples was higher than that of SK-N-MC tumor cells treated with BTEV samples (Figure 5b). Figure 6 shows confocal images of BT-474 and SK-N-MC tumor cells treated using EV samples. The treated cells were stained using DAPI and WGA-Alexa Fluor® 488 to visualize the cell nuclei and membranes [3,30,31]. The confocal images revealed that the BTEV samples were actively internalized to BT-474 tumor cells, although the SKEV samples were ineffective in interacting with BT-474 tumor cells (Figure 6a). Similarly, the SKEVs samples were efficiently internalized to SK-N-MC tumor cells, whereas the BTEV samples were poorly internalized to SK-N-MC tumor cells (Figure 6b). These results support the homing ability of EVs to their parent tumor cells, which is consistent with the results shown in Figure 4.

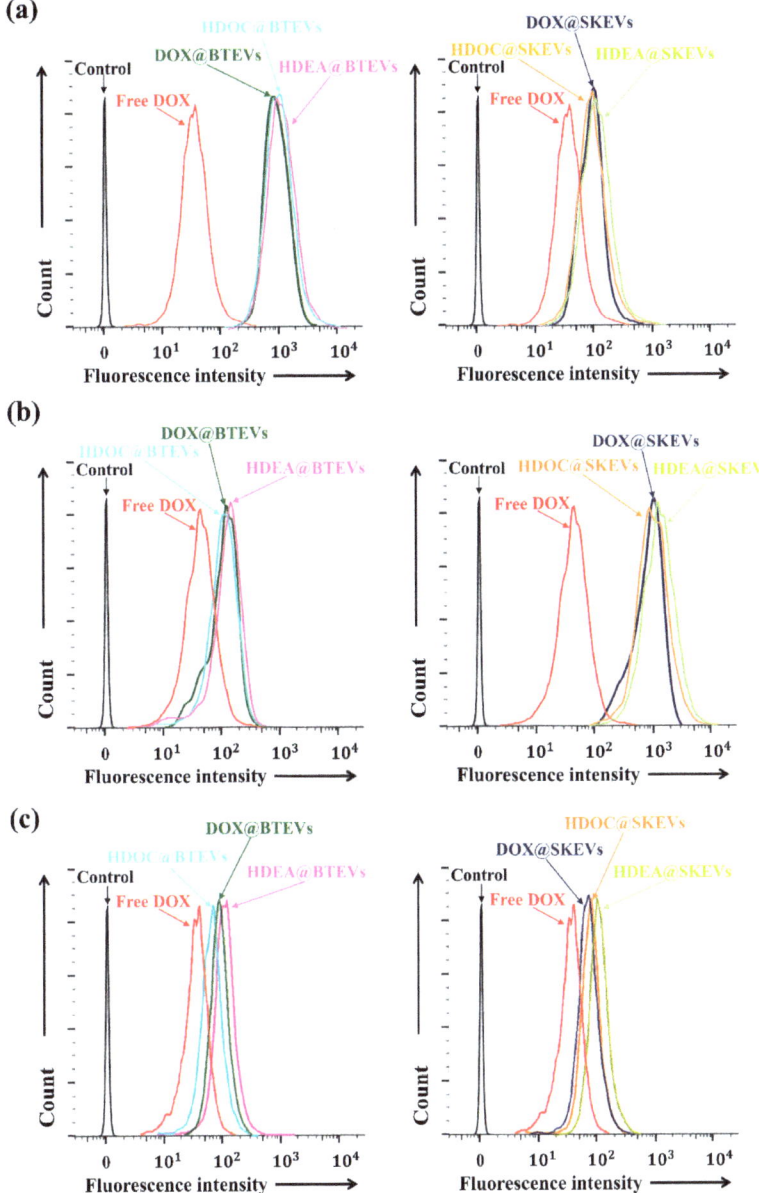

Figure 4. Flow cytometry profiles of (**a**) BT-474, (**b**) SK-N-MC and (**c**) Huh7 cells treated with free DOX (5 µg/mL) or EVs (equivalent to DOX of 5 µg/mL) for 4 h incubation at 37 °C.

To verify the cellular uptake of the EV blends for BT-474 and SK-N-MC tumor cells, we performed in vitro cell imaging studies using a confocal laser scanning microscope [3,30,31]. As shown in Figure 7a, BT-474 and SK-N-MC tumor cells were first cultured on coverslips. Subsequently, the coverslips were moved to empty cell-culture plates and then treated with each EV samples or the EV blends. As shown in Figure 7b, Ce6 dye-incorporated HDEA@BTEVs displayed strong Ce6 fluorescence in BT-474 tumor cells, although the fluorescence intensity of Ce6 was weak in SK-N-MC tumor cells. By contrast, the FITC dye-incorporated HDEA@SKEVs displayed a strong FITC fluorescence signal for SK-N-MC tumor cells, but a weak FITC fluorescence signal in BT-474 tumor cells. More importantly, the EV blends displayed a strong Ce6 fluorescence and a weak FITC fluorescence in BT-474 tumor cells, whereas a weak Ce6 fluorescence and a strong FITC fluorescence in SK-N-MC tumor cells. These results indicate that the EV blends were selectively internalized to each parent tumor cells.

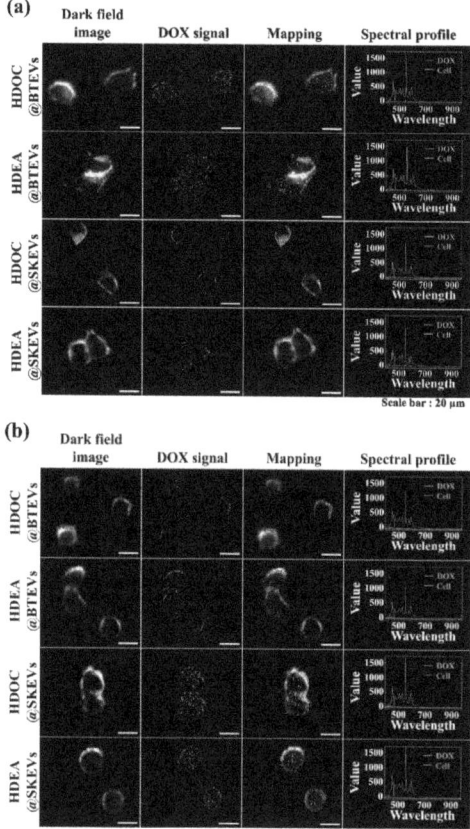

Figure 5. Hyperspectral images of (**a**) BT-474 and (**b**) SK-N-MC cells treated with EVs (equivalent to DOX of 5 µg/mL) for 4 h incubation at 37 °C.

Figure 7c shows the cytotoxicity of the HDEA@BTEVs (equivalent DOX concentration of 5 µg/mL), HDEA@SKEVs (equivalent DOX concentration of 5 µg/mL), and the EV blends (equivalent DOX concentration of 5 µg/mL) to the mixed BT-474 and SK-N-MC tumor cells (50:50, cell number ratio). The EV blends exhibited highly increased tumor cell death for mixed BT-474 and SK-N-MC tumor cells. However, the HDEA@BTEVs or HDEA@SKEVs resulted in fewer tumor cell deaths. It is assumed that the efficient uptake of the EV blends in both BT-474 and SK-N-MC tumor cells resulted in the significantly increased antitumor efficacy.

In addition, to evaluate the cytotoxicity of the EV samples, BT-474, SK-N-MC, and Huh7 tumor cells were treated using free DOX and EV samples at the equivalent DOX concentration of 5 µg/mL.

First, HDEA@BTEVs and HDOC@BTEVs exhibited relatively increased BT-474 tumor cell death compared with the SKEVs samples (HDEA@SKEVs and HDOC@SKEVs) (Figure 8a); this was likely owing to the homing ability of the BTEVs. However, the pH-insensitive HDOC@BTEVs resulted in a relatively reduced BT-474 tumor cell death, likely owing to the reduced DOX release (Figure 2). Similarly, the homing ability of the SKEVs resulted in the increased cell-cytotoxicity of the HDEA@SKEVs against SK-N-MC tumor cells (Figure 8b). However, Huh7 tumor cells treated with HDEA@BTEVs or HDEA@SKEVs did not exhibit noticeable levels of cell death. The low cellular uptake of the BTEV and SKEV samples in Huh7 tumor cells resulted in less cell-cytotoxicity for Huh7 tumor cells (Figure 8c). These results indicate that the homing ability of EVs to their parent tumor cells (Figures 4–6) and the endosomolytic activity/endosomal pH-triggered DOX releasing property of HDEA-anchored EVs (Figures 2 and 3) enabled a significantly improved tumor cell death. In addition, all EV samples without DOX showed negligible cytotoxicity up to 3×10^8 particles/mL in 24 h for incubation with BT-474, SK-N-MC, and Huh7 tumor cells (Figure 8d–f), supporting their non-toxicity.

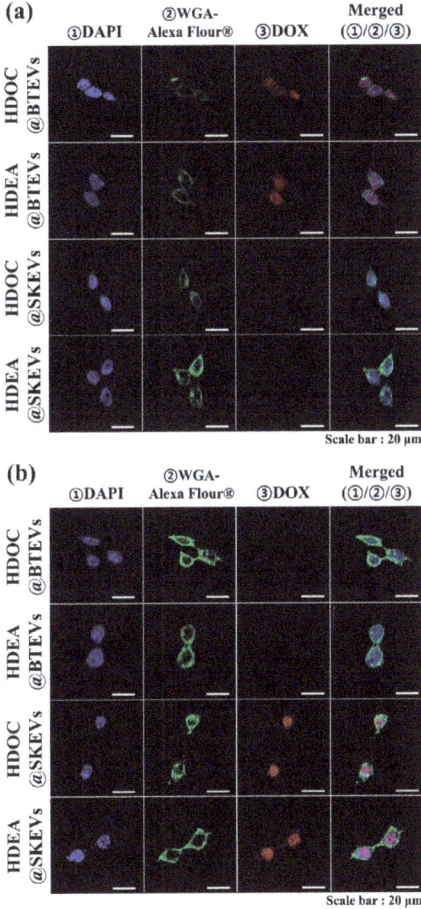

Figure 6. Confocal images of (**a**) BT-474 and (**b**) SK-N-MC cells treated with EVs (equivalent to DOX of 5 µg/mL) for 4 h incubation at 37 °C. The cells were stained using 4′,6-diamidino-2-phenylindole dihydrochloride (DAPI) and Wheat Germ Agglutinin Alexa Fluor® 488 Conjugate (WGA-Alexa Fluor®488).

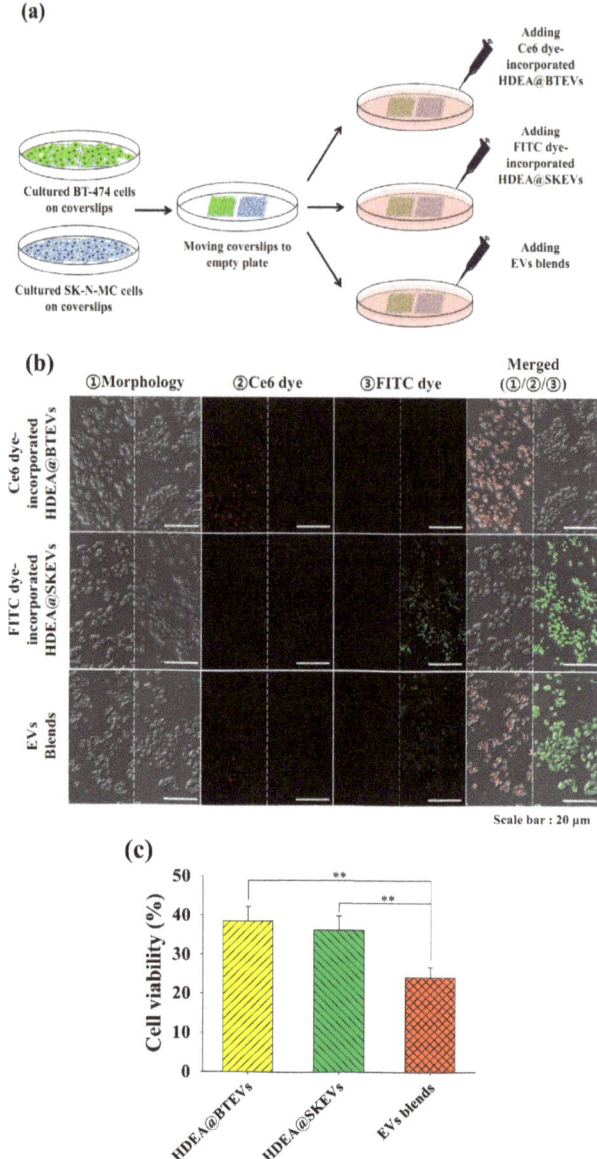

Figure 7. (a) Schematic illustration of in vitro experiments using Ce6 dye-incorporated HDEA@BTEVs, FITC dye-incorporated HDEA@SKEVs, and EV blends [Ce6 dye-incorporated HDEA@BTEVs/FITC dye-incorporated HDEA@SKEVs (50:50 wt.%)]. (b) Confocal images of BT-474 cells (left) and SK-N-MC cells (right) treated with Ce6 dye-incorporated HDEA@BTEVs, FITC dye-incorporated HDEA@SKEVs, or EV blends [Ce6 dye-incorporated HDEA@BTEVs/FITC dye-incorporated HDEA@SKEVs (50/50 wt.%)] (equivalent to EVs of 30 μg/mL) for 4 h incubation at 37 °C. (c) Cell viability determined by CCK-8 assay of tumor cells treated with EVs or EV blends [HDEA@BTEVs/HDEA@SKEVs (50/50 wt.%)] (equivalent to DOX of 5 μg/mL) for 4 h incubation at 37 °C ($n = 7$, as multiple experiments, ** $p < 0.01$ compared with each EV sample).

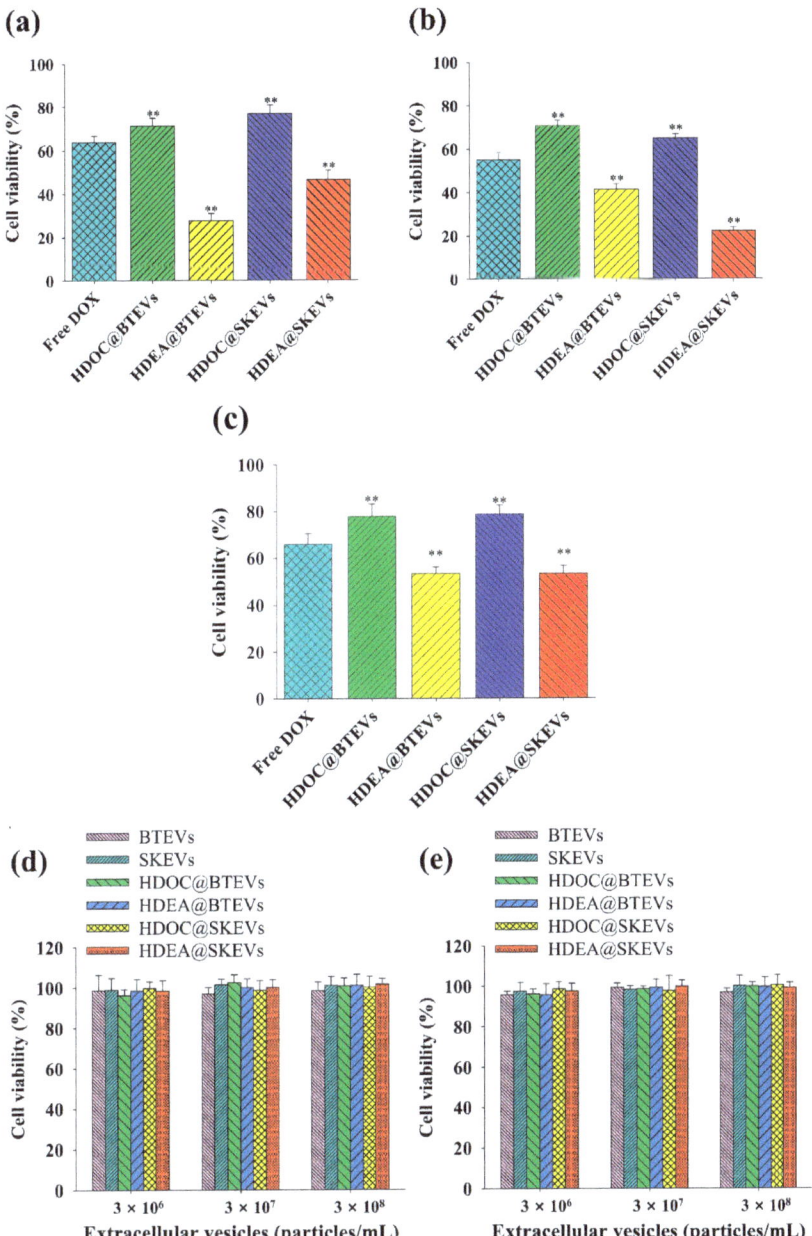

Figure 8. Cell viability determined by Cell Counting Kit-8 (CCK-8) assay of (**a**) BT-474, (**b**) SK-N-MC and (**c**) Huh7 cells treated with free DOX (5 µg/mL) or EVs (equivalent to DOX of 5 µg/mL) for 4 h incubation at 37 °C ($n = 7$, as multiple experiments), (** $p < 0.01$ compared with the free DOX). Cell viability determined by CCK-8 assay of (**d**) BT-474, (**e**) SK-N-MC, and (**f**) Huh7 cells treated with blank EVs (without DOX) for 24 h incubation at 37 °C ($n = 7$, as multiple experiments).

4. Conclusions

In this study, tumor-homing pH-sensitive EV blends were fabricated using tumor-specific EVs (extracted from SK-N-MC and BT-474 tumor cells) and pH-sensitive HDEA. HDEA and DOX were incorporated in two different EVs through sonication; subsequently, they were blended in a weight ratio of 50:50. The EV blends, comprising two different EVs, can target two different parent tumor cells owing to the EVs' homing ability. In addition, the pH-sensitive disruption of EVs owing to DEAP molecules promoted DOX release. Consequently, the EV blends killed the heterogeneous parent tumor cells effectively. Hence, we believe that EV blends with tumor cell targeting ability, the rapid release of DOX at the endosomal pH, and the enhanced antitumor effect may be novel strategies for treating various tumors.

Supplementary Materials: The following are available online at http://www.mdpi.com/1999-4923/12/4/372/s1, Figure S1. 1H-NMR analysis of HDEA. Figure S2. ^{1}H-NMR analysis of HDOC. Figure S3. TEM analysis of intact (a) BTEV or SKEV. (b) Western blot analysis of the TSG 101 (tumor susceptibility gene 101), ER-α (estrogen receptor alpha), or Tau (tau protein) in BTEVs or SKEVs.

Author Contributions: Conceptualization, E.S.L., Y.S.Y., and K.T.O.; methodology, J.P. and H.L.; investigation, J.P. and H.L.; data curation, J.P. and E.S.L.; writing—original draft preparation, E.S.L. and J.P.; writing—review and editing, E.S.L., Y.S.L., and K.T.O.; supervision, E.S.L.; funding acquisition, E.S.L. All authors have read and agreed to the published version of the manuscript.

Funding: This work was financially supported by the National Research Foundation of Korea (NRF) grant funded by the Korea government (MSIT) (grant number: NRF-2018R1A2B6000970).

Conflicts of Interest: The authors declare no competing financial interests.

References

1. Batrakova, E.V.; Kim, M.S. Using exosomes, naturally-equipped nanocarriers, for drug delivery. *J. Control. Release* **2015**, *219*, 396–405. [CrossRef] [PubMed]
2. Johnstone, R.M.; Adam, M.; Hammond, J.R.; Orr, L.; Turbide, C. Vesicle formation during reticulocyte maturation. Association of plasma membrane activities with released vesicles (exosomes). *J. Biol. Chem.* **1987**, *262*, 9412–9420. [PubMed]
3. Lee, H.; Park, H.; Noh, G.J.; Lee, E.S. pH-responsive hyaluronate-anchored extracellular vesicles to promote tumor-targeted drug delivery. *Carbohydr. Polym.* **2018**, *202*, 323–333. [CrossRef] [PubMed]
4. Luan, X.; Sansanaphongpricha, K.; Myers, I.; Chen, H.; Yuan, H.; Sun, D. Engineering exosomes as refined biological nanoplatforms for drug delivery. *Acta Pharmacol. Sin.* **2017**, *38*, 754–763. [CrossRef] [PubMed]
5. Sun, W.; Luo, J.; Jiang, H.; Duan, D.D. Tumor exosomes: A double-edged sword in cancer therapy. *Acta Pharmacol. Sin.* **2018**, *39*, 534–541. [CrossRef]
6. Pfeffer, S.R. A prize for membrane magic. *Cell* **2013**, *155*, 1203–1206. [CrossRef]
7. Milane, L.; Singh, A.; Mattheolabakis, G.; Suresh, M.; Amiji, M.M. Exosome mediated communication within the tumor microenvironment. *J. Control. Release* **2015**, *219*, 278–294. [CrossRef]
8. Chaput, N.; Théry, C. Exosomes: Immune properties and potential clinical implementations. *Semin. Immunopathol.* **2011**, *33*, 419–440. [CrossRef]
9. Harada, T.; Yamamota, H.; Kishida, S.; Kishida, M.; Awada, C.; Takao, T.; Kikuchi, A. Wnt5b-associated exosomes promote cancer cell migration and proliferation. *Cancer Sci.* **2016**, *108*, 42–52. [CrossRef]
10. Kowal, J.; Arras, G.; Colombo, M.; Jouve, M.; Morath, J.P.; Primdal-Bengtson, B.; Dingli, F.; Loew, D.; Tkach, M.; Théry, C. proteomic comparison defines novel markers to characterize heterogeneous populations of extracellular vesicle subtypes. *Proc. Natl. Acad. Sci. USA* **2016**, *113*, E968–E977. [CrossRef]
11. Frydrychowicz, M.; Kolecka-Bednarczyk, A.; Madejczyk, M.; Yasar, S.; Dworacki, G. Exosomes—Structure, Biogenesis and Biological Role in Non-Small-Cell Lung Cancer. *Scand. J. Immunol.* **2015**, *81*, 2–10. [CrossRef] [PubMed]
12. Xu, R.; Rai, A.; Chen, M.; Suwakulsiri, W.; Greening, D.W.; Simpson, R.J. Extracellular vesicles in cancer—Implications for future improvements in cancer care. *Nat. Rev. Clin. Oncol.* **2018**, *15*, 617–638. [CrossRef] [PubMed]
13. Akuma, P.; Okagu, O.D.; Udenigwe, C.C. Naturally occurring exosome vesicles as potential delivery vehicle for bioactive compounds. *Front. Sustain. Food Syst.* **2019**, *3*, 23. [CrossRef]

14. Sancho-Albero, M.; Navascués, N.; Mendoza, G.; Sebastián, V.; Arruebo, M.; Martín-Duque, P.; Santamaría, J. Exosome origin determines cell targeting and the transfer of therapeutic nanoparticles towards target cells. *J. Nanobiotechnol.* **2019**, *17*, 16. [CrossRef]
15. Liu, C.; Su, C. Design strategies and application progress of therapeutic exosomes. *Theranostics* **2019**, *9*, 1015–1028. [CrossRef]
16. Rana, S.; Yue, S.; Stadel, D.; Zöller, M. Toward tailored exosomes: The exosomal tetraspanin web contributes to target cell selection. *Int. J. Biochem. Cell Biol.* **2012**, *44*, 1574–1584. [CrossRef]
17. Tian, Y.; Li, S.; Song, J.; Ji, T.; Zhu, M.; Anderson, G.J.; Wei, J.; Nie, G. A doxorubicin delivery platform using engineered natural membrane vesicle exosomes for targeted tumor therapy. *Biomaterials* **2014**, *35*, 2383–2390. [CrossRef]
18. Hood, J.L. Post isolation modification of exosomes for nanomedicine applications. *Nanomedicine* **2016**, *11*, 1745–1756. [CrossRef]
19. Raemdonck, K.; Braeckmans, K.; Demeester, J.; de Smedt, S.C. Merging the best of both worlds: Hybrid lipid-enveloped matrix nanocomposites in drug delivery. *Chem. Soc. Rev.* **2014**, *43*, 444–472. [CrossRef]
20. Li, C.; Zhang, J.; Zu, Y.; Nie, S.; Cao, J.; Wang, Q.; Nie, S.; Deng, Z.Y.; Xie, M.; Wang, S. Biocompatible and biodegradable nanoparticles for enhancement of anti-cancer activities of phytochemicals. *Chin. J. Nat. Med.* **2015**, *13*, 641–652. [CrossRef]
21. Ding, J.; Chen, J.; Gao, L.; Jiang, Z.; Zhang, Y.; Li, M.; Xiao, Q.; Lee, S.S.; Chen, X. Engineered nanomedicines with enhanced tumor penetration. *Nano Today* **2019**, *29*, 100800. [CrossRef]
22. Coccè, V.; Franzè, S.; Brini, A.T.; Giannì, A.B.; Pascucci, L.; Ciusani, E.; Alessandri, G.; Farronato, G.; Cavicchini, L.; Sordi, V.; et al. In vitro anticancer activity of extracellular vesicles (EVs) secreted by gingival mesenchymal stromal cells primed with paclitaxel. *Pharmaceutics* **2019**, *11*, 61. [CrossRef] [PubMed]
23. Kim, S.K.; Park, H.; Lee, J.M.; Na, K.; Lee, E.S. pH-responsive starch microparticles for a tumor-targeting implant. *Polym. Adv. Technol.* **2018**, *29*, 1372–1376. [CrossRef]
24. Yu, H.S.; Lee, E.S. Honeycomb-like pH-responsive γ-cyclodextrin electrospun particles for highly efficient tumor therapy. *Carbohydr. Polym.* **2020**, *230*, 115563. [CrossRef] [PubMed]
25. Jiang, T.; Zhang, Z.; Zhang, Y.; Lv, H.; Zhou, J.; Li, C.; Hou, L.; Zhang, Q. Dual-functional liposomes based on pH-responsive cell-penetrating peptide and hyaluronic acid for tumor-targeted anticancer drug delivery. *Biomaterials* **2012**, *33*, 9246–9258. [CrossRef]
26. Park, H.; Cho, S.; Janat-Amsbury, M.M.; Bae, Y.H. Enhanced thermogenic program by non-viral delivery of combinatory browning genes to treat diet-induced obesity in mice. *Biomaterials* **2015**, *73*, 32–41. [CrossRef]
27. Park, S.Y.; Baik, H.J.; Oh, Y.T.; Oh, K.T.; Youn, Y.S.; Lee, E.S. A smart polysaccharide/drug conjugate for photodynamic therapy. *Angew. Chem. Int. Ed.* **2011**, *50*, 1644–1647. [CrossRef]
28. Oh, N.M.; Kwag, D.S.; Oh, K.T.; Youn, Y.S.; Lee, E.S. Electrostatic charge conversion processes in engineered tumor-identifying polypeptides for targeted chemotherapy. *Biomaterials* **2012**, *33*, 1884–1893. [CrossRef]
29. Kim, S.; Kwang, D.S.; Lee, D.J.; Lee, E.S. Acidic pH-stimulated tiotropium release from porous poly(lactic-co-glycolic acid) microparticles containing 3-diethylaminopropyl-conjugated hyaluronate. *Macromol. Res.* **2016**, *24*, 176–181. [CrossRef]
30. Lee, H.; Park, H.; Yu, H.S.; Na, K.; Oh, K.T.; Lee, E.S. Dendritic cell-targeted pH-responsive extracellular vesicles for anticancer vaccination. *Pharmaceutics* **2019**, *11*, 54. [CrossRef]
31. Lee, J.M.; Park, H.; Oh, K.T.; Lee, E.S. pH-Responsive hyaluronated liposomes for docetaxel delivery. *Int. J. Pharm.* **2018**, *547*, 377–384. [CrossRef] [PubMed]
32. Théry, C.; Zitvogel, L.; Amigorena, S. Exosomes: Composition, biogenesis and function. *Nat. Rev. Immunol.* **2002**, *2*, 569–579. [CrossRef] [PubMed]
33. Schageman, J.; Zeringer, E.; Li, M.; Barta, T.; Lea, K.; Gu, J.; Magdaleno, S.; Settterquist, R.; Vlassov, A.V. The complete exosome workflow solution: From isolation to characterization of RNA cargo. *Biomed. Res. Int.* **2013**, *2013*, 253957. [CrossRef] [PubMed]
34. Théry, C.; Amigorena, S.; Raposo, G.; Clayton, A. Isolation and characterization of exosomes from cell culture supernatants and biological fluids. *Curr. Protoc. Cell Biol.* **2006**, *194*, 1–29. [CrossRef]
35. Vestad, B.; Liorente, A.; Neurauter, A.; Phuyal, S.; Kierulf, B.; Kierulf, P.; Skotland, T.; Sandvig, K.; Haug, K.B.F.; Øvstebø, R. Size and concentration analyses of extracellular vesicles by nanoparticle tracking analysis: A variation study. *J. Extracell. Vesicles* **2017**, *6*, 1344087. [CrossRef]

36. Kim, M.S.; Haney, M.J.; Zhao, Y.; Mahajan, V.; Deygen, I.; Klyachko, N.L.; Inskoe, E.; Piroyan, A.; Sokolsky, M.; Okolie, O.; et al. Development of exosome-encapsulated paclitaxel to overcome MDR in cancer cells. *Nanomedicine* **2016**, *12*, 655–664. [CrossRef]
37. Lee, U.Y.; Youn, Y.S.; Park, J.; Lee, E.S. Y-Shaped ligand-driven gold nanoparticles for highly efficient tumoral uptake and photothermal ablation. *ACS Nano* **2014**, *8*, 12858–12865. [CrossRef]
38. Noh, G.; Youn, Y.S.; Lee, E.S. Preparation of iron oxide nanoparticles functionalized with Y-shaped ligands for brain tumor targeting. *J. Mater. Chem. B* **2016**, *4*, 6074–6080. [CrossRef]
39. Koo, M.; Oh, K.T.; Noh, G.; Lee, E.S. Gold nanoparticles bearing a tumor pH-sensitive cyclodextrin cap. *ACS Appl. Mater. Interfaces* **2018**, *10*, 24450–24458. [CrossRef]
40. Lee, J.O.; Oh, K.T.; Kim, D.; Lee, E.S. pH-Sensitive short worm-like micelles targeting tumors based on the extracellular pH. *J. Mater. Chem. B* **2014**, *2*, 6363–6370. [CrossRef]
41. Ahmad, I.; Perkins, W.R.; Lupan, D.M.; Selsted, M.E.; Janoff, A.S. Liposomal entrapment of the neutrophil-derived peptide indolicidin endows it with in vivo antifungal activity. *Biochim. Biophys. Acta* **1995**, *1237*, 109–114. [CrossRef]
42. Lopes, T.C.M.; Silva, D.F.; Costa, W.C.; Frézard, F.; Barichello, J.M.; Silva-Barcellos, N.M.; de Lima, W.G.; Rezende, S.A. Accelerated blood clearance (ABC) phenomenon favors the accumulation of tartar emetic in pegylated liposomes in BALB/c mice liver. *Pathol. Res. Int.* **2018**, *2018*, 9076723. [CrossRef] [PubMed]
43. Lim, C.; Kim, D.; Sim, T.; Hoang, N.H.; Lee, J.W.; Lee, E.S.; Youn, Y.S.; Oh, K.T. Preparation and characterization of a lutein loading nanoemulsion system for ophthalmic eye drops. *J. Drug Deliv. Sci. Technol.* **2016**, *36*, 168–174. [CrossRef]
44. Lee, D.J.; Oh, Y.T.; Lee, E.S. Surface charge switching nanoparticles for magnetic resonance imaging. *Int. J. Pharm.* **2014**, *471*, 127–134. [CrossRef] [PubMed]
45. Yu, H.S.; Park, H.; Tran, T.H.; Hwang, S.Y.; Na, K.; Lee, E.S.; Oh, K.T.; Oh, D.X.; Park, J. Poisonous caterpillar-inspired chitosan nanofiber enabling dual photothermal and photodynamic tumor ablation. *Pharmaceutics* **2019**, *11*, 258. [CrossRef] [PubMed]
46. Nabhan, J.F.; Hu, R.; Oh, R.S.; Cohen, S.N.; Lu, Q. Formation and release of arrestin domain-containing protein 1-mediated microvesicles (ARMMs) at plasma membrane by recruitment of TSG101 protein. *Proc. Natl. Acad. Sci. USA* **2012**, *109*, 4146–4151. [CrossRef]
47. Street, J.M.; Barran, P.E.; Mackay, C.L.; Weidt, S.; Balmforth, C.; Walsh, T.S.; Chalmers, R.T.A.; Webb, D.J.; Dear, J.W. Identification and proteomic profiling of exosomes in human cerebrospinal fluid. *J. Transl. Med.* **2012**, *10*, 5. [CrossRef]
48. Villarroya-Beltri, C.; Baixauli, F.; Mittelbrunn, M.; Fernández-Delgado, I.; Torralba, D.; Moreno-Gonzalo, O.; Baldanta, S.; Enrich, C.; Guerra, S.; Sánchez-Madrid, F. ISGylation controls exosome secretion by promoting lysosomal degradation of MVB proteins. *Nat. Commun.* **2016**, *7*, 13588. [CrossRef]
49. Jia, Y.; Chen, Y.; Wang, Q.; Jayasinghe, U.; Luo, X.; Wei, Q.; Wang, J.; Xiong, H.; Chen, C.; Xu, B.; et al. Exosome: Emerging biomarker in breast cancer. *Oncotarget* **2017**, *8*, 41717–41733. [CrossRef]
50. Dai, X.; Cheng, H.; Bai, Z.; Li, J. Breast cancer cell line classification and its relevance with breast tumor subtyping. *J. Cancer* **2017**, *8*, 3131–3141. [CrossRef]
51. Min, S.H.; Cho, J.S.; Oh, J.H.; Shim, S.B.; Hwang, D.Y.; Lee, S.H.; Jee, S.W.; Lim, H.J.; Kim, M.Y.; Sheen, Y.Y.; et al. Tau and GSK3β dephosphorylations are required for regulating Pin1 phosphorylation. *Neurochem. Res.* **2005**, *30*, 955–961. [CrossRef] [PubMed]
52. Miller, I.V.; Raposo, G.; Welsch, U.; da Costa, O.P.; Thiel, U.; Lebar, M.; Maurer, M.; Bender, H.-U.; von Luettichau, I.; Richter, G.H.S.; et al. First identification of Ewing's sarcoma-derived extracellular vesicles and exploration of their biological and potential diagnostic implications. *Biol. Cell* **2013**, *105*, 289–303. [CrossRef] [PubMed]

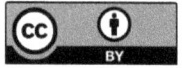

© 2020 by the authors. Licensee MDPI, Basel, Switzerland. This article is an open access article distributed under the terms and conditions of the Creative Commons Attribution (CC BY) license (http://creativecommons.org/licenses/by/4.0/).

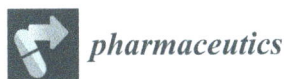

Article

Phage Display-Based Homing Peptide-Daunomycin Conjugates for Selective Drug Targeting to PANC-1 Pancreatic Cancer

Levente E. Dókus [1,2], Eszter Lajkó [3], Ivan Ranđelović [4], Diána Mező [3], Gitta Schlosser [1,2], László Kőhidai [3], József Tóvári [4] and Gábor Mező [1,2,*]

1. MTA-ELTE Research Group of Peptide Chemistry, Hungarian Academy of Sciences, 1117 Budapest, Hungary; doehabt@caesar.elte.hu (L.E.D.); schlosser@caesar.elte.hu (G.S.)
2. Institute of Chemistry, Faculty of Sciences, Eötvös Loránd University, 1117 Budapest, Hungary
3. Department of Genetics, Cell- and Immunobiology, Semmelweis University, 1089 Budapest, Hungary; lajko.eszter@med.semmelweis-univ.hu (E.L.); mezo.diana@med.semmelweis-univ.hu (D.M.); kohidai.laszlo@med.semmelweis-univ.hu (L.K.)
4. National Institute of Oncology, Department of Experimental Pharmacology, 1122 Budapest, Hungary; ivan.randel@gmail.com (I.R.); tozsi@oncol.hu (J.T.)
* Correspondence: gmezo@elte.hu; Tel.: +36-1-372-2500 (ext. 1430)

Received: 20 May 2020; Accepted: 17 June 2020; Published: 22 June 2020

Abstract: The Pancreatic Ductal Adenocarcinoma (PDAC) is one of the most aggressive and dangerous cancerous diseases, leading to a high rate of mortality. Therefore, the development of new, more efficient treatment approaches is necessary to cure this illness. Peptide-based drug targeting provides a new tool for this purpose. Previously, a hexapeptide Cys-Lys-Ala-Ala-Lys-Asn (CKAAKN) was applied efficiently as the homing device for drug-loaded nanostructures in PDAC cells. In this research, Cys was replaced by Ser in the sequence and this new SKAAKN targeting moiety was used in conjugates containing daunomycin (Dau). Five different structures were developed and tested. The results indicated that linear versions with one Dau were not effective on PANC-1 cells in vitro; however, branched conjugates with two Dau molecules showed significant antitumor activity. Differences in the antitumor effect of the conjugates could be explained with the different cellular uptake and lysosomal degradation. The most efficient conjugate was *Dau=Aoa*-GFLG-K(*Dau=Aoa*)SKAAKN-OH (conjugate 4) that also showed significant tumor growth inhibition on s.c. implanted PANC-1 tumor-bearing mice with negligible side effects. Our novel results suggest that peptide-based drug delivery systems could be a promising tool for the treatment of pancreatic cancers.

Keywords: pancreatic cancer; targeted tumor therapy; homing peptide; antitumor peptide conjugates; daunomycin; oxime linkage

1. Introduction

Pancreatic Ductal Adenocarcinoma (PDAC) is one of the most aggressive and dangerous cancerous diseases with a high mortality rate [1]. In the USA, more than 55,000 new cases were estimated in 2018 which is 3–4% of the all newly diagnosed cancer cases. Approximately 80% of these incidences will lead to death within a year [2]. The average 5-year survival rate is less than 5% [3]. The main reason for the high mortality of pancreatic cancer patients could be very poor prognosis. The early diagnosis of PDAC is still difficult, and most patients have already progressed to not operable and incurable statuses at the recognition of the disease [4]. In addition, the chemotherapy applied to treat pancreatic cancers is usually ineffective due to the fast development of resistance. Chemotherapy causes many side effects because of the low selectivity of the currently used drugs [5]. Furthermore, the hypovascularity of PDAC and a dense desmoplastic stroma that create barriers restrict drug delivery to the tumor site [6]. Therefore, the design of efficient anticancer agents against PADC is one of the most challenging tasks for scientists working on cancer research [7]. Targeted tumor therapy could be a promising strategy to overcome these drawbacks in pancreatic cancer treatment—similar to other types of cancers [8]. Targeted tumor therapy is based on targeting tumor-specific or overexpressed receptors or other cell surface compartments on tumor cells that can be recognized selectively by antibodies or small molecules like folic acid or peptides [9,10]. Drug molecules attached to these homing moieties can enter specifically into tumor cells, resulting in selective toxicity without causing toxic side effects in healthy tissues. The application of small molecule drug conjugates (SMDCs) over antibody-drug conjugate (ADCs) may have an advantage in the treatment of PDAC because SMDCs have higher tissue permeability [11].

Several homing peptides that recognize pancreatic cancer cells and could be used for drug targeting directly or as a part of nanoparticles have been described in the literature [12–15]. One of them is the CKAAKNK oligopeptide that was selected by phage display technique and which can specifically bind to tumor vessels in RIP-Tag2 transgenic mice, a prototypical mouse model of multistage pancreatic islet cell carcinoma [16]. Valetti et al. attached the CKAAKN homing peptide to a squalene (SQ) molecule via thiol-maleimide Michael addition coupling [17]. The conjugate was co-nanoprecipitated with the squalenoyl prodrug of gemcitabine (SQdFdC) resulting in nanoparticles. The construct was tested on MIA PaCa-2 human pancreatic adenocarcinoma cells, which overexpress frizzled-5 (FZD-5) receptors compared to NIH/3T3 fibroblasts. It was indicated that these cells selectively took up the nanoparticles decorated with the homing peptide by a receptor-mediated way [18]. Frizzled receptors as Wnt binding 7TM GPCRs are key players in the Wnt/β-catenin signal pathway that is commonly hyperactivated in pancreatic cancers, leading to enhanced cell proliferation [19]. In the presence of appropriate ligands, the FZD-5 receptor can be internalized, usually in a heterodimeric form [20]. Therefore, this protein is a promising target for drug targeting to tumor cells. In addition, these data indicated the efficacy of the CKAAKN peptide as a homing device—related to the Wnt-2 sequence—for targeted tumor therapy.

In our research, several SMDCs were developed, derived from the CKAAKN oligopeptide. The structure–activity relationship was investigated as well. In this work, cysteine was replaced by serine to remove the unnecessary thiol group at the conjugation site. This exchange is widely used to eliminate reactive thiol group when it is not essential for the biological activity. In addition, the substitution of Cys by Ser improves the hydrophilicity and solubility of the peptide and its conjugates. Daunomycin (Dau), as an anticancer agent was attached to the homing peptides via oxime linkage, which shows proper stability in the circulation and allows the release of an active metabolite in lysosomes [21,22]. This active metabolite contains an amino acid (Aaa) to which daunomycin is connected through an aminooxyacetyl moiety (*Dau=Aoa*-Aaa-OH). This metabolite was proved to bind to DNA; however, the binding efficacy highly depends on the type of the amino acid [22].

The PANC-1 cell line, originally derived from head pancreatic carcinoma, was applied in our studies, and has an invasive phenotype and the ability to give metastasis to the peripancreatic lymph node; thus, this cell line can be considered as an in vitro model of lymph-node-positive PDAC. The invasiveness and metastatic potential of pancreatic cancer cells has been shown to be influenced by the Wnt/β-catenin pathway. This Wnt/β-catenin pathway has also been reported as a central element of immune-escape mechanisms of pancreatic tumors by providing an environment with immune-tolerogenic cytokine and chemokine [23]. Moreover, the expression level of β-catenin, a key protein of the Wnt pathway, has been found to be well-correlated with the gemcitabine-resistance of different pancreatic cell lines, including PANC-1 cells [24]. These three characteristics of pancreatic tumor cells like PANC-1 seem to be interrelated and orchestrated by the Wnt/β-catenin pathway.

The influence of the number of drugs as well as the presence of an enzyme cleavable spacer on antitumor activity was studied in PANC-1 pancreatic cancer cells. The antitumor effect is influenced by several cellular factors; therefore, the binding, the cellular uptake and the metabolism of the conjugates were also investigated. The best compounds identified in the in vitro studies were applied in vivo experiment using subcutan (s.c.) developed PANC-1 tumor-bearing SCID mice. The results were compared with free drug administration.

2. Materials and Methods

2.1. Chemicals

All amino acid derivatives and Wang resin were purchased from Iris Biotech GmbH (Marktredwitz, Germany), whereas reagents for coupling and cleavage (N,N'-diisopropylcarbodiimide (DIC), 1,8-diazabicyclo[5.4.0]undec-7-ene (DBU), 1-hydroxybenzotriazole hydrate (HOBt), 4-(dimethylamino)pyridine (DMAP), triisopropylsilane (TIS), trifluoroacetic acid (TFA)) and ninhydrin were delivered by Sigma-Aldrich Kft. (Budapest, Hungary). Aminooxyacetic acid (Aoa) and methoxyamine were TCI (Tokyo, Japan) products. The solvents (dichloromethane (DCM), N,N-dimethylformamide (DMF), acetonitrile (CH_3CN)) for synthesis and purification were obtained from Reanal (Budapest, Hungary) or VWR International Kft. (Debrecen, Hungary). Daunomycin (Dau) was donated from IVAX (Budapest, Hungary).

2.2. Synthesis of Peptides

Peptides were synthesized manually by solid-phase peptide synthesis on Wang resin (0.25 g, 0.52 mmol/g) using the standard protocol of Fmoc/^{t}Bu strategy. The first amino acid derivative (5 equivalent to the resin capacity) was attached to the resin with a DIC coupling agent in the presence of 0.5 equivalent DMAP in DMF. The Fmoc group was removed with 2% DBU and 2% piperidine in DMF (four times; 2, 2, 5, 10 min, respectively). For the coupling of the following amino acid derivatives, DIC-HOBt mixture (3 equivalent each) were applied in DMF for 60 min. The ε-amino group of lysine used for the development of a branch was protected with 4-methyltrityl (Mtt) group that could be removed selectively next to the *tert*-butyl type protecting groups with 2% TFA and 2% TIS in DCM (7 times; 1, 1, 3, 3, 5, 10, 30 min, respectively). The aminooxyacetic acid used for the development of an oxime linkage was incorporated in its isopropylidene protected form [25] either to the N-terminus or to both N-termini (backbone and branch) of the peptides. DIC and HOBt coupling agents were used for this purpose, similar to the coupling of amino acid derivatives. The peptides were removed from the resin by cleavage with 5 mL TFA, containing 0.125 mL distilled water and 0.125 mL TIS (as scavengers). The crude product was precipitated by dry diethyl ether, dissolved in 10% acetic acid, freeze-dried and purified by RP-HPLC (Gradient I.).

2.3. Synthesis of Daunomycin Conjugates

In the first step, the isopropylidene protecting group was removed from the aminooxyacetyl moiety of the purified peptide derivatives by methoxyamine (in 1.5 M concentration) in 0.2 M NH_4OAc buffer solution (pH = 5) at RT for 2 h. The reaction took place quantitatively. The unprotected products were isolated by RP-HPLC (Gradient I.). Prior to the conjugation, the solvent was evaporated and then the rest was re-dissolved in 0.2 M NH_4OAc buffer solution (pH = 5) and 2 equivalent Dau to the peptide was added to the mixture. The reaction was carried out overnight. The reaction mixture was injected directly to the HPLC in all cases and the conjugates were separated from the excess of Dau by RP-HPLC (Gradient II.)

2.4. Reverse Phase High-Performance Liquid Chromatography (RP-HPLC)

The purification of the crude products was carried out by RP-HPLC using KNAUER 2501 HPLC system (Bad Homburg, Germany) and Phenomenex Luna (Torrance, CA, USA) C18 column (250 × 21.2 mm I.D.) with 10 μm silica (100 Å pore size). Experiments were carried out at a flow rate of 14 mL/min at room temperature. Linear gradient elution was applied. Gradient I: 0 min 5% B, 10 min 5% B, 10.1 min 20% B, 50 min 80% B. Gradient II: 0 min 20% B, 5 min 20% B, 50 min 80% B. Eluent A was 0.1% TFA in distilled water and eluent B was 0.1% TFA in CH_3CN-water (80:20, v/v). Peaks were detected at λ = 220 nm.

Analytical RP-HPLC was performed on a Waters Symmetry (WAT 045905) C18 column (150 × 4.6 mm I.D.) with 5 µm silica (100 Å pore size) as a stationary phase. A linear gradient elution was developed: 0 min 0% B; 2 min 0% B; 22 min 90% B with eluent A (0.1% TFA in water) and eluent B (0.1% TFA in acetonitrile-water (80: 20, v/v)). A flow rate of 1 mL/min was used at ambient temperature. Samples were applied dissolved in eluent A and 20 µL was injected. Peaks were detected at λ = 220 nm.

2.5. Mass Spectrometry (MS)

The identification of the peptide analogues and conjugates was achieved by electrospray ionization mass spectrometry (ESI-MS) on a Bruker Daltonics Esquire 3000 Plus (Bremen, Germany) ion trap mass spectrometer, operating in continuous sample injection at 4 µL/min flow rate. Samples were dissolved in ACN-water (50:50 v/v%) mixture containing 0.1 v/v% AcOH. Mass spectra were recorded in positive ion mode in the m/z 50–2000 range.

For the stability and metabolism studies of the conjugates, liquid chromatography–mass spectrometry (LC-MS) analyses were performed on a Q ExactiveTM Focus, high resolution and high mass accuracy, hybrid quadrupole-orbitrap mass spectrometer (Thermo Fisher Scientific, Bremen, Germany) using on-line UHPLC coupling. UHPLC separation was performed on a Dionex 3000 UHPLC system using a Supelco Ascentis C18 column (2.1 × 150 mm, 3 µm). Linear gradient elution (0 min 2% B, 1 min 2% B, 17 min 90% B) with eluent A (0.1% HCOOH in water, v/v) and eluent B (0.1% HCOOH in acetonitrile/water, 80:20, v/v) was used at a flow rate of 0.2 mL/min at 40 °C. High-resolution mass spectra were acquired in the 200–1600 m/z range. LC-MS data were analyzed by XcaliburTM software (Thermo Fisher Scientific) and with Origin Pro 8 (OriginLab Corp., Northampton, MA, USA).

2.6. Measurement of Lysosomal Degradation of Conjugates by LC-MS

Conjugates were dissolved in distilled water in 2.5 µg/µL concentration followed by dilution with 0.2 M NaOAc solution (pH = 5.03) to 0.025 µg/µL. The lysosome-homogenate was prepared from rat liver and contained proteins in 16.6 µg/µL concentration. An aliquot (20 µL) of this stock solution was further diluted with 190 µL 0.2 M NaOAc solution, therefore the final protein concentration was 0.83 µg/µL. To prepare the reaction mixture, 15 µL (0.83 µg/µL) lysosome homogenate was added to 500 µL (0.025 µg/µL) conjugate solution. Furthermore, a control reaction mixture was always prepared which contained 500 µL conjugate solution and 15 µL NaOAc solution only. The solutions were stirred on 600 rpm at 37 °C and samples (50 µL) were taken out at 0 min, 5 min, 15 min, 30 min, 1 h, 2 h, 6 h, 24 h, and 72 h. The enzymatic activity was quenched by adding 5 µL formic acid to the samples. After this procedure, samples were frozen immediately at −25 °C. Control samples were taken at 0 min, 15 min, 1 h, 6 h, 24 h and 72 h. Composition of the samples was determined by HPLC-MS as described above.

2.7. Cell Cultures

For the in vitro characterization of conjugates four different tumor cell lines were used: PANC-1 (human pancreatic carcinoma of ductal origin), Colo-205 (human colorectal adenocarcinoma), A2058 (human metastatic melanoma) obtained from the European Collection of Authenticated Cell Cultures (ECACC, Salisbury, UK) and EBC-1 (human lung squamous cell carcinoma) purchased from the Japanese Research Resources Bank (Tokyo, Japan). Normal Human Dermal Fibroblasts (NHDF; Promocell, Heidelberg, Germany) as non-tumorous control cells were also investigated in order to determine the tumor selectivity of the proposed conjugates.

Dulbecco's Modified Eagle Medium (DMEM, Lonza, Basel, Switzerland) was used for the culturing of the PANC-1, Colo-205 and EBC-1 cell lines, while the A2058 cell line was maintained in RPMI 1640 (Lonza). These basal media were supplemented with 10% fetal bovine serum

(FBS, Gibco®/Invitrogen Corporation, New York, NY, USA), L-glutamine (2 mmol/L) (Lonza) and 100 µg/mL penicillin/streptomycin (Gibco®/Invitrogen Corporation). The medium of the Colo-205 cell line also contained 4500 mg/L D-glucose (Sigma-Aldrich, St. Louis, MO, USA), while, in case of EBC-1 cells, 1% non-essential amino acids (NEAA, Gibco®/Invitrogen Corporation) and 1 mM sodium pyruvate (Sigma-Aldrich) were also added to the culturing medium. For the cultivation of NHDF cells, Promocell Fibroblast Growth Medium (Promocell, Heidelberg, Germany) was used after adding SupplementMix (supplements necessary for the optimal growth of human fibroblasts, Promocell, Heidelberg, Germany) and the aforementioned antibiotics. All cell lines were grown in a T25 culture flask (Sigma-Aldrich or Eppendorf AG, Hamburg, Germany) in an incubator providing an atmosphere of 37 °C and 5% CO_2.

2.8. Measurement of the In Vitro Cytotoxicity of Conjugates

The PANC-1 model cell line exhibits adherent properties under laboratory conditions; therefore, the potential effects of novel antitumor conjugates on cell viability were measured by impedimetry allowing the real-time detection of cell adhesion. This measurement is based on the registration of electrical resistance (impedance, Z) in alternating current (AC) field. The living cells transplanted to the gold measuring electrodes are physically insulated by phospholipid bilayer that covers them. This instrumentally measurable property changes (decreases) in response to cellular cytotoxic agents. Our measurements were performed on xCELLigence single plate (ACEA Biosciences, San Diego, CA, USA) dedicated for impedimetric analysis of cellular samples at 37 °C and 5% CO_2.

During the initial phase of the experiments—the baseline recording—a special 96-well cell culture plate, E-plate (ACEA Biosciences), equipped with measuring electrodes, was pretreated with freshly prepared cell culture medium (for 60 min; sampling frequency: 1 min). Subsequently, PANC-1 cells were plated at a cell density of 10^4 cells/well. During the 24 h incubation, the cells evenly covered the electrodes at the bottom of the wells of the E-plate. The resulting confluent cell cultures were then treated with the test substances at the following final concentrations: 10^{-6}, 10^{-5}, 10^{-4} M. Total treatment duration was 72 h and the sampling rate was 1 min (0–24 h); and then 15 min (48–72 h). In our measurements, three replicates were used, the control was the drug-free medium. The device displays the impedance change in the form of a cell index (CI), which is a relative (to the start of the experiment) and dimensionless index. The CI results were analyzed with xCELLigence RTCA 2.0 software and Origin Pro 8.0 software. Normalized CI values, expressed as a percentage of control, were used to characterize the cell viability and hence the effect of conjugates.

EBC-1 and Colo-205 model cells have weak/negligible adherent properties, and A2058 cells could not produce constant cell index values. Therefore, a colorimetric assay (alamarBlue-assay) was chosen instead of the xCELLigence system to investigate the viability of these model cells treated with the conjugates. Due to the growth characteristics of NHDF cells, alamarBlue-assay was performed also on this cell line.

The protocol for the alamarBlue-assay was similar to the method which was published earlier [26], with some minor modifications. Briefly, the cell seeding occurred on 96-well cell culture plates (Sarstedt AG, Nümbrecht, Germany) at 10^4 cells/well concentration. After a 24 h long culturing period, the treatment was carried out with the conjugates at 10^{-4}, 10^{-5} and 10^{-6} M final concentrations for 24, 48 and 72 h. In the next steps, the alamarBlue reagent (0.15 mg/mL, Sigma-Aldrich) dissolved in phosphate-buffered saline (PBS; pH = 7.2), was added to the wells. After 6 h incubation with the reagent, the fluorescence intensity of the samples was obtained by an LS-50B Luminescence Spectrometer (Perkin Elmer Ltd., Buckinghamshire, UK) or a Fluoroskan™ FL Microplate Fluorometer and Luminometer (Thermo Scientific, Waltham, MA, USA) by using the following settings: $\lambda_{ex} = 560$ nm and $\lambda_{em} = 590$ nm.

Three parallels were performed per treatment group. In the case of controls, an equivalent volume of cell culture media was added to the cell. Fluorescence intensities of the samples treated with various concentrations of conjugates were expressed as a percentage of the fluorescence of control.

2.9. Flow Cytometric Measurement of Cell Surface Binding and Internalization

Cell surface binding and internalization of the conjugates were performed by flow cytometry (FACS-Calibur, Becton Dickinson, San Jose, CA, USA) based on the detection of the fluorescence activity of Dau (λ_{ex} = 488 nm, λ_{em} = 585 nm) linked to the peptides. Studies of binding and uptake were performed on PANC-1 cells.

Cells were seeded (2.5 × 10^5 cells/mL, 900 µL/well) on 12-well plates, 24 h prior to the treatment with conjugates and free Dau. To distinguish the cell surface binding and internalization of conjugates, the cells were treated with the conjugate solutions at a final concentration of 10^{-5} M at two temperatures (37 °C and 4 °C) in parallel. After the incubation period of 30 min, cells were washed with PBS and were removed from the plate using TrypLE (Thermo Fisher Scientific, Waltham, MA, USA) cell-dissociation reagent, thus avoiding cell surface protein degradation. To stop the enzymatic dissociation, 500 µL of fresh medium was added to the wells after 3–5 min and the cells were transferred to FACS-tubes. After the centrifugation of the cell suspension, the cell pellets were resuspended in PBS (400 µL/tube) and the samples were measured by a flow cytometer.

To determine the fluorescence intensity and to evaluate the results CellQuest Pro (Becton Dickinson) and Flowing2.5.1. (Turku Center of Biotechnology, Turku, Finland) software were used. The measurement was carried out twice with two parallels per treatment group. Samples containing cells treated with fresh cell culture medium at 37 °C and 4 °C were used as negative controls. The instrument determines the relative fluorescence intensity of Dau built in the conjugates as geometric mean channel (GeoMean) value.

GeoMean values of the 4 °C and 37 °C samples were corrected with GeoMean values representing the autofluorescence of negative control samples. The fluorescence intensity of cells treated at 4 °C is proportional to the amount of conjugates bound to the cell surface, whereas the fluorescence intensity of cells treated at 37 °C is composed of the signal of conjugates internalized by the cells and those bound to the cell surface, too. The fluorescence intensity specific for the amount of conjugates internalized by the cells was calculated by subtracting GeoMean values of the cells incubated at 4 °C from GeoMean values of the samples incubated at 37 °C.

2.10. Experimental Animals

The Balb/c mice and immunodeficient SCID mice used in these studies were kept as described previously [27] and cared for according to the "Guiding Principles for the Care and Use of Animals" based upon the Helsinki Declaration, and they were approved by the local ethical committee. The permission license for breeding and performing experiments with laboratory animals: PEI/001/1738-3/2015 and PEI/001/2574-6/2015.

2.11. Acute and Chronic Toxicity Studies

Prior to the determination of in vivo antitumor activity, the acute and chronic toxicity studies of conjugate 4 (*Dau=Aoa*-GFLG-K(*Dau=Aoa*)-SKAAKN-OH) were investigated. Healthy Balb/c male mice (3 animals in each group with 29–33 g body weight) were used for these experiments. The conjugate was dissolved in sterile water for injection (Pharmamagist Kft., Budapest, Hungary) and injected in a volume of 0.1 mL/10 g body weight using the appropriate concentrations. In acute toxicity study, intraperitoneal (*i.p.*) administration of the conjugate 4 was carried out in 4 different doses: 3.125, 6.25, 12.5 and 25 mg/kg Dau-content. In chronic toxicity study, mice were treated with a dose of 10 mg/kg Dau-content of the conjugate on days 1, 3, 7, 9 and 11 (5 treatments). The toxicity was evaluated on the basis of life span, behavior and looking of the mice, as well as body weight. These parameters were followed for 14 days.

2.12. Mouse Model of Subcutaneous Human Pancreatic Cancer, Doses of Treatments and Measurements

For establishing pancreatic tumor in experimental animals, PANC-1 cells were used, which were cultured in RPMI 1640 medium (Lonza), supplemented with 10% heat-inactivated FBS (Biosera, Nuaille, France), and 1% penicillin/streptomycin (Lonza). They were cultured in sterile T175 flasks (Sarstedt AG) with a ventilation cap at 37 °C in a humidified atmosphere with 5% CO_2.

Pancreatic cancer (PANC-1) cells were injected into SCID male mice (22–34 g) subcutaneously (s.c.), 3×10^6 cells per animal in 200 µL M199 (Sigma-Aldrich) per animal. The (i.p.) administration of treatment started 10 days after cells inoculation when the average tumor volume was 36 mm^3. Four groups with 7 animals per group were established and treated. The doses and schedule were as follows: control group was treated with sterile water used for the solubilization of Dau and the conjugates, while animals in the group administered with free Dau were treated on days 10, 19 and 24 after cell inoculation with a dose of 1 mg/kg. Mice administered with the conjugate **4** were separated in two groups and treated either with a dose of 10 mg/kg Dau-content (21.6 mg/kg conjugate) or with a dose of 2 mg/kg Dau-content (4.3 mg/kg conjugate) on days 10, 13, 19, 21, 24, 28, 31, 34, 39, 42, 46, 49, 53, 56, 60, 63, 67 and 70 after cells inoculation. Animal weight and tumor volumes were measured initially when the treatment started and at periodic intervals according to the treatment schedule. A digital caliper was used to measure the longest (a) and the shortest diameter (b) of a given tumor. The tumor volume was calculated using the formula $V = ab^2 \times \pi/6$, where a and b represent the measured parameters (length and width). The experiment was terminated on day 74 after cells inoculation (day 65 of treatment). Animals treated with free Dau had to be terminated after 3 treatments on day 28 after cells inoculation (day 19 of treatment) due to significant weight-loss. Animals were sacrificed by cervical dislocation; primary tumors and livers were harvested and weighted.

2.13. Statistical Analysis

For data on the cell viability assay, a one-way ANOVA algorithm of OriginPro 8.0 (OriginLab Corporation, Northampton, MA, USA) was used to assess the significance and calculate p-values. To compare the difference for all means, a Tukey's post-hoc test was performed. In the case of the in vivo studies, statistical analyses were performed by GraphPad Prism 6 (GraphPad Software, San Diego, CA, USA) using the non-parametric Mann–Whitney test, where p-values lower or equal than 0.05 were considered statistically significant. The symbols *, **, and *** mean significant at $p \leq 0.05$, $p \leq 0.01$, and $p \leq 0.001$, respectively.

3. Results and Discussion

3.1. Synthesis and Chemical Characterization of Conjugates

Five daunomycin-peptide conjugates were prepared for targeting PDAC cells. In our research, the potential homing peptide CKAAKN derived from phage display was modified by the replacement of Cys to Ser. The Cys/Ser exchange is commonly used in peptide chemistry, because of their similar structure (only thiol group is replaced by hydroxyl group), when there is no biological function of Cys. In CKAAKN the Cys was used for conjugation through its SH group (thioether linkage). This means that the free thiol group is not necessary for the biological activity; therefore, it can be replaced by other amino acids. Using another type of conjugation (e.g., oxime bond formation) the remaining free thiol group of Cys might cause unwanted disulfide bond formation that results in by-product. In addition, the Cys/Ser substitution can increase the hydrophilicity of the peptide that improves the water solubility of the peptide–drug conjugate.

Daunomycin (Dau) was applied as a payload. It was indicated in our previous research that Dau can be attached to peptides via oxime linkage easily with good yields. The oxime linked Dau-peptide conjugates showed circa one order of magnitude lower in vitro cytotoxic effect than the free drug. It might be because of the lower DNA binding affinity of the Dau containing metabolite compared to Dau [22]. However, the oxime linked conjugates are stable in the circulation and no loss of Dau can be observed before reaching the target cells. In addition, the conjugates are significantly better tolerated in vivo. Usually, they are not toxic up to 30 mg Dau content/kg body weight, while the free Dau can be applied at 1–2 mg/kg dose as maximum tolerated dose (MTD) [28]. Furthermore, the conjugates usually show similar or higher tumor growth inhibition at 10 mg Dau content/kg than the free drug at MTD with significantly less toxic side effects [27,29]. According to our observations the oxime linked Dau-peptide conjugates prevent better also the cell proliferation and metastases in mice models.

The syntheses of homing peptides were carried out by solid-phase peptide synthesis on Wang resin, that provides free carboxyl group on the C-terminus, using Fmoc/^{t}Bu strategy. Prior to the cleavage of the peptides from resins, isopropylidene protected aminooxyacetic acid (> = Aoa-OH) was attached to the amino function(s) of peptides. The isopropylidene protecting group was cleaved from the purified peptide derivatives by 1.5 M methoxyamine in ammonium-acetate buffer at pH 5. The salt and the side products were removed by RP-HPLC. Purified peptide derivatives were linked via oxime bond to Dau overnight in ammonium-acetate buffer at pH 5 followed by an additional HPLC purification step. The synthesis route of a selected conjugate is presented on Scheme 1. Characteristics of the conjugates are given in the Tables S3–S7 with their metabolites obtained during lysosomal degradation.

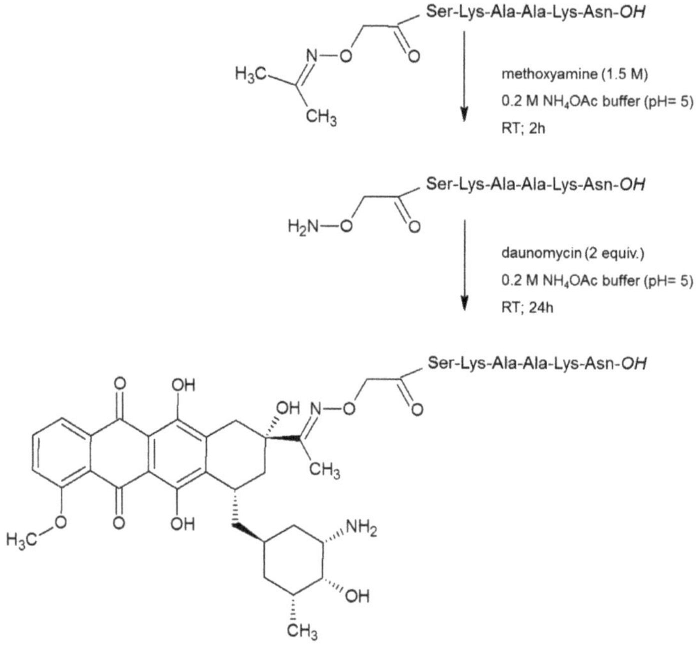

Scheme 1. Development of conjugate **1** as a representative synthesis route.

3.2. In Vitro Cytotoxicity of Conjugates

The characterization of the antitumor effect of the prepared conjugates was performed primary on PANC-1 pancreatic ductal adenocarcinoma cells. This cell line was derived from a head pancreatic carcinoma with invasive phenotype and an ability to give metastasis to peripancreatic lymph node, thus PANC-1 cell line can be considered as an in vitro model of lymph-node-positive PDAC [23]. To obtain the selectivity of the conjugates, their cytotoxicity was also measured on Colo-205 colon adenocarcinoma, A2058 metastatic melanoma and EBC-1 lung squamous cell carcinoma cell lines. Due to the different adherent and growth characteristics of these model cells, two different methods were chosen for determining the antiproliferative/cytotoxic effect of the conjugates. Measurements on PANC-1 cells were conducted by an impedimetric technique (xCELLigence System) because of its ability to establish tight adhesion and large spread area. The viability of Colo-205, A2058 and EBC-1 cells were analyzed by a colorimetric assay (alamarBlue-assay). Colo-205 cells can grow in suspension and can partly attach to a tissue culture ware. Since the xCELLigence system monitors attached cells only, and any kind of effects (e.g., cytotoxic effect) causing alteration in cell adhesion or spreading, we expected that the cytotoxic effects of conjugates on Colo-205 cells would be therefore under-detected with impedimetry. EBC-1 cells are adherent, but they have a weak spreading capacity only. Thus, the attached membrane area, which determines fundamentally the usability of impedimetry [30], is in a small range. Therefore, the impedimetric measurement is not optimal or reliable for measuring the EBC-1 cell line. In addition, CI curves of A2058 cells demonstrated that these cells were not able to form a stable plateau phase, which would be required for the treatment and for reading the concentrations having an anti-tumor effect.

To obtain cytotoxicity using impedimetry, cells were treated for 24, 48 and 72 h by the 10^{-6}, 10^{-5} and 10^{-4} M concentration solutions of the conjugates. The viability results of the 72 h treatment with conjugates at 10^{-5} M concentration are displayed in Table 1 as an example. The results show that the difference between the efficacy of the conjugates was well-observable in this concentration. The conjugates were ineffective at lower, 10^{-6} M concentration; when the conjugates were applied in a higher, 10^{-4} M concentration, most of the cells were killed after 72 h incubation.

Table 1. Characterization of the cytotoxicity of the conjugates on the PANC-1 cell line.

Code	Compounds	Viability [a] (%) at 10^{-5} M Concentration, After 72 h Incubation
1	Dau=Aoa-SKAAKN-OH	112.5 ± 5.1
2	Dau=Aoa-KSKAAKN-OH	154.2 ± 7.1
3	Dau=Aoa-GFLG-KSKAAKN-OH	105.1 ± 1.9
4	Dau=Aoa-GFLG-K(Dau=Aoa)SKAAKN-OH	0.1 ± 0.1
5	Dau=Aoa-GFLG-K(Dau=Aoa-GFLG)SKAAKN-OH	31.3 ± 1.8

[a] Cell index (CI) values of the treated cells are normalized to the CI values of the control wells and expressed as percentages. Data are given as mean values ± standard deviation (SD), (n = 3).

The linear peptide conjugate 1 did not show any antitumor effect on PANC-1 cells (Table 1) up to 10^{-5} M concentration. The connection of *Dau=Aoa* to the α-amino group of extra Lys incorporated to the N-terminus of the peptide (conjugate 2) and the presence of a Cathepsin B cleavable GFLG spacer [31] between the *Dau=Aoa* and the homing peptide (conjugate 3) did not improve the activity of conjugate 1. The modification with extra Lys was done to introduce an additional conjugation site (the ε-amino group of extra Lys), which provided the opportunity to create a branch with a second drug molecule.

The linear conjugate (3) with Gly-Phe-Leu-Gly (GFLG) spacer between the *Dau=Aoa* and the homing peptide was also used for the formation of conjugates with double Dau-content.

In contrast to the linear conjugates, the compounds with branched structure and two drug molecules decreased the cell viability significantly. Especially, conjugate 4, in which *Dau=Aoa* was attached directly to the side chain of the Lys residue used for conjugation, presented high toxicity on PANC-1 cells. Less than 1% of the cells survived a 72 h treatment at a 10^{-5} M peptide concentration (Table 1). The incorporation of an extra GFLG spacer (conjugate 5) into the branch decreased the potency of conjugate 4 (the cell viability was ca. 31% after 72 h). Nevertheless, a similar magnitude of cytotoxicity (viability: 34%) of conjugate 5 was already manifested after 24 h, while, in the case of conjugate 4, only a slight antitumor activity (viability: 91%) was observed (Figure 1A).

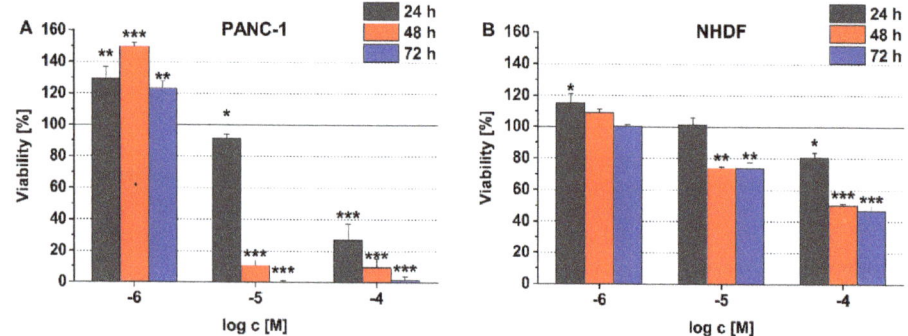

Figure 1. Comparison of the time and concentration dependent effect of conjugate **4** on (**A**) PANC-1 and (**B**) normal human dermal fibroblast (NHDF) cell viability. Data shown are mean of three parallels ± SD. The significance levels are the following: *: $p < 0.05$, **: $p < 0.01$, ***: $p < 0.005$.

It is important to note that the treatment with a conjugate could change the cell number and/or the morphology of the attached cells. In an impedimetric measurement, these changes could modify the CI and eventually the calculated viability parameter. In our previous study, the real-time curves showed a CI increase in the first 30 h of the treatment with a Dau-containing conjugate, but in the long term (40–72 h) the CI values were constantly decreased [32]. Depending on the efficacy of those conjugates, the transitional CI increase—probably as a result of morphological alterations—lasted shorter time interval and then turned into a decline of CI (cytotoxic effect) [32]. The treatment with conjugate **1** and **2** at 10^{-5} M for 72 h was not able to trigger cell death characterized by cell detachment and a decreased CI. However, our results still show that the treatment could irreversibly influence the cellular morphology (e.g., large and flat cell shape) which was manifested in increased CI values and cell viability higher than 100% (Table 1). This irreversible morphological alteration could evolve cell death by increasing incubation time and/or concentration. Real-time results of the highest concentration (10^{-4} M) of conjugate **1** and **2** support this theory. They caused an initial (0–36 h) increase in the CI values at 10^{-4} M concentration (viability after 24 h treatment: conjugate **1**: 224.1 ± 18.73%; conjugate **2**: 163.5 ± 24.3%) compared to the control. After this initial phase, the cell index values constantly decreased over the long term (after ~40 h), which represented their cytotoxic effect (viability after 24 h treatment; conjugate **1**: 17.1 ± 1.3% and conjugate **2**: 34.6 ± 9.4%).

To confirm that the different methods can be used to compare the effects of conjugates on the different model cells, the cytotoxicity of Dau was measured by both impedimetric and colorimetric methods on PANC-1 cells. In these experiments, very similar IC_{50} values—the concentration needed to decrease the cell viability by 50% (impedimetry: 1.89×10^{-7} M and colorimetry: 1.79×10^{-7} M)—were detected, which proved the suitability of these methods to evaluate the selectivity of the tested conjugates. Comparing the results of the viability measurements on different tumor cell lines, the conjugates **4** and **5** containing two drug molecules were proved to be more effective on PANC-1 cells than on melanoma (A2058), colon carcinoma (Colo-205) and lung carcinoma (EBC-1) cell lines. On the contrary, the linear conjugates (conjugates **1**, **2** and **3**), which were found to have no antitumor activity on PANC-1 cells, could exert a cytotoxic effect on the other three cell lines, especially on Colo-205 colon carcinoma cells (Table S1).

Regarding the applicability of a SMDC for targeted tumor therapy it is important to investigate whether it has no or negligible effect on healthy cells. The conjugate **4**, as the most effective conjugate on PANC-1 cells, was selected for such an experiment. The effect of conjugate **4** on NHDF cell viability is depicted in Figure 1B, in comparison with its antitumor effect on PANC-1 cells (Figure 1A). The conjugate elicited a slight cytotoxic effect on NHDF cells, but this activity proved to be much lower than in case of PANC-1 cells. After 72 h incubation with 10^{-5} M conjugate **4**, roughly 75% of

NHDF cells remained viable, while practically no viable PANC-1 cells were detectable. In the highest concentration (10^{-4} M), where most of the PANC-1 were killed already after 24 h, only 20% of NHDF cells were killed after 24 h. It seemed that the longer incubation time with conjugate **4** could not make cytotoxic effect be stronger in NHDF cells, since its time-dependent effect reached a plateau in a shorter incubation time (Figure 1B). Similar to the characteristics of the effects of conjugate **1** and **2** discussed above, the treatment with 10^{-6} M conjugate **4** resulted in cell viability values higher than 100% for PANC-1 cells. In this case as well, these results could be also due to irreversible morphological changes (e.g., large and flat cell shape) induce by conjugate **4**. The cells (so called senescent cells [33]) with altered morphology can go through apoptosis by increasing exposure time or concentration, which is recognizable in Figure 1A.

3.3. Cellular Uptake Measurements

PANC-1 cells were chosen to investigate the binding and the cellular uptake of the conjugates since these conjugates were designed for targeting pancreatic tumor cells and the most significant difference between their cytotoxic activities was also observed on this cell type.

The highest cellular uptake was detected in the case of the most cytotoxic conjugate **4** (Figure 2, Table S2). Interestingly, the binding affinity of conjugate **2** was higher compared to conjugate **4**, but its cellular uptake was lower, although different was not significant. This may be explained by the more positive character of conjugate **2** that can slightly decrease internalization. However, the difference in cellular uptake of conjugates cannot completely explain the significant difference in their biological activity. Nevertheless, some correlations between these characteristics of conjugates can be established. Conjugates **1** and **3** entered the cells less efficiently than conjugate **4**, the ability of which correlated well with the binding affinity and can explain their neutral effect on inhibition of cell viability. This negative correlation was especially significant in the case of conjugate **3** (Figure 2). The difference in the binding affinity and cellular uptake of conjugates **4** and **5** might explain their in vitro antitumor effect.

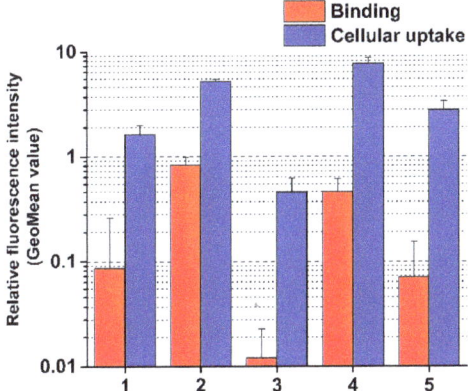

Figure 2. Binding affinity and cellular uptake of conjugates on PANC-1 cells. Binding and cellular uptake of the compounds were studied at 10^{-5} M concentration. GeoMean Data shown are mean of two parallels ± SD.

If we compared the intracellular fluorescence intensity of conjugates with that of free Dau, which served as a positive control, a two orders of magnitude difference could be observed (Table S2). This is not surprising, because the conjugates are assumed to enter the cells by receptor-mediated endocytosis, which has a lower capacity compared to the passive diffusion of free Dau. It was also previously reported that conjugation of Dau to a targeting peptide can decrease its fluorescence intensity by 90% compared to the free molecule [22]. Active metabolites released during the intracellular degradation (see in 3.4. chapter) of these constructs, have higher fluorescence than the intact conjugates.

However, 30 min incubation time used in our cellular uptake measurements is short and generate a negligible amount of metabolites only. Therefore, the fluorescence intensity originated from the intact conjugate only was detectable and evaluable in the cellular uptake measurement.

3.4. Characterization of Lysosomal Degradation of Conjugates by LC-MS

The antitumor activity of SMDCs depends on many factors, such as receptor binding, cellular uptake, stability, lysosomal degradation, the structure of the resulted metabolite and the localization of the metabolite in the cell. As was presented above, in some cases the cell viability inhibition and the cellular uptake of the conjugates correlated well, but in other cases not. Therefore, it was reasonable to study the lysosomal degradation process, which determines the formation of active metabolites and consequently the antitumor activity of SMDCs.

The conjugates were reacted with lysosome homogenate, which contains lysosomal enzymes such as various proteases, for example, Cathepsin B, that can be overproduced in cancer cells and significantly influence the degradation of the conjugates. Under this procedure the peptide bonds are cleaved by the enzymes in various positions, and thus degradation products can be identified in the reaction mixture. The identification of the degradation products was performed by the LC-MS technique. In this work, we focused on the presence and the amounts of Dau-containing metabolites, because these compounds are presumed to be responsible for the cytotoxicity of the conjugates (Tables S3–S7).

The release of free Dau was not detected from conjugates, however, various Dau-containing metabolites bearing one or a few amino acids were formed. The degradation of conjugates **1** and **2** was very fast. After 30 min, the presence of only small fragments: *Dau=Aoa-S-OH* and *Dau=Aoa-SK-OH* (Figure 3) can be detected in the case of conjugate **1** (Table S3). Because the smallest metabolite releases quite fast, the law antitumor effect can be explained either by the low cellular uptake of this metabolite or its lower binding affinity to DNA [22]. The metabolites with OH groups on the amino acids have lower binding affinity to DNA than *Dau=Aoa*-Gly-OH or H-Lys(*Dau=Aoa*)-OH. In addition, the metabolite has to diffuse out from the lysosomes that might be also prevented by its hydrophilic character.

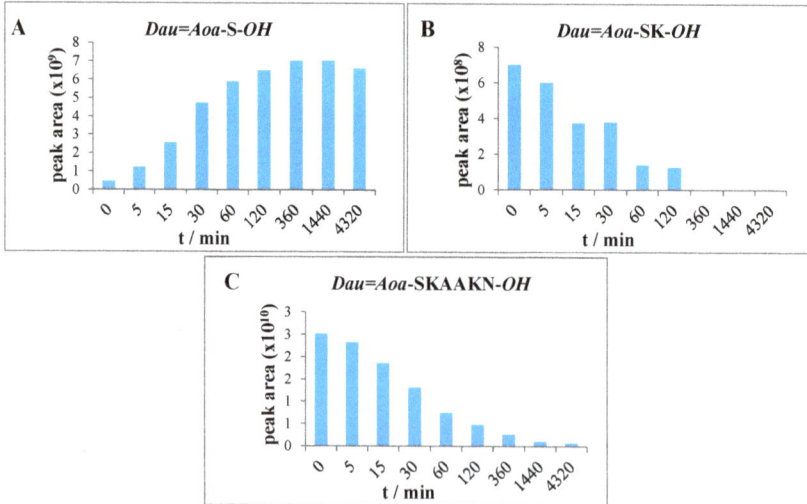

Figure 3. Time-dependent LC-MS intensity change of various molecules during the enzymatic degradation study of conjugate **1**: (**A**) the release of the smallest Dau-containing metabolite; (**B**) the intensity of the *Dau=Aoa*-SK-OH metabolite; (**C**) the time-dependent decrease in the amount of the intact conjugate **1**.

The *Dau=Aoa*-K-OH, *Dau=Aoa*-KS-OH (Figure 4) and *Dau=Aoa*-KSK-OH metabolites were detected in the case of conjugate **2** (Table S4). The results indicate that the release of the smallest metabolite was rather slow. The pK_i value of this fragment is in a basic range, that might hinder the diffusion out of the metabolite from the lysosomes as well. This observation explains the low cytotoxic effect of this conjugate—even its cellular uptake was high.

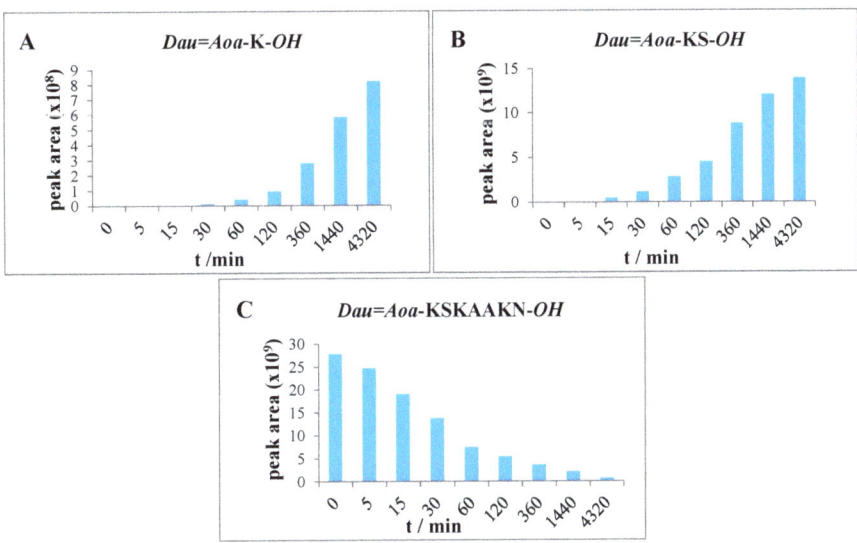

Figure 4. Time-dependent LC-MS intensity change of various molecules during the enzymatic degradation study of conjugate **2**: (**A**) the release of the smallest Dau-containing metabolite; (**B**) the intensity of the *Dau=Aoa*-KS-OH metabolite; (**C**) the time-dependent decrease in the amount of the intact conjugate **2**.

Enzymatic degradation of conjugates containing a Cathepsin B cleavable GFLG spacer (**3, 4, 5**) resulted in the formation of *Dau=Aoa*-GFL-OH; *Dau=Aoa*-GF-OH and the *Dau=Aoa*-G-OH compounds as final products of the degradation. *Dau=Aoa*-G-OH is the smallest Dau-containing metabolite, furthermore, this compound is known to have a cytotoxic effect (Tables S5–S7) [22].

Lysosomal degradation of conjugate **3** was rapid and completed within 1 h. After 0, 5, 30 and 60 min incubation, large fragments were detected lacking two or four amino acids from the C-terminus (*Dau=Aoa*-GFLGSKAA-OH, *Dau=Aoa*-GFLGKSK-OH). The detected fragments indicated that in this case, the peptidyl dipeptidase activity is predominant over the cleavage of the enzyme labile spacer. After 30 min, the presence of the two smallest fragments *Dau=Aoa*-GF-OH and *Dau=Aoa*-G-OH can be already detected. The intensity of the latter product—possessing cytotoxic property [22]—increased with increasing incubation time (Figure 5). After 72 h, only these two smallest metabolites were detected in the reaction mixture. However, the dipeptide containing fragment was still the main product.

After 72 h, the degradation of compound **4** resulted in similar products (*Dau=Aoa*-GFL-OH, *Dau=Aoa*-GF-OH and *Dau=Aoa*-G-OH) as the conjugate **3**. These metabolites originated from the cleavage of the GFLG spacer. Furthermore, additional Dau-containing metabolites could be identified in the case of conjugate **4**. After 2 h, the presence of the H-K (*Dau=Aoa*) SK-OH fragment could be detected as the main peak that was still the most intense peak after 72 h. In addition, the formation of H-K(*Dau=Aoa*)-OH (Table S6) was also observed. This compound was also shown to have DNA binding affinity similar to the *Dau=Aoa*-G-OH [22]. The time-dependent increment in the amount of these two active metabolites could be observed (Figure 6). The H-K(*Dau=Aoa*)-OH metabolite with free α-amino and the carboxyl group of Lys has a rather neutral character because of the zwitterionic structure that might help the diffusion out of the lysosomes in contrast to *Dau=Aoa*-Lys-OH. Altogether, conjugate **4** showed the highest cellular uptake and efficient release of two active Dau-containing metabolites that correlate its highest in vitro cytotoxic effect.

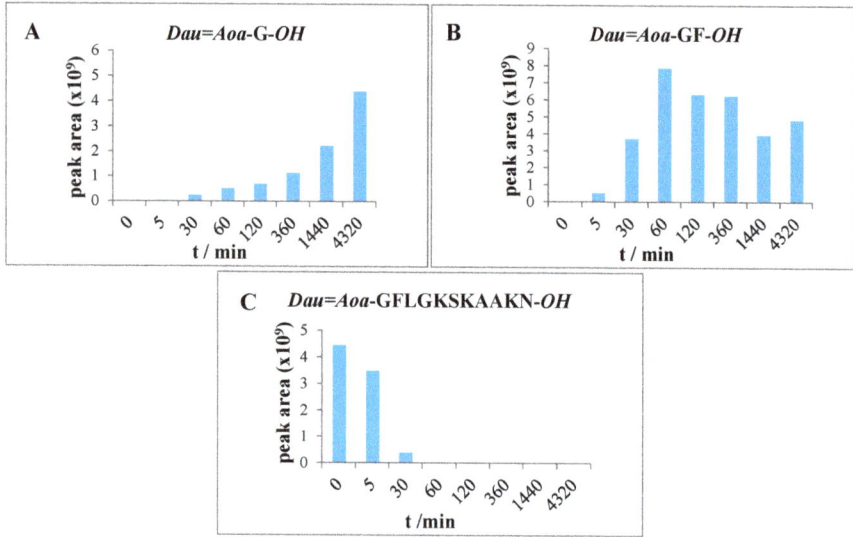

Figure 5. Time-dependent LC-MS intensity change of various molecules during the enzymatic degradation study of conjugate **3**: (**A**) the release of the smallest Dau-containing metabolite; (**B**) the intensity of the *Dau=Aoa*-GF-OH metabolite; (**C**) the time-dependent decrease in the amount of the intact conjugate **3**.

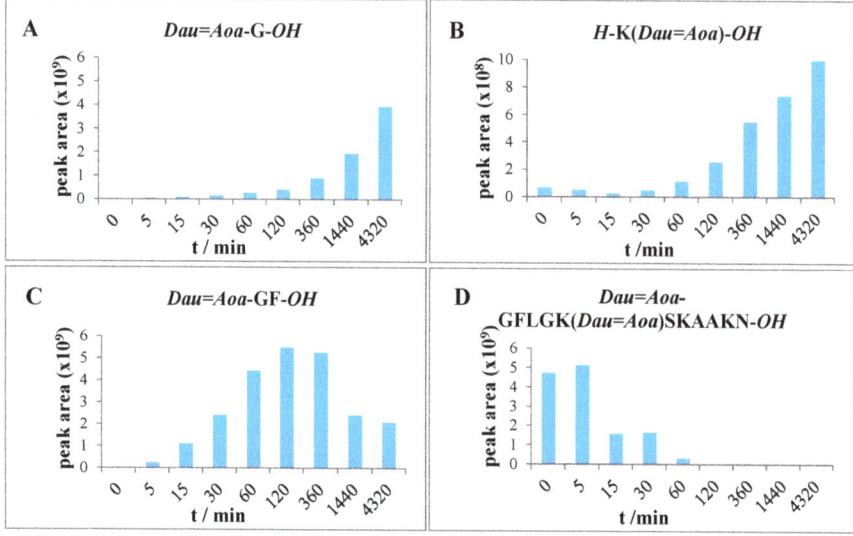

Figure 6. Time-dependent LC-MS intensity change of various molecules during the enzymatic degradation study of conjugate **4**: (**A**,**B**) the release of the two smallest Dau-containing metabolites; (**C**) the intensity of the *Dau=Aoa*-GF-OH metabolite; (**D**) the time-dependent decrease in the amount of the intact conjugate **4**.

The degradation of conjugate 5 in which both Dau are attached through GFLG spacer to the peptide backbone provided only the *Dau=Aoa-GFL-OH, Dau=Aoa-GF-OH* and *Dau=Aoa-G-OH* (Table S7) fragments that increased in time. However, the degradation of conjugate 5 was not yet complete after 72 h. In this case, a larger metabolite (H-K(*Dau=Aoa-GFLG*) SK-OH (Table S7) was still observed. The presence of this large molecular weight metabolite mentioned above suggested that the amount of the released *Dau=Aoa-G-OH* is derived rather from the N-terminus of the linear part, but its release is quite slow compared to the other conjugates (Figure 7). In comparison, compound 3 (*Dau=Aoa-GFLGKSKAAKN-OH*) was degradable by lysosomal enzymes quite fast resulting in the same metabolites, but the in vitro cytotoxic effect was much lower. This can be clearly explained by the very low binding efficiency and cellular uptake of conjugate 3. The difference in the metabolite release between compound 3 and 5 suggests that the branching cause steric hindrance for enzyme degradation. It seems that this effect is higher when the flexible GFLG spacer is in the branch (compare with conjugate 4).

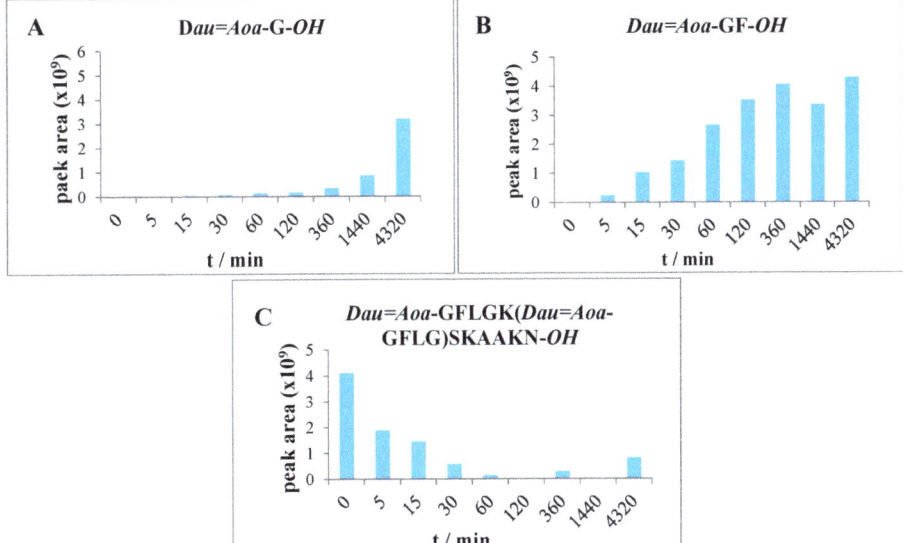

Figure 7. Time-dependent LC-MS intensity change of various molecules during the enzymatic degradation study of conjugate 5: (**A**) The release of the smallest Dau-containing metabolite; (**B**) the intensity of the *Dau=Aoa-GF-OH* metabolite; (**C**) the time-dependent decrease in the amount of the intact conjugate 5.

3.5. Acute and Chronic Toxicity Studies of Conjugate 4

The conjugate 4 (*Dau=Aoa*-GFLGK(*Dau=Aoa*)SKAAKN-OH), that was the most efficient one in vitro experiments, was selected for in vivo studies. Prior to the treatment of tumor-bearing mice, acute (single *i.p.* administration) and chronic toxicity (5 *i.p.* treatments on days 1, 3, 7, 9 and 11) studies were conducted on healthy Balb/c male mice. These experiments were continued for 14 days, and no significant changes in the body weight, the general looking and the behavior of the animals, were observed during this period of time (Figure 8). Based on the results, it was concluded that the conjugate was not toxic at the applied concentrations and can be further investigated for its in vivo antitumor activity.

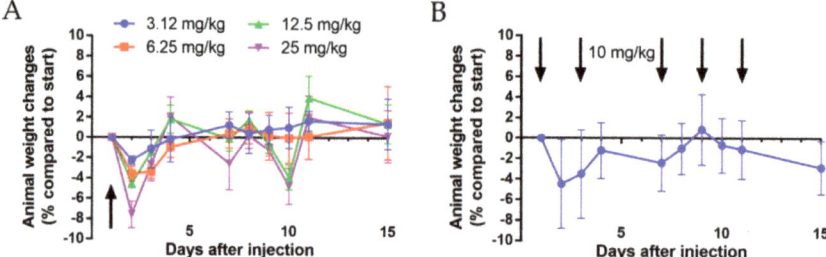

Figure 8. Animal body weight changes (percentage compared to the start of the experiment, average ± SEM). (**A**) Acute toxicity study of conjugate 4 with doses of 3.125, 6.25, 12.5 and 25 mg/kg Dau-content. (**B**) Chronic toxicity study of conjugate 4 with a dose of 10 mg/kg Dau-content, five treatments. Black arrows mean the day of treatment. Three mice per group were used for both experiments.

3.6. In Vivo Tumor Growth Inhibition of the Conjugate 4 in Pancreatic Tumor-bearing Mice

The tumor growth inhibition effect of conjugate 4 and free Dau on PANC-1 tumor-bearing SCID female mice was investigated. The free drug was applied once a week in the maximum tolerated dose of 1 mg/kg body weight while the conjugate was administered in average three times per week either in 2 mg/kg or in 10 mg/kg dose calculated for the Dau-content.

Body weight of s.c. human pancreatic cancer-bearing mice were evaluated. In comparison to the start of the experiment, the animal weight decreased significantly for 21% in the free Dau-treated group, and this group was terminated on day 28 after cell inoculation (day 19 of treatment) (Figure 9A). However, 35.7% inhibition of tumor growth (according to the tumor volume) was measured in this group, while in case of the groups treated with conjugate 4 at doses of 2 and 10 mg/kg Dau-content, the tumor growth inhibition was 6.8 and 27.9%, respectively, at this time point.

During the whole experiment, the animal weight stayed stable in conjugate 4 treated groups, with 0.8% decreasing under a dose of 2 mg/kg and 4% decrease in 10 mg/kg group. Animal weight decreased by 8.5% in the control group in comparison to the start of the experiment.

Antitumor effect of conjugate 4 was evaluated by measuring tumor volume in each group. At the end of the experiment (day 74) dose of 2 mg/kg, Dau-content inhibited tumor volume by 14%, while the dose of 10 mg/kg Dau-content inhibited significantly the tumor volume by 32.2% in comparison to the control group (Figure 9B). Interestingly, on the day 70 (day 61 of treatment), the inhibitions were 17.5%, and 39.9%, respectively, while on day 67 (day 58 of treatment) the dose of 10 mg/kg Dau-content elicited the most significant inhibition (43%) in the tumor volume compared to the control group. The data suggested that the tumor developed resistance during such a long treatment schedule.

At the end of the experiment (day 74), the animals were sacrificed and the antitumor effect of conjugate 4 was also evaluated by measuring tumor weight in each group (Figure 9C). Results showed that conjugate 4 inhibited tumor growth significantly under both doses (2 mg/kg Dau-content: 27.3%, 10 mg/kg Dau-content: 30.4%) in comparison with the tumor weight in the control group. Tumor weight depends on the content of tumor mass, necrotic cells, vessels, and general density which can differ for two tumors of the same size (same volume). Nevertheless, the correlation between the inhibition of the tumor volume and weight could be obtained at the end of the treatment with the lower dose, but the calculated SD values resulted in the significant inhibition of tumor weight ($p = 0.05$), while it was not significant for tumor volume [34]. The results indicated that the treatment with the higher dose of the conjugate might provide a higher shrinkage of tumor that could be suitable for preoperative chemotherapy.

The examination of the liver weight was carried out at the end of the experiment to determine the liver toxicity—as an indicator of toxic side effects—of conjugate 4 in s.c. human pancreatic cancer-bearing mice (Figure 9D). In the group treated with free Dau (three times with 1 mg/kg dose), the average liver/body weight ratio was significantly decreased by 29.1% compared to the control group, as well as in comparison to the groups treated with conjugate **4** (18 times with 2 or 10 mg Dau-content/kg dose); even so, the treatment period with free Dau was 46 days shorter than in case of the conjugate **4**. Average liver weight in conjugate **4** treated groups was not significantly changed in comparison to the control group.

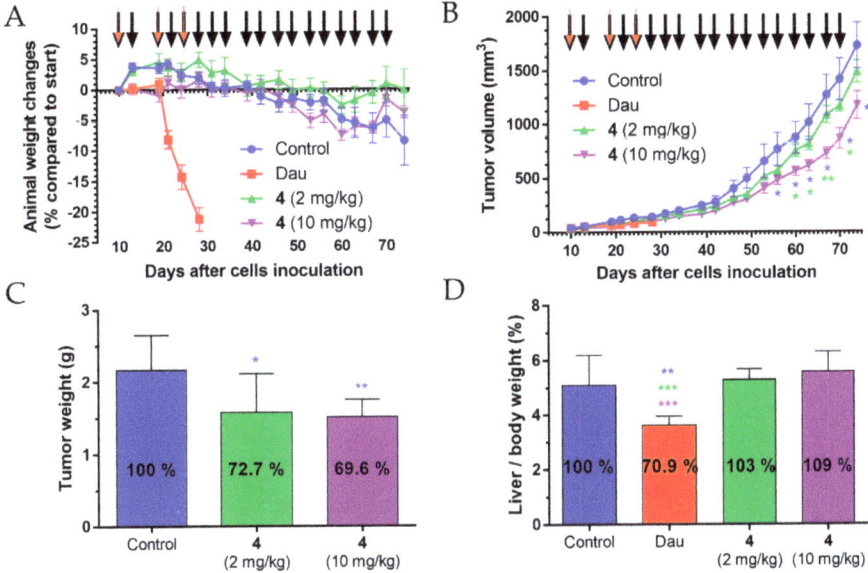

Figure 9. The effect of conjugate **4** (2 mg/kg and 10 mg/kg Dau-content, 18 treatments, black arrows) and free Dau (1 mg/kg, three treatments, red arrows) in subcutaneous PANC-1 human pancreatic carcinoma bearing mice. (**A**) Animal body weight changes (percentage compared to the start of the experiment, average ± SEM). (**B**) Tumor volume (mm^3, average ± SEM). (**C**) Tumor weight (grams, average ± SD) after termination of the experiment, 74 days subsequent to cell inoculation. (**D**) Liver weight/body weight ratio (percentage, average ± SD) after the termination of the experiment, 74 days after cell inoculation for the control and the conjugate treated groups, while 28 days after cell inoculation for the free Dau-treated group. Seven animals per group. Statistical analysis was performed by the Mann–Whitney test. *, ** and *** denote significant at $p \leq 0.05$, $p \leq 0.01$ and $p \leq 0.001$, respectively. The blue and green * denote significant difference of conjugate **4** (10 mg/kg) treated group compared to the control and conjugate **4** (2 mg/kg) groups, respectively (**B**). The blue * signifies significant difference of conjugate **4** (2 and 10 mg/kg) treated groups compared to the control (**C**). The blue, green, and purple * denotes significant difference of free Dau-treated group compared to the control and conjugate **4** (2 and 10 mg/kg) groups, respectively (**D**).

To summarize the in vivo experiments, the data indicated that conjugate **4** could inhibit the tumor growth of *s.c.* human pancreatic cancer (PANC-1)-bearing mice significantly without causing any toxic side effects. Even a low dose (2 mg/kg Dau-content) of conjugate **4** could inhibit the tumor growth significantly, without any toxicity for the animals.

4. Conclusions

In this study, our goal was to select a potential peptide–drug conjugate for efficient targeted tumor therapy against pancreatic cancer. We developed five peptide-based drug conjugates against pancreatic cancer cells (PANC-1). SKAAKN hexapeptide was applied as targeting moiety which differs only at the N-terminal amino acid of CKAAKN that was efficiently used for drug delivery in a former study. Because in our construct thiol group Cys was not used as a conjugation site, it was replaced by Ser.

Three linear conjugates with one Dau and two-branched variants with two conjugated Dau were developed. The cytotoxicity, binding and cellular uptake of the conjugates were studied on PANC-1 cells. In addition, the degradation of the conjugates in lysosome homogenate was investigated as well. It was indicated that the efficacy of these peptide–drug conjugates was influenced by various factors. Our results indicate that at the development of peptide–drug conjugates, not only the cellular uptake of the conjugates but also the effective release of the active metabolite should be taken into account. The release of active metabolites was shown to depend highly on the structure of the conjugate. The most efficient conjugate was *Dau=Aoa*-GFLGK(*Dau=Aoa*)SKAAKN-OH (conjugate 4) in the in vitro experiments, and it was selected for further in vivo studies. In contrast to the free drug, conjugate 4 did not show any toxicity during the treatment but elicited significant >30% tumor growth inhibition in PANC-1 bearing mice. The results suggested that SKAAKN peptide-based drug delivery systems could be promising constructs alone or in combination for the treatment of pancreatic cancers.

According to the results, conjugate 4 is suitable for further preclinical in vivo studies on more appropriate mice models representing better the stroma and the environment of PDAC. However, the models investigating stromal–tumor interactions are either induced (genetically modified) allograft models or patient-derived tumor xenografts (PDX). Both are very complex test tools; the use of the latter is gradually increasing, but due to the housing of special animals, the license of their use and the low efficiency of the establishment of tumors, they are not currently widespread in basic research.

Supplementary Materials: The following are available online at http://www.mdpi.com/1999-4923/12/6/576/s1, Table S1: In vitro cytotoxic effect of the prepared conjugates on various cell lines, Table S2: Relative fluorescence intensity results of binding and cellular uptake measurements on 20 PANC-1 cells, Table S3: Chemical characterization of identified fragments of conjugate 1, Table S4: Chemical characterization of identified fragments of conjugate 2, Table S5: Chemical characterization of identified fragments of conjugate 3, Table S6: Chemical characterization of identified fragments of conjugate 4, Table S7: Chemical characterization of identified fragments of conjugate 5, Figure S1–S5: HPLC chromatogram of conjugates 1–5, Figure S6–S10, Mass spectra of conjugates 1–5.

Author Contributions: Conceptualization: G.M., L.K. and J.T.; experimental design: G.M., L.K., G.S. and J.T.; investigation: L.E.D., E.L., I.R., D.M., G.S.; writing—original draft preparation: L.E.D., E.L., I.R., G.M.; writing—review and editing: G.M., L.K., G.S. and J.T.; visualization, L.E.D.; E.L.; I.R., D.M.; supervision: G.M., L.K. and J.T.; project administration: G.M.; funding acquisition: G.M., J.T. and G.S. All authors have read and agreed to the published version of the manuscript.

Funding: This research was supported by the National Research, Development and Innovation Office under grant NKFIH K119552 and NVKP_16-1-2016-0036. These studies were also supported by a grant (VEKOP-2.3.3-15-2017-00020) from the European Union and the State of Hungary, co-financed by the European Regional Development Fund. This work was completed in the ELTE Thematic Excellence Program supported by the Hungarian Ministry for Innovation and Technology. G.S. acknowledges funding by the MTA Premium Post-Doctorate Research Program of the Hungarian Academy of Sciences (HAS, MTA). The financial support from the 2019 Thematic Excellence Program (TUDFO/51757/2019-ITM) is greatly acknowledged by J.T and I.R.

Acknowledgments: The authors gratefully acknowledge the expert technical assistance provided by Zsófia Szász, Nóra Fekete and Éva Pállinger from Semmelweis University Department of Genetics, Cell- and Immunobiology.

Conflicts of Interest: The authors declare no conflict of interest.

References

1. Vincent, A.; Herman, J.; Schulick, R.; Hruban, R.H.; Goggins, M. Pancreatic cancer. *Lancet* **2011**, *378*, 607–620. [CrossRef]
2. Siegel, R.L.; Miller, K.D.; Jemal, A. Cancer Statistics, 2018. *CA Cancer J. Clin.* **2018**, *68*, 7–30. [CrossRef] [PubMed]
3. Hidalgo, M. Pancreatic cancer. *N. Engl. J. Med.* **2010**, *362*, 1605–1617. [CrossRef] [PubMed]
4. Zhang, L.; Sanagapalli, S.; Stoita, A. Challenges in Diagnosis of Pancreatic Cancer. *World J. Gastroenterol.* **2018**, *24*, 2047–2060. [CrossRef]
5. Diab, M.; Azmi, A.; Mohammad, R.; Philip, P.A. Pharmacotherapeutic strategies for treating pancreatic cancer: Advances and challenges. *Expert Opin. Pharmacother.* **2019**, *20*, 535–546. [CrossRef] [PubMed]
6. Xie, D.; Xie, K. Pancreatic cancer stromal biology and therapy. *Genes Dis.* **2015**, *2*, 133–143. [CrossRef]

7. Lei, F.; Xi, X.; Batra, S.K.; Bronich, T.K. Combination therapies and drug delivery platforms in combating pancreatic cancer. *J. Pharmacol. Exp. Ther.* **2019**, *370*, 682–694. [CrossRef]
8. Szepeshazi, K.; Schally, A.V.; Block, N.L.; Halmos, G.; Nadji, M.; Szalontay, L.; Vidaurre, I.; Abi-Chaker, A.; Rick, F.G. Powerful inhibition of experimental human pancreatic cancers by receptor targeted cytotoxic LH-RH analog AEZS-108. *Oncotarget* **2013**, *4*, 751–760. [CrossRef] [PubMed]
9. Vrettos, E.I.; Mező, G.; Tzakos, A.G. On the design principles of peptide–drug conjugates for targeted drug delivery to the malignant tumor site. *Beilstein J. Org. Chem.* **2018**, *14*, 930–954. [CrossRef]
10. Kutova, O.M.; Guriyev, E.L.; Sokolova, E.A.; Alzeibak, R.; Balalaeva, I.V. Targeted Delivery to Tumors: Multidirectional Strategies to Improve Treatment Efficiency. *Cancers* **2019**, *11*, 68. [CrossRef]
11. Zhuang, C.; Guan, X.; Ma, H.; Cong, H.; Zhang, W.; Miao, Z. Small molecule-drug conjugates: A novel strategy for cancer-targeted treatment. *Eur. J. Med. Chem.* **2019**, *163*, 883–895. [CrossRef] [PubMed]
12. Matters, G.L.; Harms, J. Utilizing peptide ligand GPCRs to image and treat pancreatic cancer biomedicines. *Biomedicines* **2018**, *6*, E65. [CrossRef] [PubMed]
13. Sanna, V.; Nurra, S.; Pala, N.; Marceddu, S.; Pathania, D.; Neamati, N.; Sechi, M. Targeted nanoparticles for the delivery of novel bioactive molecules to pancreatic cancer cells. *J. Med. Chem.* **2016**, *59*, 5209–5220. [CrossRef] [PubMed]
14. Liu, X.; Jiang, J.; Ji, Y.; Lu, J.; Chan, R.; Meng, H. Targeted drug delivery using iRGD peptide for solid cancer treatment. *Mol. Syst. Des. Eng.* **2017**, *2*, 370–379. [CrossRef] [PubMed]
15. Nishimoto, T.; Yamamoto, Y.; Yoshida, K.; Goto, N.; Ohnami, S.; Aoki, K. Development of peritoneal tumor-targeting vector by in vivo screening with a random peptide-displaying adenovirus library. *PLoS ONE* **2012**, *7*, e45550. [CrossRef] [PubMed]
16. Joyce, J.A.; Laakkonen, P.; Bernasconi, M.; Bergers, G.; Ruoslahti, E.; Hanahan, D. Stage-specific vascular markers revealed by phage display in a mouse model of pancreatic islet tumorigenesis. *Cancer Cell* **2003**, *4*, 393–403. [CrossRef]
17. Valetti, S.; Maione, F.; Mura, S.; Stella, B.; Desmaële, D.; Noiray, M.; Vergnaud, J.; Vauthier, C.; Cattel, L.; Giraudo, E.; et al. Peptide-functionalized nanoparticles for selective targeting of pancreatic tumor. *J. Control. Release* **2014**, *192*, 29–39. [CrossRef]
18. Valetti, S.; Mura, S.; Noiray, M.; Arpicco, S.; Dosio, F.; Vergnaud, J.; Desmaële, D.; Stella, B.; Couvreur, P. Peptide conjugation: Before or after nanoparticle formation? *Bioconjugate Chem.* **2014**, *25*, 1971–1983. [CrossRef]
19. Zhou, W.; Li, Y.; Gou, S.; Xiong, J.; Wu, H.; Wang, C.; Yan, H.; Liu, T. MiR-744 increases tumorigenicity of pancreatic cancer by activating Wnt/β-catenin pathway. *Oncotarget* **2015**, *6*, 37557–37569. [CrossRef]
20. Carmon, K.S.; Lin, Q.; Gong, X.; Thomas, A.; Liu, Q. LGR5 interacts and cointernalizes with Wnt receptors to modulate Wnt/β-catenin signaling. *Mol. Cell Biol.* **2012**, *32*, 2054–2064. [CrossRef]
21. Manea, M.; Leurs, U.; Orbán, E.; Baranyai, Z.; Öhlschläger, P.; Marquardt, A.; Schulcz, Á.; Tejeda, M.; Kapuvári, B.; Tóvári, J.; et al. Enhanced enzymatic stability and antitumor activity of daunomycin-GnRH-III bioconjugates modified in position 4. *Bioconjugate Chem.* **2011**, *22*, 1320–1329. [CrossRef] [PubMed]
22. Orbán, E.; Mező, G.; Schlage, P.; Csík, G.; Kulić, Z.; Ansorge, P.; Fellinger, E.; Möller, H.M.; Manea, M. In vitro degradation and antitumor activity of oxime bond-linked daunomycin-GnRH-III bioconjugates and DNA-binding properties of daunomycin-amino acid metabolites. *Amino Acids* **2011**, *41*, 469–483. [CrossRef]
23. Argentiero, A.; De Summa, S.; Di Fonte, R.; Iacobazzi, R.M.; Porcelli, L.; Da Vià, M.; Brunetti, O.; Azzariti, A.; Silvestris, N.; Solimando, A.G. Gene Expression Comparison between the Lymph Node-Positive and -Negative Reveals a Peculiar Immune Microenvironment Signature and a Theranostic Role for WNT Targeting in Pancreatic Ductal Adenocarcinoma: A Pilot Study. *Cancers (Basel)* **2019**, *11*, 942. [CrossRef] [PubMed]
24. Zhang, Q.; Meng, X.K.; Wang, W.X.; Zhang, R.M.; Zhang, T.; Ren, J.J. The Wnt/β-catenin signaling pathway mechanism for pancreatic cancer chemoresistance in a three-dimensional cancer microenvironment. *Am. J. Transl. Res.* **2016**, *8*, 4490–4498. [PubMed]
25. Enyedi, K.N.; Tóth, S.; Szakács, G.; Mező, G. NGR-peptide–drug conjugates with dual targeting properties. *PLoS ONE* **2017**, *12*, e0178632. [CrossRef] [PubMed]
26. Bárány, P.; Oláh, R.S.; Kovács, I.; Czuczi, T.; Szabó, C.L.; Takács, A.; Lajkó, E.; Láng, O.; Kőhidai, L.; Schlosser, G.; et al. Ferrocene-containing impiridone (ONC201) hybrids: Synthesis, DFT modelling, in vitro evaluation, and structure-activity relationships. *Molecules* **2018**, *23*, E2248. [CrossRef]

27. Ranđelović, I.; Schuster, S.; Kapuvári, B.; Fossati, G.; Steinkühler, C.; Mező, G.; Tóvári, J. Improved In Vivo Anti-Tumor and Anti-Metastatic Effect of GnRH-III-Daunorubicin Analogs on Colorectal and Breast Carcinoma Bearing Mice. *Int. J. Mol. Sci.* **2019**, *20*, E4763. [CrossRef]
28. Szabó, I.; Manea, M.; Orbán, E.; Csámpai, A.; Bősze, S.; Szabó, R.; Tejeda, M.; Gaál, D.; Kapuvári, B.; Przybylski, M.; et al. Development of an oxime bond containing daunorubicin-gonadotropin-releasing hormone-III conjugate as a potential anticancer drug. *Bioconjugate Chem.* **2009**, *20*, 656–665. [CrossRef]
29. Kiss, K.; Biri-Kovács, B.; Szabó, R.; Ranđelović, I.; Enyedi, K.N.; Schlosser, G.; Orosz, Á.; Kapuvári, B.; Tóvári, J.; Mező, G. Sequence modification of heptapeptide selected by phage display as homing device for HT-29 colon cancer cells to improve the anti-tumour activity of drug delivery systems. *Eur. J. Med. Chem.* **2019**, *176*, 105–116. [CrossRef]
30. Wegener, J.; Keese, C.R.; Giaever, I. Electric cell-substrate impedance sensing (ECIS) as a noninvasive means to monitor the kinetics of cell spreading to artificial surfaces. *Exp. Cell Res.* **2000**, *259*, 158–166. [CrossRef]
31. Peterson, J.J.; Meares, C.F. Cathepsin Substrates as Cleavable Peptide Linkers in Bioconjugates, Selected Selected from a Fluorescence Quench Combinatorial Library. *Bioconjugate Chem.* **1998**, *9*, 618–626. [CrossRef] [PubMed]
32. Lajkó, E.; Hegedüs, R.; Mező, G.; Kőhidai, L. Apoptotic effects of drug targeting conjugates containing different GnRH analogs on colon carcinoma cells. *Int. J. Mol. Sci.* **2019**, *20*, E4421. [CrossRef] [PubMed]
33. Van Deursen, J.M. The role of senescent cells in ageing. *Nature* **2014**, *509*, 439–446. [CrossRef] [PubMed]
34. McLean, M.; Wallace, H.L.; Sharma, A.; Hill, H.C.; Sabel, M.S.; Egilmez, N.K. A BALB/c murine lung alveolar carcinoma used to establish a surgical spontaneous metastasis model. *Clin. Exp. Metastasis* **2004**, *21*, 363–369. [CrossRef] [PubMed]

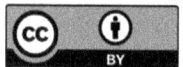

© 2020 by the authors. Licensee MDPI, Basel, Switzerland. This article is an open access article distributed under the terms and conditions of the Creative Commons Attribution (CC BY) license (http://creativecommons.org/licenses/by/4.0/).

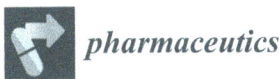

Article

Preclinical Evaluation of the GRPR-Targeting Antagonist RM26 Conjugated to the Albumin-Binding Domain for GRPR-Targeting Therapy of Cancer

Ayman Abouzayed [1,†], Hanna Tano [2,†], Ábel Nagy [2], Sara S. Rinne [1], Fadya Wadeea [1], Sharmishtaa Kumar [2], Kristina Westerlund [2], Vladimir Tolmachev [3,4], Amelie Eriksson Karlström [2,†] and Anna Orlova [1,4,5,*,†]

1. Department of Medicinal Chemistry, Uppsala University, 751 83 Uppsala, Sweden; Ayman.Abouzayed@ilk.uu.se (A.A.); sara.rinne@ilk.uu.se (S.S.R.); Fadya.Wadeea.6129@student.uu.se (F.W.)
2. Department of Protein Science, School of Engineering Sciences in Chemistry, Biotechnology and Health, KTH Royal Institute of Technology, AlbaNova University Center, 106 91 Stockholm, Sweden; htano@kth.se (H.T.); abelna@kth.se (Á.N.); shakum@kth.se (S.K.); krw@kth.se (K.W.); ameliek@kth.se (A.E.K.)
3. Department of Immunology, Genetics and Pathology, Uppsala University, 751 85 Uppsala, Sweden; vladimir.tolmachev@igp.uu.se
4. Research Centrum for Oncotheranostics, Research School of Chemistry and Applied Biomedical Sciences, Tomsk Polytechnic University, Tomsk 634050, Russia
5. Science for Life Laboratory, Uppsala University, 751 05 Uppsala, Sweden
* Correspondence: anna.orlova@ilk.uu.se
† These authors contribute equally to this paper.

Received: 28 September 2020; Accepted: 14 October 2020; Published: 16 October 2020

Abstract: The targeting of gastrin-releasing peptide receptors (GRPR) was recently proposed for targeted therapy, e.g., radiotherapy. Multiple and frequent injections of peptide-based therapeutic agents would be required due to rapid blood clearance. By conjugation of the GRPR antagonist RM26 (D-Phe-Gln-Trp-Ala-Val-Gly-His-Sta-Leu-NH$_2$) to an ABD (albumin-binding domain), we aimed to extend the blood circulation of peptides. The synthesized conjugate DOTA-ABD-RM26 was labelled with indium-111 and evaluated in vitro and in vivo. The labelled conjugate was stable in PBS and retained specificity and its antagonistic function against GRPR. The half-maximal inhibitory concentration (IC$_{50}$) of ^{nat}In-DOTA-ABD-RM26 in the presence of human serum albumin was 49 ± 5 nM. [^{111}In]In-DOTA-ABD-RM26 had a significantly longer residence time in blood and in tumors (without a significant decrease of up to 144 h pi) than the parental RM26 peptide. We conclude that the ABD-RM26 conjugate can be used for GRPR-targeted therapy and delivery of cytotoxic drugs. However, the undesirable elevated activity uptake in kidneys abolishes its use for radionuclide therapy. This proof-of-principle study justified further optimization of the molecular design of the ABD-RM26 conjugate.

Keywords: prostate cancer; gastrin-releasing peptide receptor; RM26; albumin-binding domain; targeted therapy; gastrin-releasing peptide receptors (GRPR) antagonist

1. Introduction

Prostate cancer is one of the most commonly diagnosed and deadliest cancers in men worldwide [1]. A lot of research has been focused on identifying novel prostate cancer cell targets, raising the sensitivity towards diagnosing prostate cancer, including detection of distant metastases, and expanding the therapeutic options for patients.

The gastrin-releasing peptide receptor (GRPR), a G-protein coupled receptor, is a member of the bombesin receptor family. GRPR is normally expressed in different organs such as the pancreas and the stomach [2], and is overexpressed in various cancers, including prostate and breast cancers. GRPR overexpression in prostate cancer is androgen dependent and is found in 63–100% of primary prostate cancer samples and in more than 50% of lymph node and bone metastases, but not in hyperplastic and benign prostate cells [3,4]. Overexpression of GRPR is high in the early stages of prostate cancer (but decreases with disease progression when tumors dedifferentiate into higher grade) and in androgen-insensitive and spread metastatic lesions [5–7].

These findings established GRPR as an important target for diagnostic imaging of prostate cancer and, possibly, for therapeutic use. A limited clinical study in patients with prostate cancer ($n = 11$) reported high sensitivity, specificity, and accuracy (88%, 81% and 83%, respectively) in the detection of primary lesions, and a sensitivity of 70% for the detection of metastatic lymph nodes [8]. Numerous bombesin analogues have been developed to target GRPR [9], but antagonists have recently been favored over agonists for receptor targeting [10]. Activation by agonists causes receptor downregulation [11] and is accompanied by physiological actions that are not limited to cell proliferation [12].

RM26 (D-Phe-Gln-Trp-Ala-Val-Gly-His-Sta-Leu-NH$_2$) is an extensively studied GRPR antagonist [13]. It binds to GRPR with high affinity and shows favorable pharmacokinetics when linked to different macrocyclic chelators using PEG linkers [14–16]. In clinics, [^{68}Ga]Ga-NOTA-PEG$_3$-RM26 has recently been evaluated for GRPR imaging in patients with prostate and breast cancers. [^{68}Ga]Ga-NOTA-PEG$_3$-RM26 could efficiently detect primary tumors and distant metastases, and was well tolerated by patients [17–19].

Other GRPR antagonists have demonstrated inhibition of cell proliferation in vitro, and multiple injections of therapeutic doses of the GRPR antagonist RC-3095 in a phase I trial were well tolerated; however, no follow-up studies were reported [20]. Antagonists to GRPR labelled with lutetium-177 were evaluated in preclinical studies on mice bearing prostate cancer xenografts, demonstrating a promising therapeutic efficacy with extended survival of the mice receiving the radiolabelled peptide [21,22]. The GRPR antagonist [^{177}Lu]Lu-RM2 was studied for the treatment of patients with metastatic castration-resistant prostate cancer by delivering at least one therapy cycle of the GRPR-targeting radioligand [23]. The therapy was deemed safe with no reported adverse effects and with the pancreas being the dose-limiting organ. However, due to rapid blood clearance of the labelled peptide, multiple frequent injections are required to deliver an appropriate dose to the tumor.

Extending the biological half-life of the GRPR-targeting ligand is a way to minimize the number of injections and to prolong the bioavailability of the ligand for binding to tumor cells. One approach of extending the biological half-life is by conjugating an albumin-binding domain (ABD) that would extend the biological half-life of the targeting agent. The engineered albumin-binding domain ABD035, derived from streptococcal protein G, has a femtomolar affinity for human serum albumin (HSA) [24]. ABD035 and related variants have been conjugated to several proteins for increases in vivo half-life, and the conjugates were considered safe and non-immunogenic, and have also been used in clinical studies with no reported adverse effects [25].

In this study, we aimed to develop and perform preclinical evaluation of the GRPR antagonist RM26 conjugated to ABD035 and assess the possibility for using the ligand in GRPR-targeting therapy for cancer treatment. The chelator DOTA (1,4,7,10-tetraazacyclododecane-1,4,7,10-tetraacetic acid) was coupled to the N-terminus of ABD for radiolabeling with indium-111 for in vitro and in vivo characterization. DOTA is a convenient chelator for stable coordination of indium-111, an isotope with relatively long half-life of 2.6 d that allows for the examination of biodistribution over several days.

2. Materials and Methods

Prostate carcinoma cell line PC-3 (GRPR positive) was purchased from ATCC, Manassas, VA, USA. The cells were maintained in RPMI-1640 media supplemented with 10% fetal bovine serum (FBS), 1% penicillin–streptomycin (PEST) (100 IU/mL penicillin, 100 µg/mL streptomycin), and 1% 2 mM L-glutamine (L-Glut), all purchased from Biochrom AG, Berlin, Germany, and incubated at 37 °C in 5% carbon dioxide gas and 95% air.

The activity content was measured using a 2840 automated gamma counter Wizard^{2TM} (PerkinElmer, Waltham, MA, USA). Instant thin-layer chromatography (ITLC) results were analyzed using Cyclone® Plus (PerkinElmer). Statistical analyses were performed by unpaired, two-tailed t-tests using GraphPad Prism 8 for Windows (GraphPad Software, San Diego, CA, USA); p values below 0.05 were considered significant.

2.1. General Peptide Synthesis

Peptides were produced by solid phase peptide synthesis (SPPS) with a fully automated microwave-assisted synthesis instrument (Biotage®-Initiator Alstra, Uppsala, Sweden). The amino acid monomers were Fmoc-protected, and as solid support, a Rink amide ChemMatrix resin (Biotage®) was used. Amino acids were purchased from Advanced Chemtech (Louisville, KY, USA), Novabiochem (St. Louis, MO, USA) and Sigma Aldrich (St. Louis, MO, USA). For a scale of 0.1 mmol peptide, 200 mg of resin was used. The resin loading was 0.5 mmol/g, and a five-times molar excess of amino acid was used in each cycle. For the coupling reaction, equimolar concentrations of DIC (*N,N*-diisopropylcarbodiimide, Sigma Aldrich, St. Louis, MO, USA)/Oxyma (ethyl (2Z)-2-cyano-2-hydroxyiminoacetate, Merck, Kenilworth, NJ, USA) (1:1) were used to activate the amino acids. Double coupling steps were applied for selected amino acid residues.

The temporary protecting group Fmoc was cleaved with 20% piperidine (Sigma Aldrich) in NMP (1-methyl-2-pyrrolidone, Merck). The non-reacted amino groups were capped with acetic anhydride (Honeywell Fluka, Charlotte, NC, USA)/DIEA (*N,N*-diisopropylethylamine, Sigma Aldrich) after each round of coupling. The amino acid side chains were protected with the following protecting groups: tBu (*tert*-butyl) for Ser and Tyr; Pbf (2,2,4,6,7-pentamethyldihydrobenzofuran-5-sulfonyl) for Arg; Trt (trityl) for Asn and His; Boc (*tert*-butyloxycarbonyl for Lys; and OtBu (*tert*-butyl ester) for Glu and Asp. The orthogonal protecting group Mtt (4-methyltrityl) was used for selected Lys residues.

2.1.1. Synthesis of DOTA-ABD-Cl

The 46 amino acid ABD was synthesized by SPPS as described in the previous paragraph. Double coupling steps were applied for selected amino acid residues: Asn9, Lys14, Tyr15, Tyr21, Arg23 and Asn26. A DOTA chelator (DOTA-tris(tBu)ester, CheMatech) was manually coupled to the N-terminus using DIC/Oxyma (1:1)-activated coupling chemistry. After the conjugation of DOTA, the Mtt-protected Lys14 was manually deprotected by 10 × 2 min treatment of the peptide–resin with a reaction solution of DCM/TFA/TIS (dichloromethane, VWR (Radnor, PA, USA)/trifluoroacetic acid, Alfa Aesar, Kandel, Germany)/triisopropylsilane, Sigma Aldrich) at a 94:1:5 ratio. The deprotected Lys residue was acylated with chloroacetic acid (Sigma Aldrich) (10 equivalents) in the presence of *N,N*-dicyclohexylcarbodiimide (DCC, Aldrich) (5 equivalents) as an activator and DIEA (10 equivalents) as a base for 1 h at room temperature. All manual coupling and deprotection steps were monitored by ninhydrin tests and repeated if necessary.

The final product was cleaved from the resin, and the side chains were deprotected with a mixture of TFA/TIS/H$_2$O 95:2.5:2.5 for 3 h. The crude peptide was extracted with H$_2$O/*tert*-butyl-methyl ether (Merck) with a 1:1 ratio, and the water phase containing the peptide was lyophilized. The correct molecular weight was confirmed after the synthesis by MALDI-TOF mass spectrometry (MALDI TOF/TOF analyzer, Sciex, (Applied Biosystems, Foster City, CA, USA).

2.1.2. Synthesis of RM26

The bombesin analogue RM26 was synthesized by SPPS as described above. Fmoc-statine was incorporated without side chain protection. After the synthesis of the first nine amino acids, the PEG_4 linker (Fmoc-15-amino-4,7,10,13-tetraoxapentadecacanoic acid, ChemScene, Chemtronica AB, Sollentuna, Sweden) and the N-terminal thiol group-containing mercaptopropionic acid (S-trityl-β-mercaptopropionic acid, Peptides International, Gardner, MA, USA) were coupled manually to the RM26 peptide (D-Phe-Gln-Trp-Ala-Val-Gly-His-Sta-Leu-NH_2) in sequential steps. The coupling and deprotection steps were monitored by ninhydrin tests and repeated if necessary. As a last step of the synthesis, a final piperidine deprotection was performed in order to reverse possible acylation of the statine side chain. After the final cleavage from the resin using a mixture of TFA/TIS/H_2O/EDT 94:1:2.5:2.5 and an ether extraction step, the correct product was analyzed and verified with MALDI-TOF.

2.1.3. Purification of DOTA-ABD-Cl and RM26

DOTA-ABD-Cl and RM26 were purified by reversed-phase HPLC (RP-HPLC) (Agilent 1200 series, Agilent Technologies, Santa Clara, CA, USA) on a semi-preparative column (5 μm, 9.4 × 250 mm Zorbax 300SB-C_{18}, Agilent Technologies). A gradient of 20–60% acetonitrile in H_2O with 0.1% TFA was used as the mobile phase. The total running time was 30 min with a flow rate of 3 mL/min, and a 40 °C column temperature was applied in order to maximize the degree of separation. The peaks were collected and analyzed by MALDI-TOF to identify the correct product. The fractions containing the correct product were pooled and lyophilized.

2.1.4. Conjugation of DOTA-ABD-Cl to RM26

Purified DOTA-ABD-Cl and RM26 were conjugated through formation of an alkyl thioester between the chloroacetyl and thiol functional groups on the two molecules. The reaction was performed as described by Lindgren, et al. [26] in a ligation buffer containing 10 mM EDTA (ethylenediaminetetraacetic acid) in phosphate buffered saline (PBS, 60%, pH 8) with acetonitrile as co-solvent (40%). The pH of the reaction was set to 8–8.5 with NaOH (5%). A two times molar excess of RM26 was used. The total peptide concentration was approximately 2 mg/mL. To avoid the formation of disulfide-linked RM26 dimers and to reduce dimers already present in the solution, TCEP (tris(2-carboxyethyl)phosphine) (10 mM TCEP for 0.2–1 mg/mL protein) was added to RM26 prior to the conjugation reaction.

The final product was purified by reversed-phase high-performance liquid chromatography (RP-HPLC) with a gradient of 20–60% acetonitrile in H_2O with 0.1% TFA as the mobile phase over 30 min with a flow rate of 3 mL/min and 40 °C column temperature. The peaks were collected and analyzed by MALDI-TOF mass spectrometry, and the correct molecular weight was confirmed with electrospray ionization-mass spectrometry (ESI-MS) (Thermo Ultimate3000, Thermo Fisher Scientific, Waltham, MA, USA, Bruker Impact II, Bruker Daltonics, Billerica, MA, USA). The purity of the conjugate was analyzed with an analytical RP-HPLC column (3.5 μm, 4.6 × 150 mm Zorbax 300SB-C_{18}, Agilent Technologies) using the same conditions as described for the purification of the product. The protein concentration of the samples used for surface plasmon resonance (SPR) analysis and circular dichroism (CD) spectroscopy was determined by quantitative amino acid analysis (Alphalyse, Odense, Denmark).

2.1.5. Expression and Purification of Recombinant ABD Control Protein

Methods for expression and purification of recombinant ABD can be found in detail in the Supplementary Materials Information. In brief, ABD035 was expressed as a thioredoxin fusion protein using the pET32a expression vector in BL21 (DE3) star *Escherichia coli* cells. After overnight autoinduction, the cells were lysed by sonication, and the His_6-tagged fusion protein was purified using immobilized-metal ion chromatography (IMAC) purification. Following enterokinase-His$_6$ (Sino Biological, Beijing, China) cleavage, the now untagged ABD035 protein was purified by collecting the unretarded flow-through from a second IMAC round. The purity and molecular weight of the purified ABD035 were confirmed using MALDI-TOF and SDS-PAGE.

2.2. Circular Dichroism

The secondary structures of ABD035, DOTA-ABD-Cl and DOTA-ABD-RM26 were determined by circular dichroism spectroscopy (Chirascan, Applied Photophysics, Leatherhead, UK). All CD spectra were obtained at 20 °C using a protein concentration of 0.2 mg/mL in 20 mM potassium phosphate buffer with 100 mM KCl pH 7.4. To estimate the percentage of helicity in each construct, the measured ellipticity (θ_{obs}) was first converted to the mean residue ellipticity (MRE) using the following formula MRE = $\theta_{obs}/10 \times l \times C \times n$, where l is the pathlength in cm, C is the peptide concentration in the molar, and n is the number of residues in each construct. From the mean residue ellipticity at 222 nm, MRE$_{222}$, the fraction helix, F_H, was calculated using the following formula, $F_H = (MRE_{222} - [\theta]_C)/([\theta]_H - [\theta]_C)$. $[\theta]_H$ and $[\theta]_C$ are given by $[\theta]_H = 40{,}000 \times (1 - (2.5/n) + 100 \times T$, and $[\theta]_C = 640 - 45 \times T$. T is given in °C, here 20, and n is the number of residues in each construct (Scholtz 1991).

2.3. Surface Plasmon Resonance (SPR) Experiments

The interaction between DOTA-ABD-RM26 and HSA was investigated using Biacore T200 (GE Healthcare Life Sciences, Uppsala, Sweden). HSA was immobilized to 660 RU at a dextran surface on a Series S Sensor Chip CM5 chip (GE Healthcare Life Sciences, Uppsala, Sweden). Immobilization was performed using standard (1-ethyl-3-(3-dimethylamino) propyl carbodiimide, hydrochloride/N-hydroxysuccinimide (EDC/NHS) amine coupling procedures. After immobilization of the ligand, remaining unreacted NHS esters were deactivated by injection of 1 M ethanolamine. One surface was activated followed by deactivation and used as a reference, and another surface was immobilized with L1CAM-Fc (Sino Biological) as a control in all SPR experiments. All runs were performed with phosphate buffered saline with 0.5% Tween®-20 (PBST), pH 7.4 as running buffer. DOTA-ABD-RM26 at seven concentrations (0.27, 0.82, 2.47, 7.4, 22.2, 66.7 and 200 nM) was injected onto HSA for 150 sec at a flow rate of 30 µL/min. Dissociation was allowed for 7200 s (2 h) followed by surface regeneration by injection of 10 mM HCl. As comparison, unconjugated ABD035 and DOTA-ABD-Cl were injected to the surface at the same concentrations, using the same flow rate, association time and dissociation time. Kinetic parameters were calculated using a 1:1 Langmuir binding model in the Biacore T200 Evaluation software. All runs were performed in duplicates.

2.4. Radiolabeling and In Vitro Stability of DOTA-ABD-RM26

The DOTA-ABD-RM26 conjugate was radiolabeled with indium-111 by adding [^{111}In]InCl$_3$ (2.3–19.7 MBq) to 14–21 µg of DOTA-ABD-RM26 (2–3 nmol) and 80 µL of ammonium acetate buffer (0.2 M, pH 5.5). The reaction mixture was incubated at 85 °C for 30 min, and the radiochemical yield was determined by radio ITLC using 0.2 M citric acid buffer for elution. The radiolabeled conjugate was purified using NAP-5 size-exclusion columns. The labelling stability was tested by adding 1000-fold molar excess of EDTA or PBS to [^{111}In]In-DOTA-ABD-RM26, and the percentage of indium-111 release was determined using radio ITLC at 1, 4 and 24 h at room temperature. For some of the experiments, HSA was bound to the purified [^{111}In]In-DOTA-ABD-RM26 by adding 10-fold molar excess of HSA and allowing the conjugation to proceed for 1 h at room temperature.

Parental peptide DOTA-RM26 was labelled with indium-111 according to previously described procedure [14] with quantitative yield (determined by HPLC) and used in experiments without purification.

2.5. In Vitro Specificity Assay

The in vitro specificity assay was performed on PC-3 cells (GRPR positive). One day before the experiment, the cells (5×10^5 cells/well) were plated on 6-well plates. At the time of the assays, the cells were washed, and 500 nM/well of DOTA-ABD-RM26 in the presence of HSA or 250 nM/well of DOTA-RM26 were added to the blocked wells in triplicates. The blocking was allowed to proceed for 10 min at room temperature; then, 20 nM/well of [^{111}In]In-DOTA-ABD-RM26 plus HSA was added to non-blocked wells and to the wells blocked with either DOTA-ABD-RM26 plus HSA or DOTA-RM26. The dishes were incubated for 1 h at 37 °C followed by washing the cells and treatment with trypsin–EDTA to the cells detached. The cells were then collected, and the radioactivity content was measured using a gamma counter.

2.6. Competitive Binding (IC_{50}) Assay

PC-3 cells (5×10^5 cells/well) were plated on 12-well plates one day before the competitive binding assays. Three conjugates (^{nat}In-DOTA-RM26, ^{nat}In-DOTA-ABD-RM26 and ^{nat}In-DOTA-ABD-RM26 with addition of HSA) were used to compete with [^{111}In]In-NOTA-PEG$_4$-RM26 for GRPR. DOTA-RM26 and DOTA-ABD-RM26 were loaded with stable indium by adding 3-fold molar excess of InCl$_3$ to each conjugate, and the reactions proceeded as described earlier. On the day of the experiment, the cells were washed, and 1 nM of [^{111}In]In-NOTA-PEG$_4$-RM26 was added to each well along with a series of concentrations ranging between 0–10 µM of the competing conjugate. The dishes were incubated at 4 °C for 5 h. The cells were then washed and treated with trypsin–EDTA until cell detachment. The cells were collected, and the radioactivity content was measured using a gamma counter.

2.7. Cellular Processing Assay

For the cellular processing assay, PC-3 cells (5×10^5 cells/well) were plated on 35×10 mm dishes two days before the experiment. On the day of the experiment, the cells were washed, and 20 nM/well of [^{111}In]In-DOTA-ABD-RM26 plus HSA were added. At predetermined time points of 1, 2, 4, 8 and 24 h, the cells were washed, and the dishes were placed on ice. The membrane-bound fraction was separated by adding 1 mL of 0.2 M glycine buffer containing 0.15 M NaCl and 4 M urea (pH 2) and incubation on ice for 5 min. The solution was collected, and the cells were washed with more glycine buffer that was collected as well. To collect the cells and determine the internalized fraction, 0.5 mL of 1 M NaOH was added followed by incubation at 37 °C for 30 min. The cells were scraped, and the solution was collected after washing with additional 1 M NaOH. The radioactivity content was then measured on a gamma counter.

2.8. In Vivo Targeting Specificity and Biodistribution Studies

All animal studies were approved by the Ethics Committee for Animal Research in Uppsala, Sweden, following the national legislation on protection of laboratory animals (4/16, 26 February 2016).

BALB/c nu/nu female mice were implanted subcutaneously with PC-3 cells in PBS (6.5×10^6 cells/mouse) on the hind leg. Tumor size was 0.4 ± 0.2 g at the time of the experiment (2–3 weeks following implantations). A group of four mice was used per data point.

One group of mice was intravenously injected with 40 pmol (30 kBq in 100 µL PBS) of [^{111}In]In-DOTA-ABD-RM26 and another group was injected with the same amount and activity of [^{111}In]In-DOTA-ABD-RM26 along with 10 nmol of DOTA-ABD-RM26 to test the in vivo targeting specificity for [^{111}In]In-DOTA-ABD-RM26. The mice were euthanized at 72 h post injection (pi).

To study the biodistribution over time, four groups of mice were injected with 40 pmol (30 kBq in 100 µL PBS) of [^{111}In]In-DOTA-ABD-RM26 and euthanized at predetermined time points of 1, 24, 72 and 144 h pi. A group of mice was injected with 40 pmol (30 kBq in 100 µL PBS) of [^{111}In]In-DOTA-RM26 and euthanized at 1 h pi. After euthanization, the organs of interest were collected and weighed, and the radioactivity content was measured on a gamma counter.

3. Results

3.1. Peptide Synthesis, Purification and Conjugation

The syntheses of DOTA-ABD-Cl and RM26 were successfully performed in an automated SPPS system using microwave-assisted coupling and Fmoc chemistry. Double-coupling steps for the selected amino acids were introduced in order to increase the yield. Final modifications were performed manually. Following the final TFA cleavage and ether extraction of both peptides, RP-HPLC was performed to purify the crude peptides. The crude purities of DOTA-ABD-Cl and RM26 after the syntheses were 40% and 45%, respectively. The purified products were used as starting material for the conjugation reaction (Figure 1).

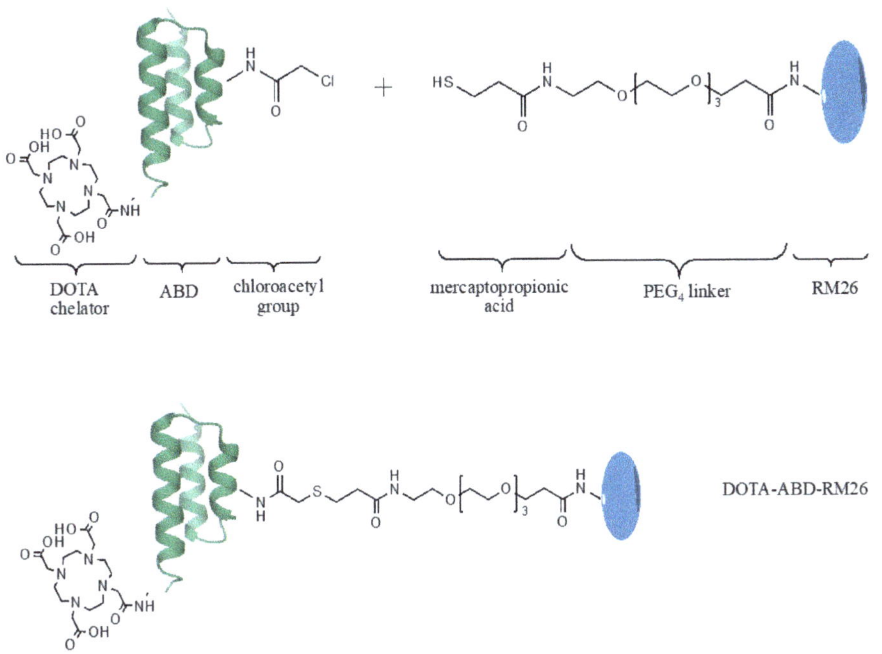

Figure 1. Schematic protocol for production of the DOTA-ABD-RM26 conjugate.

During the different steps of the synthesis, the peptides and the final products were analyzed, and the correct molecular weights were confirmed with MALDI-MS (Table 1; Figures S1–S3). The conjugation reaction was performed based on a previously developed protocol [26]. After the successful crosslinking of the peptides, another HPLC purification step was performed where the peaks containing the conjugate were collected and analyzed (Figure S4). The molecular weight of the final product was confirmed by ESI-MS (Table 1; Figure S5), and the high purity of the conjugate (98%) was assessed by analytical HPLC. The correct size and purity of recombinantly produced ABD035 were verified by SDS-PAGE (Figure S6) and MALDI-MS (Table 1; Figure S7).

Table 1. Peptides and proteins used in the study.

Name	Peptide Sequences [a]	Theoretical MW (Da)	Experimental MW (Da)
RM26	Mercaptopropionyl-[PEG$_4$]-D-Phe-Gln-Trp-Ala-Val-Gly-His-Sta-Leu-NH$_2$	1448.7	1446 [b]
ABD035	AMALAEAKVLAN RELDKYGVSDFY KRLINKAKTVEGV EALKLHILAALP	5383.4	5367 [b]
DOTA-ABD-Cl	[DOTA]-LAEAKVLANRELDK (ClAc)YGVSDFYKRLINKAKT VEGVEALKLHILAALP-NH$_2$	5571.9	5555 [b]
DOTA-ABD-RM26	[DOTA]-LAEAKVLANRELDK (RM26)YGVSDFYKRLI NKAKTVEGVEAL KLHILAALP-NH$_2$	6984.2	6989 [b] 6983.9 [c]

[a] RM26 amino acid sequence shown in three-letter code, and ABD amino acid sequences shown in one-letter code. PEG$_4$ = 15-amino-4,7,10,13-tetraoxapentadecacanoic acid. DOTA = 1,4,7,10-tetraazacyclododecane -1,4,7,10-tetraacetic acid. [b] Analyzed by MALDI-MS. [c] Analyzed by ESI-MS.

3.2. Characterization of Synthesized Conjugate

Circular dichroism: The CD spectra of both DOTA-ABD-Cl and the control protein ABD035 displayed a characteristic alpha-helical pattern with minima at 208 nm and 222 nm (see Figure 2A). The CD spectrum of the DOTA-ABD-RM26 conjugate indicated a contribution of both random coil and alpha-helix, with a signal minimum at approximately 205 nm and a dip at 222 nm. The melting temperature was estimated to be 50 °C for the synthetic constructs DOTA-ABD-Cl and DOTA-ABD-RM26, and 54 °C for the recombinant control protein ABD035 (Figure 2B). CD spectra collected at 20 °C after thermal unfolding suggest that all proteins refold after heating.

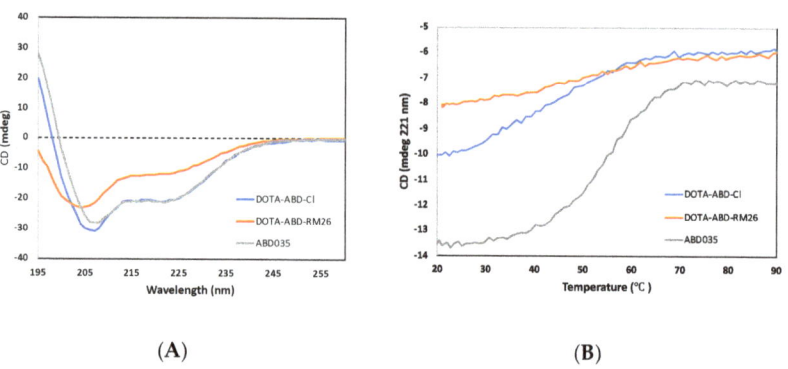

(A)   (B)

Figure 2. Circular dichroism (CD) spectra (A) and thermal melting curves (B) of DOTA-ABD-RM26, DOTA-ABD-Cl and ABD035.

SPR analyses: According to the SPR analysis of the interaction between DOTA-ABD-RM26 and HSA, the conjugation of RM26 and DOTA to ABD had a limited impact on the binding of ABD035 to HSA at room temperature (Figure 3). The K_D (equilibrium dissociation constant) for DOTA-ABD-RM26 binding to HSA is similar to that of the control protein ABD035 alone for binding to HSA (Table 2). SPR sensorgrams for each construct are to be found in Supplementary Information Figures S8–S10. As presented in Figure 3, the dissociation rate is the fastest for DOTA-ABD-Cl among the three constructs, while the unmodified ABD035 has the slowest dissociation rate.

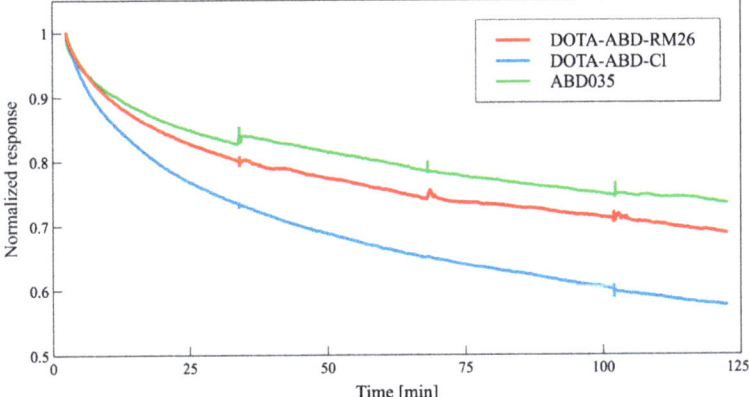

Figure 3. Surface plasmon resonance (SPR) sensorgrams illustrating the relative responses of DOTA-ABD-RM26, DOTA-ABD-Cl and ABD035 binding to HSA at 200 nM. Responses are normalized to the starting point of the dissociation to allow for comparison of dissociation phases for the three constructs.

Table 2. Kinetic constants for ABD variants binding to human serum albumin (HSA) determined by SPR.

Construct	k_a (1/Ms)	k_d (1/s)	K_D (M)
ABD035	2.5×10^6	5.4×10^{-5}	2.2×10^{-11}
DOTA-ABD-Cl	3.0×10^6	3.8×10^{-4}	1.3×10^{-10}
DOTA-ABD-RM26	7.9×10^6	6.6×10^{-5}	8.3×10^{-11}

3.3. Radiolabelling of DOTA-ABD-RM26 and Stability of the Labelled Conjugate

DOTA-ABD-RM26 was radiolabelled with indium-111 with good radiochemical yield (63 ± 3%) determined by ITLC. After purification on a size-exclusion column, the radiochemical purity of [^{111}In]In-DOTA-ABD-RM26 was higher than 99.5%. The purified [^{111}In]In-DOTA-ABD-RM26 was stable in PBS with minimal release of indium-111 within 24 h incubation (0.9 ± 0.2%). However, there was noticeable release of indium-111 when challenged with 1000-*fold* molar excess of EDTA—15 ± 1% release after 24 h incubation.

3.4. In Vitro Characterization of [^{111}In]In-DOTA-ABD-RM26

The binding specificity of [^{111}In]In-DOTA-ABD-RM26 toward GRPR: the in vitro binding specificity assay (Figure 4A) showed significantly decreased cell-associated activity when GRPR-expressing PC-3 cells were preincubated with 250 nM of RM26 or 500 nM of DOTA-ABD-RM26 in the presence of HSA. This demonstrated that the GRPR antagonist retained specific binding toward GRPR after conjugation with ABD. This also confirmed that the conjugate bound to HSA retained binding to GRPR.

Cellular processing: The cellular processing of [^{111}In]In-DOTA-ABD-RM26 was studied on GRPR-expressing PC-3 cells in the presence of 10-fold molar excess of HSA (Figure 4B). Internalization of the radiolabelled conjugate was slow, and after 24 h of incubation, no more than 27% of cell-associated activity was internalized, which corroborated the antagonistic nature of RM26.

Competitive binding: The half-maximal inhibitory concentration (IC$_{50}$) for ^{nat}In-DOTA-ABD-RM26 was 30 ± 3 nM and 49 ± 5 nM in the presence of 10-fold molar excess of HSA, which demonstrated that binding of albumin to the ABD-containing conjugate did not influence the binding to GRPR (Figure 5). The half-maximal inhibitory concentration for ^{nat}In-DOTA-RM26 measured in the same setting was 4.5 ± 0.7 nM.

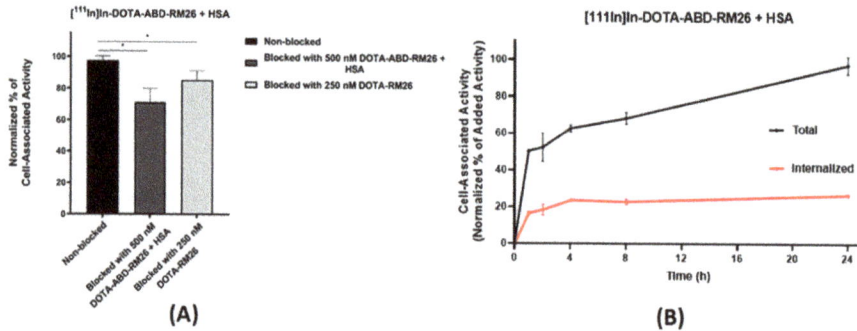

Figure 4. (**A**) In vitro binding specificity. (**B**) Cellular processing under continuous incubation at 1, 2, 4, 8 and 24 h. The error bars represent the standard deviation ($n = 3$). * indicates a significant difference with a p value < 0.05.

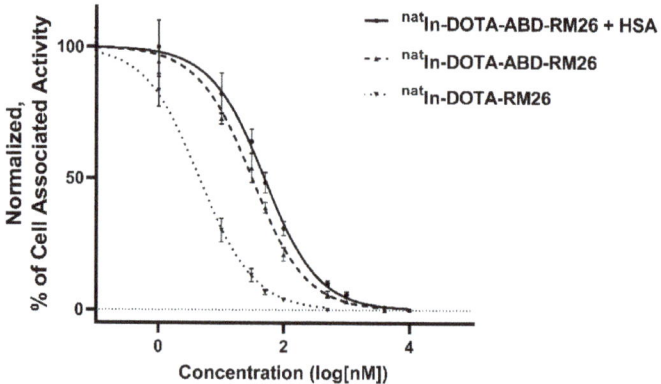

Figure 5. Half-maximal inhibitory concentration (IC$_{50}$). The error bars represent the standard deviation ($n = 3$).

3.5. In Vivo Characterization of [^{111}In]In-DOTA-ABD-RM26

In vivo targeting specificity: The in vivo targeting specificity of [^{111}In]In-DOTA-ABD-RM26 to GRPR was studied in mice bearing PC-3 xenografts and demonstrated significant reduction of activity uptake in tumors when 10 nmol of non-labelled DOTA-ABD-RM26 was co-injected with the labelled conjugate (5 ± 2% ID/g) and compared with the group injected with 40 pmol of [^{111}In]In-DOTA-ABD-RM26 (10 ± 1% ID/g) (Figure 6). The activity uptake in the spleen and stomach was slightly but significantly lower in the blocked group than in the non-blocked group.

Biodistribution of [^{111}In]In-DOTA-ABD-RM26: The biodistribution of [^{111}In]In-DOTA-ABD-RM26 1 h pi showed the highest activity concentration in blood (32 ± 4% ID/g) and an elevated uptake in kidneys (35 ± 6% ID/g) (Figure 7). The activity uptake in PC-3 tumors was 7 ± 2% ID/g at this time point. At 24 h pi, the activity uptake in blood decreased more than 3-fold, while the activity uptake in tumors increased almost 2-fold to 11 ± 2% ID/g. At this time point, activity uptake in the lungs decreased 2-fold, but activity uptake remained stable in the majority of the other studied organs, except bones, where it increased significantly from 3.3 ± 0.4% ID/g at 1 h pi to 4.4 ± 0.5% ID/g at 24 h pi.

With time, the activity concentration in blood continued to decrease, and the activity uptake in the kidney was reduced 2-fold 6 d pi. The tumor activity uptake remained stable within the observation period (144 h pi 10 ± 1% ID/g). The activity uptake in the majority of the other organs remained stable, except the lungs and intestine where it continuously decreased.

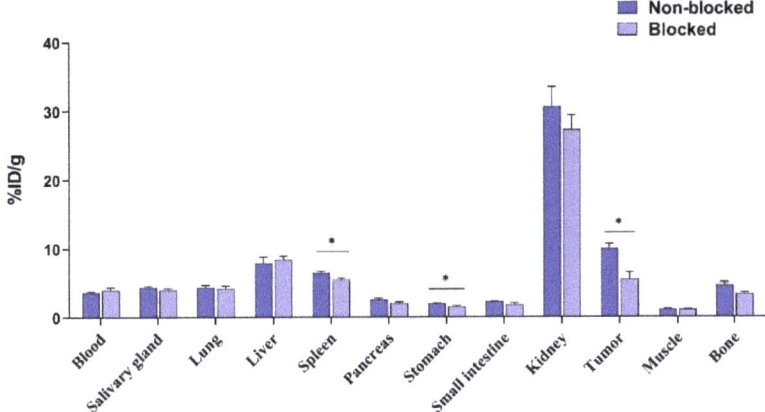

Figure 6. In vivo targeting specificity at 72 h pi. The error bars represent the standard deviation. * indicates a significant difference with a p value < 0.05.

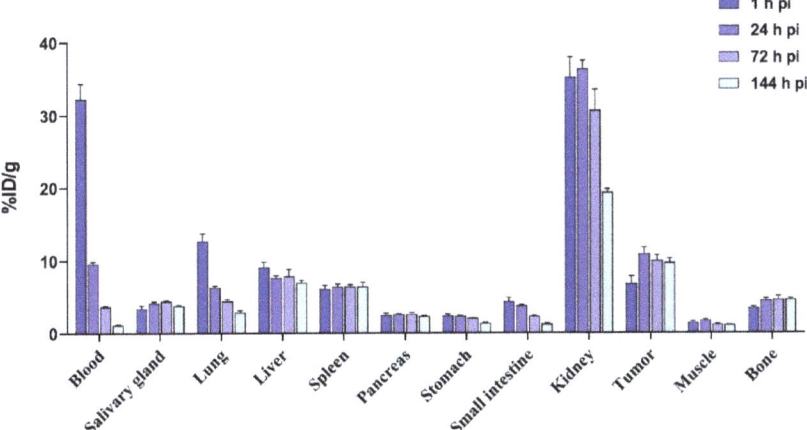

Figure 7. Biodistribution of [^{111}In]In-DOTA-ABD-RM26 at 1, 24, 72 and 144 h pi. The error bars represent the standard deviation.

The biodistribution of [^{111}In]In-DOTA-ABD-RM26 was compared with that of [^{111}In]In-DOTA-RM26 1 h pi to evaluate the impact of ABD coupling on the biodistribution pattern and tumor targeting of RM26, as shown in Figure 8. The uptake in the pancreas (GRPR-expressing tissue) and tumor were on the same level for both radiolabelled conjugates. The activity uptake of [^{111}In]In-DOTA-ABD-RM26 was significantly higher than that of [^{111}In]In-DOTA-RM26 in all other studied organs and tissues. Activity concentration in blood was over 100-fold higher for the GRPR-targeting peptide coupled to ABD (32 ± 4% ID/g for [^{111}In]In-DOTA-ABD-RM26 compared with 0.27 ± 0.04% ID/g for [^{111}In]In-DOTA-RM26).

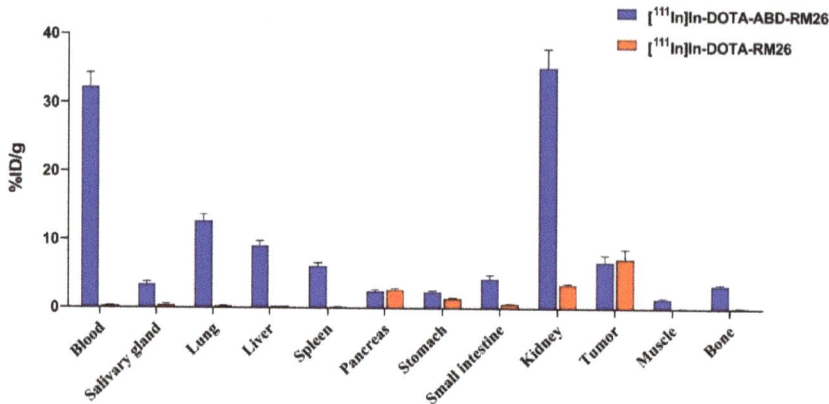

Figure 8. Comparison between biodistribution of [^{111}In]In-DOTA-ABD-RM26 and [^{111}In]In-DOTA-RM26 at 1 h pi. The error bars represent the standard deviation.

4. Discussion

Prostate cancer remains a challenge with high incidence and mortality rates. Several molecular targets associated with prostate cancer cells have been identified with the main focus aimed at prostate specific membrane antigen (PSMA)-targeting [27]. Targeting PSMA has demonstrated its utility in prostate cancer patient management both for diagnostic and radionuclide targeted therapy. However, other targets need to be evaluated for the treatment of prostate cancer, since not all tumors overexpress PSMA [28]. GRPR has emerged as an important target in a number of cancers including prostate cancer [20]. Targeting GRPR in oligometastatic prostate cancer could improve therapy output in early stages of prostate cancer. GRPR antagonists have been used for imaging GRPR-expressing tumors demonstrating high sensitivity and safety [8,17–19,29]. Recent clinical studies have commenced evaluating GRPR antagonists for treating patients with metastatic castration-resistant prostate cancer showing promising results [23].

Radiolabelled GRPR-targeting antagonistic peptides have demonstrated high and specific uptake in GRPR lesions and a rapid blood clearance which is favorable to diagnostic imaging shortly after administration, but for targeted radiotherapy, multiple injections would be required. The aim of this study was to develop a GRPR-targeting ligand based on a GRPR antagonist and an ABD that would have prolonged blood circulation time and, therefore, increase the tumor uptake of the ligand. This therapeutic construct could further be coupled to a cytotoxic agent (drug or therapeutic radionuclide) and used for targeting therapy of cancer. This approach would facilitate therapy by minimizing the number of injections and by improving delivery of cytotoxic agent to tumors.

To extend the circulatory half-life of the RM26 analogue targeting the GRPR receptor, a construct was designed with the peptide conjugated to an ABD (see Figure 1). Since the C-terminus of RM26 is important for receptor binding [30], the N-terminus of the peptide was modified for crosslinking to ABD. These modifications included the addition of a PEG$_4$ linker as a spacer between the two molecules and a terminal thiol-containing mercaptopropionic acid residue for the conjugation to ABD via a thioether bond. ABD was functionalized with a chloroacetyl group at the Lys residue in position 14. Position 14 was chosen for conjugation as helices two and three of ABD are responsible for the interaction with HSA, and by coupling RM26 to the first helix of ABD, it was hypothesized that the HSA binding would not be impaired. In an earlier study, it has been shown that this position in ABD is suitable for conjugation of short peptides, without disrupting HSA binding [26]. The chelator DOTA was coupled to the N-terminus of ABD for the purpose of coordinating radionuclides for in vitro and in vivo experiments.

The designed conjugate, entitled DOTA-ABD-RM26, was successfully labelled with indium-111, a radiometal with relatively long half-life (2.81 d), allowing for studies of the biodistribution pattern of the labelled conjugate over several days. We noticed that both labelling yield and stability of the new conjugate were moderate when challenged with EDTA. Together this could mean sterical hindrance in building the In-DOTA cage complex, because usually this complex is very stable [31]. The new GRPR-binding conjugate retained both specific targeting to the receptor and antagonistic feature despite the bulky modification (the total molecular weight of albumin-ABD-RM26 construct is approximately 60-fold higher than for RM26). However, both coupling of ABD and further interaction of the conjugate with albumin negatively affected binding to GRPR, decreasing the IC_{50} value for ABD-RM26 towards GRPR. Further, the apparent affinity of ABD-RM26 toward HSA was slightly compromised (see Table 2). In the literature, affinity measurements of ABD035 have indicated higher affinity for HSA with a K_D of about 120 fM [25]. However, the very slow off-rates make it difficult to calculate the kinetic parameters, and the results presented herein should be seen as a comparison of the relative affinities of the ABD constructs rather than exact values. The obtained results confirm that the conjugation of RM26 and DOTA only marginally affects the binding of ABD035 to HSA, and that high affinity to HSA is retained, with an estimated K_D of 83 pM for DOTA-ABD-RM26 binding to HSA. A folded protein typically gives rise to a defined CD spectrum, while unfolding or partially unfolding the protein leads to changes in secondary structure, which results in changes in the CD spectrum. Far-UV CD spectra on DOTA-ABD-Cl and ABD035 are typical of helical proteins, while ABD-RM26 is partially unfolded (Figure 2A). According to helix–coil theory [32], ABD035 is about 75% helical (36 out of 49 residues in helical conformation), and DOTA-ABD-Cl is about 60% helical (27 out of 46 residues in helical conformation), while ABD-RM26 is only about 33% helical (18 out of 56 residues in helical conformation). A helicity of 75% for ABD035 is in agreement with a solution NMR structure of the serum albumin binding domain G148–GA3, which show a helicity of about 80% in the same region [33].

While data from our SPR measurements indicate that conjugation of DOTA and RM26 has a minimal impact on ABD binding to HSA at 25 °C, the CD spectra display lower helicity of DOTA-ABD-RM26 than ABD and DOTA-ABD-Cl under the tested conditions. When determining melting point for the three constructs, we found that T_m is approximately 50–54 °C for all constructs. However, as a consequence of the low amplitude for the melting curve of DOTA-ABD-RM26, the melting temperature can only be roughly estimated for this conjugate. Our data showed that DOTA-ABD-RM26 had low helicity at 42 °C in the tested conditions during CD measurements. This could have an impact on experiments performed in vivo. However, bombesin has previously been shown to form alpha-helical structures upon interaction with lipids and membranes [34]. Hence, the conditions used for measurements of T_m and secondary structure by CD might not be fully representative of the biophysical properties of DOTA-ABD-RM26 when interacting with GRPR or HSA in vivo.

Despite compromised affinity to GRPR, the new conjugate bound to GRPR specifically in mice bearing PC-3 xenografts. The in vivo targeting specificity was evaluated at 72 h pi so that the radioligand could be appropriately cleared from blood and other non-targeting organs. It is interesting to note that while activity uptake decreased 2-fold in xenografts with high GRPR expression, the uptake in other GRPR-expressing tissues (pancreas and organs of GI tract) decreased only marginal. Lower GRPR expression in these organs than in xenografts together with relatively moderate affinity of the new conjugate to GRPR (IC_{50} 49 ± 5 nM vs 4.5 ± 0.7 nM for parental peptide DOTA-RM26) could explain this observation.

The utilized approach for extension of blood circulation of a GRPR-targeting peptide by conjugation to ABD resulted in significantly slower blood clearance of the targeting agent. The activity concentration in blood 1 h pi was as high as 32 ± 4% ID/g and decreased only 3.5-fold at 24 h pi. Such extension would not be possible for the relatively small ABD-RM26 conjugate (7 kDa) without interaction with albumin in blood circulation [35–37]. High activity concentration in blood contributed to elevated activity uptake in non-targeted organs (see Figure 8). Contrastingly, in targeted organs (pancreas and intestines) and GRPR expressing xenografts, activity uptake was equal both for ABD-coupled and parental RM26. We could speculate that the initially bulky ABD-RM26/albumin complex has limited tissue penetration in comparison with the small RM26 peptide. However, the high concentration of labelled conjugate in blood overcame this limitation, and activity uptake in tumors increased up to 24 h pi, while RM26 reached maximum activity uptake at 1 h pi (with 80% of maximum uptake reaching 30 min pi, data for [^{177}Lu]Lu-DOTAGA-RM26 [21]).

The activity uptake in tumors increased by 50% from 1 to 24 h pi; this demonstrated the presence of an intact radiolabelled conjugate in blood circulation capable of binding. This could be evidence that the ABD-fused GRPR antagonist escaped neprilysin activity in blood circulation. This is of special importance for targeting therapy. Furthermore, the activity uptake in tumors remained stably high up to 6 d pi, which dramatically differentiated this conjugate from small antagonistic peptides targeting GRPR. Typically, activity uptake in tumors decreases 2-4-fold within 24 h pi and continues to decrease further with time [21,22,38].

However, the in vivo study also showed a very high activity uptake in kidneys, higher than that in tumors at all studied time points. This high renal uptake was unexpected because conjugation of ABD to small proteins has been shown to decrease renal reabsorption dramatically, e.g., renal activity uptake decreased 30-fold for anti-HER2 affibody molecules when coupled to ABD and was below 5% ID/g at a peak 24 h pi [35,39]. The GRPR antagonist RM26 exhibited low renal reabsorption: for RM26 labelled with lutetium-177, the highest activity uptake in kidneys was found to be at 30 min pi and dropped 2-fold during the next 30 min [21]. Thus, neither RM26 nor ABD have a tendency to accumulate in the kidneys. The high renal reabsorption of ABD-RM26 conjugate at later time points could be explained by corrupted affinity to albumin allowing the construct to retain in blood circulation due to high albumin availability, but directing the dissociated fraction to renal clearance. The uptake in other organs such as the liver and bone was also elevated up to 144 h pi, and this can be a consequence of the radiolabel instability in vivo.

In this study, we hypothesized that conjugation of GRPR antagonist RM26 with ABD would facilitate GRPR-targeting therapy by minimizing the number of injections, increasing and prolonging the uptake of targeting agent in tumors, and keeping the healthy organs at a safe level of exposure to cytotoxic agents, especially to radiation. This study was a proof-of-principle that this approach is suitable for the development of therapeutic agents. This conjugate could be used for inhibition of GRPR-driven cell proliferation or delivering cytotoxic agents to GRPR-overexpressing tumors following previously reported concepts [20,40]. Particularly, high renal and hepatic accumulation of the anti-HER2 affibody-ABD conjugate bearing cytotoxic maytansine derivate MC-DM1 did not cause any morphological differences or signs of injury in kidneys and livers, while it demonstrated significant therapeutic effects in a preclinical therapy experiment [41]. However the unfavorable renal reabsorption abolished the possibility of using this conjugate for radionuclide therapy, which is in fact only one type of targeting therapies, due to the high absorbed dose to the kidneys, the critical organ for radio-targeting therapy. One approach is to redesign the conjugate with the aim of improving the biodistribution profile, as the position of the ABD could alter the properties of the conjugate, as previously demonstrated [42].

5. Conclusions

In conclusion, we herein report a successful conjugation of a GRPR antagonist and an albumin-binding domain that retained GRPR-targeting in vivo and, due to binding to albumin, resulted in a high and stable tumor uptake over several days. The developed conjugate could be used for targeted delivery of cytotoxic drugs to GRPR-expressing tumors and to keep a high therapeutic concentration of the GRPR-targeting antagonistic agent for inhibition therapy. However, this conjugate is not suitable for radionuclide therapy, and further research with the aim of improving the biodistribution profile of the ABD-RM26 conjugate is desirable.

Supplementary Materials: The following are available online at http://www.mdpi.com/1999-4923/12/10/977/s1, Figure S1: MALDI-MS spectrum of DOTA-ABD-Cl after RP-HPLC purification; Figure S2: MALDI-MS spectrum of RM26 after RP-HPLC purification; Figure S3: MALDI-MS spectrum of DOTA-ABD-RM26 after RP-HPLC purification; Figure S4: RP-HPLC elution profiles of the DOTA-ABD-RM26 conjugation reaction; Figure S5: ESI-MS spectrum of DOTA-ABD-RM26 after RP-HPLC purification; Figure S6: SDS-PAGE analysis of recombinant ABD035; Figure S7: MALDI-MS spectrum of recombinant ABD035; Figure S8: SPR sensorgram of ABD035 injected to surface with HSA at six different concentrations; Figure S9: SPR sensorgram of DOTA-ABD035-RM26 binding to HSA at seven different concentrations; Figure S10: SPR sensorgram of DOTA-ABD035-Cl binding to HSA at seven different concentrations.

Author Contributions: Conceptualization, A.O., V.T., and A.E.K.; methodology, A.O., and A.E.K.; investigation, AA, S.S.R., F.W., A.O., H.T., Á.N. and S.K.; resources, A.O., A.E.K.; writing—original draft preparation, A.A., H.T. and Á.N.; writing—review and editing, A.A., H.T., Á.N., S.K., K.W., S.S.R., F.W., V.T., A.O., and A.E.K.; visualization, A.A., H.T. and Á.N.; project administration, A.O.; A.E.K.; funding acquisition, A.O., V.T. and. A.E.K. All authors have read and agreed to the published version of the manuscript.

Funding: The project was funded by the Swedish Agency for Innovation VINNOVA (2019/00104), the Swedish Cancer Society (Cancerfonden: CAN 2017/425 (AO), 2018/436 (VT), 19 0212 Pj 01H (AEK)), and the Swedish Research Council (Vetenskapsrådet: 2019-00986 (AO), 2015-02353 (VT) and 2016-05207 (AEK)).

Conflicts of Interest: The authors declare no conflict of interest.

References

1. Bray, F.; Ferlay, J.; Soerjomataram, I.; Siegel, R.L.; Torre, L.A.; Jemal, A. Global cancer statistics 2018: GLOBOCAN estimates of incidence and mortality worldwide for 36 cancers in 185 countries. *CA Cancer J. Clin.* **2018**, *68*, 394–424. [CrossRef]
2. Xiao, D.; Wang, J.; Hampton, L.L.; Weber, H.C. The human gastrin-releasing peptide receptor gene structure, its tissue expression and promoter. *Gene* **2001**, *264*, 95–103. [CrossRef]
3. Markwalder, R.; Reubi, J.C. Gastrin-releasing peptide receptors in the human prostate: Relation to neoplastic transformation. *Cancer Res.* **1999**, *59*, 1152–1159. [PubMed]
4. Ananias, H.J.; van den Heuvel, M.C.; Helfrich, W.; de Jong, I.J. Expression of the gastrin-releasing peptide receptor, the prostate stem cell antigen and the prostate-specific membrane antigen in lymph node and bone metastases of prostate cancer. *Prostate* **2009**, *69*, 1101–1108. [CrossRef] [PubMed]
5. Körner, M.; Waser, B.; Rehmann, R.; Reubi, J.C. Early over-expression of GRP receptors in prostatic carcinogenesis. *Prostate* **2014**, *74*, 217–224. [CrossRef] [PubMed]
6. Beer, M.; Montani, M.; Gerhardt, J.; Wild, P.J.; Hany, T.F.; Hermanns, T.; Müntener, M.; Kristiansen, G. Profiling gastrin-releasing peptide receptor in prostate tissues: Clinical implications and molecular correlates. *Prostate* **2012**, *72*, 318–325. [CrossRef] [PubMed]
7. Manyak, M.J. Indium-111 capromab pendetide in the management of recurrent prostate cancer. *Expert Rev. Anticancer Ther.* **2008**, *8*, 175–181. [CrossRef]
8. Kähkönen, E.; Jambor, I.; Kemppainen, J.; Lehtiö, K.; Grönroos, T.J.; Kuisma, A.; Luoto, P.; Sipilä, H.J.; Tolvanen, T.; Alanen, K.; et al. In vivo imaging of prostate cancer using [68Ga]-labeled bombesin analog BAY86-7548. *Clin. Cancer Res.* **2013**, *19*, 5434–5443. [CrossRef]
9. Reynolds, T.J.S.; Smith, C.J.; Lewis, M.R. Peptide-Based Radiopharmaceuticals for Molecular Imaging of Prostate Cancer. *Adv. Exp. Med. Biol.* **2018**, *1096*, 135–158.
10. Schroeder, R.P.J.; Müller, C.; Reneman, S.; Melis, M.L.; Breeman, W.A.P.; de Blois, E.; Bangma, C.H.; Krenning, E.P.; van Weerden, W.M.; de Jong, M. A standardised study to compare prostate cancer targeting efficacy of five radiolabeled bombesin analogues. *Eur. J. Nucl. Med. Mol. Imaging* **2010**, *37*, 1386–1396. [CrossRef]
11. Millar, J.B.; Rozengurt, E. Chronic desensitization to bombesin by progressive down-regulation of bombesin receptors in Swiss 3T3 cells. Distinction from acute desensitization. *J. Biol. Chem.* **1990**, *265*, 12052–12058.
12. Casanueva, F.F.; Perez, F.R.; Casabiell, X.; Camiña, J.P.; Cai, R.Z.; Schally, A.V. Correlation between the effects of bombesin antagonists on cell proliferation and intracellular calcium concentration in Swiss 3T3 and HT-29 cell lines. *Proc. Natl. Acad. Sci. USA* **1996**, *93*, 1406–1411. [CrossRef] [PubMed]
13. Mitran, B.; Tolmachev, V.; Orlova, A. Radiolabeled GRPR Antagonists for Imaging of Disseminated Prostate Cancer. Influence of Labeling Chemistry on Targeting Properties. *Curr. Med. Chem.* **2020**, *27*, 1–22.

14. Mitran, B.; Varasteh, Z.; Selvaraju, R.K.; Lindeberg, G.; Sörensen, J.; Larhed, M.; Tolmachev, V.; Rosenström, U.; Orlova, A. Selection of optimal chelator improves the contrast of GRPR imaging using bombesin analogue RM26. *Int. J. Oncol.* **2016**, *48*, 2124–2134. [CrossRef] [PubMed]
15. Varasteh, Z.; Rosenström, U.; Velikyan, I.; Mitran, B.; Altai, M.; Honarvar, H.; Rosestedt, M.; Lindeberg, G.; Sörensen, J.; Larhed, M.; et al. The effect of mini-PEG-based spacer length on binding and pharmacokinetic properties of a 68Ga-labeled NOTA-conjugated antagonistic analog of bombesin. *Molecules* **2014**, *19*, 10455–10472. [CrossRef]
16. Varasteh, Z.; Mitran, B.; Rosenström, U.; Velikyan, I.; Rosestedt, M.; Lindeberg, G.; Sörensen, J.; Larhed, M.; Tolmachev, V.; Orlova, A. The effect of macrocyclic chelators on the targeting properties of the 68Ga-labeled gastrin releasing peptide receptor antagonist PEG2-RM26. *Nucl. Med. Biol.* **2015**, *42*, 446–454. [CrossRef]
17. Zhang, J.; Niu, G.; Fan, X.; Lang, L.; Hou, G.; Chen, L.; Wu, H.; Zhu, Z.; Li, F.; Chen, X. PET Using a GRPR Antagonist 68Ga-RM26 in Healthy Volunteers and Prostate Cancer Patients. *J. Nucl. Med.* **2018**, *59*, 922–928. [CrossRef]
18. Zang, J.; Mao, F.; Wang, H.; Zhang, J.; Liu, Q.; Peng, L.; Li, F.; Lang, L.; Chen, X.; Zhu, Z. 68Ga-NOTA-RM26 PET/CT in the Evaluation of Breast Cancer: A Pilot Prospective Study. *Clin. Nucl. Med.* **2018**, *43*, 663–669. [CrossRef]
19. Zang, J.; Liu, Q.; Sui, H.; Guo, H.; Peng, L.; Li, F.; Lang, L.; Jacobson, O.; Zhu, Z.; Mao, F.; et al. Combined 68Ga-NOTA-Evans Blue Lymphoscintigraphy and 68Ga-NOTA-RM26 PET/CT Evaluation of Sentinel Lymph Node Metastasis in Breast Cancer Patients. *Bioconjug. Chem.* **2020**, *31*, 396–403. [CrossRef] [PubMed]
20. Cornelio, D.B.; Roesler, R.; Schwartsmann, G. Gastrin-releasing peptide receptor as a molecular target in experimental anticancer therapy. *Ann. Oncol.* **2007**, *18*, 1457–1466. [CrossRef]
21. Mitran, B.; Rinne, S.S.; Konijnenberg, M.W.; Maina, T.; Nock, B.A.; Altai, M.; Vorobyeva, A.; Larhed, M.; Tolmachev, V.; de Jong, M.; et al. Trastuzumab cotreatment improves survival of mice with PC-3 prostate cancer xenografts treated with the GRPR antagonist 177Lu-DOTAGA-PEG2-RM26. *Int. J. Cancer* **2019**, *145*, 3347–3358. [CrossRef]
22. Dumont, R.A.; Tamma, M.; Braun, F.; Borkowski, S.; Reubi, J.C.; Maecke, H.; Weber, W.A.; Mansi, R. Targeted radiotherapy of prostate cancer with a gastrin-releasing peptide receptor antagonist is effective as monotherapy and in combination with rapamycin. *J. Nucl. Med.* **2013**, *54*, 762–769. [CrossRef]
23. Kurth, J.; Krause, B.J.; Schwarzenböck, S.M.; Bergner, C.; Hakenberg, O.W.; Heuschkel, M. First-in-human dosimetry of gastrin-releasing peptide receptor antagonist [177Lu]Lu-RM2: A radiopharmaceutical for the treatment of metastatic castration-resistant prostate cancer. *Eur. J. Nucl. Med. Mol. Imaging* **2020**, *47*, 123–135. [CrossRef] [PubMed]
24. Jonsson, A.; Dogan, J.; Herne, N.; Abrahmsén, L.; Nygren, P.Å. Engineering of a femtomolar affinity binding protein to human serum albumin. *Protein Eng. Des. Sel.* **2008**, *21*, 515–527. [CrossRef]
25. Frejd, F.Y.; Kim, K.T. Affibody molecules as engineered protein drugs. *Exp. Mol. Med.* **2017**, *49*, e306. [CrossRef]
26. Lindgren, J.; Refai, E.; Zaitsev, S.V.; Abrahmsén, L.; Berggren, P.O.; Karlström, A.E. A GLP-1 receptor agonist conjugated to an albumin-binding domain for extended half-life. *Biopolymers* **2014**, *102*, 252–259. [CrossRef]
27. Czarniecki, M.; Mena, E.; Lindenberg, L.; Cacko, M.; Harmon, S.; Radtke, J.P.; Giesel, F.; Turkbey, B.; Choyke, P.L. Keeping up with the prostate-specific membrane antigens (PSMAs): An introduction to a new class of positron emission tomography (PET) imaging agents. *Transl. Urol.* **2018**, *7*, 831–843. [CrossRef]
28. Sheikhbahaei, S.; Afshar-Oromieh, A.; Eiber, M.; Solnes, L.B.; Javadi, M.S.; Ross, A.E.; Pienta, K.J.; Allaf, M.E.; Haberkorn, U.; Pomper, M.G.; et al. Pearls and pitfalls in clinical interpretation of prostate-specific membrane antigen (PSMA)-targeted PET imaging. *Eur. J. Nucl. Med. Mol. Imaging* **2017**, *44*, 2117–2136. [CrossRef]
29. Minamimoto, R.; Hancock, S.; Schneider, B.; Chin, F.T.; Jamali, M.; Loening, A.; Vasanawala, S.; Gambhir, S.S.; Iagaru, A. Pilot Comparison of 68Ga-RM2 PET and 68Ga-PSMA-11 PET in Patients with Biochemically Recurrent Prostate Cancer. *J. Nucl. Med.* **2016**, *57*, 557–562. [CrossRef] [PubMed]
30. Mervic, M.; Moody, T.W.; Komoriya, A. A structure function study of C-terminal extensions of bombesin. *Peptides* **1991**, *12*, 1149–1151. [CrossRef]
31. Wadas, T.J.; Wong, E.H.; Weisman, G.R.; Anderson, C.J. Coordinating Radiometals of Copper, Gallium, Indium, Yttrium, And Zirconium for Pet and Spect Imaging of Disease. *Chem. Rev.* **2010**, *110*, 2858–2902. [CrossRef] [PubMed]

32. Scholtz, J.M.; Qian, H.; York, E.J.; Stewart, J.M.; Baldwin, R.L. Parameters of helix-coil transition theory for alanine-based peptides of varying chain lengths in water. *Biopolymers* **1991**, *31*, 1463–1470. [CrossRef] [PubMed]
33. Johansson, M.U.; Frick, I.M.; Nilsson, H.; Kraulis, P.J.; Hober, S.; Jonasson, P.; Linhult, M.; Nygren, P.Å.; Uhlén, M.; Björck, L.; et al. Structure, specificity, and mode of interaction for bacterial albumin-binding modules. *J. Biol. Chem.* **2002**, *277*, 8114–8120. [CrossRef] [PubMed]
34. Cavatorta, P.; Farruggia, G.; Masotti, L.; Sartor, G.; Szabo, A.G. Conformational flexibility of the hormonal peptide bombesin and its interaction with lipids. *Biochem. Biophys. Res. Commun.* **1986**, *141*, 99–105. [CrossRef]
35. Tolmachev, V.; Orlova, A.; Pehrson, R.; Galli, J.; Baastrup, B.; Andersson, K.; Sandström, M.; Rosik, D.; Carlsson, J.; Lundqvist, H.; et al. Radionuclide therapy of HER2-positive microxenografts using a 177Lu-labeled HER2-specific Affibody molecule. *Cancer Res.* **2007**, *67*, 2773–2782. [CrossRef]
36. Kelly, J.M.; Amor-Coarasa, A.; Ponnala, S.; Nikolopoulou, A.; Williams, C.; DiMagno, S.G.; Babich, J.W. Albumin-Binding PSMA Ligands: Implications for Expanding the Therapeutic Window. *J. Nucl. Med.* **2019**, *60*, 656–663. [CrossRef]
37. Garousi, J.; von Witting, E.; Borin, J.; Vorobyeva, A.; Altai, M.; Vorontsova, O.; Konijnenberg, M.W.; Oroujeni, M.; Orlova, A.; Tolmachev, V.; et al. Radionuclide Therapy Using ABD-fused ADAPT Scaffold Protein: Proof of Principle. *Biomaterials* **2020**, in press.
38. Dalm, S.U.; Bakker, I.L.; de Blois, E.; Doeswijk, G.N.; Konijnenberg, M.W.; Orlandi, F.; Barbato, D.; Tedesco, M.; Maina, T.; Nock, B.A.; et al. 68Ga/177Lu-NeoBOMB1, a Novel Radiolabeled GRPR Antagonist for Theranostic Use in Oncology. *J. Nucl. Med.* **2017**, *58*, 293–299. [CrossRef]
39. Orlova, A.; Jonsson, A.; Rosik, D.; Lundqvist, H.; Lindborg, M.; Abrahmsen, L.; Ekblad, C.; Frejd, F.Y.; Tolmachev, V. Site-specific radiometal labeling and improved biodistribution using ABY-027, a novel HER2-targeting affibody molecule-albumin-binding domain fusion protein. *J. Nucl. Med.* **2013**, *54*, 961–968. [CrossRef]
40. Safavy, A.; Raisch, K.P.; Khazaeli, M.B.; Buchsbaum, D.J.; Bonner, J.A. Paclitaxel Derivatives for Targeted Therapy of Cancer: Toward the Development of Smart Taxanes. *J. Med. Chem.* **1999**, *42*, 4919–4924. [CrossRef]
41. Altai, M.; Liu, H.; Ding, H.; Mitran, B.; Edqvist, P.H.; Tolmachev, V.; Orlova, A.; Gräslund, T. Affibody-derived drug conjugates: Potent cytotoxic molecules for treatment of HER2 over-expressing tumors. *J. Control. Release* **2018**, *288*, 84–95. [CrossRef] [PubMed]
42. Altai, M.; Leitao, C.D.; Rinne, S.S.; Vorobyeva, A.; Atterby, C.; Ståhl, S.; Tolmachev, V.; Löfblom, J.; Orlova, A. Influence of Molecular Design on the Targeting Properties of ABD-Fused Mono- and Bi-Valent Anti-HER3 Affibody Therapeutic Constructs. *Cells* **2018**, *7*, 164. [CrossRef] [PubMed]

Publisher's Note: MDPI stays neutral with regard to jurisdictional claims in published maps and institutional affiliations.

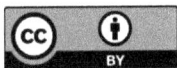

© 2020 by the authors. Licensee MDPI, Basel, Switzerland. This article is an open access article distributed under the terms and conditions of the Creative Commons Attribution (CC BY) license (http://creativecommons.org/licenses/by/4.0/).

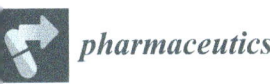

Review

Therapeutic Approaches for Metastases from Colorectal Cancer and Pancreatic Ductal Carcinoma

Adriana G. Quiroz-Reyes [1], Jose F. Islas [1], Paulina Delgado-Gonzalez [1], Hector Franco-Villarreal [2] and Elsa N. Garza-Treviño [1,*]

[1] Biochemistry and Molecular Medicine Department, School of Medicine, Universidad Autonoma de Nuevo Leon, Monterrey 64460, Mexico; he.franco@althian.com (A.G.Q.-R.); jose.islasc@uanl.mx (J.F.I.); paulina.delgadogn@uanl.edu.mx (P.D.-G.)
[2] Althian Clinical Research, Monterrey 64000, Mexico; dr.hectorfranco@gmail.com
* Correspondence: elsa.garzatr@uanl.edu.mx

Abstract: Metastasis is the process of dissemination of a tumor, whereby cells from the primary site dislodge and find their way to other tissues where secondary tumors establish. Metastasis is the primary cause of death related to cancer. This process warrants changes in original tumoral cells and their microenvironment to establish a metastatic niche. Traditionally, cancer therapy has focused on metastasis prevention by systematic treatments or direct surgical re-sectioning. However, metastasis can still occur. More recently, new therapies direct their attention to targeting cancer stem cells. As they propose, these cells could be the orchestrators of the metastatic niche. In this review, we describe conventional and novel developments in cancer therapeutics for liver and lung metastasis. We further discuss the resistance mechanisms of targeted therapy, the advantages, and disadvantages of diverse treatment approaches, and future novel strategies to enhance cancer prognosis.

Keywords: lung metastasis; liver metastasis; cancer stem cells; cancer treatments and progression biomarkers

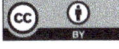

1. Introduction

Metastasis is an inefficient process in which cells from the primary tumor spread by releasing circulating tumor cells (CTCs) into the vasculature towards a distant organ to colonize it, establishing metastasis. A process where only 0.01% of the cells that enter the circulation can successfully reestablish a new metastasis, and while this seems highly inefficient, it is more often than not a fatal step in cancer progression [1,2]. Cancer stem cells (CSC) are the subpopulation of cells responsible for promoting angiogenesis, local invasion, distant metastasis, and resistance to apoptosis. Moreover, epithelial tumor cells (mature population) gain invasiveness and migratory abilities through the process of epithelial–mesenchymal transition (EMT), which is where a complex network of interconnected factors and pathways meet, such as transforming growth factor-β (TGFβ), epidermal growth factor (EGF), insulin-like growth factor (IGF), WNT, Hedgehog, and Notch pathways, all of which regulate and promote CSC growth [3–5]. The spread of CSC from the primary tumor to a secondary site is a process highly dependent on signaling cues, such as hypoxia, acidic pH, and/or glucose deprivation [6]. However, only one out of 500 CSC will survive in the circulation, even though mechanisms to protect CSC from elimination by the immune system exist as the secretion of IL-4 and CD200, which represents an important role in immune escape [7]. CSC in the bloodstream or otherwise in the lymphatic system can cluster together with stromal cells (fibroblasts, endothelial, tumor-infiltrated myeloid cells, or pericytes) for improved metastasis potential. Endothelial cells (ECs) in healthy established vessels remain quiescent for years. Under certain conditions, such as hipoxia or inflammation, as occurs in pathologies such as cancer and wounds, they can rapidly switch to an angiogenic state and start to form new blood vessels by interaction with pericytes [8–10]. Once an angiogenic switch is turned on, factors (VEGF, PDGF, TNF-α, and IL-8) inside the tumor promote growth and metastasis [11,12]. A majority of ECs in the tumor vasculature are tumor-derived ECs (TECs) retain remain distinct from cancer cells, by are not immortal and their ontological endothelial identity permit participate in making up the lining of neoangiogenic vasculatures in the TME and accelerating tumor progression [13,14]. Circulating tumor endothelial cells (CTECs) with a mature phenotype, derived from vessel wall turnover, play an important role in tumor initiation, progression, metastasis, and neovascularization [15]. Moreover, it has been found clusters of endothelial cells expressing endothelial markers as vimentin and other lineage markers, such as FN1, SERPINE1, and FOXC1, that improve the survival of cancer stem cells and promote their dissemination [15]. Increased CTECs in cancer patients have a worse prognosis, indicated as potential biomarkers of angiogenesis and metastasis, and can express PDL-1 that permit the evaluation of immunotherapy efficacy [16].

Once CSC attaches and develops with success, a pre-metastatic niche will form. Pre-metastatic niches additionally require exosomes or exosomal-like extracellular vesicles (ECV) from entrained bone marrow-derived cells and macrophages to start changes in the cells. Ideally building an effective microenvironment that serves as a fertile niche for tumor cell growth [8–10]. Researchers estimate that between 20% and 54% of malignant tumors develop metastasis. Primarily at lymph nodes, with the liver and lungs as the second most common sites of metastasis [17]. Colorectal cancer, the third most frequent neoplasm, can progress to the liver (40–50%) and lung (10–20%) depending on the primary tumor's stage. Clinical data show that median survival is just 5–20 months without treatment [18]. Meanwhile, pancreatic ductal adenocarcinoma (PDAC) is one of the most aggressive cancers with high metastatic potential. At the time of PDAC diagnosis, approximately 50% of patients present metastatic disease with 19–39% affected in the lungs and >50% in the liver. The median survival time is around 6–11 months in patients with metastatic pancreatic cancer [19]. Interestingly, several studies have reported that isolated lung metastases are associated with better survival outcomes than patients with other solitary metastatic organs [20–22]. In what follows, we will discuss differences between the cascade of events in primary tumors which promote the establishment of pre-niche and niche metastasis.

2. Why Liver Metastasis?

The physiological functions of the liver are related to the metabolism of nutrients absorbed by the gastrointestinal tract and the detoxification of dangerous molecules present in the circulation. These functions are responsible for a delicate balance between immune tolerance and immune response. Their correct functioning requires normal cytoarchitecture of the hepatic lobules. This cytoarchitecture includes polarized hepatocytes and an intricate network of discontinuous capillaries (sinusoids) and bile ducts. Important cell types in the lobule are Kupffer cells (KCs), a type of specialized macrophages that take up and destroy foreign material, and hepatic stellate cells (HSCs), which are involved in the response to liver damage. HSCs are found in the space of Disse, which separates hepatocytes from sinusoids [23]. Due to the total blood volume that circulates through the liver, about 30% of blood volume per minute, it is the preferred organ for metastasis development [24]. The portal vein is a vessel that carries blood from the gastrointestinal tract, gallbladder, pancreas, and spleen to the liver. The right portal vein is the continuation of the main portal vein, while it separates the left portal vein from the main portal vein at an acute angle [25]. This explains why the segment of the right lobe liver is the main target of metastases. Also, the blood circulation in the colon and proximal rectum drain through the hepatic portal system, while the blood of the distal rectum goes to the lung. This vascular organization correlates with the fact that colorectal cancer prefers liver metastasis, with the lung as the second favored metastatic site [26]. However, to allow hepatic metastasis development, the liver must present damage. There are several hypotheses regarding the pro-metastatic state consequent to cirrhosis, steatosis, and nonalcoholic fatty liver disease. Some authors state that altered hepatic cytoarchitecture creates an unfavorable environment [27]. Others report that these alterations slow the passage of neoplastic cells through the microcirculation and enhance cellular-vascular contact and stress micro thrombotic phenomena through the expression of adhesion molecules, facilitating metastasis [28]. Chronic inflammation that results from receiving nutrients, toxins, and microorganisms via the portal vein from the gut can activate HSCs or produce oxidative stress that leads to liver injury creating a microenvironment favorable for the increased growth of metastases [27]. Also, organotropism is regulated by multiple factors, organ-specific niches, and the interaction between tumor cells and the host microenvironment [29].

Factors Crucial for the Formation of Liver Metastasis

Pre-niche is formed by the preconditions in specific organs in terms of nutrients, extracellular matrix, and immune cells necessary to generate fertile soil before the arrival of CTC, which increases the success of metastasis establishment, as shown in Figure 1 [30].

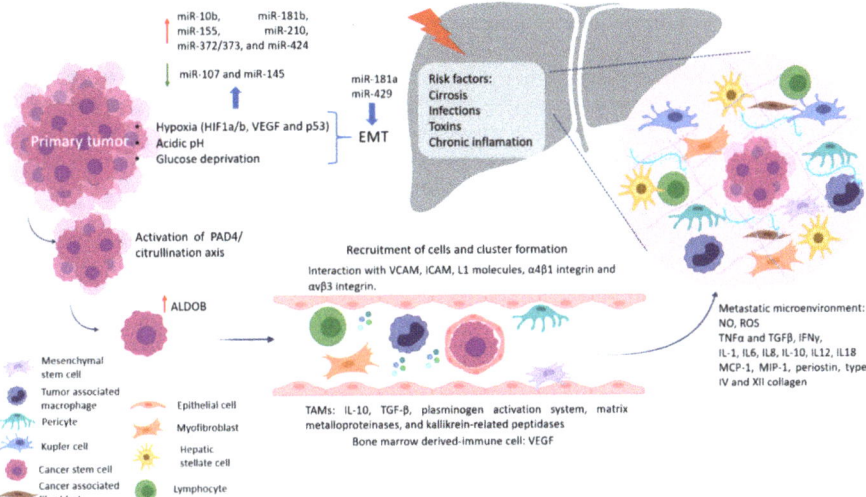

Figure 1. Liver metastases process. Development of liver metastases involves changes in tumor cell metabolism, as well as EMT and is induced by inflammatory cytokines, miRNAs, hypoxia, and pH. These factors allow for dissemination of CSC. Growth factors promote survival of cells in the blood and the lymphatic circulation, these cells form clusters (fibroblasts, endothelial, tumor-infiltrated myeloid cells, or pericytes) in order to arrive to hepatic tissue. Also, liver metastasis niche is improved by damage inducers, that activate HSCs, KCs, CAFs, myofibroblast, TAMs or produce oxidative stress and cytokines production promoting CSC establishment and growth.

After that, primary tumors can induce stromal cell remodeling of the extracellular matrix which takes care of cell organization. To increase the survival of CTC from the hostile microenvironment, they usually form CTC clusters. Interactions between cancer cells and endothelial cells with an endothelial layer, and the underlying basement membrane VCAM, ICAM, or L1 molecules, expressed by the vascular endothelium, in interaction with $\alpha 4\beta 1$ integrin and $\alpha v\beta 3$ integrin, play a central role in leukocyte recruitment to develop this process [28,31]. Other tumor-recruited cells such as cancer-associated fibroblasts (CAFs), stromal myofibroblast, endothelial cells, pericytes, diverse immune cells, mesenchymal stem cells (MSCs), and tumor-associated macrophages (TAMs) contribute to tumor growth and serve as a prerequisite for tumor cell invasion and metastasis [8,30]. For example, during the early stages of tumor development, cytotoxic immune cells such as natural killer (NK) and CD8+ T cells recognize and eliminate the more immunogenic cancer cells. High levels of tumor-infiltrated T cells indicate a good prognosis in many solid tumors, while high levels of macrophage infiltration correlate with a worse prognosis. TAMs promote tumor progression in different ways, such as secreting cytokines like IL-10 and TGF-β, which induce immunosuppression and impair poor response by cytotoxic lymphocytes T and dendritic cell maturation [32]. Also, TAMs release a plethora of extracellular matrix (ECM) remodeling factors (plasminogen activation system, matrix metalloproteinases, and kallikrein-related peptidases), affecting the composition, structure, and elasticity of the ECM and the availability of growth factors, creating conduits for the migration of tumor cells [32]. Metastasis-associated macrophages (MAMs), in murine CRC models, have been shown to increase the extravasation of tumor cells and help in their survival by secreting growth factors and concomitantly inhibiting cytotoxic T cells [33]. Some key mediators in regulating immune responses are myeloid-derived suppressor cells (MDSC) which express CD11b+ and CD33+. CD11b is a subunit of the integrin adhesion molecule, which expresses in bone marrow-derived immune cells. CD11b was reported to promote myeloid cell migration to the tumor microenvironment, which secreted cytokines related to tumor growth and angiogenesis. Researchers relate the expansion of MDSCs to tumorigenesis in CRC, and the density of CD33+ MDSCs in the microenvironment was a negative prognostic factor in CRC patients. Recently reported higher expression (lymphocytes CD3+) in primary tumor than in hepatic metastases, while CD33 had higher expression in hepatic metastases than in primary tumor. In turn, CD33+ showed that more immunosuppression of cells in the liver may contribute to the poor response to immunotherapy [34–36]. Although to date, some cell types have been associated with better or worse prognoses of primary tumors, unlike in metastasis where there are many other factors involved, such as the treatment they are receiving, this may change the microenvironment and therefore favor the progression of the disease. In most patients, physicians do not focus the treatment used on destroying the cells responsible for tumor chemoresistance and progression, and therefore this approach is being increasingly included in patients with already advanced stages, increasing their survival. MicroRNAs (miRNAs or miR) are short 18–22 nucleotide non-coding RNAs that control several processes by regulating gene expression. miRNAs can bind directly to mRNAs forming miRNA-mRNA complexes at the 3′UTR, where they recruit the ribonucleotide silencing complex (RiSC) and undergo either deadenylation and degradation via CAF1 and PABP, or transcriptional repression [8,37–41]. Colon cancer metastasis regulation has been a widely studied topic; in particular, the study of miR which acts as oncogenes have gained track in the last couple of decades. Cancer alters miRNA expression as stress and other microenvironmental factors changed through cancer's development [42]. Factors involved in tumor progression and the development of metastasis include hypoxia, which in CRC is very common and becomes more aggressive, invasive, and resistance to chemo- and radiotherapy. It associates with the activation of transcription factors involved in the maintenance of EMT/CSC phenotypes and enrichment of $CD44^{high}$, $CD24^{low}$ or $ALDH^{high}$ CSC population [43,44]. Non-coding RNAs play critical roles in the response to hypoxia in various cancers as miR-10b, miR-181b, miR-155, miR-210, miR-372/373, and miR-424 become upregulated under hypoxia [45]. A recent review by Gonzalez-Villareal in colorectal cancer metastasis emphasized EMT regulation, with members of the miR-200 family upregulated by Ascl2 as key regulators. Moreover, miR-199a downregulation and miR-210 and miR-21 upregulation are also associated with EMT enhancing HIF-1α/VEGF expression [30]. An EMT major driver is hypoxia, which involves HIF1a/b, VEGF, and p53, all of which downregulate miR-107 and miR-145, negatively correlating with p70S6K1 [46]. Increase expression of miR-210 via HIF-1α downregulates ephrin A3, which results in decreased migration, with an increase in glucose metabolism stimulating tumor growth [47–49]. Particularly in liver metastasis, p53 mutations, such as R175, G245, R248, R249, R273, and R282, produce gain-of-function and typically translocate with p63 (DNp63a) and p73 to promote TGF-β by RhoA or BRAF. miR-527/665 suppresses KSRP and miR-198, switching off SMAD4 and TGF-βR2 [50–52]. Malignant cells have glucose consumption rates about 200 times higher than normal cells; hence, their energy has more to do with the Warburg effect. According to this model, cancer cells get energy from lactate, free fatty acids, and ketones generated from the activation of anaerobic glycolytic and autophagic programs. Several authors have proposed that CSCs possess unique metabolic features when compared with the differentiated bulk of tumor cells, and with normal stem cells which allow CSC maintenance and dissemination. This might represent an effective approach to ablate the cells at the origin of the cancer. Their nutrients become linked via metabolic networks, enhancing the ability of cancer cells to survive and seed in a certain environment. Researchers have shown that liver metastasis regulation has a dependency on miR-885 overexpression by targeting CPEB2 and vWF. Significantly, these targets involve insulin regulation via insulin-like factor growth protein 5. IGFBP5 has been shown to regulate cell growth, differentiation, apoptosis, and metastasis. Yet, oxidative phosphorylation, due to hypoxic conditions, remains a preferred energy source [30,53]. Implied in this alternative energy metabolism is creatine kinase brain-type (CKB), necessary to produce phosphocreatine and maintain ATP levels, which are secreted into the microenvironment by the downregulation of miR-483 and miR-551a [54]. In liver metastasis of CRC, researchers observed an enhancement of fructose metabolism via the upregulation of enzyme aldolase B (ALDOB), hence providing extra fuel for metastatic outgrowth [55]. Thus, as the metabolic center of the entire organism, the liver appears to provide a unique milieu enabling or forcing cancer cells to assume specific metabolic activities for colonization. It involves molecular pathways for liver colonization, including nitric oxide and ROS, and the expression of adhesion molecules such as selectins and integrins. Also involved are phagocytosis, cytokines, such as TNFα and TGFβ, interferon gamma (IFNγ), interleukins (IL-1, IL6, IL8, IL-10, IL12, and IL18), growth factor monocyte chemoattract protein-1 (MCP-1), and macrophage inflammatory protein (MIP-1) released by KCs and HSCs [56]. Proinflammatory cytokines such as IL-6, preparing a permissive inflammatory pre-metastatic niche where circulating CRC cells can home and survive, colonize, and eventually form micro and macro metastasis. IL-6 then activates signal transducer and activator of transcription 3 (STAT3) signaling in hepatocytes, which produces serum amyloid A protein (SAA) that orchestrates the formation of a pro-metastatic niche in the liver. It has been reported that S1PR1–STAT3 upregulation in tumor cells induces IL-6, which activates S1PR1–STAT3 in MDSCs in the liver, leading to pre-metastatic niche formation prior to CRC cell arrival [57]. Expression of fibronectin and granulin by macrophages stimulates HSC for differentiation into myofibroblasts, whose release periostin, creates a fibrotic environment in the liver that sustains tumor growth [58]. Similarly, human hepatic sinusoidal endothelial cells in vitro express macrophage migration inhibitory factor (MIF-1), which improves EMT, migration, proliferation, and apoptotic resistance in CRC cells. Finally, angiopoietin-like 6 protein from the liver sinusoidal endothelial cells (LSEC) induces liver colonization of CRC cells and correlates with CRC progression in in vitro models [59].

Recent works reported that type XII collagen was the most significantly upregulated collagen in cancer liver metastasis (CLM) and that there was a difference with the ECM of the CRC. Collagens that are present in metastatic disease were COL10A1, COL12A1, COL 14A1, and COL15A1. Also, collagen type IV has a strong association with liver metastasis in CRC. One important miR is miR-19, which inhibits Transglutaminase-2, a critical crosslinking enzyme of the ECM, hence inducing invasiveness [60,61]. Another tumor suppressor miR is miR-155 which acts over several important regulators such as CTHRC1 and TP53, involved in tumor intravastation [62–64]. Moreover, miR-155, alongside miR-21, miR-1827, miR-145, and miR-34a, activate Wnt/b-catenin signaling. Additionally miR135a/b, miR-494, and miR-19a suppress APC and directly activate Wnt [65]. Wnt regulation is paramount during metastasis, as described in this review. Another study by Ji et al. confirmed that miR-181a promotes EMT by hindering WIF-. Furthermore, miR-429, was shown to impede apoptosis and induce EMT by targeting SOX2 [66]. The potential targeting of miR-429 would then lead to apoptosis. This could be critical to "kill off" metastatic cells, although research is warranted in order to have precise control as not to lead a systemic proapoptotic process. Some factors influencing liver metastasis on CRC were found, but we know that tumor cells themselves, stromal cells, and the interaction between CRC cells and their microenvironment, all contribute to hepatic invasion. Until now, we have known much about the establishment of the pre-metastatic niche but little about the metastatic niche itself. Therefore, the search for mechanisms and possible therapeutic targets that can reverse or change the prognosis of the disease is currently being continued since most patients at the time of diagnosis already arrive in very advanced stages of the disease, when the approach to treatment is more complex than just treating the primary tumor and preventing metastasis. Next, the management of patients with liver and lung metastases in two neoplasms that are on the rise without hereditary history will be reviewed.

3. Lung Metastasis

The lungs are one of the most complex organs in the human body. Their function is to exchange oxygen from the external environment with carbon dioxide from the cardiovascular system. Its role in the development of metastasis can result after physical trauma that induces local inflammation (smokers, asthma, obstructive pulmonary disease, or pneumonia) and tissue damage, creating a favorable environment that attracts metastatic cells from distant sites. Also, it has been reported that lung inflammation in smokers or in people with lung diseases such as asthma, chronic obstructive pulmonary disease, and infections, such as pneumonia, are risk factors for lung metastases. Some factors related to the migration of cells and vascular permeability are CCL2, S100A8, and SAA3. Upregulation of fibronectin colocalized with LOX, and higher levels of expression of VCAM-1, a receptor for VLA-4 in patient samples of metastatic tumor nodules in the lungs and bone, have been found [67]. The pro-metastatic effect played by exposure to smoking is related to the activation of the ubiquitin-chemokine receptor type 4 (CXCR4) pathway, high tissue levels of E-selectin, activation of the nuclear factor kappa-light-chain-enhancer of activated B cells (NFκB), signaling in pneumocytes, increased chemokine ligand 2 (CCL2) expression, and macrophage infiltration in the lung microenvironment. Moreover, lung alveolar cells induce chemokine secretion, which recruits neutrophils. The latter, through the synthesis of arachidonate 5-lipoxygenase (ALOX5)-dependent leukotriene, may promote survival and proliferation of leukotriene B4-expressing metastatic clones [17]. Inflamed lungs recruit neutrophils to release Cathepsin G and neutrophil elastase and destroy the protein Thrombospondin 1 (Tsp-1), which protects lung tissue from metastasis. Another alternative, but not mutually exclusive, is that micro-metastatic foci are already present at the time of physical injury [68]. Therefore, it is believed that lung metastases depend on circulatory system involvement, which flows into the pulmonary arterial system through the subclavian vein via the thoracic duct from the lymph nodes invaded by tumor cells [69]. More recently, DPC4 loss is shown to be associated with EMT, tumor progression, and the presence pulmonary metastases [70].

Factors Crucial for the Formation of Lung Metastasis

Factors produced by cells in pre-niche can support survival and growth of disseminated tumor cells were in Figure 2. The interstitial space is the main site for lung metastasis, which is adjacent to the terminal bronchioles. Bronchioalveolar stem cells (BASC) are situated in the terminal bronchioles and present pro-surfactant apoprotein-C (SP-C), a marker for alveolar type II (AT2) cells, and CC10, a marker for club cells—both are related with the lung pre-metastatic niche. Bone marrow cells, club cells, and alveolar macrophages are also present in pre-metastatic lung [67].

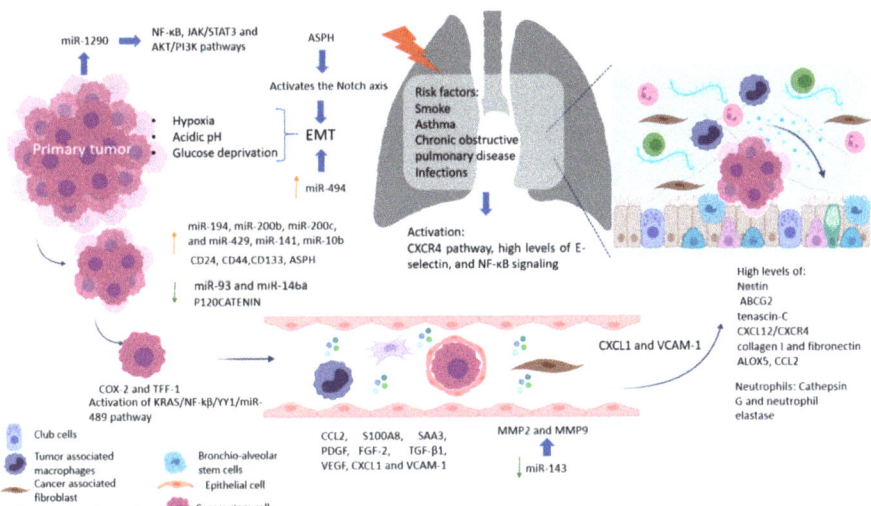

Figure 2. Lung metastases process. Tumor cell dissemination to lungs results after tissue damage that induces local inflammation and improves metastatic environment. club cells, alveolar cells recruit neutrophils, CAFs, TAMs, MSCs, and form a protective niche for help to CSC. In addition, metastases are promoted by CXCR4 signaling, miRNAs, growth factors, hypoxia, pH and glucose metabolism. Deposition of tenascin-C, collagen I, fibronectin and particular metalloproteases 2 and 9 after cancer cells dissemination to the lung in and important feature for CSC and tumor outgrowth.

Besides promoting the outgrowth of tumor cells, some microenvironmental components can suppress metastasis formation. Bone morphogenic protein (BMP) signaling is an example of an active process that can render tumor cells dormant in the lung. BMPs belong to the TGF-β family in the lungs, but not in the bone or brain. Endogenous BMP4 generated by epithelial cells and mesenchymal cells confers dormancy on metastasizing tumor cells [67]. The involvement of the tumor microenvironment contributes to invasion and chemoresistance, where the extracellular matrix, CAFs, activated pancreatic stellate cells (PSC), MSCs, and TAMs form a protective niche for CSC [21]. The origin of CSC in the pulmonary metastatic niche has been associated with the tumor microenvironment to support cell persistence and maintenance of the undifferentiated state characterized by the expression of markers such as CD24, CD44, and CD133, which are identified as resistant to treatment markers and CSC. For example, one miRNA recently studied in PDAC was miR-93, known to have implications in lung metastasis. miR-93 seems to regulate microtubule dynamics by controlling the expression of YES1, CRMP2, and MAPRE1. Dysregulation of these proteins consequently leads to growth by faults in G2/M cell cycle progression [39,71]. As cross-regulation is crucial in metastasis, recent research suggests that EGF and miR-146a have a reverse dependency in metastasis, since miR-146a levels diminish as metastasis develops. A study by Mess et al. found that highly metastatic pancreatic cells are distinct in their overexpression of miR-194, miR-200b, miR-200c, and miR-429, all of which work in concert to target the tumor suppressor gene EP300 and mutations in CREBBP [72,73]. The role of these miR-200 family members, including miR-141, is critical in EMT facilitating invasion. Likewise, miR-494 is important in EMT by targeting PTEN and TGF-β/SMAD pathways [74]. In contrast, functional studies have currently found that both miR-141 and miR-429 inhibit tumor development [75–78]. Researchers have also found that miR-10b increases invasiveness in metastasis by effecting EGF and TGF-β signaling through SMAD regulation implicating reduction of miR-323-3p and miR-193a, a decrease of both miRNAs enhances colonization by PANC-1 cells. Out of the many targets regulated by miR-10b both HOXD10 and KFL4 have implications in the control of matrix metalloproteinases -2,-9,-14 and E-Cadherin which involve extracellular matrix remodeling, helping promote angiogenesis development. Therefore, it is suitable to point out that miR-10b is a likely therapeutic target [79]. Interestingly, miR-10b is a metastatic regulator in both pancreatic and colorectal cancer, and other cancers such as lung cancer [80,81]. Therefore, a proposal would be a reactivation of miR-323-3p to control epithelial-mesenchymal transition and reduce PANC-1 cell growth [82–84]. In lung metastasis, nestin and ABCG2 levels are elevated [85,86] and associated with the formation of spheroids that are characteristic of CSCs. Loss of P120CATENIN has been associated with lung metastasis [85,87]. Aspartate-β-hydroxylase (ASPH) is an enzyme that can propagate an aggressive phenotype characterized by EMT, invasion, degradation or remodeling of the extracellular matrix, angiogenesis, stem and colonization to distant sites. ASPH works by activating the Notch axis. ASPH stabilizes Notch receptors, JAG ligands and the ADAM regulator improve interactions between receptors and Notch ligands, activate the Notch cascade, positively regulate the genes responsible for EMT, and recently, in PDAC models, their expression in lung metastases [88]. Pancreatic CSC has been reported to require platelet-derived growth factor (PDGF) for proliferation and induction of migration. Also, basic fibroblast growth factor (FGF-2) and TGF-β1 are required for component synthesis. Other factors are involved in the interaction of cancer cells and CSC include cyclooxygenase (COX)-2 and as the conditioned environment of cancer cells increases, COX-2 expression and CSC proliferation, and Trefoil factors (TFF)-1, whose expression stimulates the proliferation and migration of CSC [89]. The arrival of cancer cells to the lung generates a series of changes that help create mature metastatic niches. One of them is the deposition of the ECM component tenascin-C after dissemination of cancer cells to the lung which is important for metastatic outgrowth. For example, one important signaling axis in pancreatic cancer metastasis is the KRAS/NF-kb/YY1/miR-489. Recently, researchers found that KRAS activation (90% of pancreatic cancers) leads to miR-489, which exerts control over the ECM. When KRAS activates it signals YY1, suppresses miR-489, a suppressor of metastasis, leading to a signaling cascade that activates ADAM9 and MMP7 promoting migration [90]. Also involved with KRAS regulation is miR-143 which downregulates the activity of MMP2, and MMP9. Recent therapeutic research showed that restoring either miR-143 or miR-145 significantly inhibited pancreatic metastasis [73,80]. Another study by Ta et al. showed that NF-kβ, constitutively active in pancreatic cancer patients, is promoted by miR-1290, relates to the expression of IKK1 [91], and is implicated in the downregulation of miR-146a, suggesting its role as a tumor suppressor in most cancers. Meanwhile, miR-27a becomes highly upregulated and could be a target for therapeutics during metastasis. Moreover, it targets Sprouty2 which antagonizes the RAS/MAPK signaling pathway [92]. miR-27a can induce the suppression of PHLPP2, leading to stimulation of the AKT/GSK3β pathway, reducing the expression of FOXO1 and upregulating Bcl-2, which leads to minimizing cell damage [93] with less reduced damage. Apoptosis signaling is further reduced as miR-320 and miR-365 become upregulated, particularly miR-365 targets SHC-1 and blocks the pro-apoptotic regulator BAX [94]. Also, miR-1290 is responsible for downregulating the suppression of cytokine signaling 4, which leads to the activation of both JAK/STAT3 and AKT/PI3K pathways (proliferation) [95]. In addition, these patients have elevated levels of miR-31-5p, miR-101-3p, miR-34a-3p, miR-21-5p, and miR-155. Interestingly, both miR-1290 and miR-1246. because of their detectability in serum, are being studied as potential biomarkers [91,96]. In metastasis, miR-34a is found downregulated since it is a direct target of TP53 to reduce pro-inflammatory cytokines. Its restoration could be key in tumor suppression [97,98]. CXCL1/2-expressing tumor cells can recruit CD11b+ Gr1+ bone marrow cells and CXCL1/2 expression promotes lung metastasis and may contribute to metastatic niche formation after tumor cell dissemination [67]. Coculture of CSC with a subpopulation of endoglin-expressing pancreatic cancer cells (CD105) has been reported to increase the proportion of CD105-positive cancer cells and these cells present higher migration activity compared to CD105-negative cells. Additionally, the CXCL12/CXCR4 axis is implicated in the homing of cancer cells to metastatic sites which have been reported associated with melanoma and breast cancer. CXCL1 modulates the tumor microenvironment (macrophages, fibroblasts, neutrophils, and osteoclasts). Higher levels of CXCL1 are associated with tumor size, advancing stage, depth of invasion, and patient survival in liver metastasis of colorectal and hepatocellular cancer. Promotion of lung metastasis also is induced by secretion of CXCL1 and VCAM-1 expression and this regulates trans-endothelial migration of cancer cells. Elevated circulating levels of VEGF and CXCL1 are predictive of liver and lung metastasis, respectively, making them interesting as a therapeutic target for improved patient care and the prevention of many deaths from cancer [99]. Although we know a lot of factors that are involved in the establishment of the metastatic pre-niche, we still have much to discover about the niche that promotes the progression of metastasis and the best therapeutic targets or biomarkers of clinical response according to the progression of the disease. The treatment approaches and their advantages will be reviewed together with the differences observed between metastases in lung and liver and between CRC and the pancreas.

4. Biomarkers in Metastatic Cancer

Important biomarkers of prognostic significance reported in metastatic disease in PDAC and CRC are shown in Table 1. Prognostic factors before therapy that influence success and survival in resection of lung metastases are demographics (age, gender), primary tumor characteristics (stage, histology, origin), and lung metastases characteristics (number, size of lesions, the coexistence of liver disease, lymph nodes involved) [100].

Table 1. Biomarkers of lung and liver metastasis.

Biomarker	Characteristic	Reference
Serum amyloid A (SAA)	-Main acute phase proteins expressed in the liver. -Circulating levels correlate with cancer progression and poor survival. -SAA3 in PDAC is associated with fewer differentiated tumors, greater migration, and the number of CD133+ CSCs.	[101]
Thrombospondin-2	-Detection of liver metastases. -Monitor therapy response.	[101]
DPC4	-Prognostic marker in PDAC and CRC. -Promotes EMT. -DPC4 loss is associated with metastatic disease.	[101]
ASPH	-Prognostic factor of PDAC. -Upregulated in metastatic PDAC.	[101]
Oncostatin M (OSM)	-Elevated in the serum of PC patients. -Associated with highly aggressive metastatic cancers, increased risk of tumor recurrence, and poor prognosis.	[101]
Non-alcoholic fatty liver disease fibrosis score (NFS)	-Includes age, diabetes/hyperglycemia, BMI, platelet count, albumin, and AST/ALT ratio. -Predicts survival in liver metastases.	[101]
Carcinoembrionary antigen (CEA)	-Predicts survival in liver metastasis during treatment.	[101]

Recently aneuploidy, leading to genomic instability is known to be the most common characteristic of malignant cells, was detected on CD31+ CTECs, together with their counterpart CD31- circulating tumor cells (CTCs), together they constitute a unique pair of cellular circulating tumor biomarkers [13,102,103]. In addition, the basic helix loop helix factor Twist1 seem to be activated by hypoxia, by this effect it can induce differentiation of tumor cells into endothelial cells and promote tumor-derived vascular formation [104]. Moreover, recent studies showed that TECs could improve tumor angiogenesis by enhancing EGFR expression, by increasing its proliferation, and losing ErbB3 expression, hence inhibiting proliferation [103]. However, recent reports propose that the co-detection of CTC and CTEC subtypes can be used to predict and evaluate therapeutic effectiveness of anti-angiogenic treatments [13]. Therefore, in this field, it is necessary to continue studying comprehensively CTECs to find novel molecular target in preventing angiogenesis and development metastasis.

Other factors that influence survival are disease-free time before metastases, and different histologic characteristics of the primary and secondary tumors [100]. This indicates that a combination of clinical features and metabolic molecules improves sensitivity and specificity parameters for the establishment of accurate biomarkers. Nowadays, when liver metastases are detected in patients with advanced cancer, surgery is still the first choice. However, most of the patients with metastasis lesions at diagnosis are not suitable for surgery, and immunotherapy may improve tumor elimination and increase survival time in cancer patients. We start by addressing the highly aggressive and notoriously lethal pancreatic cancer and its metastasis. From a clinical perspective, pancreatic cancer is a highly aggressive malignancy capable of disseminating to other tissues.

Characteristically, pancreatic cancer has the potential to metastasize quickly to various locations such as the lung and liver, yet if detected early, several treatment options are available including surgery (best scenario), chemotherapy, radiotherapy, and more recently immunotherapy [77,82,83,105]. While these treatments continue to be at the forefront, a full understanding of the underlying mechanisms of how metastasis develops and novel achievements are being sought. The available regional treatments for liver metastases from CRC include surgical resection, thermal ablation, regional hepatic intraarterial chemotherapy, chemoembolization, radioembolization, and radiation therapy (RT) including stereotactic RT, as shown in Table 2 [100,101].

Table 2. Conventional treatment for metastatic CCR and PDAC.

Treatment	Advantages	Limitations	Reference
Surgical resection	-Gold standard for liver metastases. -5-year survival of 33% in CRC liver metastases. -5-year survival is 27% in PDAC liver metastases. -Surgical mortality rate is <5%. The 5-year survival of 43% (21–62%) in PC lung metastases. -Better outcome in PDAC (40%) lung metastases.	-Limited liver resection. -Relapse occurred in 75% of patients in the first 2 years after surgery. -Liver resection is not available for all patients in PC. -5-year survival of 19.8% in PDAC lung multiple metastases.	[21,100,101,106]
Thermal ablation	-5-year overall survival of 19.9–70% in CRC lung metastases and 25–55% in liver metastases. -Minimal invasiveness, safety, equivalent local control, and survival to lung resection.	-More suitable for small-volume tumors (diameter ≤ 3 cm). -Aiming at a tumor-free margin of > 10 mm. -Recurrence of 46% after thermal ablation.	[107–109]
Regional hepatic chemotherapy	-Overall survival of 6 to 12 months. -Alternative for patients unable to hepatic resection or those with poor prognostic features. -Allows chemotherapy administration for a longer time. -10–20% of unresectable patients become resectable with chemotherapy -Reduction in CEA.	-70% of patients have residual metastases. -Pump placement by surgery.	[100,110,111]
Radiation	-Tumor volumes decrease in liver metastases. -Option for unresectable disease and for medically inoperable patients. -Survival is 70%, 46%, and 46% at 6, 12, and 18 months using selective internal radiation therapy (SIRT). -Local controlled disease is >70% using stereotactic body radiation therapy (SBRT).	-Requires chemotherapy for better response. -Tumor diameter of less than 6 cm.	[112,113]

5. Novel Strategies for Liver and Lung Metastasis Treatment

5.1. Immunotherapy

Immunotherapy is a therapeutic strategy that has been extended to a wide variety of cancers. In this strategy, the immune system is stimulated by different mechanisms to facilitate cancer cell elimination. It uses peptides such as cytokines, growth factors, antibodies, cells, and immune checkpoint regulators to improve immune performance [114].

5.2. Immune Checkpoint

Cancer cells take advantage of tolerant immune regulatory mechanisms to evade elimination by T cells. Several immune checkpoints have been identified as targets that are presented in cancer stem cells as CD28/CD80 (CD86), ICOS (CD278)/ICOSL, CD27/CD70 GITR/GITRL, or co-inhibitors, such as PD-1/PDL-1 (PD-L2), BTLA/HVEM, CTLA4/CD80 (CD86), B7H3, B7H4, B7H5/HVEM, LAG3/MHC II, TIM3/GAL9, TIGIT/Nectin-2, or IDO, as shown in Table 3. An important target in immunotherapy is programmed death receptor-1/ligand-1 (PD-1/PD-1L), which are members of the CD28 and B7 families, and participate in the induction of tolerance through the regulation of T-cell activity. PD-L1 (also known as CD274 or B7H1) and B7H3 have been identified as promoters of the CSC-like phenotype, EMT, tumor cell proliferation, metastases, and resistance to therapy. However, tumoral cells take advantage of this mechanism for immune evasion and improve survival. In some cases of CRC, this strategy has demonstrated a complete response. The U.S. Food and Drug Administration (FDA) has approved three PD-1 inhibitors (nivolumab, pembrolizumab, and cemiplimab) and three PD-L1 inhibitors (atezolizumab, durvalumab, and avelumab) for the treatment of different types of cancer.

Table 3. Immune checkpoint targets.

Molecule	Characteristics	Reference
ICOS (CD28)/ICOSL	-ICOS: ICOSL pathway provides key positive second signals that promote T cell activation, differentiation and effector responses, and T cell-dependent B cell responses.	[115]
CD27/CD70	-Ligation of CD27 by CD70 induces strong ubiquitination of TRAF and the activation of both canonical and non-canonical nuclear factor-kB (NF-kB) pathways. -Reduced regulatory CD4 T-cell numbers -CD70 is expressed in most primary human breast carcinomas and that its expression selectively correlates with lung metastasis.	[116,117]
GITR/GITRL	GITR enhances T-cell proliferation and that the absence of GITR is protective in several inflammatory disease models, which is attributed to an impaired effector T-cell function of T cells	[116]
PD-1/PDL-1 (PD-L2)	Members of CD28 and B7 families Induce tolerance by regulation of T-cell	[118]
BTLA/HVEM	BTLA may specifically downregulate Th1-mediated inflammatory responses Exerts inhibitory effects on B and T lymphocytes	[115]
CTLA4/CD80 (CD86)	An inhibitory, co-stimulatory molecule which interferes with the process of T cell activation Natural ligands of CTLA-4 are CD80 (B7-1) and CD86 (B7-2), which are both expressed by antigen-presenting cells (APCs).	[119]
B7H3	Tumor cell immune evasion promotes angiogenesis by upregulating VEGFA	[120]
B7H4	molecular biomarker associated with tumor progression and prognosis	[121]
B7H5/HVEM	Sub-expression of B7H5 is correlated with metastases and poor prognosis	[122]
LAG3/MHC II	Negatively regulates T-cell function, contributing to tumor escape.	[123]
TIM3/GAL9	Associated with immunosuppression and worse clinical outcome in multiple cancers.	[124]
TIGIT/Nectin-2	Inhibition of NK cell activation.	[125]
Indoleamine 2,3-dioxygenase (IDO)	Tolerance and suppressing T cell responses to MHC mismatched allografts, tumors, and self-antigens.	[115]

The combination of nivolumab and ipilimumab also appears to improve overall survival (OS) and progression-free survival (PFS) in patients with metastatic CRC and has an acceptable safety profile [118]. In patients with CRC, it has been demonstrated that a subgroup can benefit from immune checkpoint inhibitors. For example, Le et al. in a phase II clinical trial, after the administration of pembrolizumab, showed a partial objective response rate of 40% for DNA mismatch repair deficiency (dMMR) in CRC patients. Nivolumab was approved in 2017 for metastatic colorectal cancer (mCRC) refractory to fluoropyrimidine, oxaliplatin, and irinotecan with high microsatellite instability (MSI-H) and dMMR, in a dose of 3 mg/kg every two weeks. It achieved objective response rates (ORR) of (31%) and only 12% of patients presented secondary effects like fatigue, diarrhea, and pruritus. Currently, more questions than answers remain, including when to start treatment, the optimal sequence, and the optimal duration of treatment. What is certain is that the effectiveness of the treatment is only initial since as time passes immunological tolerance occurs that entails a mechanism of evasion of the immune system and therefore, a null therapeutic effect. It is also necessary to have more molecular tools or biomarkers to have a more precise evaluation of the expected response and the proper management of adverse effects and more multiple clinical trials that are in progress. An alternative in the field of immunotherapy is the granulocyte-macrophage colony-stimulating factor (GM-CSF) because it can enhance T cell proliferation and cytokine secretion of IFN-γ and IL-2. In CRC, GM-CSF improves the antibody response to CEA and inhibits metastasis [118]. Also, pancreatic cancer cells secrete GM-CSF, which can inhibit T-cell antitumoral activity by releasing IL-6 and IL-8. Whole-cell and antigen-specific vaccines have been developed. The first whole-cell vaccine was GVAX, which has GM-CSF. GVAX has been evaluated in metastatic CRC patients with or without chemotherapy showing an overall survival of 2.3 and 4.3 months with less toxic effects than conventional treatment [126]. Gene therapy has been applied for immunotherapy as encapsulation and delivery of plasmids DNA (pDNAs). Encoding PD-L1 and CXCL12 in a lipid calcium phosphate vector induces local expression in metastatic liver, reducing lymphoid structures associated with liver metastasis, progression, and immune evasion in CRC. This is a transitory expression. However, it can recruit CD8+ T-cell and activation in the metastatic niche. In murine models, this strategy improves survival by more than 70% [127]. B7H3 is a marker expressed on immune cells (such as APCs or macrophages) and tumor cells, and it has inhibitory roles on T cells, contributing to tumor cell immune evasion by immune tolerance. Some studies report that the upregulation of B7-H3 is closely related to lymph node metastasis in patients with CRC. Blocking B7H3 with a monoclonal antibody reduces the number of cancer-initiating cells and is, therefore, a potential new biomarker and therapeutic target for CRC. Furthermore, based on in vitro and in vivo experiments, it was shown that B7H3 in CRC cells positively regulates the expression of VEGFA and angiogenesis by activating the NF-κB pathway. Combination therapy of the B7H3 inhibitor 3E8 with bevacizumab inhibits tumor growth in mouse xenograft models. As such, combination therapy with B7H3 blocking and anti-angiogenesis compounds is expected to be applied for the clinical treatment of tumors. On the other hand, this strategy has also been shown to present activity in pancreatic cancer animal models, inhibiting the infiltration of CAFs that play a common role in immunosuppression by preventing the infiltration of T cells into tumors. When CAFs are depleted, these mice are susceptible to the antitumoral effects of both anti-CTLA-4 and anti-PD-1 antibodies. In pancreatic cancer there is a strong anti-inflammatory response by T helper type 17 (Th17) cells, T helper type 2 (Th2) cells, and reduction of APCs. There is also upregulation of immunoinhibitory receptors, such as CTLA-4 and PD-1, which improve therapeutic performance [126].

5.3. Vaccines

Vaccines in cancer immunotherapy are based on cancer metabolites that can induce a strong immune response by activation of T cells, and usually employ a vector for delivery. Dendritic cells (DCs) are the most important potent antigen-presenting cells in vivo, which prominently express costimulatory molecules that are uniquely able to induce primary immune responses. Most clinical trials using DC-vaccines are based on DC loaded with lysates of isolated CSCs. Recently, it has been reported by Li et al. that DC vaccination using lung CSC antigens induced MHC expression, cytokine production, lymphocyte infiltration, and long-term protection against prostate cancer. CD90+ HepG2 cells were fused with DCs as a CD90+ HepG2/DC vaccine. CD90+ is one of multiple antigens for CSC which by a fusion process with DC can present antigens to T cells, activating T cells to be cytolysis-specific CTLs to eliminate CSC. Also, DCs with CD44 or EpCAM peptides enhanced T cell stimulation thus resulting in the induction of cell cytotoxicity against human breast cancer and HCC [128] A CSC lysate has been used as a DC vaccine (Panc-1 and ALDH^{high}) and has the ability to induce proliferation of T cell lymphocytes and B cells (IgG) which are capable of reducing tumor growth, the development of lung metastases, and increasing survival. Other immunotherapy alternatives in pancreatic cancer consist of a live-attenuated *Listeria monocytogenes* vaccine vector, which expresses mesothelin, a tumor-associated antigen expressed in a wide number of pancreatic cancers. This molecule activates mesothelin-specific T cells to eliminate cancer cells; patients with pancreatic cancer who underwent treatment with the vaccine had markedly prolonged survival [129]. This strategy has great benefits, such as generating scalable standardized vaccines by promoting humoral immunity-immunological memory with low toxic effects (compared with recombinant proteins or antibodies). However, to have the expected activity, it requires the co-stimulation of molecules and molecular signals that induce the clonal expansion of effector cells, which can sometimes be an obstacle to obtaining the desired effect.

5.4. Cell Therapy

Cancer progression is generally associated with impaired antitumor immunity and recruitment of regulatory cell populations to the tumor microenvironment. Cellular immunotherapy refers to the administration of living cells to a patient; this type of immunotherapy can be active, where the cells can stimulate an antitumor response in the patient (dendritic cells), or it can be passive, known as adoptive cell transfer (ACT), when the cells directly attack tumor cells. The cells that are mainly used are T lymphocytes, NK, and NKT, which are autologous or allogenic with or without modification. We summarize the recent research on cellular immunotherapy for destroyed CSC in CRC and pancreatic cancer [101,118].

5.5. Active Therapy

Success partial in CRC has recently been achieved with this therapy, as it has increased tumoral expression of an HLA-class I-associated β2- microglobulin molecule, an indicator of CD8+ T cell activity. In this study, three of 15 patients with metastatic CRC had stabilization or partial remission [118]. Although it turns out to be a promising approach, there is a more efficient strategy in which DCs are loaded with peptides, proteins, or mRNAs, controlling with greater precision the immune response generated. Autologous dendritic cells showed an anti-tumor effect in metastatic liver tumors in a phase II clinical trial [130]. Bagheri V et al. loaded DC with total gastric CSC mRNA expressing markers CD44, CD54, and EpCAM. These DC were able to induce expression of the IFN-γ gene and generate a cytotoxic effect after a 12-day coculture with T lymphocytes. Recent studies proposed the transformation of somatic cells into stem cells (iPS) by DC with transcription factor overexpression of CSC (NANOG, OKT4a, SOX2, c-MYC, and KLF4). For example, DCs loaded with NANOG peptides can generate immunological memory after vaccination and help the immune system to manage the plasticity of the CSC [28]. This strategy is quite promising since it is a specific target that will mainly affect CSC. Therefore, it will probably immunologically protect and expect to avoid the development of metastasis from CRC and pancreatic cancer. Allogeneic CD34+ hematopoietic stem cell transplantation is commonly employed in the treatment of blood-related malignancies after a regimen of lymphodepleting drugs. However, CD34+ stem cells play an important role during liver development and regeneration. Thus, we hypothesized that some human liver carcinomas (HLCs) might be derived from transformed CD34+ stem cells. We determined that a population of CD34+ stem cells functioned as liver CSCs (LCSCs). They were proposed as a marker of disease progression.

5.6. Passive Therapy

Natural killer (NK) cells participate in the innate immune response by targeting virus-infected, transformed, and allogeneic cells by NK cell receptors that are activated or inactivated to eliminate altered cells [131]. These receptors include NKp30, NKp44, NKp46, DNAX-activating molecule-I (DNAM-I), which can recognize ligands such as MICA, MICB, and a group of ULBPs. The ability of NKT cells in targeting CSC in colon adenocarcinoma lesions has been demonstrated. This is mainly due to higher expression of NKp30 and NKp44, both ligands of CSC for NKT cells [132]. The liver is the main site of CRC metastasis and shows an increased level of immature NKT cells, which indicates that NKT cells could be used as a strategy for cancer treatment [131]. Entolimod is a pharmacologically optimized flagellin derivative that can activate vertebral Toll-like receptor 5, and consequently activate the NF-kβ pathway. Moreover, this activation can inhibit the growth of tumoral cells expressing TLR5 while protecting normal tissues from radiation and ischemia-reperfusion injuries. It has been found that NK cells are critical for the activity of entolimod against liver metastases [131]. In another liver metastasis murine model, the alteration of commensal gut bacteria by antibiotics (vancomycin, neomycin, and primaxin) increases hepatic CXCR6+ NK cells in metastatic tumors. These NK cells also generate more interferon-γ (IFN-γ) [133]. Besides NK cells, T cells are also used in immunotherapy. Tregs (regulatory T cells) also benefit CRC patients as T cells marked with FoxP3+ in CRC correlate with patient survival and no development of metastases. Adoptive transfer of lymph node derived CD4+ TH1 cells in stage IV CRC patients improve complete remission of the disease. Adoptive T-cell transfer is T lymphocytes that are genetically modified ex vivo to express chimeric antigen receptors and recognize specific membrane proteins expressed on tumor cells [129]. This engineering of T-cells expressing chimeric antigen receptors (CARs) is another immunotherapy strategy. CARs are antigen-specific heavy and light chain antibodies genetically attached to cytoplasmic signaling molecules, such as 4-1BB, OX40, Luk, and TCR ζ-chain, which activate T cell cytotoxic activity without peptide presentation. This type of therapy is important when MHC class I is reduced. CAR T-cell technology was described more than twenty years ago and was a success with complete remission in hematological malignancies (B cells target) [118]. Modification of T cells for specific recognition of CEA, which has been widely identified in colorectal tumors, helps patients with advanced-stage CRC [118]. However solid tumors, such as breast, colorectal, prostate, and kidney, have not been nearly as successful. This strategy of treatment with CAR-T cells has significant limitations, accessibility, safety, and cost. A phase I clinical trial of immunotherapy for liver metastasis showed that patients receiving CAR-T cells modified with an anti-CEA receptor had increased necrosis or fibrosis in metastasis biopsies and a serum CEA decrease of 37%. Those patients were refractory to conventional therapy and showed more abundant levels of CAR-T cells in liver metastases than in normal liver. However, another study of CAR-T cells (HITM-SIT) showed the safety and activity of CAR-T infused by hepatic artery cells followed by selective radiotherapy (SIRT). In Table 4 are included some new strategies used for immunotherapy in liver and lung metastasis.

Table 4. Strategies of immunotherapy liver and lung metastasis cancer.

Strategy	Drug	Advances	Clinical Trials	Reference
Anti-PD-L1	Nivolumab Pembrolizumab	-Nivolumab has an objective response rate of 31% in metastatic CRC. -Pembrolizumab has a response rate of 40%.	NCT03307603 NCT03832621 NCT04030260 NCT04575922 NCT02834052 NCT03265080	[118,134]
	Atezolizumab Durvalumab Avelumab	-Suppress metastatic colonization on CRC cells. -Reduction of CEA levels.	NCT03721653 NCT03256344 NCT03555149 NCT03193190 NCT03435107 NCT02734160 NCT03563144	[118,134, 135]
GM-CSF Vaccine	GVAX	-Enhance T cell proliferation and secretion of IFN γ and IL-2. -Overall survival of 2.3 and 4.3 months. -Less toxic effects.	NCT01417000 NCT00777441 NCT02004262	[118,176]
Anti-B7H3	Monoclonal antibody (3E8) and bevacizumab MGC018 DS-7300a	-Reduce CSC number. -Inhibits tumor growth and angiogenesis. -Depletion of cancer-associated fibroblasts.	NCT03729596 NCT04145622	[120,136]
Dendritic Cells (DC) Vaccines	DC loaded with lysates of CSC Peptides: CD90, CD54, CD44, EpCAM, Panc-1, ALDH, mRNA	-Induction of MHC expression, cytokine production (IFN γ), lymphocyte infiltration, proliferation T, and B lymphocytes.	NCT02615574 NCT02503150 NCT00176761 NCT00558051 NCT00868114 NCT01410968	[128,130, 137]
Mesothelin Vaccine	Live-attenuated *Listeria monocytogenes* vaccine	-Activates mesothelin T cells in PC.	NCT03122106 NCT03956056	[129]
DC Expressing CSC Transcription Factors	NANOG, OKT4a, SOX2, c-MYC, KLF4	-Cellular immunological memory.	NCT00103142	[138]
Natural Killer Cells	Recognition of receptors in CSC: NKp30, NKp44	-Targeting of CSC.	NCT03008499	[131]
CAR-T Cells	Chimeric antigen receptors for specific proteins Anti-mesothelin Anti-CEA	-Increase in cell death. -Serum CEA decrease.	NCT01897415 NCT01583686 NCT02416466	[129]

5.7. miRNA and siRNA

Therapies based on oligonucleotides are directed at target tumor suppressor genes and oncogenes in cancer cells to improve apoptosis and reduce cancer cell invasion. Oligonucleotide-based therapies include mRNA, siRNA, miRNA, and non-coding RNA [139]. KITENIN (KAI1 C-terminal interacting tetraspanin) is a member of the tetraspanin protein family that interacts with the C-terminal cytoplasmatic domain of KAI1. In CRC, KITENIN increases migration and invasiveness by recruiting Dishevelled (Dvl) and protein kinase Cδ (PKCδ); in contrast, its knockdown inhibits tumor metastasis by distorting actin arrangement and decreasing AP-1 target genes, such as MMP-1, MMP-3, and CD44. Intravenous administration of KITENIN shRNA reduces tumor growth and liver metastasis development in murine models of CRC [140]. An enhancer of zest homolog 2 (EZH2), a member of the Polycomb group (PcG) protein family, contributes to CRC acting as an oncogene. The sub-expression of EZH2 impairs the ability of CRC cancer cells to invade other sites and improves its apoptosis [141]. EZH2 is a target of miR-506. However, its expression is downregulated in CRC tissues. Overexpression of this miRNA significantly inhibits cell proliferation and metastasis of CRC by modulating the Wnt/β-catenin signaling pathway [142]. miR-155 is overexpressed in several cancers such as CRC; its overexpression is associated with poor prognosis and improves cell migration. HuR (ELAVL1) is a nuclear RNA binding protein (RBP) that has been associated with an increase of cell division by improving stabilization of COX-2, cyclin A, MMP-9, EGFR, and c-fos. HuR also promotes pro-inflammatory and angiogenic factors, such as TNF-α and VEGF, and is related to the migration process of cancer cells. Targeting miR-155-5p reduced HuR expression and migration of CRC cells by a union to 3-UTR in HuR mRNA [130]. miR-3653 expression is downregulated in CRC cells and tissues, which in turn improves metastasis. However, its overexpression is associated with less CRC cell migration and invasion, showing tumor suppression activity by inhibiting epithelial–mesenchymal transition. This is mediated by its binding to Zeb2 3′UTR [142]. A clinical trial (NCT03480152) used mRNA vaccination with epitopes from immunogenic neoantigens, predicted neoantigens, and mutations in tumor suppressor or driver genes for CRC liver metastasis [130]. For now, miRNAs can be used as a tool for diagnosis, prognosis, and as a therapeutic target as is mentioned in Table 5. Treatment can inhibit CSC functions and enhance sensitivity to conventional treatments and these results significantly improve the course of the disease. However, there is a coincidence in some cases microRNAs activate signaling pathways changes during cancer stages and when only one target of treatment is used it cannot considerably affect progression by inducing a resistance mechanism. For now, they turn out to be ideal candidates since they are specific to a cell type representing an ideal treatment for future research in the field.

Table 5. Novel miRNAs from CSC as target therapy.

miRNA	Disease	Characteristics	
miR-93	Pancreatic adenocarcinoma and lung metastases	Regulates microtubule dynamics by controlling YES1, CRMP2, and MAPRE1 expression.	[39,71]
miR-146a	Pancreatic adenocarcinoma and lung metastases	Diminishes in metastasis.	[72,73]
miR-200 family members: miR-194, miR-200b, miR-200c, and miR-429	Pancreatic adenocarcinoma	EMT facilitating invasion, targeting PTEN, EP300, and TGF-b/SMAD pathways.	[72–74]
miR-141 and miR-429	Pancreatic adenocarcinoma	Inhibit tumor development.	[75–78]
miR-10b	Pancreatic adenocarcinoma	Increases invasiveness in metastasis by the effect of EGF and TGF-β signaling.	[82–84]

5.8. Gene Therapy

Gene therapy implies the administration of a gene sequence to counteract a defect in target cells or eliminate a phenotype. Polo-like kinase 1 (PLK1) is a protein overexpressed in multiple human tumors as CRC. In general, PLKs have functions in mitosis ensuring the fidelity of checkpoint controls [130,143]. However, PLK1 es a biomarker of prognosis in CRC and is considered an oncogene of cell cycle progression. Thus, a siRNA has been developed against PLK1 encapsulated in lipid nanoparticles (TKM-080301), which has been used in a clinical trial for CRC liver metastases [143]. The administration of certain gene sequences for targeting liver metastases has been improved in recent decades. Rexin-G is a dominant-negative form of cyclin G1 released by non-replicable retroviral vector injection into the hepatic artery. Clinical trials are employing this strategy in CRC liver metastases and gemcitabine-refractory pancreatic cancer [143]. Rexin-G displays a cryptic collagen-binding motif on its gp70 surface membrane for targeting abnormal signature (SIG) proteins in the TME and encodes a dominant-negative mutant construct (dnG1) of human cyclin G1 (CCNG1), which in turn enters proliferating cancer cells and fibroblasts, and blocks the cell division cycle generating apoptosis [144]. Other viral gene therapies for metastatic pancreatic cancers are oncolytic adenovirus expressing IL-12 in combination with chemotherapy, vaccines of virus expressing CEA, mucin-1, and a triad of costimulatory molecules (TRICOM) (PANVAC-VF). This strategy is combined with GM-CSF at the vaccination site [144]. Recent studies have evaluated the use of CRISPR/Cas9 to replace native TCR which increases antigen sensitivity and specificity. Also, it can be used to knock out HLA from allogeneic cells to reduce the cost, time, and resources required to generate CAR T cells for every patient. Although it is still under investigation, the CART-cell strategy for solid tumors, probably in the next years, will be a great option to destroy solid tumors and prevent metastasis progression. Gene therapy in clinical practice is a viable alternative for monogenic diseases and cancer when standard treatments do not have good results. The design of new experimental vectors, increased efficiency, specificity of delivery systems, and a better understanding of the induction of the inflammatory response may balance improved safety expanding techniques in clinical applications. However, the knowledge and experience gained from a careful evaluation of the toxicity of these technologies also allow significant advances in the application of these methods. Therefore, gene therapy, like any new technology, needs more enlightening preclinical studies. In the future, there is a promise to apply these techniques in combination with other strategies and a greater percentage of clinical trials to evaluate its therapeutic potential.

5.9. Nanomedicine

Nanomedicine presents several advantages over chemotherapy such as enhanced permeability and retention in tumors, easy surface modification for tumor targeting by conjugating molecules, controlled drug release, the facility of structural and morphological modification, and the integration of various drugs [145]. Nanoparticles have diameters of 10 to 1000 nm. These systems have specific properties that modify the fate of the nanoparticle and loaded drug. Its application in cancer therapy has been widely explored and optimized for delivery systems for cytotoxic molecules. Nanoparticles can be developed from multiple elements, such as lipids, polymers, and carbon. Frugs can be loaded by different principles such as physical entrapment, covalent linking, and surface adhesion, which is selected according to drug properties as an active conformation. Attaching targeting moieties includes antibodies, nucleic acids, peptides, recombinant proteins, and aptamers [146]. However, the main interest in nanomedicine is that nanoparticles can be capable of eliminating cancer cells while avoiding toxicity in normal tissues [145]. Nanoparticles of chitosan-tripolyphosphate (CS-TPP) charged with IL12 have been developed for liver metastasis. This technology was able to release IL-12 in a sustained and acid-responsive way, with low toxicity compared to intravenous free administration, and improve recruitment and tumor infiltration of NK cells. This reduces the number and volume of CRC liver metastasis foci with a lower drug concentration than free IL-12 (0.1 µg/mg) [145]. NK012 polymeric micelle of SN38 (PEG-PGA) is a nanoparticle used in the treatment of cell lung cancer and metastatic CRC that is in a phase II trial [146]. Folic acid has tumor tissue specificity and is non-immunogenic. Linked in nanoparticles, folic acid has a high binding affinity to receptors expressed on tumor cells. There have been developing systems of RNA nanoparticles to carry therapeutic modules and folic acid ligands for specific CRC cell targeting. RNA packaging of bacteriophage phi29 DNA is used [147]. Melittin peptide presents immunomodulatory effects. In one study, nanoparticles were conjugated with α-melittin modulate liver stellate cells to become APCs, affecting cytotoxicity and generating a pro-inflammatory microenvironment to eliminate tumoral cells by infiltration of T and NK cells. Moreover, intravenous administration of α-melittin nanoparticles blocks metastasis formation and prolongs survival in liver metastases models [148]. There is a commercial compound based on nanoparticles, Onivyde, which is liposomal irinotecan (PEGylated) for metastatic pancreatic cancer. This drug was approved by the FDA in 2015, and allows prolonged circulation of irinotecan with reduced toxicity [146]. Nanoparticles are a very effective drug, protein, or nucleic acid delivery system. They present the advantages of high drug concentrations and specific targeting of cancer cells. However, their use against CSC is still complicated since, although an expected cytotoxic effect has been demonstrated in vitro in an in vivo model, accessibility in the tumor and the microenvironment play a role in the effectiveness of this therapeutic strategy. Furthermore, the current markers are not specific, and their expression level can change depending on the microenvironment. The current aim in this field is to develop multifunctional nanoparticles that can load multiple drugs simultaneously and that do not present long-term toxicity. To achieve this, a greater understanding of CSC and the metastatic niche is required in order to use this information to provide more efficient therapeutic strategies.

6. Conclusions

Cancer is typically detected late, at a time when the disease is in advanced clinical stages and many times, although detected in early stages, the disease can develop metastases. So far, there has been a greater understanding of the growth factors, cytokines, changes in the microenvironment, cells, microRNAs, and signaling pathways that orchestrate the premetastatic niche. However, much remains to be understood about the key regulatory mechanisms for the establishment of the metastatic niche and which of these can be used as biomarkers or therapeutic targets. Some markers and signaling pathways that coincide in lung and liver metastasis can be used to direct treatment or biomarkers used for diagnosis. Moreover, the results were very different even using a similar treatment approach. CSCs have taken a central role since they are characterized as the main cells responsible for metastasis and resistance to conventional treatments. A great effort has been made in recent years with various approaches to improve the diagnosis and treatment of cancer patients. One of the areas that continue to be one of the main approaches is immunotherapy, where to date, there is more and more clinical trials evaluating therapeutic targets using properties of CSC. In this work, we highlight the main findings and strategies used to treat patients with the most frequent metastases, which are liver and lung. In addition, we show that several groups seek to adopt strategies such as gene therapy, nanoparticles with peptides, or microRNA against CSC markers as targets with promising results. However, in this sense, it is still necessary to have specific markers and greater knowledge of mechanisms that allow CSCs to change expression depending on the microenvironment and therefore it is proposed that the disease, for now, is attacked by different targets to prevent resistance mechanisms from developing in the short term. The long-term effect of these strategies is still unknown, and therefore, we continue to evaluate the scope of these strategies in in vitro and in vivo models. Another important problem is that few biomarkers allow evaluating the response to treatment. Survival may change in some patients since the patient is sometimes expected to improve with the therapeutic strategies used but patients do not have the economic resources to carry out treatment completely as expected. On the other hand, it is necessary to better define the characterization of patients who are candidates for treatment, since in some patients, the clinical significance is not so relevant, and if they present significant side effects, they represent a high cost for families. Hopefully, the combination of some of the therapies and different biomarkers, genetics, and metabolites can contribute in the future to offer an effective and accessible treatment to change the course of metastatic disease and at the same time be specific for every patient's needs.

Author Contributions: A.G.Q.-R. conducted the literature analysis, wrote and discussed the revised manuscript of this review and designed the images; J.F.I. wrote, analyzed, and corrected the manuscript; P.D.-G. and H.F.-V. conducted the literature analysis and wrote part of the text; E.N.G.-T. supervised, directed, and edited the manuscript. All authors have read and agreed to the published version of the manuscript.

Funding: This research received no external funding.

Institutional Review Board Statement: Not applicable.

Informed Consent Statement: Not applicable.

Data Availability Statement: Data sharing not applicable.

Acknowledgments: Special thanks to Sergio Lozano for reviewing this manuscript.

Conflicts of Interest: All authors indicated no potential conflicts of interest in publishing this manuscript.

References

1. Valastyan, S.; Weinberg, R.A. Tumor Metastasis: Molecular Insights and Evolving Paradigms. *Cell* **2011**, *147*, 275–292. [CrossRef] [PubMed]
2. Quail, D.F.; Joyce, J.A. Microenvironmental regulation of tumor progression and metastasis. *Nat. Med.* **2013**, *19*, 1423–1437. [CrossRef] [PubMed]
3. Kuşoğlu, A.; Avcı, Ç.B. Cancer stem cells: A brief review of the current status. *Gene* **2019**, *681*, 80–85. [CrossRef] [PubMed]
4. Rodriguez-Aznar, E.; Wiesmüller, L.; Sainz, J.B.; Hermann, P.C. EMT and Stemness—Key Players in Pancreatic Cancer Stem Cells. *Cancers* **2019**, *11*, 1136. [CrossRef] [PubMed]
5. Tsubakihara, Y.; Moustakas, A. Epithelial-Mesenchymal Transition and Metastasis under the Control of Transforming Growth Factor β. *Int. J. Mol. Sci.* **2018**, *19*, 3672. [CrossRef] [PubMed]
6. Mendoza, M.; Khanna, C. Revisiting the seed and soil in cancer metastasis. *Int. J. Biochem. Cell Biol.* **2009**, *41*, 1452–1462. [CrossRef] [PubMed]
7. Codony-Servat, J.; Rosell, R. Cancer stem cells and immunoresistance: Clinical implications and solutions. *Transl. Lung Cancer Res.* **2015**, *4*, 689–703.
8. Garza Treviño, E.N.; González, P.D.; Valencia Salgado, C.I.; Martinez Garza, A. Effects of pericytes and colon cancer stem cells in the tumor microenvironment. *Cancer Cell Int.* **2019**, *19*, 1–12. [CrossRef]

9. Plaks, V.; Kong, N.; Werb, Z. The Cancer Stem Cell Niche: How Essential is the Niche in Regulating Stemness of Tumor Cells? *Cell Stem Cell* **2015**, *16*, 225–238. [CrossRef]
10. Ren, J.; Ding, L.; Zhang, D.; Shi, G.; Xu, Q.; Shen, S.; Wang, Y.; Wang, T.; Hou, Y. Carcinoma-associated fibroblasts promote the stemness and chemoresistance of colorectal cancer by transferring exosomal lncRNA H19. *Theranostics* **2018**, *8*, 3932–3948. [CrossRef]
11. Hida, K.; Maishi, N.; Annan, D.A.; Hida, Y. Contribution of Tumor Endothelial Cells in Cancer Progression. *Int. J. Mol. Sci.* **2018**, *19*, 1272. [CrossRef] [PubMed]
12. Salazar, N.; Zabel, B.A. Support of Tumor Endothelial Cells by Chemokine Receptors. *Front. Immunol.* **2019**, *10*, 147. [CrossRef] [PubMed]
13. Lin, P.P. Aneuploid Circulating Tumor-Derived Endothelial Cell (CTEC): A Novel Versatile Player in Tumor Neovascularization and Cancer Metastasis. *Cells* **2020**, *9*, 1539. [CrossRef] [PubMed]
14. Wei, Y.F.; Yang, Q.; Zhang, Y.; Zhao, T.J.; Liu, X.M.; Zhong, J.; Ma, J.; Chen, Y.X.; Zhao, C.; Li, J.X. Plumbagin restrains hepatocellular carcinoma angiogenesis by suppressing the migration and invasion of tumor-derived vascular endothelial cells. *Oncotarget* **2017**, *8*, 15230–15241. [CrossRef]
15. Cima, I.; Kong, S.L.; Sengupta, D.; Tan, I.B.; Phyo, W.M.; Lee, D.; Hu, M.; Iliescu, C.; Alexander, I.; Goh, W.L.; et al. Tumor-derived circulating endothelial cell clusters in colorectal cancer. *Sci. Transl. Med.* **2016**, *8*, 345ra89. [CrossRef]
16. Zhang, L.; Zhang, X.; Liu, Y.; Zhang, T.; Wang, Z.; Gu, M.; Li, Y.; Wang, D.D.; Li, W.; Lin, P.P. PD-L1+ aneuploid circulating tumor endothelial cells (CTECs) exhibit resistance to the checkpoint blockade immunotherapy in advanced NSCLC patients. *Cancer Lett.* **2020**, *469*, 355–366. [CrossRef]
17. Stella, G.M.; Kolling, S.; Benvenuti, S.; Bortolotto, C. Lung-seeking metastases. *Cancers* **2019**, *11*, 1010. [CrossRef]
18. Jahanafrooz, Z.; Hashemzaei, M. Colon cancer therapy by focusing on colon cancer stem cells and their tumor microenvironment. *J. Cell. Phys.* **2019**, *235*, 4153–4166. [CrossRef]
19. Kulke, M.H. Metastatic Pancreatic Cancer. *Curr. Treat. Options Oncol.* **2002**, *3*, 449–457. [CrossRef]
20. Oweira, H.; Petrausch, U.; Helbling, D.; Schmidt, J.; Mannhart, M.; Mehrabi, A.; Schöb, O.; Giryes, A.; Decker, M.; Abdel-Rahman, O. Prognostic value of site-specific metastases in pancreatic adenocarcinoma: A Surveillance Epidemiology and End Results database analysis. *World J. Gastroenterol.* **2017**, *23*, 1872–1880. [CrossRef]
21. Bellon, E.; Gebauer, F.; Tachezy, M.; Izbicki, J.R.; Bockhorn, M. Pancreatic cancer and liver metastases: State of the art. *Update Surg.* **2016**, *68*, 247–251. [CrossRef] [PubMed]
22. Deeb, A.; Haque, S.-U.; Olowokure, O. Pulmonary metastases in pancreatic cancer, is there a survival influence? *J. Gastrointest. Oncol.* **2015**, *6*, E48–E51. [PubMed]
23. Trefts, E.; Gannon, M.; Wasserman, D.H. The Liver. *Curr Biol.* **2017**, *27*, R1147–R1151. [CrossRef] [PubMed]
24. Zarour, L.R.; Anand, S.; Billingsley, K.G.; Bisson, W.H.; Cercek, A.; Clarke, M.F.; Coussens, L.M.; Gast, C.E.; Geltzeiler, C.B.; Hansen, L.; et al. Colorectal Cancer Liver Metastasis: Evolving Paradigms and Future Directions. *Cell. Mol. Gastroenterol. Hepatol.* **2017**, *3*, 163–173. [CrossRef]
25. Carneiro, C.; Brito, J.; Bilreiro, C.; Barros, M.; Bahia, C.; Santiago, I.; Caseiro-Alves, F. All about portal vein: A pictorial display to anatomy, variants and physiopathology. *Insights Imaging* **2019**, *10*, 38. [CrossRef]
26. Riihimäki, M.; Hemminki, A.; Sundquist, J.; Hemminki, K. Patterns of metastasis in colon and rectal cancer. *Sci. Rep.* **2016**, *6*, 29765. [CrossRef]
27. Rossetto, A.; De Re, V.; Steffan, A.; Ravaioli, M.; Miolo, G.; Leone, P.; Racanelli, V.; Uzzau, A.; Baccarani, U.; Cescon, M. Carcinogenesis and Metastasis in Liver: Cell Physiological Basis. *Cancers* **2019**, *11*, 1731. [CrossRef]
28. Bendas, G.; Borsig, L. Cancer Cell Adhesion and Metastasis: Selectins, Integrins, and the Inhibitory Potential of Heparins. *Int. J. Cell Biol.* **2012**, *2012*, 1–10. [CrossRef]
29. Yuzhalin, A.E.; Gordon-Weeks, A.; Tognoli, M.L.; Jones, K.; Markelc, B.; Konietzny, R.; Fischer, R.; Muth, A.; O'Neill, E.; Thompson, P.R.; et al. Colorectal cancer liver metastatic growth depends on PAD4-driven citrullination of the extracellular matrix. *Nat. Commun.* **2018**, *9*, 1–15. [CrossRef]
30. Gonzalez-Villarreal, C.A.; Quiroz-Reyes, A.G.; Islas, J.F.; Garza-Treviño, E.N. Colorectal Cancer Stem Cells in the Progression to Liver Metastasis. *Front. Oncol.* **2020**, *10*, 1–17. [CrossRef]
31. Winkler, J.; Abisoye-Ogunniyan, A.; Metcalf, K.J.; Werb, Z. Concepts of extracellular matrix remodelling in tumour progression and metastasis. *Nat. Commun.* **2020**, *11*, 1–19. [CrossRef] [PubMed]
32. Gonzalez, H.; Hagerling, C.; Werb, Z. Roles of the immune system in cancer: From tumor initiation to metastatic progression. *Genes Dev.* **2018**, *32*, 1267–1284. [CrossRef] [PubMed]
33. Cortese, N.; Soldani, C.; Franceschini, B.; Barbagallo, M.; Marchesi, F.; Torzilli, G.; Donadon, M. Macrophages in Colorectal Cancer Liver Metastases. *Cancers* **2019**, *11*, 633. [CrossRef] [PubMed]
34. Goh, C.; Narayanan, S.; Hahn, Y.S. Myeloid-derived suppressor cells: The dark knight or the joker in viral infections? *Immunol. Rev.* **2013**, *255*, 210–221. [CrossRef]
35. Zhang, Q.-Q.; Hu, X.-W.; Liu, Y.-L.; Ye, Z.-J.; Gui, Y.-H.; Zhou, D.-L.; Qi, C.-L.; He, X.-D.; Wang, H.; Wang, L.-J. CD11b deficiency suppresses intestinal tumor growth by reducing myeloid cell recruitment. *Sci. Rep.* **2015**, *5*, 15948. [CrossRef]

36. Zhou, S.-N.; Pan, W.-T.; Pan, M.-X.; Luo, Q.-Y.; Zhang, L.; Lin, J.-Z.; Zhao, Y.-J.; Yan, X.-L.; Yuan, L.-P.; Zhang, Y.-X.; et al. Comparison of Immune Microenvironment Between Colon and Liver Metastatic Tissue in Colon Cancer Patients with Liver Metastasis. *Dig. Dis. Sci.* **2020**, 1–9. [CrossRef]
37. Islas, J.F.; Moreno-Cuevas, J.E. A MicroRNA Perspective on Cardiovascular Development and Diseases: An Update. *Int. J. Mol. Sci.* **2018**, *19*, 2075. [CrossRef]
38. Nguyen, L.S.; Fregeac, J.; Bole-Feysot, C.; Cagnard, N.; Iyer, A.; Anink, J.J.; Aronica, E.; Alibeu, O.; Nitschke, P.; Colleaux, L. Role of miR-146a in neural stem cell differentiation and neural lineage determination: Relevance for neurodevelopmental disorders. *Mol. Autism* **2018**, *9*, 1–12. [CrossRef]
39. Vila-Navarro, E.; Fernandez-Castañer, E.; Rovira-Rigau, M.; Raimondi, G.; Vila-Casadesus, M.; Lozano, J.J.; Soubeyran, P.; Iovanna, J.; Castells, A.; Fillat, C.; et al. MiR-93 is related to poor prognosis in pancreatic cancer and promotes tumor progression by targeting microtubule dynamics. *Oncog.* **2020**, *9*, 1–14. [CrossRef]
40. Fabian, M.R.; Mathonnet, G.; Sundermeier, T.; Mathys, H.; Zipprich, J.T.; Svitkin, Y.V.; Rivas, F.; Jinek, M.; Wohlschlegel, J.; Doudna, J.A.; et al. Mammalian miRNA RISC Recruits CAF1 and PABP to Affect PABP-Dependent Deadenylation. *Mol. Cell* **2009**, *35*, 868–880. [CrossRef]
41. Liu, H.; Lei, C.; He, Q.; Pan, Z.; Xiao, D.; Tao, Y. Nuclear functions of mammalian MicroRNAs in gene regulation, immunity and cancer. *Mol. Cancer* **2018**, *17*, 1–14. [CrossRef] [PubMed]
42. Sun Lee, Y.; Dutta, A. MicroRNAs in cancer. *Annu. Rev. Pathol.* **2009**, *4*, 199–227. [CrossRef]
43. Muz, B.; De La Puente, P.; Azab, F.; Azab, A.K. The role of hypoxia in cancer progression, angiogenesis, metastasis, and resistance to therapy. *Hypoxia* **2015**, *3*, 83–92. [CrossRef] [PubMed]
44. Shibue, T.; Weinberg, R.A. EMT, CSCs, and drug resistance: The mechanistic link and clinical implications. *Nat. Rev. Clin. Oncol.* **2017**, *14*, 611–629. [CrossRef]
45. Huang, X.; Zuo, J. Emerging roles of miR-210 and other non-coding RNAs in the hypoxic response Non-coding RNAs—Critical Regulators of Gene Function. *Acta Biochim. Biophys. Sin.* **2014**, *46*, 220–232. [CrossRef]
46. Cho, H.-S.; Han, T.-S.; Hur, K.; Ban, H.S. The Roles of Hypoxia-Inducible Factors and Non-Coding RNAs in Gastrointestinal Cancer. *Genes* **2019**, *10*, 1008. [CrossRef]
47. Al Tameemi, W.; Dale, T.P.; Al-Jumaily, R.M.K.; Forsyth, N. Hypoxia-Modified Cancer Cell Metabolism. *Front. Cell Dev. Biol.* **2019**, *7*, 4. [CrossRef]
48. Soon, P.; Kiaris, H. MicroRNAs in the tumour microenvironment: Big role for small players. *Endocr. Relat. Cancer* **2013**, *20*, R257–R267. [CrossRef]
49. Graham, R.M.; Frazier, D.P.; Thompson, J.W.; Haliko, S.; Li, H.; Wasserlauf, B.J.; Spiga, M.-G.; Bishopric, N.H.; Webster, K.A. A unique pathway of cardiac myocyte death caused by hypoxia-acidosis. *J. Exp. Biol.* **2004**, *207*, 3189–3200. [CrossRef]
50. Vasilaki, E.; Morikawa, M.; Koinuma, D.; Mizutani, A.; Hirano, Y.; Ehata, S.; Sundqvist, A.; Kawasaki, N.; Cedervall, J.; Olsson, A.-K.; et al. Ras and TGF-β signaling enhance cancer progression by promoting the ΔNp63 transcriptional program. *Sci. Signal.* **2016**, *9*, ra84. [CrossRef]
51. Tsilimigras, D.I.; Ntanasis-Stathopoulos, I.; Bagante, F.; Moris, D.; Cloyd, J.M.; Spartalis, E.; Pawlik, T.M. Clinical significance and prognostic relevance of KRAS, BRAF, PI3K and TP53 genetic mutation analysis for resectable and unresectable colorectal liver metastases: A systematic review of the current evidence. *Surg. Oncol.* **2018**, *27*, 280–288. [CrossRef] [PubMed]
52. AshokKumar, P.; Divya, T.; Kumar, K.; Dineshbabu, V.; Velavan, B.; Sudhandiran, G. Colorectal carcinogenesis: Insights into the cell death and signal transduction pathways: A review. *World J. Gastrointest. Oncol.* **2018**, *10*, 244–259. [CrossRef] [PubMed]
53. Chae, Y.C. Cancer stem cell metabolism: Target for cancer therapy. *BMB Rep.* **2018**, *51*, 319–326. [CrossRef] [PubMed]
54. De Francesco, E.M.; Sotgia, F.; Lisanti, M.P. Cancer stem cells (CSCs): Metabolic strategies for their identification and eradication. *Biochem. J.* **2018**, *475*, 1611–1634. [CrossRef]
55. Bu, P.; Chen, K.-Y.; Xiang, K.; Johnson, C.; Crown, S.B.; Rakhilin, N.; Ai, Y.; Wang, L.; Xi, R.; Astapova, I.; et al. Aldolase B-Mediated Fructose Metabolism Drives Metabolic Reprogramming of Colon Cancer Liver Metastasis. *Cell Metab.* **2018**, *27*, 1249–1262. [CrossRef]
56. Paschos, K.A. Natural history of hepatic metastases from colorectal cancer—pathobiological pathways with clinical significance. *World J. Gastroenterol.* **2014**, *20*, 3719–3737. [CrossRef]
57. Lin, Q.; Ren, L.; Jian, M.; Xu, P.; Li, J.; Zheng, P.; Feng, Q.; Yang, L.; Ji, M.; Wei, Y.; et al. The mechanism of the premetastatic niche facilitating colorectal cancer liver metastasis generated from myeloid-derived suppressor cells induced by the S1PR1–STAT3 signaling pathway. *Cell Death Dis.* **2019**, *10*, 1–18. [CrossRef]
58. Nielsen, S.R.; Quaranta, V.; Linford, A.; Emeagi, P.; Rainer, C.; Santos, A.; Ireland, L.; Sakai, T.; Sakai, K.; Kim, Y.-S.; et al. Macrophage-secreted granulin supports pancreatic cancer metastasis by inducing liver fibrosis. *Nat. Cell Biol.* **2016**, *18*, 549–560. [CrossRef]
59. Hu, C.-T.; Guo, L.-L.; Feng, N.; Zhang, L.; Zhou, N.; Ma, L.-L.; Shen, L.; Tong, G.-H.; Yan, Q.-W.; Zhu, S.-J.; et al. MIF, secreted by human hepatic sinusoidal endothelial cells, promotes chemotaxis and outgrowth of colorectal cancer in liver prometastasis. *Oncotarget* **2017**, *6*, 22410–22423. [CrossRef]
60. Liu, Y.; Liu, R.; Yang, F.; Cheng, R.; Chen, X.; Cui, S.; Gu, Y.; Sun, W.; You, C.; Liu, Z.; et al. miR-19a promotes colorectal cancer proliferation and migration by targeting TIA1. *Mol. Cancer* **2017**, *16*, 1–17. [CrossRef]

61. Cellura, D.; Pickard, K.; Quaratino, S.; Parker, H.; Strefford, J.; Thomas, G.; Mitter, R.; Mirnezami, A.; Peake, N. miR-19–Mediated Inhibition of Transglutaminase-2 Leads to Enhanced Invasion and Metastasis in Colorectal Cancer. *Mol. Cancer Res.* **2015**, *13*, 1095–1105. [CrossRef] [PubMed]
62. Jablonska, E.; Gorniak, P.; Prusisz, W.; Kiliszek, P.; Szydlowski, M.; Sewastianik, T.; Bialopiotrowicz, E.; Polak, A.; Prochorec-Sobieszek, M.; Szumera-Cieckiewicz, A.; et al. MiR-155 Amplifies AKT and NFkB Signaling By Targeting Multiple Regulators of BCR Signal in DLBCL. *Blood* **2015**, *126*, 2455. [CrossRef]
63. Ling, X.; Yao, D.; Kang, L.; Zhou, J.; Zhou, Y.; Dong, H. Involment of RAS/ERK1/2 signaling and MEF2C in miR-155-3p inhibition-triggered cardiomyocyte differentiation of embryonic stem cell. *Oncotarget* **2017**, *8*, 84403–84416. [CrossRef] [PubMed]
64. Liu, F.; Song, D.; Wu, Y.; Liu, X.; Zhu, J.; Tang, Y. MiR-155 inhibits proliferation and invasion by directly targeting PDCD4 in non-small cell lung cancer. *Thorac. Cancer* **2017**, *8*, 613–619. [CrossRef]
65. Balacescu, O.; Sur, D.; Cainap, C.; Vișan, S.; Cruceriu, D.; Manzat-Saplacan, R.; Muresan, M.-S.; Balacescu, L.; Lisencu, C.; Irimie, A. The Impact of miRNA in Colorectal Cancer Progression and Its Liver Metastases. *Int. J. Mol. Sci.* **2018**, *19*, 3711. [CrossRef] [PubMed]
66. Huang, S.; Tan, X.; Zhongcheng, H.; Chen, Z.; Lin, P.; Fu, W. microNA biomarkers in colorectal cancer liver metastasis. *J. Cancer* **2018**, *9*, 3867–3873. [CrossRef] [PubMed]
67. Maru, Y. The lung metastatic niche. *J. Mol. Med.* **2015**, *93*, 1185–1192. [CrossRef]
68. El Rayes, T.; Catena, R.; Lee, S.; Stawowczyk, M.; Joshi, N.; Fischbach, C.; Powell, C.A.; Dannenberg, A.J.; Altorki, N.K.; Gao, D.; et al. Lung inflammation promotes metastasis through neutrophil protease-mediated degradation of Tsp-1. *Proc. Natl. Acad. Sci. USA* **2015**, *112*, 16000–16005. [CrossRef]
69. Font-Clos, F.; Zapperi, S.; La Porta, C.A.M. Blood Flow Contributions to Cancer Metastasis. *iScience* **2020**, *23*, 101073. [CrossRef]
70. Shin, S.H.; Kim, H.J.; Hwang, D.W.; Lee, J.H.; Song, K.B.; Jun, E.; Shim, I.K.; Hong, S.-M.; Kim, H.J.; Park, K.M.; et al. The DPC4/SMAD4 genetic status determines recurrence patterns and treatment outcomes in resected pancreatic ductal adenocarcinoma: A prospective cohort study. *Oncotarget* **2017**, *8*, 17945–17959. [CrossRef]
71. Yang, G.; Sau, C.; Lai, W.; Cichon, J.; Li, W. miR-93-directed down-regulation of DAB2 defines a novel oncogenic pathway in lung cancer. *Oncogene* **2014**, *33*, 4307–4315. [CrossRef]
72. Chen, Z.; Zhang, S.; Guo, C.; Li, J.; Sang, W. Downregulation of miR-200c protects cardiomyocytes from hypoxia-induced apoptosis by targeting GATA-4. *Int. J. Mol. Med.* **2017**, *39*, 1589–1596. [CrossRef] [PubMed]
73. Srivastava, S.K.; Arora, S.; Singh, S.; Bhardwaj, A.; Averett, C.; Singh, A.P. MicroRNAs in pancreatic malignancy: Progress and promises. *Cancer Lett.* **2014**, *347*, 167–174. [CrossRef] [PubMed]
74. Zhang, J.; Zhu, Y.; Hu, L.; Yan, F.; Chen, J. miR-494 induces EndMT and promotes the development of HCC (Hepatocellular Carcinoma) by targeting SIRT3/TGF-β/SMAD signaling pathway. *Sci. Rep.* **2019**, *9*, 7213. [CrossRef] [PubMed]
75. Yin, J.; Bai, Z.; Song, J.; Yang, Y.; Wang, J.; Han, W.; Zhang, J.; Meng, H.; Ma, X.; Yang, Y.; et al. Differential expression of serum miR-126, miR-141 and miR-21 as novel biomarkers for early detection of liver metastasis in colorectal cancer. *Chin. J. Cancer Res.* **2014**, *26*, 95–103.
76. Lee, S.Y.; Ju, M.K.; Jeon, H.M.; Lee, Y.J.; Kim, C.H.; Park, H.G.; Han, S.I.; Kang, H.S. Oncogenic Metabolism Acts as a Prerequisite Step for Induction of Cancer Metastasis and Cancer Stem Cell Phenotype. *Oxidative Med. Cell. Longev.* **2018**, *2018*, 1–28. [CrossRef] [PubMed]
77. Zhang, X.; Ren, D.; Wu, X.; Lin, X.; Ye, L.; Lin, C.; Wu, S.; Zhu, J.; Peng, X.; Song, L. miR-1266 Contributes to Pancreatic Cancer Progression and Chemoresistance by the STAT3 and NF-κB Signaling Pathways. *Mol. Ther. Nucleic Acids* **2018**, *11*, 142–158. [CrossRef]
78. Zhao, Y.; Dong, Q.; Li, J.; Zhang, K.; Qin, J.; Zhao, J.; Sun, Q.; Wang, Z.; Wartmann, T.; Jauch, K.W.; et al. Targeting cancer stem cells and their niche: Perspectives for future therapeutic targets and strategies. *Semin. Cancer Biol.* **2018**, *53*, 139–155. [CrossRef]
79. Sheedy, P.; Medarova, Z. The fundamental role of miR-10b in metastatic cancer. *Am. J. Cancer Res.* **2018**, *8*, 1674–1688.
80. Vychytilova-Faltejskova, P.; Pesta, M.; Radova, L.; Liska, V.; Daum, O.; Kala, Z.; Svoboda, M.; Kiss, I.; Capoor, M.N. Genome-wide microRNA Expression Profiling in Primary Tumors and Matched Liver Metastasis of Patients with Colorectal Cancer. *Cancer Genom. Proteom.* **2016**, *13*, 311–316.
81. Abdelmaksoud-Dammak, R.; Chamtouri, N.; Triki, M.; Saadallah-Kallel, A.; Ayadi, W.; Charfi, S.; Khabir, A.; Ayadi, L.; Sallemi-Boudawara, T.; Mokdad-Gargouri, R. Overexpression of miR-10b in colorectal cancer patients: Correlation with TWIST-1 and E-cadherin expression. *Tumor Biol.* **2017**, *39*, 1–9. [CrossRef] [PubMed]
82. Khan, M.A.; Zubair, H.; Srivastava, S.K.; Singh, S.; Singh, A.P. Insights into the Role of microRNAs in Pancreatic Cancer Pathogenesis: Potential for Diagnosis, Prognosis, and Therapy. In *microRNA: Cancer*; Springer: Cham, Germany, 2015; pp. 71–87. [CrossRef]
83. Fang, C.; Dai, C.-Y.; Mei, Z.; Jiang, M.-J.; Gu, D.-N.; Huang, Q.; Tian, L. microRNA-193a stimulates pancreatic cancer cell repopulation and metastasis through modulating TGF-β2/TGF-βRIII signalings. *J. Exp. Clin. Cancer Res.* **2018**, *37*, 1–16. [CrossRef] [PubMed]
84. Wang, C.; Liu, P.; Wu, H.; Cui, P.; Li, Y.; Liu, Y.; Liu, Z.; Gou, S. MicroRNA-323-3p inhibits cell invasion and metastasis in pancreatic ductal adenocarcinoma via direct supression of SMAD2 and SMAD3. *Oncotarget* **2016**, *7*, 14912–14924. [CrossRef] [PubMed]

85. Lanfranca, M.P.; Thompson, J.K.; Bednar, F.; Halbrook, C.; Lyssiotis, C.; Levi, B.; Frankel, T.L. Metabolism and Epigenetics of Pancreatic Cancer Stem Cells. *Semin. Cancer Biol.* **2019**, *57*, 19–26. [CrossRef] [PubMed]
86. Matsuda, Y.; Yoshimura, H.; Ueda, J.; Naito, Z.; Korc, M.; Ishiwata, T. Nestin delineates pancreatic cancer stem cells in metastatic foci of NOD/Shi-scid IL2Rγ(null) (NOG) mice. *Am. J. Pathol.* **2014**, *184*, 674–685. [CrossRef]
87. Reichert, M.; Bakir, B.; Moreira, L.; Pitarresi, J.R.; Feldmann, K.; Simon, L.; Suzuki, K.; Maddipati, R.; Rhim, A.D.; Schlitter, A.M.; et al. Regulation of Epithelial Plasticity Determines Metastatic Organotropism in Pancreatic Cancer. *Dev. Cell* **2018**, *45*, 696–711.e8. [CrossRef]
88. Ogawa, K.; Lin, Q.; Li, L.; Bai, X.; Chen, X.; Chen, H.; Kong, R.; Wang, Y.; Zhu, H.; He, F.; et al. Prometastatic secretome trafficking via exosomes initiates pancreatic cancer pulmonary metastasis. *Cancer Lett.* **2020**, *481*, 63–75. [CrossRef]
89. Apte, M.V.; Pothula, S.P.; Wilson, J.S.; Apte, M.V. Pancreatic cancer and its stroma: A conspiracy theory. *World J. Gastroenterol.* **2014**, *20*, 11216–11229. [CrossRef]
90. Yuan, P.; He, X.H.; Rong, Y.F.; Cao, J.; Li, Y.; Hu, Y.P.; Liu, Y.; Li, D.; Lou, W.; Liu, M.F. KRAS/NF-kb/YY1/miR489 Signaling Axis Controls Pancreatic Cancer Metastasis. *Mol. Cell. Pathobiol.* **2016**, *28*, 100–111.
91. Ta, N.; Huang, X.; Zheng, K.; Zhang, Y.; Gao, Y.; Deng, L.; Zhang, B.; Jiang, H.; Zheng, J. miRNA-1290 Promotes Aggressiveness in Pancreatic Ductal Adenocarcinoma by Targeting IKK1. *Cell. Physiol. Biochem.* **2018**, *51*, 711–728. [CrossRef]
92. Ma, Y.; Yu, S.; Zhao, W.; Lu, Z.; Chen, J. miR-27a regulates the growth, colony formation and migration of pancreatic cancer cells by targeting Sprouty2. *Cancer Lett.* **2010**, *298*, 150–158. [CrossRef] [PubMed]
93. Zhang, J.; Cao, Z.; Yang, G.; You, L.; Zhang, T.; Zhao, Y.-P. MicroRNA-27a (miR-27a) in Solid Tumors: A Review Based on Mechanisms and Clinical Observations. *Front. Oncol.* **2019**, *9*, 893. [CrossRef] [PubMed]
94. Hamada, S.; Masamune, A.; Miura, S.; Satoh, K.; Shimosegawa, T. MiR-365 induces gemcitabine resistance in pancreatic cancer cells by targeting the adaptor protein SHC1 and pro-apoptotic regulator BAX. *Cell. Signal.* **2014**, *26*, 179–185. [CrossRef] [PubMed]
95. Xiao, X.; Yang, D.; Gong, X.; Mo, D.; Pan, S.; Xu, J. miR-1290 promotes lung adenocarcinoma cell proliferation and invasion by targeting SOCS4. *Oncotarget* **2018**, *9*, 11977–11988. [CrossRef] [PubMed]
96. Wei, J.; Yang, L.; Wu, Y.-N.; Xu, J. Serum miR-1290 and miR-1246 as Potential Diagnostic Biomarkers of Human Pancreatic Cancer. *J. Cancer* **2020**, *11*, 1325–1333. [CrossRef]
97. Hidalgo-Sastre, A.; Lubeseder-Martellato, C.; Engleitner, T.; Steiger, K.; Zhong, S.; Desztics, J.; Öllinger, R.; Rad, R.; Schmid, R.M.; Hermeking, H.; et al. Mir34a constrains pancreatic carcinogenesis. *Sci. Rep.* **2020**, *10*, 9654. [CrossRef]
98. Zhou, R.; Yuan, P.; Wang, Y.; Hunsberger, J.G.; Elkahloun, A.G.; Wei, Y.; Damschroder-Williams, P.; Du, J.; Chen, G.; Manji, H.K. Evidence for Selective microRNAs and Their Effectors as Common Long-Term Targets for the Actions of Mood Stabilizers. *Neuropsychopharmacology* **2009**, *34*, 1395–1405. [CrossRef]
99. Chao, C.; Lee, C.; Chang, T.; Chen, P.; Liu, J. CXCL1/CXCR2 Paracrine Axis Contributes to Lung Metastasis in Osteosarcoma. *Cancers* **2020**, *12*, 459. [CrossRef]
100. Stewart, C.L.; Warner, S.; Ito, K.; Raoof, M.; Wu, G.X.; Lu, W.P.; Kessler, J.; Kim, J.Y.; Fong, Y. Cytoreduction for Colorectal Metastases: Liver, Lung, Peritoneum, Lymph Nodes, Bone, Brain. When Does it Palliate, Prolong Survival, and Potentially Cure. *Curr Probl Surg.* **2018**, *55*, 330–379. [CrossRef]
101. Pfannschmidt, J.; Muley, T.; Hoffmann, H.; Dienemann, H. Prognostic factors and survival after complete resection of pulmonary metastases from colorectal carcinoma: Experiences in 167 patients. *J. Thorac. Cardiovasc. Surg.* **2003**, *126*, 732–739. [CrossRef]
102. Garza Treviño, E.N.; Delgado-Gonzalez, P.; Valencia Salgado, C.I.; Ortega Garcia, J.L. Pericytes Relationship with Cancer Stem Cells in the Colon. *Curr. Tissue Microenviron. Rep.* **2020**, *1*, 187–198. [CrossRef]
103. Amin, D.N.; Hida, K.; Bielenberg, D.R.; Klagsbrun, M. Tumor Endothelial Cells Express Epidermal Growth Factor Receptor (EGFR) but not ErbB3 and Are Responsive to EGF and to EGFR Kinase Inhibitors. *Cancer Res.* **2006**, *66*, 2173–2180. [CrossRef] [PubMed]
104. Chen, H.F.; Wu, K.J. Endothelial transdifferentiation of tumor cells triggered by the Twist1-Jagged1-KLF4 axis: Relationship between cancer stemness and angiogenesis. *Stem Cells Int.* **2016**, *2016*. [CrossRef] [PubMed]
105. Schizas, D.; Charalampakis, N.; Kole, C.; Economopoulou, P.; Koustas, E.; Gkotsis, E.; Ziogas, D.C.; Psyrri, A.; Karamouzis, M.V. Immunotherapy for pancreatic cancer: A 2020 update. *Cancer Treat. Rev.* **2020**, *86*, 102016. [CrossRef] [PubMed]
106. Sahin, I.H.; Elias, H.; Chou, J.F.; Capanu, M.; O'Reilly, E.M. Pancreatic adenocarcinoma: Insights into patterns of recurrence and disease behavior. *BMC Cancer* **2018**, *18*, 769. [CrossRef]
107. Liu, J.; Xi, L.; Yu, Y.; Chen, N.; Wang, S.; Sun, P.; Liu, A.; Zhang, X.; Gong, W.; Zhang, X.; et al. Thermal ablation for colorectal pulmonary metastases: A meta-analysis. *Int. J. Clin. Exp. Med.* **2018**, *11*, 11521–11534.
108. Puijk, R.S.; COLLISION Trial Group; Ruarus, A.H.; Vroomen, L.; Van Tilborg, A.A.J.M.; Scheffer, H.J.; Nielsen, K.; De Jong, M.C.; De Vries, J.J.J.; Zonderhuis, B.M.; et al. Colorectal liver metastases: Surgery versus thermal ablation (COLLISION)—A phase III single-blind prospective randomized controlled trial. *BMC Cancer* **2018**, *18*, 821. [CrossRef]
109. Gurusamy, K.S.; Corrigan, N.; Croft, J.; Twiddy, M.; Morris, S.; Woodward, N.; Bandula, S.; Hochhauser, D.; Napp, V.; Pullan, A.; et al. Liver resection surgery versus thermal ablation for colorectal LiVer MetAstases (LAVA): Study protocol for a randomised controlled trial. *Trials* **2018**, *19*, 105. [CrossRef]
110. Dizon, D.S.; Schwartz, J.; Kemeny, N. Regional Chemotherapy: A Focus on Hepatic Artery Infusion for Colorectal Cancer Liver Metastases. *Surg. Oncol. Clin. N. Am.* **2008**, *17*, 759–771. [CrossRef]

111. Ammori, J.B.; Kemeny, N.E. Regional Hepatic Chemotherapies in Treatment of Colorectal Cancer Metastases to the Liver. *Semin. Oncol.* **2010**, *37*, 139–148. [CrossRef]
112. Welsh, J.S.; Kennedy, A.S.; Thomadsen, B. Selective internal radiation therapy (SIRT) for liver metastases secondary to colorectal adenocarcinoma. *Int. J. Radiat. Oncol.* **2006**, *66*, S62–S73. [CrossRef] [PubMed]
113. Robin, T.P.; Raben, D.; Schefter, T. A Contemporary Update on the Role of Stereotactic Body Radiation Therapy (SBRT) for Liver Metastases in the Evolving Landscape of Oligometastatic Disease Management. *Semin. Radiat. Oncol.* **2018**, *28*, 288–294. [CrossRef] [PubMed]
114. Riley, R.S.; June, C.H.; Langer, R.; Mitchell, M.J. Delivery technologies for cancer immunotherapy. *Nat. Rev. Drug Discov.* **2019**, *18*, 175–196. [CrossRef] [PubMed]
115. Greenwald, R.J.; Freeman, G.J.; Sharpe, A.H. THE B7 FAMILY REVISITED. *Annu. Rev. Immunol.* **2005**, *23*, 515–548. [CrossRef]
116. Nolte, M.A.; Van Olffen, R.W.; Van Gisbergen, K.P.J.M.; Van Lier, R.A.W. Timing and tuning of CD27-CD70 interactions: The impact of signal strength in setting the balance between adaptive responses and immunopathology. *Immunol. Rev.* **2009**, *229*, 216–231. [CrossRef]
117. Liu, L.; Yin, B.; Yi, Z.; Liu, X.; Hu, Z.; Gao, W.; Yu, H.; Li, Q. Breast cancer stem cells characterized by CD70 expression preferentially metastasize to the lungs. *Breast Cancer* **2018**, *25*, 706–716. [CrossRef]
118. Zumwalt, T.J.; Goel, A. Immunotherapy of Metastatic Colorectal Cancer: Prevailing Challenges and New Perspectives. *Curr. Color. Cancer Rep.* **2015**, *11*, 125–140. [CrossRef]
119. De Vos, L.; Grünwald, I.; Bawden, E.G.; Dietrich, J.; Scheckenbach, K.; Wiek, C.; Zarbl, R.; Bootz, F.; Landsberg, J.; Dietrich, D. The landscape of CD28, CD80, CD86, CTLA4, and ICOS DNA methylation in head and neck squamous cell carcinomas. *Epigenetics* **2020**, *15*, 1195–1212. [CrossRef]
120. Dong, P.; Xiong, Y.; Yue, J.; Hanley, S.J.B.; Watari, H. B7H3 As a Promoter of Metastasis and Promising Therapeutic Target. *Front. Oncol.* **2018**, *8*, 264. [CrossRef]
121. Piao, L.; Yang, Z.; Jin, J.; Ni, W.; Qi, W.; Xuan, Y. B7H4 is associated with stemness and cancer progression in esophageal squamous cell carcinoma. *Hum. Pathol.* **2018**, *80*, 152–162. [CrossRef]
122. Chen, Q.; Wang, J.; Chen, W.; Zhang, Q.; Wei, T.; Zhou, Y.; Xu, X.; Bai, X.; Liang, T. B7-H5/CD28H is a co-stimulatory pathway and correlates with improved prognosis in pancreatic ductal adenocarcinoma. *Cancer Sci.* **2019**, *110*, 530–539. [CrossRef] [PubMed]
123. Shapiro, M.; Herishanu, Y.; Katz, B.-Z.; Dezorella, N.; Sun, C.; Kay, S.; Polliack, A.; Avivi, I.; Wiestner, A.; Perry, C. Lymphocyte activation gene 3: A novel therapeutic target in chronic lymphocytic leukemia. *Haematology* **2017**, *102*, 874–882. [CrossRef] [PubMed]
124. Li, X.; Chen, Y.; Liu, X.; Zhang, J.; He, X.; Teng, G.; Yu, D. Tim3/Gal9 interactions between T cells and monocytes result in an immunosuppressive feedback loop that inhibits Th1 responses in osteosarcoma patients. *Int. Immunopharmacol.* **2017**, *44*, 153–159. [CrossRef] [PubMed]
125. Deuss, F.A.; Gully, B.S.; Rossjohn, J.; Berry, R. Recognition of nectin-2 by the natural killer cell receptor T cell immunoglobulin and ITIM domain (TIGIT). *J. Biol. Chem.* **2017**, *292*, 11413–11422. [CrossRef]
126. Reha, J.; Katz, S.C. Regional immunotherapy for liver and peritoneal metastases. *J. Surg. Oncol.* **2017**, *116*, 46–54. [CrossRef]
127. Goodwin, T.J.; Shen, L.; Hu, M.; Li, J.; Feng, R.; Dorosheva, O.; Liu, R.; Huang, L. Liver Specific Gene Immunotherapies Resolve Immune Suppressive Ectopic Lymphoid Structures of Liver Metastases and Prolong Survival. *Biomaterials* **2017**, *141*, 260–271. [CrossRef]
128. Choi, Y.J.; Park, S.-J.; Park, Y.-S.; Park, H.S.; Yang, K.; Heo, K. EpCAM peptide-primed dendritic cell vaccination confers significant anti-tumor immunity in hepatocellular carcinoma cells. *PLoS ONE* **2018**, *13*, e0190638. [CrossRef]
129. Ko, A.H. Progress in the Treatment of Metastatic Pancreatic Cancer and the Search for Next Opportunities. *J. Clin. Oncol.* **2015**, *33*, 1779–1786. [CrossRef]
130. Strebhardt, K.; Ullrich, A. Targeting polo-like kinase 1 for cancer therapy. *Nat. Rev. Cancer* **2006**, *6*, 321–330. [CrossRef]
131. Burdelya, L.G.; Brackett, C.M.; Kojouharov, B.; Gitlin, I.I.; Leonova, K.I.; Gleiberman, A.S.; Aygun-Sunar, S.; Veith, J.; Johnson, C.; Haderski, G.J.; et al. Central role of liver in anticancer and radioprotective activities of Toll-like receptor 5 agonist. *Proc. Natl. Acad. Sci. USA* **2013**, *110*, E1857–E1866. [CrossRef]
132. Tallerico, R.; Todaro, M.; Di Franco, S.; Maccalli, C.; Garofalo, C.; Sottile, R.; Palmieri, C.; Tirinato, L.; Pangigadde, P.; La Rocca, R.; et al. Human NK Cells Selective Targeting of Colon Cancer–Initiating Cells: A Role for Natural Cytotoxicity Receptors and MHC Class I Molecules. *J. Immunol.* **2013**, *190*, 2381–2390. [CrossRef] [PubMed]
133. Ma, C.; Han, M.; Heinrich, B.; Fu, Q.; Zhang, Q.; Sandhu, M.; Agdashian, D.; Terabe, M.; Berzofsky, J.A.; Fako, V.; et al. Gut microbiome–mediated bile acid metabolism regulates liver cancer via NKT cells. *Science* **2018**, *360*, eaan5931. [CrossRef] [PubMed]
134. Ghatalia, P.; Nagarathinam, R.; Cooper, H.; Geynisman, D.M.; El-Deiry, W.S. Mismatch repair deficient metastatic colon cancer and urothelial cancer: A case report of sequential immune checkpoint therapy. *Cancer Biol. Ther.* **2017**, *18*, 651–654. [CrossRef] [PubMed]
135. Toyoshima, Y.; Kitamura, H.; Xiang, H.; Ohno, Y.; Homma, S.; Kawamura, T.; Takahashi, N.; Kamiyama, T.; Tanino, M.; Taketomi, A. IL6 Modulates the Immune Status of the Tumor Microenvironment to Facilitate Metastatic Colonization of Colorectal Cancer Cells. *Cancer Immunol. Res.* **2019**, *7*, 1944–1957. [CrossRef]
136. Yang, S.; Wei, W.; Zhao, Q. B7-H3, a checkpoint molecule, as a target for cancer immunotherapy. *Int. J. Biol. Sci.* **2020**, *16*, 1767–1773. [CrossRef]

137. Bagheri, V.; Abbaszadegan, M.R.; Memar, B.; Motie, M.R.; Asadi, M.; Mahmoudian, R.A.; Gholamin, M. Induction of T cell-mediated immune response by dendritic cells pulsed with mRNA of sphere-forming cells isolated from patients with gastric cancer. *Life Sci.* **2019**, *219*, 136–143. [CrossRef]
138. Wefers, C.; Schreibelt, G.; Massuger, L.F.A.G.; De Vries, I.J.M.; Torensma, R. Immune Curbing of Cancer Stem Cells by CTLs Directed to NANOG. *Front. Immunol.* **2018**, *9*, 1412. [CrossRef]
139. Hwang, J.-E.; Shim, H.-J.; Park, Y.-K.; Cho, S.-H.; Bae, W.-K.; Kim, D.-E.; Kim, K.-K.; Chung, I.-J. Intravenous KITENIN shRNA Injection Suppresses Hepatic Metastasis and Recurrence of Colon Cancer in an Orthotopic Mouse Model. *J. Korean Med. Sci.* **2011**, *26*, 1439–1445. [CrossRef]
140. Zhang, Y.; Lin, C.; Liao, G.; Liu, S.; Ding, J.; Tang, F.; Wang, Z.; Liang, X.; Li, B.; Wei, Y.; et al. MicroRNA-506 suppresses tumor proliferation and metastasis in colon cancer by directly targeting the oncogene EZH2. *Oncotarget* **2015**, *6*, 32586–32601. [CrossRef]
141. Al-Haidari, A.; Algaber, A.; Madhi, R.; Syk, I.; Thorlacius, H. MiR-155-5p controls colon cancer cell migration via post-transcriptional regulation of Human Antigen R (HuR). *Cancer Lett.* **2018**, *421*, 145–151. [CrossRef]
142. Zhu, W.; Luo, X.; Fu, H.; Liu, L.; Sun, P.; Wang, Z. MiR-3653 inhibits the metastasis and epithelial-mesenchymal transition of colon cancer by targeting Zeb2. *Pathol. Res. Pract.* **2019**, *215*, 152577. [CrossRef] [PubMed]
143. Kamimura, K.; Yokoo, T.; Abe, H.; Terai, S. Gene Therapy for Liver Cancers: Current Status from Basic to Clinics. *Cancers* **2019**, *11*, 1865. [CrossRef] [PubMed]
144. Chawla, S.P.; Bruckner, H.; Morse, M.A.; Assudani, N.; Hall, F.L.; Gordon, E.M. A Phase I-II Study Using Rexin-G Tumor-Targeted Retrovector Encoding a Dominant-Negative Cyclin G1 Inhibitor for Advanced Pancreatic Cancer. *Mol. Ther. Oncolytics* **2019**, *12*, 56–67. [CrossRef] [PubMed]
145. He, Q.; Guo, S.; Qian, Z.; Chen, X. Development of individualized anti-metastasis strategies by engineering nanomedicines. *Chem. Soc. Rev.* **2015**, *44*, 6258–6286. [CrossRef]
146. Arshad, U.; Sutton, P.A.; Ashford, M.B.; Treacher, K.E.; Liptrott, N.J.; Rannard, S.P.; Goldring, C.E.; Owen, A. Critical considerations for targeting colorectal liver metastases with nanotechnology. *Wiley Interdiscip. Rev. Nanomed. Nanobiotechnol.* **2019**, *12*, e1588. [CrossRef]
147. Rychahou, P.; Haque, F.; Shu, Y.; Zaytseva, Y.; Weiss, H.L.; Lee, E.Y.; Mustain, W.; Valentino, J.; Guo, P.; Evers, B.M. Delivery of RNA Nanoparticles into Colorectal Cancer Metastases Following Systemic Administration. *ACS Nano* **2015**, *9*, 1108–1116. [CrossRef]
148. Yu, X.; Chen, L.; Liu, J.; Dai, B.; Xu, G.; Shen, G.; Luo, Q.; Zhang, Z. Immune modulation of liver sinusoidal endothelial cells by melittin nanoparticles suppresses liver metastasis. *Nat. Commun.* **2019**, *10*, 1–14. [CrossRef]

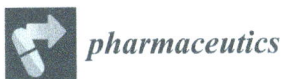

Article

Anti-Cancer Activity of As$_4$O$_6$ and its Efficacy in a Series of Patient-Derived Xenografts for Human Cervical Cancer

Joseph J. Noh [1,†], Myeong-Seon Kim [2,†], Young-Jae Cho [3,†], Soo-Young Jeong [1], Yoo-Young Lee [1], Ji-Yoon Ryu [3], Jung-Joo Choi [3], Illju Bae [4], Zhaoyan Wu [4], Byoung-Gie Kim [1,*], Jae Ryoung Hwang [3,*] and Jeong-Won Lee [1,*]

[1] Division of Gynecologic Oncology, Department of Obstetrics and Gynecology, Samsung Medical Center, Sungkyunkwan University School of Medicine, Seoul 06351, Korea; josephnoh.medicine@gmail.com (J.J.N.); sy1130.jeong@samsung.com (S.-Y.J.); yooyoung.lee@samsung.com (Y.-Y.L.)
[2] Department of Obstetrics and Gynecology, St. Vincent's Hospital, Catholic University of Korea, Seoul 16247, Korea; mseon.kim@outlook.com
[3] Research Institute for Future Medicine, Samsung Medical Center, Sungkyunkwan University School of Medicine, Seoul 06351, Korea; yj35.cho@sbri.co.kr (Y.-J.C.); jiyoon.ryu@sbri.co.kr (J.-Y.R.); jungjoo.choi@samsung.com (J.-J.C.)
[4] Chemas Co., Ltd., Seoul 06163, Korea; cjsbij@gmail.com (I.B.); pineapple97531@gmail.com (Z.W.)
* Correspondence: bksong.kim@samsung.com (B.-G.K.); jr3143.hwang@sbri.co.kr (J.R.H.); garden.lee@samsung.com (J.-W.L.); Tel.: +82-2-3410-1382 (J.-W.L.); Fax: +82-2-3410-0630 (J.-W.L.)
† These authors contributed equally as co-first authors.

Received: 23 September 2020; Accepted: 16 October 2020; Published: 19 October 2020

Abstract: Purpose: To investigate the anti-cancer effects of tetraarsenic hexoxide (TAO, As$_4$O$_6$) in cervical cancer cell lines and in a series of patient-derived xenograft (PDX) mouse models. Methods: Human cervical cancer cell lines, including HeLa, SiHa and CaSki, and human umbilical vein endothelial cells (HUVECs), were used to evaluate the anti-cancer activity of TAO. Cellular proliferation, apoptosis, and enzyme-linked immunosorbent assay (ELISA) for matrix metallopeptidase 2 (MMP-2) and 9 (MMP-9) were assessed. The tumor weights of the PDXs that were given TAO were measured. The PDXs included primary squamous cell carcinoma, primary adenocarcinoma, recurrent squamous cell carcinoma, and recurrent adenocarcinoma. Results: TAO significantly decreased cellular proliferation and increased apoptosis in cervical cancer cell lines and HUVEC. The functional studies on the cytotoxicity of TAO revealed that it inhibited the activation of Akt and vascular endothelial growth factor receptor 2 (VEGFR2). It also decreased the concentrations of MMP-2 in both cervical cancer cell lines and HUVECs. Active caspase-3 and p62 were both increased by the treatment of TAO, indicating increased rates of apoptosis and decreased rates of autophagy, respectively. In vivo studies with PDXs revealed that TAO significantly decreased tumor weight for both primary squamous cell carcinoma and adenocarcinoma of the cervix. However, this anti-cancer effect was not seen in PDXs with recurrent cancers. Nevertheless, the combination of TAO with cisplatin significantly decreased tumor weight in PDX models for both primary and recurrent cancers. Conclusions: TAO exerted inhibitory effects on angiogenesis, cellular migration, and autophagy, and it showed stimulatory effects on apoptosis. Overall, it demonstrated anti-cancer effects in animal models for human cervical cancer.

Keywords: cervical cancer; tetraarsenic hexoxide; patient-derived xenograft; autophagy; cisplatin

1. Introduction

Cervical cancer is one of the most common cancers among women worldwide, with almost half a million new cases occurring in each year. In 2015, 526,000 women were diagnosed with cervical cancer and the estimated number of deaths caused by the disease was 239,000 [1]. Cervical cancer patients are prone to developing pelvic recurrence or distant metastasis. A 10–20% recurrence rate has been reported following primary surgery or radiotherapy in women with stage IB–IIA cervical cancer with no evidence of lymph node involvement, while up to 70% of patients with nodal metastases were reported to relapse [2,3]. Because of the unfavorable prognosis of the disease and its high recurrence rate, cervical cancer continues to be a major public health problem, despite widespread screening methods [4]. Various treatment modalities including chemotherapy and radiotherapy have been developed, but none have demonstrated promising results thus far. In order to develop a new approach to improve the prognosis of cervical cancer, researchers have started to investigate various non-chemotherapeutic agents, such as arsenic trioxide (As_2O_3) and tetraarsenic hexoxide (As_4O_6, TAO).

Arsenic is a naturally occurring substance that has been used as a medicinal agent for more than 2400 years to treat a variety of medical conditions ranging from infectious disease to cancer [5]. It is stable in dry air, but the surface oxidizes slowly in moist air to give a bronze tarnish and, finally, a black covering to the element. When heated in the air, it ignites to form arsenic trioxide and tetraarsenic hexoxide. In traditional Chinese medicine, arsenic trioxide is recorded in the Compendium of Materia Medica as having therapeutic benefits. Because of the toxic side effects and the introduction of modern radiotherapy and chemotherapy, Western medicine has abandoned the use of arsenic as a treatment for cancer. However, its therapeutic effect on leukemia has initiated a re-awakening of interest in arsenic compounds. Studies have demonstrated that TAO induces apoptosis in hematopoietic and non-hematopoietic tumor cells, eventually gaining approval from the U.S. Food and Drug Administration (FDA) to treat acute promyelocytic leukemia (APL) [6]. The molecular formula of the drug substance in the solid state is As_2O_3 (molecular weight of 197.84 g mol^{-1}). Because arsenic trioxide is poorly soluble in pure water, inactive ingredients, such as sodium hydroxide, are added to increase its solubility. Under normal conditions (room temperature and atmospheric pressure), solid arsenic trioxide is present in the form of As_4O_6 (dimeric As_2O_3) and only dissociates into monomeric As_2O_3 above 800 °C. Upon dissolution of arsenic trioxide in aqueous media, both As_2O_3 and As_4O_6 are converted into the same arsenic species. It is hypothesized that its anti-cancer effects are mediated by the induction of cellular differentiation, tumor cell apoptosis, degradation of specific transcripts, inhibition of tumor cell growth, modulation of redox balance, and abrogation of vascular networks that cause blood flow to shut down, subsequently causing cell necrosis [7–10]. In an effort to add further evidence to the body of literature suggesting the anti-cancer effects of TAO, the present study was designed to demonstrate the effectiveness of TAO in a series of patient-derived xenografts (PDXs) for cervical cancer, including primary and recurrent patients.

2. Materials and Methods

2.1. Cell Lines and Tetraarsenic Hexoxide

Three different cervical cancer cell lines, SiHa (*Homo sapiens* uterine cervix, squamous cell carcinoma: HTB-35), HeLa (*Homo sapiens* uterine cervix, adenocarcinoma: CCL-2), CaSki (*Homo sapiens* uterine cervix, derived from metastatic site of small intestine, epidermoid carcinoma: CRL-1550), and human umbilical vein endothelial cells (HUVECs, CRL-1730) were obtained (American Type Culture Collection, Manassas, VA, USA). Cells were maintained in Dulbecco's modified eagle medium (DMEM), minimal essential medium (MEM), and Roswell Park Memorial Institute (RPMI) medium containing 10% fetal bovine serum (FBS) with 100 units/mL penicillin and 100 µg/mL streptomycin (Invitrogen, Carlsbad, CA, USA) for HeLa, SiHa, and CaSki, respectively. They were grown at 37 °C in a 5% CO_2 incubator. HUVECs were grown in an endothelial cell growth medium 2 (EGM-2) bullet kit (Lonza, Basel, Switzerland). TAO was obtained from CHEMAS (Seoul, South Korea). A 1%

concentration of TAO solution in distilled water was made by heating for 4 h at 90–100 °C and was then filtered through a 0.2 μm filter.

2.2. MTT (3-(4,5-Dimethylthiazol-2-yl)-2,5-diphenyltetrazolium bromide) Assay

For assaying cell viability, cells were plated with 3000–4000 cells/well onto a 96-well plate in triplicate and then treated with the indicated amount of TAO for 72 h at 37 °C in a 5% CO_2 incubator. After the drug treatment, cells were incubated with 5 mg/mL MTT (3-(4,5-Dimethylthiazol-2-yl)-2,5-diphenyltetrazolium bromide, M2128, Sigma-Aldrich, St. Louis, MO, USA) solution in 1X phosphate-buffered saline (PBS) for 4 h in a 37 °C incubator. The MTT crystal was dissolved in dimethyl sulfoxide (DMSO, D1370, Duchefa Biochemie, Haarlem, The Netherlands), and cell viability was measured at 540 nm by spectrometry.

2.3. Western Blot Analysis

Cells were plated with 200,000 cells/well on a 6-well plate. The cells were treated with TAO at concentrations indicated in the text for 48 h. Cellular protein was lysed by incubating for 20 min on ice in radioimmunoprecipitation assay (RIPA) buffer containing 1X protease inhibitor mix (P-8340, Sigma-Aldrich, St. Louis, MO, USA) and 1 mmol/L of phenylmethylsulfonyl fluoride (PMSF, P-7626, Sigma-Aldrich, St. Louis, MO, USA). Protein concentrations were determined using the Bio-Rad protein assay (Bio-Rad Laboratories, Hercules, CA, USA), and proteins were separated by sodium dodecyl sulfate-polyacrylamide gel electrophoresis (SDS-PAGE), then were electrotransferred to a polyvinylidene difluoride (PVDF) membrane. After blocking membranes with 5% non-fat dry milk in PBS, membranes were incubated with primary antibodies overnight at 4 °C. After several washes, blots were incubated with secondary antibodies (GeneTex, Irvine, CA, USA) for 1 h. After an additional wash, light development was initiated by adding enhanced chemiluminescence (ECL) reagents (Amersham PLC, Buckinghamshire, United Kingdom). Primary antibodies for studying phosphorylated Akt (Ser473, #9271), Akt (#9272), and VEGFR2 (#2479) were obtained from Cell Signal Technology (Danvers, MA, USA), and β-actin (sc-47778) was obtained from Santa Cruz Biotechnology (Dallas, TX, USA). Phosphorylated-vascular endothelial growth factor receptor 2 (VEGFR2, ab5473) and p62 (ab56416) were obtained from Abcam (Cambridge, UK), and anti-LC3 antibody (NB100-2220) was purchased from Novus Biologicals (Centennial, CO, USA).

2.4. ELISA (Enzyme-Linked Immunosorbent Assay) for MMP-2 (Matrix Metallopeptidase 2) and 9

For the enzyme-linked immunosorbent assay (ELISA), media was collected from the cells in culture and transferred to a 96-well plate for matrix metallopeptidase 2 (MMP-2, MMP200) or MMP-9 (DMP900) specific ELISAs using a Quantikine ELISA Kit (R&D Systems, Minneapolis, MN, USA) according to the manufacturer's instructions. A standard curve using each recombinant protein provided in the kit was run with each assay, and the concentration of each protein was determined by the standard curve.

2.5. Caspase-3 Assay

Cell death was assessed using an active caspase-3 assay kit (KHO1091, Invitrogen, Carlsbad, CA, USA). Cells (2×10^5/well) were plated in a 6-well plate and treated with TAO as indicated for 48 h. After TAO treatment, cells were lysed in RIPA buffer, and 50 ug of total protein was used for the caspase-3 assay according to the manufacturer's instructions.

2.6. Treatment of VEGF to Cervical Cancer Cell Lines and HUVEC

Cells (2×10^5/well) were plated in a 6-well plate and treated with TAO in the growth media as indicated for 48 h. Human vascular endothelial growth factor (VEGF165, H9166) was purchased from Peprotech (Rocky Hill, NJ, USA) and was dissolved in 1X PBS containing 0.1% bovine serum albumin (BSA, A-3294, Sigma-Aldrich, St. Louis, MO, USA) to make a 100 µg/mL solution. VEGF was introduced into the growth media containing TAO overnight before lysis of the cells.

2.7. Animal Study Using Cell Lines and PDX (Patient-Derived Xenograft) Models for Cervical Cancer

To establish the SiHa cell line xenograft tumor, female BALB/c nude mice were purchased from Orient Bio (Seongnam, South Korea). Autoclaved water and food were available to the mice ad libitum. The same SiHa cell line that was used for in vitro experiments was employed. It was cultured in MEM containing 10% FBS. A total of 2×10^6 cells were inoculated subcutaneously in 200 µL of Hanks' Balanced Salt Solution (HBSS, Biocompare, San Francisco, CA, USA) into the flank of the animals bilaterally. Tumor growth was measured twice a week. The volume of tumors was calculated using a standard formula (length × width^2 × 0.52), and growth curves were drawn.

To establish PDX models of cervical cancer, surgically removed patient tumor specimens were reduced to small pieces (less than 2–3 mm), implanted into the subrenal capsules of the left kidneys of BALB/c nude mice, and propagated by serial transplantation [11,12]. The clinical information of the patients is provided in Supplementary Table S1 and Supplementary Figures S1–S5. The mice used in these experiments were 6 to 8-weeks old. TAO (8 mg/kg) or PBS was intraperitoneally injected into the model mice once a week for the subsequent 3–4 weeks. For combination therapy with cisplatin, the model mice were either given intraperitoneal cisplatin (4 mg/kg) once a week alone or cisplatin (same dosage) in addition to TAO injections. The mice were then sacrificed and tumors were imaged and weighed. The mice ($n = 10$ per group) were monitored daily for tumor development and sacrificed when any appeared moribund. We recorded the body weight, tumor weight, and number of tumor nodules. Tumors were fixed in formalin and embedded in paraffin or snap-frozen in optimal cutting temperature (OCT) compound (Sakura Finetek Japan, Tokyo, Japan) in liquid nitrogen. This study was reviewed and approved by the Institutional Animal Care and Use Committee (IACUC) of the Samsung Biomedical Research Institute (protocol number H-A9-003). The IACUC is accredited by the Association for the Assessment and Accreditation of Laboratory Animal Care International (AAALAC International) and abides by the guidelines of the Institute of Laboratory Animal Resources (ILAR). Study of the PDX model for cervical cancers was approved by the Samsung Medical Center Institutional Review Board (IRB file number 2010-04-004) and experiments were performed in accordance with the approved guidelines and regulations.

2.8. Statistical Analysis

The Mann–Whitney U test was used to compare differences between the groups in both in vitro and in vivo assays. All statistical tests were two-sided, and P values less than 0.05 were considered to be statistically significant. SPSS software (Version 17.0; SPSS, Chicago, IL, USA) was used for all statistical analyses.

3. Results

3.1. Effects of TAO on Cell Viability, Apoptosis, and Cell Line Xenograft

In order to see the effects of TAO on cell viability, an MTT assay was performed in cervical cancer cell lines, including SiHa, HeLa, CaSki, and HUVECs. In all three cervical cancer cell lines and HUVECs, cell viability decreased as the concentration of TAO increased (Figure 1A). The IC$_{50}$ of TAO on SiHa, CaSki, and HUVEC at 72 h was 3 µM, and the IC$_{50}$ of HeLa was 0.6 µM (Table 1). The levels of active caspase-3 were also measured with Western blot. It was shown that active caspase-3 increased as the concentration of TAO increased, suggesting an increase of cellular apoptosis in all three cancer cell lines and HUVECs (Figure 1B). Mice bearing SiHa cell tumors were treated with TAO, which was injected intraperitoneally at 8 mg/kg body weight per injection, once a week. Calculated tumor volume was significantly smaller in animal models that were injected with TAO in comparison to those injected 0.9% sodium chloride control solution (Figure 1C).

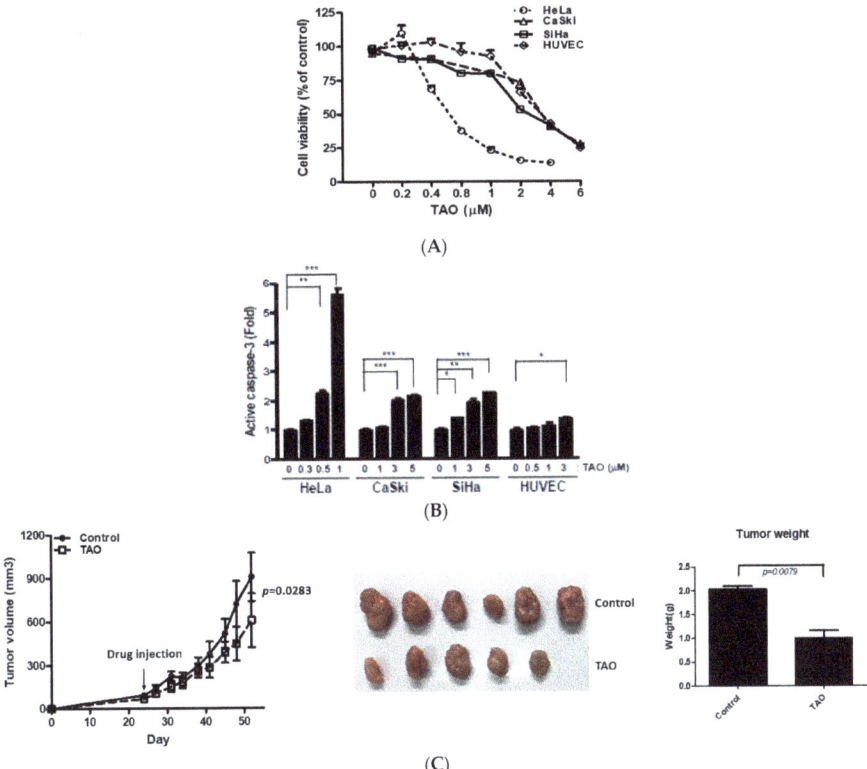

Figure 1. (**A**) Cellular metabolic activities in cervical cancer cell lines and human umbilical vein endothelial cells (HUVECs) measured by MTT assay. Decreasing cell viability with increasing concentration of tetraarsenic hexoxide (TAO) is shown; (**B**) Increasing levels of active caspase-3 are shown in cervical cancer cell lines and HUVECs as the concentration of TAO increases; (**C**) Significant difference is observed in tumor volumes between the mice bearing SiHa cells treated with TAO vs. 0.9% sodium chloride solution. The days represent post-implantation of tumor cells. TAO or 0.9% sodium chloride solution was injected once the tumor grew to a certain volume, which was about 85.5 mm^3 in the present experiments. The mean weight of the treatment group vs. control group shows a statistically significant difference. * p-value < 0.05, ** p-value < 0.01, *** p-value < 0.001.

Table 1. IC$_{50}$ values of TAO on HeLa, CaSki, SiHa cell lines and HUVEC measured by MTT (3-(4,5-dimethyl-thiazol-2-yl)-2,5-Diphenyl-tetrazolium bromide) assay at 72 h after the treatment.

Types of Cell Lines	IC50 (μM)
HeLa	0.6
CaSki	3.0
SiHa	3.0
HUVEC	3.0

3.2. Effects of TAO on MMP-2 and MMP-9

MMP-2 and MMP-9 were measured by ELISA to examine the inhibitory effects of TAO on extracellular matrix degradation and presumably cancer metastasis (Figure 2). The reduction of MMP-2 was observed by the treatment of TAO in SiHa cell lines. Compared to the expression levels of MMP-2 in SiHa cells that were neither treated by TAO nor VEGF, TAO reduced MMP-2 by about

80%. When SiHa cell lines were treated by both TAO and VEGF, the levels of MMP-2 also decreased significantly. Similar patterns were observed in HeLa and CaSki cell lines. The reduction of MMP-2 was observed by the treatment of TAO. Compared to the expression levels of MMP-2 in each cancer cell line that was not treated by either TAO or VEGF, TAO reduced MMP-2 by about 40% in HeLa and 60% in CaSki cell lines. When CaSki cell lines were treated with VEGF alone, MMP-2 was also reduced, but the reduction was not statistically significant. However, when they were treated with VEGF and TAO together, they showed approximately 25% additional reduction of MMP-2. When HeLa cell lines were treated with VEGF alone, MMP-2 increased by about 5%. However, when they were treated with VEGF and TAO together, they showed 50% reduction in MMP-2. When HUVECs were treated with VEGF, MMP-2 increased by more than 50%. However, the levels of MMP-2 significantly decreased when it was treated with TAO and VEGF together. When HUVECs were treated with TAO without VEGF, MMP-2 was also reduced by about 60%. The extent of reactivity to VEGF seemed to differ among cancer cell lines. However, it was evident that TAO reduced the expression levels of MMP-2, regardless of the seemingly different reactivity of cell lines to VEGF. We could not measure MMP-9 in cancer cell lines as it seemed that MMP-9 was too low to be detected in these cell lines.

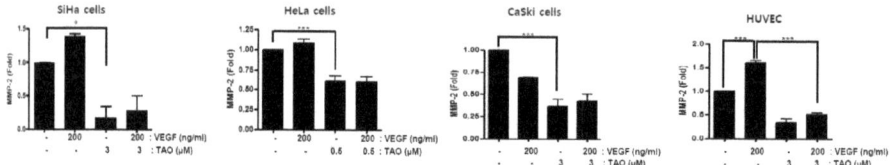

Figure 2. The concentrations of MMP-2 by enzyme-linked immunosorbent assay (ELISA). The treatment of TAO significantly decreased the concentrations of MMP-2 in all cervical cancer cell lines and HUVECs. The co-administration of vascular endothelial growth factor (VEGF) and TAO did not change the inhibitory effects of TAO on MMP-2, whereas the treatment of VEGF only mildly increased the concentrations of MMP-2 in SiHa and HeLa cell lines and HUVECs. * p-value < 0.05, *** p-value < 0.001.

3.3. Effects of TAO on the Activation of Akt

Akt (also known as protein kinase B (PKB)) is a serine/threonine protein kinase. Akt plays an important role in intracellular signaling pathways that are involved in glucose metabolism, apoptosis, cell proliferation, DNA transcription, and cell migration. It promotes cancer cell invasion by increasing motility and metalloproteinase production [13]. Western blot analysis of Akt and phosphorylated-Akt (p-Akt) were performed after the treatment of cervical cancer cell lines with TAO for 48 h. The results demonstrated that the levels of p-Akt decreased dose-dependently with the treatment of TAO in all HeLa, SiHa, and CaSki cell lines and HUVECs, suggesting the inhibitory effects of TAO (Figure 3A). The levels of total Akt, however, were not affected by the treatment of TAO and remained constant in all cancer cell lines and HUVECs as the concentration of TAO treatment increased.

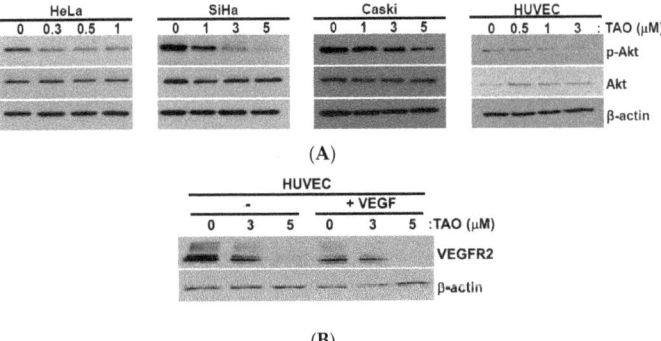

Figure 3. (**A**) Western blot analysis of Akt and phosphorylated-Akt (p-Akt) in the cell lines 48 h after the treatment of TAO with varying concentrations. The treatment of TAO decreases the phosphorylation of Akt. (**B**) Western blot analysis of vascular endothelial growth factor receptor 2 (VEGFR2), demonstrating that the treatment of TAO in HUVECs results in decreased concentration of VEGFR2. The same pattern of observation is seen in HUVEC, both with and without the treatment by vascular endothelial growth factor (VEGF).

3.4. Effects of TAO on VEGF-Related Signaling Pathway

HUVECs are known to be sensitive to vascular endothelial growth factor (VEGF). There are three receptor types of the VEGF signaling pathway, and VEGF receptor 2 (VEGFR2) is the major one among them. When the signal is initiated by VEGF, VEGFR2 is auto-phosphorylated, and the corresponding pathway is activated. To investigate the inhibiting effects of TAO on angiogenesis, we studied the response of VEGFR2 in HUVEC to TAO.

HUVECs were treated with TAO for 24 h, followed by Western blot analysis. As the concentration of TAO increased, the expression levels of VEGFR2 decreased. The same results were seen when the concurrent treatment of VEGF was performed (Figure 3B). These findings suggest that TAO suppresses the expression of VEGFR2, thereby exerting its inhibitory effects on the signaling pathway that is related to angiogenesis, regardless of the presence of signaling molecules.

3.5. Effects of TAO on Autophagy

To determine if TAO was involved in the autophagy pathway, p62, an intermediate of autophagy, and LC3, an autophagy marker protein, were analyzed by Western blot (Figure 4). It was shown that p62 increased with the treatment of TAO in all three cervical cancer cell lines. This implies that autophagy was reduced in the cell lines by TAO. The treatment of TAO also increased the concentrations of p62 in HUVECs. Conversion of LC3-I to LC3-II, a phosphatidylethanolamine-conjugated form of LC3-I, is a marker for autophagy activation. When autophagy is inhibited, LC3-II cannot be degraded by autolysosome and thereby accumulates in the cytoplasm. In cervical cancer cell lines and HUVECs, the accumulation of LC3-II was observed as the concentration of TAO increased, suggesting its inhibitory effects on autophagy.

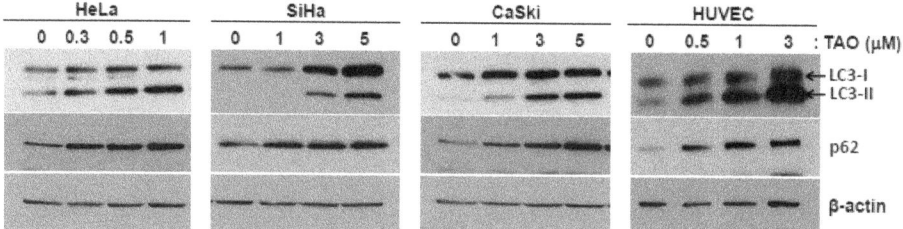

Figure 4. Western blot analysis of autophagy-related proteins in cervical cancer cell lines and HUVECs. The conversion of LC3-II increases as the concentration of TAO increases. Increasing concentrations of p62 are seen as concentrations of TAO increase, suggesting the inhibitory effects of TAO on autophagy.

3.6. Effects of TAO in Patient-Derived Xenograft (PDX) Mouse Models

Patient-derived xenograft (PDX) mouse models of invasive squamous cell carcinoma, adenocarcinoma, recurrent squamous cell carcinoma, and recurrent adenocarcinoma of the uterine cervical cancer were examined. Ten mice were treated with TAO (experimental group), while another 10 mice did not receive the treatment (control group). The mean tumor weight of the control group was measured. In the analysis of primary invasive squamous cell carcinoma PDX, the mean tumor weight of the control group was 2.31 g, while the mean tumor weight of the experimental group was 1.03 g (2.31 ± 1.52 vs. 1.03 ± 0.59, $p = 0.0232$), showing a statistically significant difference between the two groups (Figure 5). The same results were obtained in the PDX mouse models of adenocarcinoma. The mean tumor weight of the control group was 0.44 g, while the mean tumor weight of the treatment group was 0.30 g, with a statistical difference between the two groups (0.44 ± 0.18 vs. 0.30 ± 0.11, $p = 0.036$). The mean tumor weight of the control group in the analysis of recurrent squamous cell carcinoma was 4.43 g, and the mean tumor weight of the experimental group was 3.89 g (4.43 ± 2.17 vs. 3.89 ± 1.33, $p > 0.05$). No statistical difference was observed between the two groups in the recurrent squamous cell carcinoma models. The same experiments were also performed for recurrent adenocarcinoma. The mean tumor weight of the control group was 1.45 g, and the mean tumor weight of the experimental group was 1.41 g (1.45 ± 0.77 vs. 1.41 ± 0.68, $p > 0.05$). Recurrent tumors seemed to have gained resistance to cytotoxic agents and did not respond to the treatment of TAO. The terminal deoxynucleotidyl transferase dUTP nick end labeling (TUNEL) assay was performed to measure DNA fragmentation generated during apoptosis, as described previously [14]. While TUNEL positive cells increased significantly in the tumors of mouse models treated with TAO in primary squamous cell carcinoma and adenocarcinoma, this observation was not seen in the mouse models of recurrent diseases. The Ki-67 protein, a cellular marker for proliferation, was measured in the tumors of the mouse models as well [15]. As seen in Figure 5, the amount of Ki-67 positive cells significantly decreased after the treatment of TAO in primary cancer models, while it did not change in recurrent cancer models.

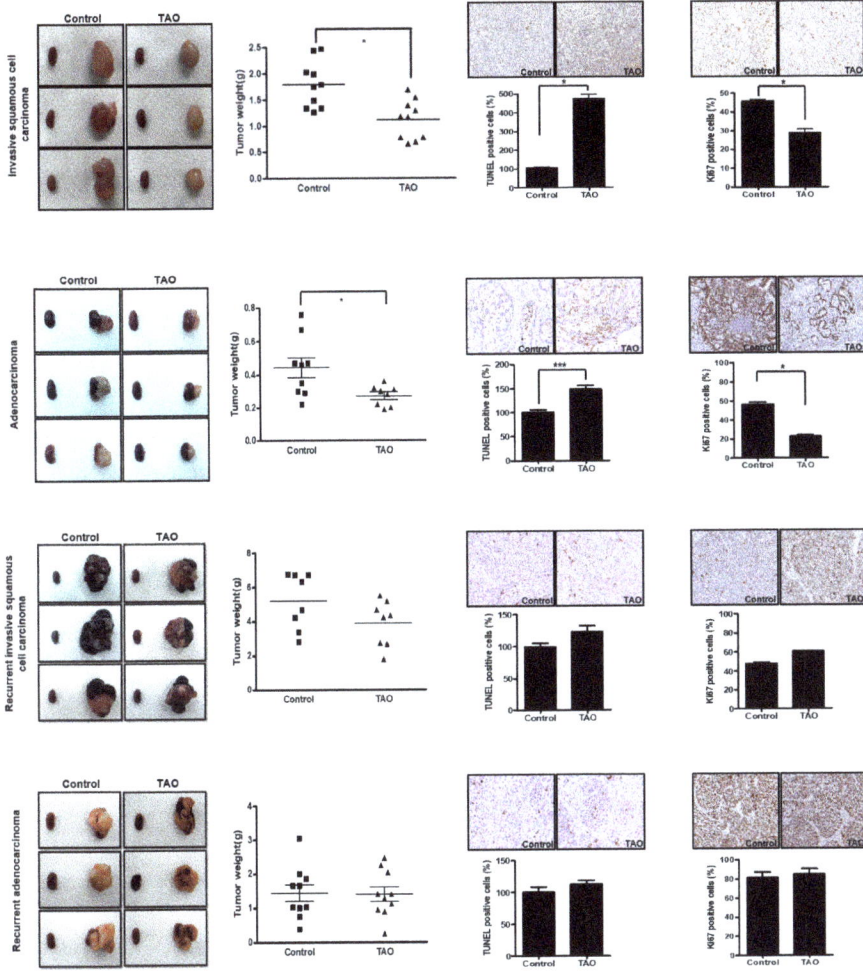

Figure 5. Gross appearance of xenograft from mouse models with primary invasive squamous cell carcinoma, adenocarcinoma, recurrent invasive squamous cell carcinoma, and recurrent adenocarcinoma of the cervix. The tumors of the control group (**left**) vs. the TAO-treated (8 mg/kg) experimental group (**right**) are shown, demonstrating statistically significant differences of tumor weight between the two groups in the primary cancer models. However, this difference is not seen in recurrent cancer models. The TUNEL assay and Ki-67 assay also show the anti-cancer effects of TAO in primary cancer models, while these effects are not seen in recurrent cancer models. * p-value < 0.05, *** p-value < 0.001.

3.7. Effects of Combination of TAO with Cisplatin in PDX Mouse Models

In order to investigate the potential synergistic effects of TAO in addition to conventional cytotoxic agent cisplatin, mouse models were assigned to one of the four groups: control, cisplatin alone, TAO alone, or cisplatin plus TAO. When mouse models with primary invasive squamous cell carcinoma were evaluated, the mean tumor weight of the mouse models that were given cisplatin plus TAO was significantly less than the other three groups (0.94 ± 0.56 vs. 1.84 ± 0.95 vs. 1.30 ± 0.38 vs. 1.61 ± 0.60 g in cisplatin plus TAO, control, cisplatin alone, and TAO alone groups, respectively, p = 0.0315). The same patterns of the synergistic anti-cancer effects of TAO with cisplatin were observed in the mouse models generated from recurrent squamous cell carcinoma and recurrent adenocarcinoma (Figure 6). The TUNEL assay and Ki-67 assay were also performed. The synergistic effects of TAO with cisplatin were observed not only in primary cancer models but also in recurrent cancer models.

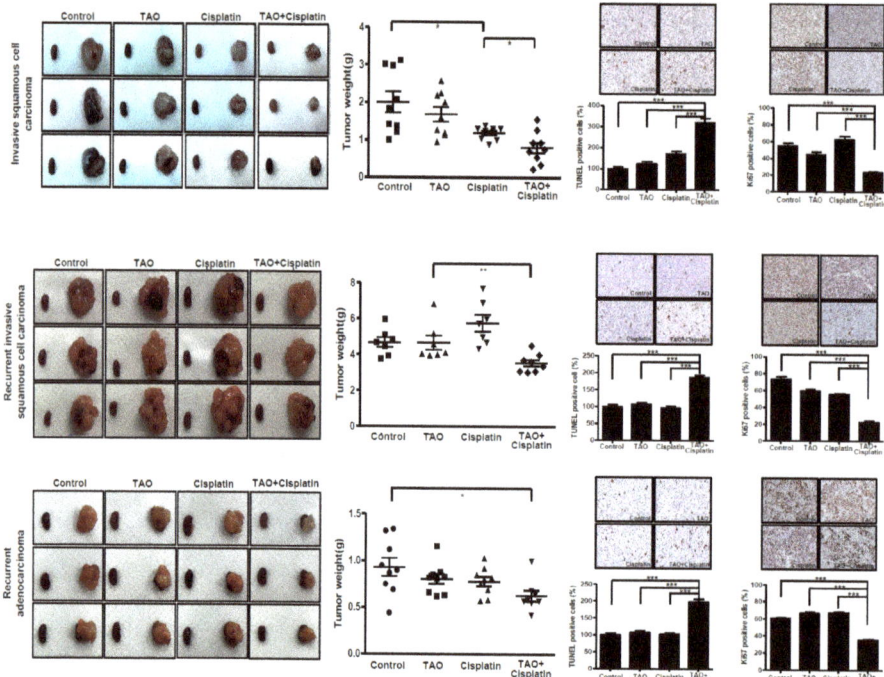

Figure 6. Gross appearance of xenograft from mouse models receiving PBS, TAO (8 mg/kg), cisplatin (4 mg/kg), and TAO plus cisplatin (8 mg/kg of TAO and 4 mg/kg of cisplatin) in order from left to right. Significant reductions of tumor weight in mouse models given TAO plus cisplatin are observed in primary invasive squamous cell carcinoma as well as in recurrent invasive squamous cell carcinoma and adenocarcinoma. The TUNEL assay and Ki-67 assay results also support the synergistic effects of TAO with cisplatin, both in primary and recurrent cancer models. * p-value < 0.05, ** p-value < 0.01, *** p-value < 0.001.

4. Discussion

The present study demonstrated that TAO has anti-cancer effects in patient-derived xenograft mouse models of cervical cancer in vivo, and these results were supported by the experiments with cervical cancer cell lines in vitro. Although the exact mechanisms by which TAO exerts its inhibitory effects on cancer cells is yet to be fully defined, we herein established evidence that it is involved in the regulation of autophagy and angiogenesis of cancer cells to a certain extent. To our knowledge, no previous studies have shown such effects of TAO.

Cervical cancer carries a significant burden on patients, the medical field, and society. Despite widespread screening programs and available vaccinations, it remains one of the most difficult types of cancer to conquer, especially in developing countries. Cervical cancer carries a poor prognosis, and the current standard treatment modalities, especially for advanced stages, do not yield promising clinical results. Although bevacizumab has demonstrated improved survival rates and overall response rates in recurrent cervical cancer in a clinical trial, which has consequently permitted its use as the current standard treatment regimen, further studies to develop efficient and innovative treatment approaches are urgently needed [16].

Preclinical studies have provided some potential therapeutic benefits of TAO on cervical cancer. Studies have shown that it induces cell cycle arrest in the G1 or G2/M phase and suppresses the secretion of MMP-2, which is consistent with the results of the present study. TAO has also been shown to inhibit the phosphorylation of Akt, an upstream signaling protein in MMP-2 and 9 expressions in both cervical cancer cell lines and HUVECs [17]. TAO may also inhibit angiogenesis via downregulation of VEGFR2 expression. In the present study, TAO was shown to inhibit VEGF-induced MMP-2 expression in HUVEC. Because tumor cell metastasis is a complex cascade of events involving multiple steps such as proliferation, adhesion, and migration of cells, an attempt to understand the exact alterations caused by TAO in these intricate relations of different mechanisms is demanding, and there are also other possible mechanisms facilitated within the intricate network of regulatory effects.

Hypoxia and lack of nutrition are a hallmark of cancer tissue, and cancer cells often activate autophagy to evade such conditions. Therefore, autophagy has been considered as one of the survival pathways that growing cancer cells adopt, and its inhibition has been studied for treatment modalities of cancer. The present study demonstrates that the treatment of TAO increases the expression of p62, which normally decreases as the rate of autophagy increases. Although further investigations are warranted to delineate the exact mechanisms of how TAO inhibits autophagy, the evidence shown in the present study provides support for the potential efficacy of TAO as a cancer treatment agent by inducing autophagy. The effects of TAO on the cellular process of autophagy in normal tissue should also be studied because non-specific and global inhibition of autophagy may lead to unwanted clinical consequences.

The interaction of TAO with conventional chemotherapeutic agents and its additive or subtractive effects should also be evaluated. It has been illustrated that arsenic trioxide has a synergistic effect in combination with cisplatin in ovarian cancer cells [18]. Another research group reported the potential synergistic effects of TAO with cisplatin in cervical cancer cells [19,20]. They also reported that the combination of cisplatin with TAO was more effective than the combination of cisplatin with paclitaxel in cervical cancer [20]. The present study suggested the inhibitory effects of TAO on angiogenesis as a possible explanation for the observed results. We also found that the combination of TAO with cisplatin was more effective than cisplatin alone in the PDX mouse model. This effect was seen even in the mouse models with recurrent tumors. Taken together, these results offer further support for the use of TAO in cancer treatment, possibly as a combined regimen with chemotherapeutic agents with previously revealed clinical efficacy.

The lack of significant reduction of cancer tissue in the PDX models of recurrent cervical cancer compared to the substantial decrease in naïve cancer tissue from the TAO treatment is noteworthy. It is thought that the mechanisms by which cells gain resistance to conventional chemotherapeutic agents contribute to the lack of inhibitory effects of TAO seen in recurrent cancer models, and further investigations are necessary.

The strengths of the present study include the utilization of different histology of cervical cancer, such as squamous cell carcinoma, adenocarcinoma, and recurrent cervical cancer. It also employs experiments with cell lines to understand the changes in multiple signaling pathways caused by TAO, as well as xenograft mouse models to validate the eventual consequences of it. One of the limitations of the present study is that it did not evaluate the effects of human papillomavirus (HPV) infection status of tumor cells. Cervical cancer is unique in that most malignant cells are caused by HPV infection. Although TAO has been shown to induce apoptosis of various cancer cell lines, including both HPV-infected and non-infected cells, the mechanisms by which it induces apoptosis may be different [21].

In conclusion, the present study shows that TAO has anti-tumor effects in various types of treatment-naïve cervical cancer cell lines, including squamous cell carcinoma and adenocarcinoma, and these effects are presumably due to its inhibitory effects on autophagy, angiogenesis, and the induction of apoptosis. The potential usefulness of TAO for cervical cancer treatment is thus suggested. Clinical trials of TAO are also suggested to further explore the potential use of TAO in cancer treatment.

Supplementary Materials: The following are available online at http://www.mdpi.com/1999-4923/12/10/987/s1, Figure S1: T2 sagittal magnetic resonance imaging (MRI) of the cancer lesion that was used to generate the patient-derived xenograft (PDX) I. Figure S2: T2 sagittal MRI of the cancer lesion that was used to generate the PDX II. Figure S3: T2 sagittal MRI of the cancer lesion that was used to generate the PDX III. Figure S4: T2 transverse MRI of the cancer lesion that was used to generate the PDX IV (top). Figure S5: T2 transverse MRI of the cancer lesion that was used to generate the PDX V (top). Table S1: Clinical information of the patients for patient-derived xenograft (PDX).

Author Contributions: Conceptualization, J.-W.L.; methodology, J.R.H. and B.-G.K.; investigation, Y.-J.C., S.-Y.J., Y.-Y.L., J.-Y.R., J.-J.C., and Z.W.; writing, J.J.N. and M.-S.K.; funding acquisition, I.B. All authors have read and agreed to the published version of the manuscript.

Funding: This research was funded by the National Research Foundation of Korea (NRF) grant funded by the Korean government (Ministry of Education, Science and Technology, MEST) (2016R1A2B3006644), the National Research Foundation of Korea (NRF) grant funded by the Korean government (Ministry of Science and Information Technology, MSIT) (2020R1C1C1007482), and a grant from CHEMAS Co., Ltd.'s development project for research (Korea).

Conflicts of Interest: The authors declare no conflict of interest. Wu Zhaoyan is a full-time employee of Chemas company. He is a full-tile researcher and has contributed to the experiment. The funders had no role in the design of the study, in the collection, analyses, or interpretation of data or any other process of the publication.

References

1. Altobelli, E.; Rapacchietta, L.; Profeta, V.F.; Fagnano, R. HPV-vaccination and cancer cervical screening in 53 WHO European Countries: An update on prevention programs according to income level. *Cancer Med.* **2019**, *8*, 2524–2534. [CrossRef] [PubMed]
2. Stehman, F.B.; Bundy, B.N.; DiSaia, P.J.; Keys, H.M.; Larson, J.E.; Fowler, W.C. Carcinoma of the cervix treated with radiation therapy. I. A multi-variate analysis of prognostic variables in the Gynecologic Oncology Group. *Cancer* **1991**, *67*, 2776–2785. [CrossRef]
3. Delgado, G.; Bundy, B.; Zaino, R.; Sevin, B.U.; Creasman, W.T.; Major, F. Prospective surgical-pathological study of disease-free interval in patients with stage IB squamous cell carcinoma of the cervix: A Gynecologic Oncology Group study. *Gynecol. Oncol.* **1990**, *38*, 352–357. [CrossRef]
4. Chan, C.K.; Aimagambetova, G.; Ukybassova, T.; Kongrtay, K.; Azizan, A. Human Papillomavirus Infection and Cervical Cancer: Epidemiology, Screening, and Vaccination-Review of Current Perspectives. *J. Oncol.* **2019**, *2019*, 3257939. [CrossRef] [PubMed]
5. Vernhet, L.; Allain, N.; Le Vee, M.; Morel, F.; Guillouzo, A.; Fardel, O. Blockage of multidrug resistance-associated proteins potentiates the inhibitory effects of arsenic trioxide on CYP1A1 induction by polycyclic aromatic hydrocarbons. *J. Pharmacol. Exp. Ther.* **2003**, *304*, 145–155. [CrossRef]
6. Zhang, X.W.; Yan, X.J.; Zhou, Z.R.; Yang, F.F.; Wu, Z.Y.; Sun, H.B.; Liang, W.X.; Song, A.X.; Lallemand-Breitenbach, V.; Jeanne, M.; et al. Arsenic trioxide controls the fate of the PML-RARalpha oncoprotein by directly binding PML. *Science* **2010**, *328*, 240–243. [CrossRef]
7. Dai, J.; Weinberg, R.S.; Waxman, S.; Jing, Y. Malignant cells can be sensitized to undergo growth inhibition and apoptosis by arsenic trioxide through modulation of the glutathione redox system. *Blood* **1999**, *93*, 268–277. [CrossRef]
8. Zhu, X.H.; Shen, Y.L.; Jing, Y.K.; Cai, X.; Jia, P.M.; Huang, Y.; Tang, W.; Shi, G.Y.; Sun, Y.P.; Dai, J.; et al. Apoptosis and growth inhibition in malignant lymphocytes after treatment with arsenic trioxide at clinically achievable concentrations. *J. Natl. Cancer Inst.* **1999**, *91*, 772–778. [CrossRef]
9. Kim, J.H.; Lew, Y.S.; Kolozsvary, A.; Ryu, S.; Brown, S.L. Arsenic trioxide enhances radiation response of 9 L glioma in the rat brain. *Radiat. Res.* **2003**, *160*, 662–666. [CrossRef] [PubMed]
10. Lew, Y.S.; Brown, S.L.; Griffin, R.J.; Song, C.W.; Kim, J.H. Arsenic trioxide causes selective necrosis in solid murine tumors by vascular shutdown. *Cancer Res.* **1999**, *59*, 6033–6037. [PubMed]
11. Heo, E.J.; Cho, Y.J.; Cho, W.C.; Hong, J.E.; Jeon, H.K.; Oh, D.Y.; Choi, Y.L.; Song, S.Y.; Choi, J.J.; Bae, D.S.; et al. Patient-Derived Xenograft Models of Epithelial Ovarian Cancer for Preclinical Studies. *Cancer Res. Treat.* **2017**, *49*, 915–926. [CrossRef] [PubMed]
12. Oh, D.Y.; Kim, S.; Choi, Y.L.; Cho, Y.J.; Oh, E.; Choi, J.J.; Jung, K.; Song, J.Y.; Ahn, S.E.; Kim, B.G.; et al. HER2 as a novel therapeutic target for cervical cancer. *Oncotarget* **2015**, *6*, 36219–36230. [CrossRef]

13. Kim, D.; Kim, S.; Koh, H.; Yoon, S.O.; Chung, A.S.; Cho, K.S.; Chung, J. Akt/PKB promotes cancer cell invasion via increased motility and metalloproteinase production. *FASEB J.* **2001**, *15*, 1953–1962. [CrossRef] [PubMed]
14. Kyrylkova, K.; Kyryachenko, S.; Leid, M.; Kioussi, C. Detection of apoptosis by TUNEL assay. *Methods Mol. Biol.* **2012**, *887*, 41–47. [CrossRef] [PubMed]
15. Bullwinkel, J.; Baron-Luhr, B.; Ludemann, A.; Wohlenberg, C.; Gerdes, J.; Scholzen, T. Ki-67 protein is associated with ribosomal RNA transcription in quiescent and proliferating cells. *J. Cell. Physiol.* **2006**, *206*, 624–635. [CrossRef] [PubMed]
16. Tewari, K.S.; Sill, M.W.; Long, H.J., 3rd; Penson, R.T.; Huang, H.; Ramondetta, L.M.; Landrum, L.M.; Oaknin, A.; Reid, T.J.; Leitao, M.M.; et al. Improved survival with bevacizumab in advanced cervical cancer. *N. Engl. J. Med.* **2014**, *370*, 734–743. [CrossRef] [PubMed]
17. Woo, S.H.; Park, M.J.; An, S.; Lee, H.C.; Jin, H.O.; Lee, S.J.; Gwak, H.S.; Park, I.C.; Hong, S.I.; Rhee, C.H. Diarsenic and tetraarsenic oxide inhibit cell cycle progression and bFGF- and VEGF-induced proliferation of human endothelial cells. *J. Cell. Biochem.* **2005**, *95*, 120–130. [CrossRef]
18. Zhang, N.; Wu, Z.M.; McGowan, E.; Shi, J.; Hong, Z.B.; Ding, C.W.; Xia, P.; Di, W. Arsenic trioxide and cisplatin synergism increase cytotoxicity in human ovarian cancer cells: Therapeutic potential for ovarian cancer. *Cancer Sci.* **2009**, *100*, 2459–2464. [CrossRef]
19. Mi Byun, J.; Hoon Jeong, D.; Sim Lee, D.; Ran Kim, J.; Nam Kim, Y.; Jeong Jeong, E.; Sung, M.; Bok Lee, K.; Tae Kim, K. Inhibition of Cell Growth and Apoptosis in CaSki, Cervical Cancer Cell Line by Arsenic Compounds. *Obstet. Gynecol. Sci.* **2010**, *53*, 616–625.
20. Byun, J.M.; Jeong, D.H.; Lee, D.S.; Kim, J.R.; Park, S.G.; Kang, M.S.; Kim, Y.N.; Lee, K.B.; Sung, M.S.; Kim, K.T. Tetraarsenic oxide and cisplatin induce apoptotic synergism in cervical cancer. *Oncol. Rep.* **2013**, *29*, 1540–1546. [CrossRef]
21. Wang, H.; Gao, P.; Zheng, J. Arsenic trioxide inhibits cell proliferation and human papillomavirus oncogene expression in cervical cancer cells. *Biochem. Biophys. Res. Commun.* **2014**, *451*, 556–561. [CrossRef] [PubMed]

Publisher's Note: MDPI stays neutral with regard to jurisdictional claims in published maps and institutional affiliations.

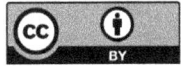

© 2020 by the authors. Licensee MDPI, Basel, Switzerland. This article is an open access article distributed under the terms and conditions of the Creative Commons Attribution (CC BY) license (http://creativecommons.org/licenses/by/4.0/).

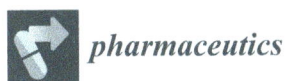

Article

Enhanced Antisense Oligonucleotide Delivery Using Cationic Liposomes Grafted with Trastuzumab: A Proof-of-Concept Study in Prostate Cancer

Guillaume Sicard [1], Clément Paris [2], Sarah Giacometti [1], Anne Rodallec [1], Joseph Ciccolini [1], Palma Rocchi [2,*] and Raphaëlle Fanciullino [1]

[1] SMARTc Unit, CRCM Inserm U1068, Aix Marseille University, 13007 Marseille, France; guillaume.sicard@univ-amu.fr (G.S.); sarah.giacometti@univ-amu.fr (S.G.); anne.rodallec@univ-amu.fr (A.R.); joseph.ciccolini@univ-amu.fr (J.C.); raphaelle.fanciullino@univ-amu.fr (R.F.)
[2] CNRS, INSERM, Institut Paoli-Calmettes, CRCM, Aix Marseille University, 13007 Marseille, France; clement.paris@inserm.fr
* Correspondence: palma.rocchi@inserm.fr

Received: 13 November 2020; Accepted: 27 November 2020; Published: 29 November 2020

Abstract: Prostate cancer (PCa) is the second most common cancer in men worldwide and the fifth leading cause of death by cancer. The overexpression of TCTP protein plays an important role in castration resistance. Over the last decade, antisense technology has emerged as a rising strategy in oncology. Using antisense oligonucleotide (ASO) to silence TCTP protein is a promising therapeutic option—however, the pharmacokinetics of ASO does not always meet the requirements of proper delivery to the tumor site. In this context, developing drug delivery systems is an attractive strategy for improving the efficacy of ASO directed against TCTP. The liposome should protect and deliver ASO at the intracellular level in order to be effective. In addition, because prostate cancer cells express Her2, using an anti-Her2 targeting antibody will increase the affinity of the liposome for the cell and optimize the intratumoral penetration of the ASO, thus improving efficacy. Here, we have designed and developed pegylated liposomes and Her2-targeting immunoliposomes. Mean diameter was below 200 nm, thus ensuring proper enhanced permeation and retention (EPR) effect. Encapsulation rate for ASO was about 40%. Using human PC-3 prostate cancer cells as a canonical model, free ASO and ASO encapsulated into either liposomes or anti-Her2 immunoliposomes were tested for efficacy in vitro using 2D and 3D spheroid models. While the encapsulated forms of ASO were always more effective than free ASO, we observed differences in efficacy of encapsulated ASO. For short exposure times (i.e., 4 h) ASO liposomes (ASO-Li) were more effective than ASO-immunoliposomes (ASO-iLi). Conversely, for longer exposure times, ASO-iLi performed better than ASO-Li. This pilot study demonstrates that it is possible to encapsulate ASO into liposomes and to yield antiproliferative efficacy against PCa. Importantly, despite mild Her2 expression in this PC-3 model, using a surface mAb as targeting agent provides further efficacy, especially when exposure is longer. Overall, the development of third-generation ASO-iLi should help to take advantage of the expression of Her2 by prostate cancer cells in order to allow greater specificity of action in vivo and thus a gain in efficacy.

Keywords: liposomes; immunoliposomes; antisense oligonucleotides; prostate cancer

1. Introduction

Prostate cancer (PCa) is the second most common cancer in men worldwide with 1.3 million new cases in 2018. PCa is the fifth leading cause of death by cancer with more than 360,000 deaths in

2018, despite a decrease in its incidence by 6% over 2005–2009 [1,2]. At initial diagnosis, treatment depends on the stage based on Gleason score, the patient's characteristics and the PSA level [3,4]. Surgical treatment, i.e., prostatectomy, is the standard of care, but patients with advanced disease (i.e., stages III or IV, high Gleason score) are precluded. The first-line therapy for advanced PCa is castration therapy which consists in androgen deprivation since it is a hormone-sensitive cancer [5]. After a period of therapeutic response, usually 1–3 years, patients will ultimately become resistant to the therapy and develop metastases. A new approach is therefore needed for these castration-resistant PCa (CRPCa) patients.

The overexpression of the TCTP protein plays an important role in PCa and most particularly in CRPCa [6]. Indeed, this protein is involved in progression of the disease and therapeutic failure. The interactions between TCTP and p53 and their negative feedback regulation loop are responsible for progression and invasion of PCa [7,8]. Recently, antisense technology has emerged as a promising strategy in cancer [9]. The principle of this approach is the sequence-specific binding of an antisense oligonucleotide (ASO) to target mRNA, thus preventing gene translation [10]. The development of an ASO directed against TCTP seems therefore to be an interesting strategy [11]. The shutting down of TCTP by ASO is expected to restore apoptosis and sensitivity to hormone-therapy and chemotherapy of cancer cells. ASOs are only active after cell uptake, and therefore, a carrier is necessary to help them pass the membranes. In this context, developing carriers to transport ASO is an attractive strategy, especially since nanoparticles are increasingly considered to stretch the efficacy/toxicity balance of a variety of anticancer agents or payloads [12–14]. Various other technological approaches such as the direct pegylation of compounds [15] or using Nab conjugates [16] or antibody–drug conjugates [17,18] illustrate this major trend to develop drug carriers in oncology today. One of the critical points when developing nanoparticles is based on their size being <200 nm. Nanoparticles leave the vascular compartment and accumulate in the interstitial space next to the tumor. This phenomenon is called passive targeting or the enhanced permeability and retention (EPR) effect [19].

Our study is based upon this double trend of encapsulation and use of therapeutic monoclonal antibodies to improve the specificity of nanoparticles against tumors. The conjunction of these two concepts results in a new nanoparticle, the antibody nanoconjugate (ANC), more commonly called the immunoliposome [20,21]. In this study, we present the early development steps of an innovative stealth liposomal ASO nanoparticle targeting prostate cancer through anti-Her2 functionalization [22] (Figure 1).

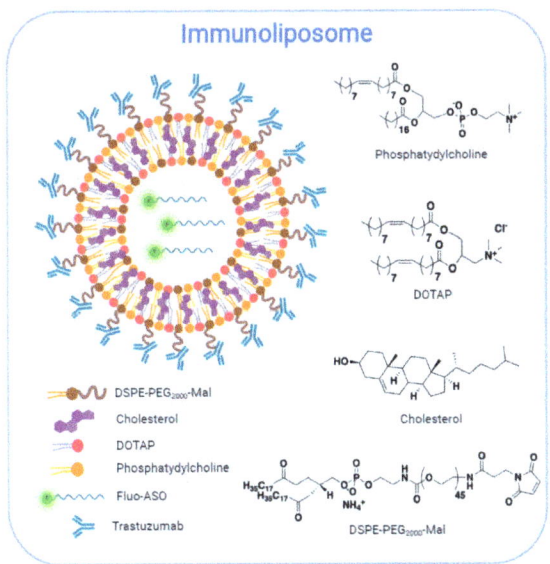

Figure 1. Schematic representation of the immunoliposome structure and composition.

2. Materials and Methods

2.1. Cell Lines

Experiments were carried on canonical human prostate cancer cell line PC-3 (American Type Culture Collection, Rockville, MD, USA) Cells were cultured in RPMI supplemented with 10% FBS, 1% penicillin and 0.16% kanamycin and grown in a humidified 5% CO_2 incubator at 37 °C. Cells were regularly authenticated in terms of cell viability, morphology and doubling time. For Her2 characterization, breast cancer cell lines, i.e., MDA231, MDA 453 and SKBR3, were used (American Type Culture Collection, Manassas, VA, USA).

2.2. Drugs and Chemicals

1,2-distearoyl-*sn*-glycero-3-phosphoethanolamine-N-(aleimide(polyethyleneglycol)-2000) (Mal-PEG) and 1,2-dioleoyl-3-trimethylammoniumpropane (DOTAP) were purchased from COGER (Paris, France). Egg yolk phosphatidylcholine (PC) and cholesterol (Chol) were purchased from Sigma (St-Quentin-Fallavier, France). ASO was purchased from Eurofins (Les Ullis, France). 2-iminothiolane (Traut's reagent) and Draq5 were purchased from Fisher Scientific (Illkirch-Graffenstaden, France). QuantiBRITE phycoerythrin (PE) and PE Mouse Anti-Human Her-2/neu were purchased from BD Biosciences (San Jose, CA, USA). Trastuzumab (Herceptin) was kindly given by Genentech (South San Francisco, CA, USA). All other reagents were of analytical grade.

2.3. ASO Stability in Solvents

ASO stability in three solvents, i.e., NaCl 0.9%, water and methanol, was tested over one month.
HPLC detection was performed on an HPLC (Agilent 1260, Agilent, Les Ulis, France). The HPLC column Xbrige OST C18 2.5 μm 4.6 × 50 mm (Waters, Guyancourt, France) was equilibrated at a flow rate of 0.8 mL/min. Eluant A contained 0.1 M TEAA (Triethylammonium acetate) in 5% ACN (acetonitrile) in water and eluant B contained ACN. The elution gradient was 0 to 45% in 10 min. ASO was detected at the wavelength of 260 nm. Ninety microliters of ASO in NaCl 0.9% and ASO

in water were directly injected. For ASO in MeOH, 100 µL of sample was evaporated to dryness; the sample was resuspended in water, and then 90 µL was injected.

2.4. Pegylated Liposome Preparation

Two different compositions of liposomes were studied: formulation 1, using DOTAP, Mal-PEG and Chol, and formulation 2, using DOTAP, PC, Mal-PEG and Chol.

Both compositions were prepared using the classic thin-film method [23]. Briefly, lipids were dissolved in methanol as organic solvent. Methanol was then removed by rotary evaporation (Laborota 4003, Heidolph Instruments, Schwabach, Germany) at 38 °C under vacuum to avoid further toxicity. After 30 min, a thin lipid film was obtained. To remove the residual solvent, lipid film was dried under a stream of nitrogen for 2 h at room temperature. The film was then hydrated with a 5% v/v dextrose solution in water for formulation 1 or a 0.9% v/v sodium chloride solution in water for formulation 2, and then multilamellar vesicle (MLV) liposomes were obtained. Extrusion step was performed to reduce and homogenize liposomes in size through two 0.1 µm and two 0.08 µm polycarbonate pore membranes (Nucleopore, Whatman, Maidstone, UK) using LipoFast LF-50, and then small unilamellar vesicle (SUV) liposomes were obtained [24].

For each formulation, liposomes (i.e., ASO-Li-1 for formulation 1 and ASO-Li-1 for formulation 2) and immunoliposomes (i.e., ASO-iLi-1 and ASO-iLi-2) were generated.

2.5. Pegylated Immunoliposome Preparation: Encapsulation Strategies

Different encapsulation strategies were tested with both formulations.

With formulation 1, ASO was introducing in methanol with lipids during the thin lipid film formation. Extraction from liposome was performed by 100 µL methanol for 100 µL liposome.

With formulation 2, three different strategies were tested. First, ASO was included in aqueous solvent, i.e., sodium chloride 0.9%, during the hydration step of the lipidic film. ASO was also included in preformed liposomes by contact using other strategies, namely soft agitation by rotation at 38 °C or fast agitation using bar magnet at 38 °C.

Besides, a new extraction technique was used with a chloroform–methanol solution (1:2 ratio) [25]. For each 100 µL of liposome solution, we added 375 µL of chloroform–methanol solution. Then, 125 µL of chloroform was added to the sample and vortexed. Afterward, 125 µL of MilliQ water was added to the sample and vortexed again. Finally, the sample was centrifugated at 1500× g for 90 s. The topper phase contained the ASO freed from the lipids. The entire aqueous phase was recuperated, evaporated and reconstituted with 100 µL of MilliQ water.

2.6. Pegylated Immunoliposome Preparation: Antibody Engraftment

Trastuzumab engraftment was performed from previously obtained liposome, generating immunoliposome.

The engraftment was carried out by maleimide–thiol conjugation after having previously derivatized the trastuzumab with thiol function. To this end, trastuzumab was first dissolved in a 0.1 M sodium phosphate-buffered saline (PBS), pH 8.0, containing 5 mM ethylene diamine tetra-acetic acid, and mixed under constant shaking for 2 h at room temperature with a Traut's reagent solution at 1:10 molar ratio (Traut's/trastuzumab). Thiolated trastuzumab was then directly mixed with the pegylated liposomes at 1:127 molar ratio (trastuzumab/MAL-PEG).

The mixture was kept under constant shaking at 4 °C overnight. Unbound trastuzumab and free ASO were removed from the liposomal solution using 6000× g centrifugation on MWCO 300 KDa Vivaspin (VWR, Fontenay-sous-Bois, France) [26].

2.7. Size and Polydispersity Study

Size and polydispersity index (PDI) of liposomes and immunoliposomes were measured by dynamic light scattering (DLS). Analysis parameters were as follows: medium: PBS solution, viscosity of water: 0.8937, temperature: 25 °C, dielectric constant: negative but not used in these measurements, nanoparticles: liposomes, refractive index of water: 1.333 cP, detection angle: 173°, wavelength: 632.8 nm, software for analysis of data: Zetasizer Nano software v3.30.

Liposomes and immunoliposomes were diluted in a PBS solution and then analyzed by a Zetasizer Nano S (Malvern Instruments, Malvern, UK). Liposomal preparations were considered unimodal for a PDI < 0.2. The measures were performed extemporaneously after liposome formation for both formulations in triplicate.

Stability study was performed at 7, 14 and 28 days after liposome formation.

2.8. ASO Encapsulation Rate

ASO encapsulation rate was only determined for formulation 2 by fluorescence (495/520 nm). After grafting ASO with FITC in 3′ (Eurofins, Les Ullis, France), ASO–FITC encapsulation rate was determined by measuring the FITC fluorescence at 520 nm (PHERAstar FSX, BMG Labtech, Ortenberg, Germany) [27]. All the measures were performed in triplicate.

2.9. Quantification of HER2 on Cells

Flow cytometry analysis allowed measuring the expression of Her2 on the surface of PC-3 cells [28].

As previously described [29], QuantiBRITE PE (BD Biosciences, San Jose, USA) was used to estimate the absolute number of Her2 receptors on cell membranes. About 100,000 cells of PC-3 were incubated under saturated conditions with PE Mouse Anti-Human HER-2/neu (BD Biosciences, San Jose, USA) for 30 min at 4 °C before being rinsed with PBS. IgG2a-PE anti-mouse antibodies (Fisher Scientific, Illkirch, France) were used for isotopic control. Analysis was then immediately performed on Gallios Beckman Coulter. Assuming our anti-HER-2 PE antibody has a 1:1 fluorochrome/antibody ratio, PE median fluorescence intensity (MFI) was measured for all cell lines and reported on a log–log graph with MFI vs. PE molecules, after subtracting isotopic control MFI. All the measures were performed in triplicate.

2.10. In Vitro Assays

Spheroids were obtained with PC-3 cells seeded with 20% methylcellulose solution on a 96-well U-bottom plate for at least 24 h before the experiment began. Different drug concentrations and scheduling conditions were tested on 5000-cell spheroids. Viability was assessed by bioluminescence assay. The cell viability in bioluminescence was determined on PC-3 cells using luminescent cell viability assay (CellTiter-Glo, Promega, Madison, WI, USA) and bioluminescence reading (PHERAstar FSX; BMG Labtech, Ortenberg, Germany). Cellular uptake was observed using confocal microscopy (TCS SP2 Leica) coupled to a digital camera.

Using 5000-cell spheroids, we determined nontoxic concentrations of lipid treated on day 1 and day 8 with viability determined in bioluminescence at day 15.

Subsequently, in a first protocol, we tested one nontoxic concentration of lipid (i.e., 8 nM) following day 3 and day 10 (after spheroid formation) treatment schedule with viability assay on day 15 or only at day 3 with viability assay at day 15. Encapsulated ASO concentration (i.e., after lipidic film formation) at 150 nM was tested. Cells were exposed to treatment for four hours on Day 3 and/or day 10. After four hours of exposure, treatment was removed and replaced by supplemented RPMI.

In a second protocol, using 5000-cell spheroids, we tested two nontoxic concentrations of lipid (i.e., 2 and 8 nM) following day 3 and day 10 treatment schedule with viability assay on day 15. Encapsulated ASO concentration (i.e., after lipidic film formation) at 150 nM was tested. Empty liposomes and immunoliposomes, for each nontoxic lipid concentration, were used as control.

2.11. Statistical Analysis

Formulation experiments were performed at least in triplicate and data were represented as mean ± SD or ±standard error of the mean. Statistical analyses were performed on MedCalc 17.2.1. Software (MedCalc, Acacialaan, Belgium).

In vitro experiment was performed at least in triplicate and data were represented as mean ± SD or ±standard error of the mean. All statistical analyses were performed with car [30] and multcomp [31] packages of the software R [32].

3. Results

3.1. ASO Stability in Solvents

ASO stability has been studied in three different solvents. Sodium chloride 0.9% solution was tested because it was used during the hydration step of the lipidic film during liposome formation, water was used because lyophilized ASO was reconstituted with it and methanol was the organic solvent used for lipid dissolution before lipid film formation and for liposome extraction.

Results show that ASO is stable in the three solvents over 32 days. Thus, formulation tests can be carried out by including ASO in the organic phase (methanol) or in the hydration solvent (NaCl 0.9%) without fear of deterioration of the ASO (Figure 2).

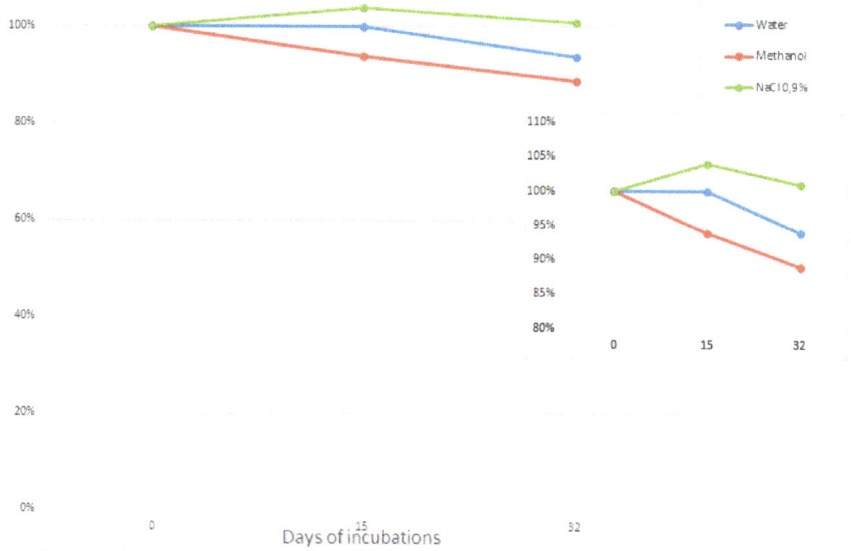

Figure 2. Normalized percentage of full antisense oligonucleotide (ASO) length over time for three solvents.

3.2. Size and Polydispersity

We have developed two lipidic compositions: DOTAP/Mal-PEG/Chol (29:2:69) and DOTAP/Mal-PEG/PC/Chol (20:20:58:2) respectively for ASO-Li-1/ASO-iLi-1 and ASO-Li-2/ASO-iLi-2. Size and PDI are summarized in Table 1.

Table 1. Size and polydispersity index (PDI) comparison for both formulations of liposomes and immunoliposomes.

Formulation	Size (nm) ± SD	PDI ± SD
ASO-Li-1	127.7 ± 4.8	0.161 ± 0.03
ASO-iLi-1	139.6 ± 1.8	0.183 ± 0.06
ASO-Li-2	145.6 ± 4.1	0.080 ± 0.01
ASO-iLi-2	154.1 ± 9.4	0.090 ± 0.03

We observed a statistically significant difference in size between ASO-Li-1 and ASO-iLi-1 ($p = 0.016$) and ASO-Li-2 and ASO-iLi-2 ($p = 0.032$, Student's t-test).

Stability study was performed on days 7, 14 and 28 after liposome formation. For formulation 1, size showed an increase both for ASO-Li-1 ($p = 0.007$, Student's t-test) and ASO-iLi-1 ($p = 0.002$, Student's t-test). Given these results, stability study was not performed on days 14 and 28.

For formulation 2, size showed no difference from first measures ($p = 0.838$ for ASO-Li-2 and $p = 0.838$ for ASO-iLi-2, one-way ANOVA testing). Results for size and PDI monitoring over time are summarized in Table 2.

Table 2. Size and PDI comparison over time for formulation 2.

Formulation	Day 7		Day 14		Day 28	
	Size (nm) ± SD	PDI ± SD	Size (nm) ± SD	PDI ± SD	Size (nm) ± SD	PDI ± SD
ASO-Li-1	150.7 ± 6.1	0.16 ± 0.03	not performed			
ASO-iLi-1	166.9 ± 6.4	0.18 ± 0.07	not performed			
ASO-Li-2	148.3 ± 8.4	0.07 ± 0.01	148.2 ± 5.3	0.08 ± 0.03	150.4 ± 4.7	0.11 ± 0.05
ASO-iLi-2	151.6 ± 1.0	0.06 ± 0.01	154.4 ± 3.4	0.08 ± 0.03	162.3 ± 1.0	0.10 ± 0.03

3.3. Pegylated Immunoliposome Preparation: Encapsulation Strategies

ASO–FITC was encapsulated into liposomes composed of DOTAP/Mal-PEG/PC/Chol in the molar ratio 20:20:58:2. Mean encapsulation rates of ASO–FITC were 21.14 ± 7.65% for fast agitation, 42.88 ± 3.80% for soft agitation and 39.00 ± 2.16% combined hydration solvent and soft agitation (Figure 3). No significant difference appears between the two formulations using soft agitation $p = 0.484$). Whether ASO was introduced in organic or in hydrophilic phase had no influence on ASO encapsulation.

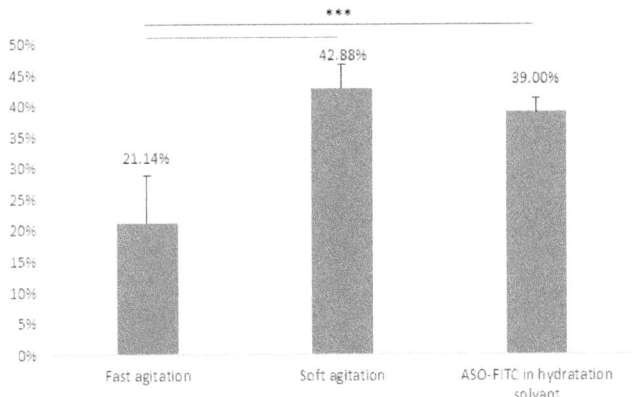

Figure 3. Influence of different strategies on encapsulation rate (***, 0; **, 0.001; * 0.01).

3.4. Quantification of Her2 on Cells

PC-3 cells were found to express $12 \times 10^3 \pm 0.5 \times 10^3$ Her2 receptors per cell. This was next compared to the expression of Her2 receptor on breast cancer cells MDA-MB-231, MDA-MB-453 and SKBR3 (reference cells for Her2 expression), as shown in Figure 4.

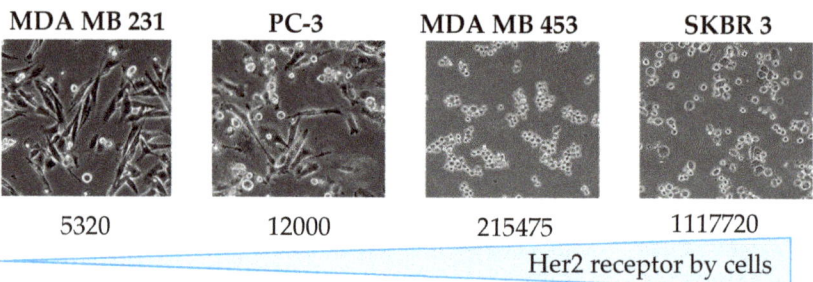

Figure 4. Comparison of Her2 receptors on cell surface for MDA-MB-231, PC-3, MDA-MB-453 and SKBR3.

3.5. 3D In Vitro

3.5.1. Lipidic Antiproliferative Activity

For both liposomes and immunoliposomes and for both formulations, the nontoxic concentration in empty liposomes was observed for lipid concentrations <10 nM for PC-3 cells treated at days 1 and 8 with viability determined in bioluminescence at day 15 (Figure 5). These results agree with those obtained in 2D (data not shown).

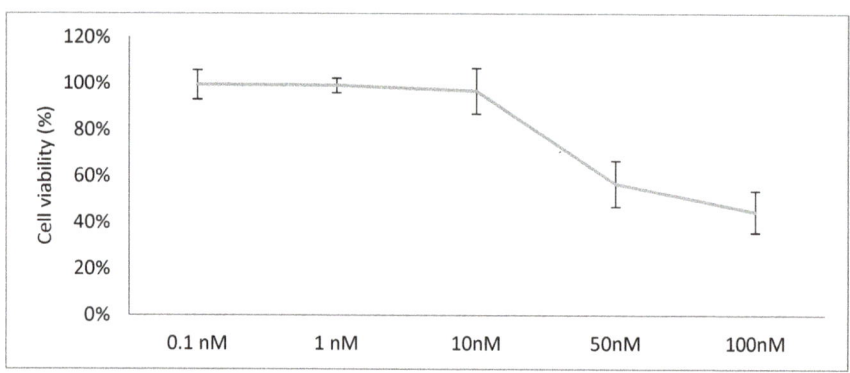

Figure 5. Cell viability (%) of PC-3 when exposed to Empty-Li-2.

Following these results, we decided to work with formulation 2 at two nontoxic lipid concentrations (2 and 8 nM) and an encapsulated ASO at 150 nM. Encapsulation rate for each batch was 41 ± 6%.

3.5.2. Liposomal Antiproliferative Activity

All the measures were performed in triplicate; these protocols (protocols 1 and 2) are summarized in Figures 6 and 7.

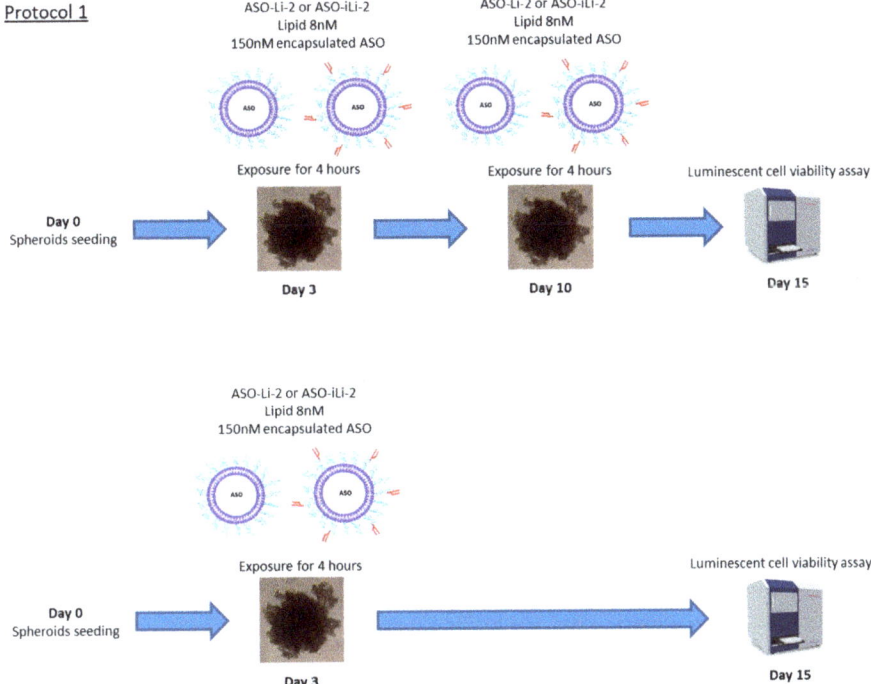

Figure 6. Protocol 1: liposomal antiproliferative activity with short exposition time. 3D in vitro assessment with spheroid treatment protocol 1. All the measures were performed in triplicate.

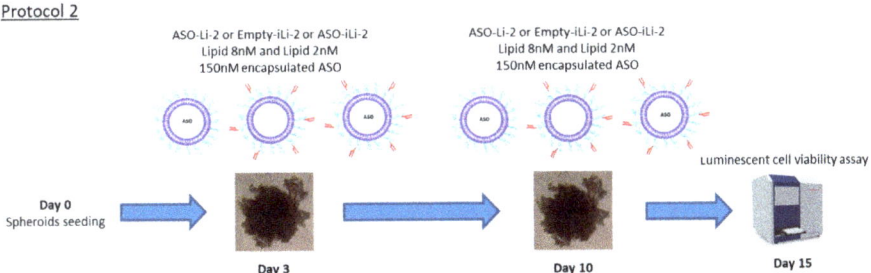

Figure 7. Protocol 2: liposomal antiproliferative activity with long exposition time. 3D in vitro assessment with spheroid treatment protocol 2. All the measures were performed in triplicate.

Empty liposomes and immunoliposomes showed no in vitro cytotoxicity (data not shown). Results of cytotoxic studies with protocol 1 are summarized in Figure 8. Greater cytotoxicity was observed in PCa exposed to liposomes with both treatment schemes. No effect was detected with ASO-iLi-2 at 8 nM with both schedules.

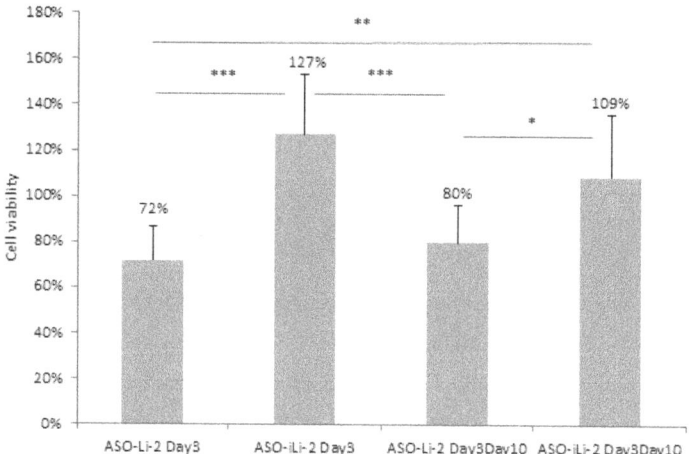

Figure 8. Cell viability (%) of 5000 PC-3 cell spheroids when exposed to ASO-Li-2 at 8 nM and ASO-iLi-2 at 8 nM for 4h at day 3 and days 3–10 (***, 0; **, 0.001; * 0.01).

Results of cytotoxic studies with protocol 2 at low lipid concentration are summarized in Figure 9. Greater cytotoxicity was observed in PCa exposed to immunoliposomes encapsulated with 150 nM of ASO and to lipid concentration of 2 nM ($p = 0.039$). No cytotoxic effect on PCa cells was detected after ASO-Li-2 treatment at low lipid concentration.

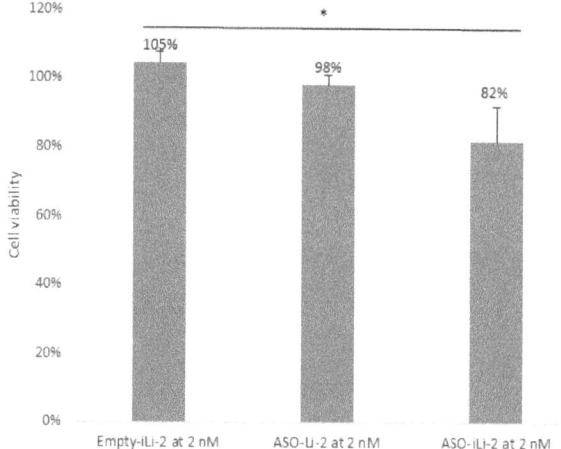

Figure 9. Cell viability (%) of 5000 PC-3 cell spheroids when exposed to Empty-iLi-2 at 2 nM, ASO-Li-2 at 2 nM and ASO-iLi-2 at 2 nM (***, 0; **, 0.001; * 0.01).

Results of cytotoxic studies with protocol 2 at high lipid concentration are summarized in Figure 10. A greater cytotoxicity was observed in PCa exposed to immunoliposomes encapsulated 150 nM of ASO ($p = 0.0041$ vs. Empty-iL-2 and $p = 0.0039$ vs. ASO-Li-2).

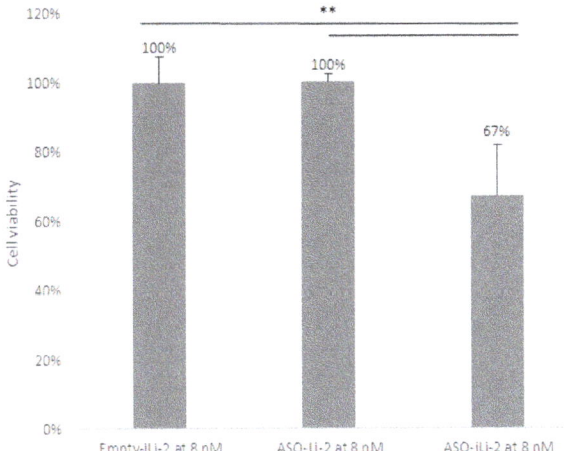

Figure 10. Cell viability (%) of 5000 PC-3 cell spheroids when exposed to Empty-iLi-2 at 8 nM, ASO-Li-2 at 8 nM and ASO-iLi-2 at 8 nM (***, 0; **, 0.001; * 0.01).

Cell viability results obtained were confirmed by microscopic observation (Figure 11). Observations were made on days 1 (24 h after cell seeding), 8 and 15.

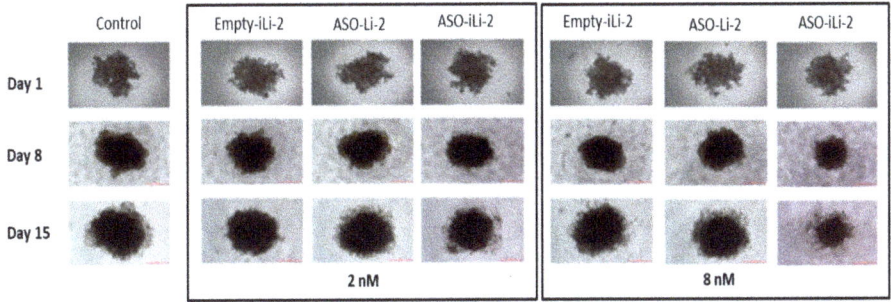

Figure 11. Spheroid (5000 cells) microscopy observations.

Microscopy observations were consistent with bioluminescence ones. On day 15, spheroids treated with ASO-iLi-2 at 8 nM seemed to present more cellular death than control and other treatment conditions.

4. Discussion

ASOs are a promising approach in oncology, and more particularly in CRPCa with the development of ASO targeting TCTP.

While ASO has shown its efficacy in vitro, cellular uptake has proven to be much more challenging. In this respect, we have here studied a new encapsulated formulation of ASO, designed to penetrate in cells. In this work, we have developed innovative second- and third-generation liposomal formulations encapsulating ASO, so as to enhance cellular penetration and effectiveness in PCa cells [33–36].

Pegylated immunoliposomes, thanks to their stealthiness and size compatible with the EPR effect, provide a unique opportunity for both passive and active targeting of tumors. To this end, liposomal formulations must take into account two important parameters: the nature of the ASO (i.e., its hydrophilic nature and its anionic character) and the necessity of a diameter below 200 nm for EPR effect. Here, anti-Her2 trastuzumab was used as a targeting agent because Her2 is frequently expressed in several cancers such as breast cancer or gastric/gastroesophageal cancers [37].

We found that the level of Her2 expression in PC-3 was relatively low, so previous work on MDA-MB231 cells with even a lower level of target expression than PC-3 showed promising results in our laboratory. Still, the rationale for targeting Her2 on PC-3 cells could be questioned here. Because the PC-3 cells are the cells mostly used as an experimental model for CRPa [38,39], they were considered as a fully suitable model for evaluating the usefulness of transporting ASOs with immunoliposomes in prostate cancer, especially because we have demonstrated previously that higher efficacy with trastuzumab-grafted liposomes was not necessarily correlated to a high level of Her2 expression.

The innovative nature of this approach consisted in the combination of the advantages of a small diameter (i.e., <150 nm) of lipid–nucleic acid nanoparticles, improving ASO drug delivery through passive targeting, with the advantages of active targeting (i.e., anti-Her2) [40–42]. Prostate tumors are highly vascularized tumors, thus making this tumor eligible for EPR effects [43,44].

Previous studies have highlighted the complexity of defining optimal formulations yielding acceptable encapsulation rates with other hydrophilic active agents such as siRNA [45]. In our study, the difficulty was to combine acceptable encapsulation rates with small-sized nanoparticles while allowing trastuzumab engraftment.

In the present study, we showed that is it possible to design ASO liposomes and immunoliposomes. We have developed two different liposomal formulations showing good performances in terms of size, encapsulation rate and stability. DOTAP is a cationic lipid used to optimize liposome stability and increase anionic oligonucleotide ASO encapsulation rate. Chol and PC are neutral lipids frequently used for liposome formulation. The two tested formulations differ by PC presence in order to increase liposome stability. Finally, Mal-PEG is a common stealth agent used for all kinds of nanoparticles [46,47].

We worked with two nontoxic lipid concentrations (2 nM and 8 nM) and an encapsulated ASO at 150 nM. Indeed, lipid concentration plays a major role in liposome stability and leakage from the membrane. Low cholesterol concentration decreases stability and increases drug release [48]. Testing two lipid concentration levels allowed differences in cytotoxic effect to be highlighted.

Moreover, cholesterol affects the plasticity of the liposomal membrane; i.e., increasing cholesterol decreases the plasticity and increases the rigidity of the membranes [49]. Cholesterol was therefore a critical component because, for hydrophilic components such as ASO, membrane rigidity determines the release rate of the content [50].

A significant difference was found between formulations using fast agitation and the two other formulations ($p < 0.001$). This difference can be explained by destabilization and weakening of liposomes during fast agitation.

Following these results, we decided to work with formulation 2 composed of DOTAP/Mal-PEG/PC/Chol in the molar ratio 20:20:58:2. The encapsulation rate for each batch was 41 ± 6%.

Liposomes and immunoliposomes were compared in terms of physical characteristics, size suitable for EPR effect and encapsulation rates. The extraction of the ASO was optimized using a chloroform–methanol mixture. Finally, soft agitation with thin-film method was selected as the best encapsulation method, yielding encapsulation rates of about 50%, i.e., twice as much as the other methods we tested.

However, for the present proof-of-concept study, aiming at demonstrating that encapsulating ASOs in lipidic carriers helps to increase their efficacy, we decided to work on freshly prepared batches, rather than trying to improve shelf-stability.

Antiproliferative assays were performed on PCa-3 cells using both 2D and 3D models. Spheroids (i.e., 3D) are considered as a better model for evaluating the efficacy of nanoparticles [51]; however, 2D models were useful for determining IC50s of free ASO and free trastuzumab, as well as for determining the nontoxic concentrations of blank liposomes. These preliminary results on 2D models helped us to determine the concentrations (i.e., 2 and 8 nM) to be used for the 3D testing without confounding factors such as the direct toxic effect of overly concentrated lipids.

When using 3D models, the antiproliferative activity of free ASO was low and fully in line with that already described in the literature, thus confirming the need to provide ASO with a carrier to further increase its efficacy. Empty liposomes and blank immunoliposomes did not show antiproliferative activity. In 3D culture, the nontoxic concentration in lipids was confirmed to be 10 nM.

For free drugs (i.e., free ASO and free trastuzumab), no efficacy was observed in 3D models (data not shown). These data confirmed that ASO needs to be encapsulated to be efficient. We subsequently developed two processing protocols taking into account the preliminary data available [22].

Regardless of the short exposition time (4 h) and delayed exposure (i.e., day 3 and days 3 and 10), we observed a significant superiority in the efficacy of the liposomes as compared to the immunoliposomes. On the other hand, in these conditions of brief exposure, the treatment of PCa cells by immunoliposomes did not show any efficacy.

This scheduling was previously used in 2D models with PC-3 and already showed an effect in downregulation of TCTP expression and cell viability when using lipid-conjugated ASO carrier [12]. However, with our liposomes and immunoliposomes, these results were not confirmed. This loss of efficacy for immunoliposomes encapsulating ASO could come from this incubation time being too short to allow proper interaction between trastuzumab and Her2 receptors on PC-3 cells, preventing the efficient intracellular release of ASO. Indeed, the presence of the grafted antibody in the bilayer of the nanoparticle causes steric hindrance and is probably accompanied by a longer cellular uptake, resulting in a delayed release of ASO at the cellular level and limiting its efficacy.

In protocol 2 with extended exposure time, no significant differences were found between liposome-encapsulated ASO and empty liposome at all lipid concentrations. We have demonstrated significantly superior efficacy of ASO-iLi-2 at any lipid concentration for long exposure times when compared to liposome treatment.

In addition, for long exposure times, we have demonstrated significantly superior efficacy of ASO-iLi-2 at 8 nM lipid concentration when compared to ASO-Li-2 treatment.

Trastuzumab, therefore, seems to play a critical role in the active targeting of PC-3 cells, despite their low expression level of Her2. Indeed, free trastuzumab showed no efficacy in 3D models. Thus, the greater antiproliferative efficacy achieved with immunoliposomes as compared with liposomes encapsulating ASO cannot be directly related to some kind of direct trastuzumab cytotoxicity. Instead, better targeting of cancer cells by passive and active targeting due to a better distribution of the immunoliposomes in the core of the spheroid could explain this increase in efficacy.

Moreover, the differences in efficacy observed between immunoliposomes used at 2 and 8 nM can be explained by differences in the membrane plasticity of the carriers. Indeed 2 nM immunoliposomes contain less cholesterol than 8 nM immunoliposomes, and consequently, the membrane is less rigid, resulting in a possible leaking process due to poor stability. Conversely, the lipid concentration of 8 nM immunoliposomes allows better protection and subsequently also better intracellular penetration of ASO into cancer cells.

The challenge of this work was to highlight the possibility of encapsulating the ASO into lipidic nanoparticles so as to increase its efficacy. For both the developed liposomes and immunoliposomes, we have demonstrated that lipidic nanoparticles are suitable for encapsulating ASOs in terms of size, short-term stability and encapsulation rates. Results showed that both liposomes and immunoliposomes performed better than free ASO, thus suggesting that encapsulating ASO could help to increase its cytotoxicity. Because nanoparticles do not aim at changing the pharmacology of a drug, but rather aim at affecting the delivery and pharmacokinetics, we hypothesize here that lipids containing ASO could help carry the payload inside tumors.

5. Conclusions

In this proof-of-concept study, we have demonstrated that it is possible to increase the efficacy of ASO in the canonical PC-3 model for prostate cancer by using lipid carriers. Interestingly, immunoliposomes targeting Her2 have presented the most promising efficacy on 3D spheroids, provided that incubation time was long enough, despite a low expression of Her2 in PC-3 cells. Conversely, short exposure times led to higher efficacy of liposomes as compared with immunoliposomes. This difference could come from the steric hindrance of the immunoliposomes requiring a delay in the release of ASO, thus making it a more suitable candidate for long-exposure schedules. Overall, this work suggests that shifting from standard intratumoral administration of oligonucleotides to systemic administration is feasible, provided that a suitable vehicle is developed.

Poor stability of encapsulated ASO obliged us to use extemporaneously prepared batches; however, this weakness could be fixed in the future, i.e., by lyophilization of the nanoparticles so as to enhance shelf-stability.

Author Contributions: Conceptualization, G.S. and R.F.; resources, C.P. and A.R.; supervision, P.R.; visualization, J.C.; funding acquisition, S.G. All authors have read and agreed to the published version of the manuscript.

Funding: This research received no external funding.

Conflicts of Interest: The authors declare no conflict of interest.

References

1. Litwin, M.S.; Tan, H.-J. The Diagnosis and Treatment of Prostate Cancer: A Review. *JAMA* **2017**, *317*, 2532–2542. [CrossRef] [PubMed]
2. Bray, F.; Ferlay, J.; Soerjomataram, I.; Siegel, R.L.; Torre, L.A.; Jemal, A. Global cancer statistics 2018: GLOBOCAN estimates of incidence and mortality worldwide for 36 cancers in 185 countries. *CA Cancer J. Clin.* **2018**, *68*, 394–424. [CrossRef] [PubMed]
3. Epstein, J.I.; Zelefsky, M.J.; Sjoberg, D.D.; Nelson, J.B.; Egevad, L.; Magi-Galluzzi, C.; Andrew, J.; Parwani, A.V.; Reuter, V.E.; Fine, S.W.; et al. A Contemporary Prostate Cancer Grading System: A Validated Alternative to the Gleason Score. *Eur. Urol.* **2016**, *69*, 428–435. [CrossRef] [PubMed]
4. Jayaram, A.; Attard, G. Diagnostic Gleason score and castration-resistant prostate cancer. *Ann. Oncol.* **2016**, *27*, 962–964. [CrossRef]
5. Katsogiannou, M.; Ziouziou, H.; Karaki, S.; Andrieu, C.; Henry de Villeneuve, M.; Rocchi, P. The hallmarks of castration-resistant prostate cancers. *Cancer Treat. Rev.* **2015**, *41*, 588–597. [CrossRef]
6. Baylot, V.; Karaki, S.; Rocchi, P. TCTP Has a Crucial Role in the Different Stages of Prostate Cancer Malignant Progression. *Results Probl. Cell Differ.* **2017**, *64*, 255–261.
7. Rho, S.B.; Lee, J.H.; Park, M.S.; Byun, H.-J.; Kang, S.; Seo, S.-S.; Kim, J.-Y.; Park, S.-Y. Anti-apoptotic protein TCTP controls the stability of the tumor suppressor p53. *FEBS Lett.* **2011**, *585*, 29–35. [CrossRef]
8. Amson, R.; Pece, S.; Lespagnol, A.; Vyas, R.; Mazzarol, G.; Tosoni, D.; Colaluca, I.; Viale, G.; Rodrigues-Ferreira, S.; Wynendaele, J.; et al. Reciprocal repression between P53 and TCTP. *Nat. Med.* **2011**, *18*, 91–99. [CrossRef]
9. Stahel, R.A.; Zangemeister-Wittke, U. Antisense oligonucleotides for cancer therapy—An overview. *Lung Cancer* **2003**, *41*, 81–88. [CrossRef]
10. Geary, R.S.; Norris, D.; Yu, R.; Bennett, C.F. Pharmacokinetics, biodistribution and cell uptake of antisense oligonucleotides. *Adv. Drug Deliv. Rev.* **2015**, *87*, 46–51. [CrossRef]
11. Baylot, V.; Katsogiannou, M.; Andrieu, C.; Taieb, D.; Acunzo, J.; Giusiano, S.; Fazli, L.; Gleave, M.; Garrido, C.; Rocchi, P. Targeting TCTP as a New Therapeutic Strategy in Castration-resistant Prostate Cancer. *Mol. Ther.* **2012**, *20*, 2244–2256. [CrossRef] [PubMed]
12. Karaki, S.; Benizri, S.; Mejías, R.; Baylot, V.; Branger, N.; Nguyen, T.; Vialet, B.; Oumzil, K.; Barthélémy, P.; Rocchi, P. Lipid-oligonucleotide conjugates improve cellular uptake and efficiency of TCTP-antisense in castration-resistant prostate cancer. *J. Control. Release* **2017**, *258*, 1–9. [CrossRef] [PubMed]
13. Fanciullino, R.; Ciccolini, J. Liposome-encapsulated anticancer drugs: Still waiting for the magic bullet? *Curr. Med. Chem.* **2009**, *16*, 4361–4371. [CrossRef] [PubMed]
14. Bitounis, D.; Pourchez, J.; Forest, V.; Boudard, D.; Cottier, M.; Klein, J.-P. Detection and analysis of nanoparticles in patients: A critical review of the status quo of clinical nanotoxicology. *Biomaterials* **2016**, *76*, 302–312. [CrossRef]
15. Pasut, G.; Veronese, F.M. State of the art in PEGylation: The great versatility achieved after forty years of research. *J. Control. Release* **2012**, *161*, 461–472. [CrossRef]

16. Montero, A.J.; Adams, B.; Diaz-Montero, C.M.; Glück, S. Nab-paclitaxel in the treatment of metastatic breast cancer: A comprehensive review. *Expert Rev. Clin Pharmacol.* **2011**, *4*, 329–334. [CrossRef]
17. Prabhu, S.; Boswell, C.A.; Leipold, D.D.; A Khawli, L.; Li, D.; Lu, D.; Theil, F.-P.; Joshi, A.; Lum, B.L. Antibody delivery of drugs and radionuclides: Factors influencing clinical pharmacology. *Ther. Deliv.* **2011**, *2*, 769–791. [CrossRef]
18. Adair, J.R.; Howard, P.W.; Hartley, J.A.; Williams, D.G.; Chester, K.A. Antibody-drug conjugates—A perfect synergy. *Expert Opin. Biol. Ther.* **2012**, *12*, 1191–1206. [CrossRef]
19. Greish, K. Enhanced permeability and retention (EPR) effect for anticancer nanomedicine drug targeting. *Methods Mol. Biol.* **2010**, *624*, 25–37.
20. Mamot, C.; Ritschard, R.; Wicki, A.; Stehle, G.; Dieterle, T.; Bubendorf, L.; Hilker, C.; Deuster, S.; Herrmann, R.; Rochlitz, C. Tolerability, safety, pharmacokinetics, and efficacy of doxorubicin-loaded anti-EGFR immunoliposomes in advanced solid tumours: A phase 1 dose-escalation study. *Lancet Oncol.* **2012**, *13*, 1234–1241. [CrossRef]
21. Lehtinen, J.; Raki, M.; Bergström, K.A.; Uutela, P.; Lehtinen, K.; Hiltunen, A.; Pikkarainen, J.; Liang, H.; Pitkänen, S.; Määttä, A.; et al. Pre-Targeting and Direct Immunotargeting of Liposomal Drug Carriers to Ovarian Carcinoma. *PLoS ONE* **2012**, *7*, e41410. [CrossRef] [PubMed]
22. Rodallec, A.; Brunel, J.-M.; Giacometti, S.; Maccario, H.; Correard, F.; Mas, E.; Ornetto, C.; Savina, A.; Bouquet, F.; Lacarelle, B.; et al. Docetaxel-trastuzumab stealth immunoliposome: Development and in vitro proof of concept studies in breast cancer. *Int. J. Nanomed.* **2018**, *13*, 3451–3465. [CrossRef] [PubMed]
23. Bangham, A.D.; Standish, M.M.; Watkins, J.C. Diffusion of univalent ions across the lamellae of swollen phospholipids. *J. Mol. Biol.* **1965**, *13*, 238–252. [CrossRef]
24. Fanciullino, R.; Mollard, S.; Correard, F.; Giacometti, S.; Serdjebi, C.; Iliadis, A.; Ciccolini, J. Biodistribution, tumor uptake and efficacy of 5-FU-loaded liposomes: Why size matters. *Pharm. Res.* **2014**, *31*, 2677–2684. [CrossRef]
25. Eg, B.; Wj, D. A rapid method of total lipid extraction and purification. *Can. J. Biochem. Physiol.* **1959**, *37*, 911–917.
26. Soema, P.C.; Willems, G.-J.; Jiskoot, W.; Amorij, J.-P.; Kersten, G.F. Predicting the influence of liposomal lipid composition on liposome size, zeta potential and liposome-induced dendritic cell maturation using a design of experiments approach. *Eur. J. Pharm. Biopharm.* **2015**, *94*, 427–435. [CrossRef] [PubMed]
27. Oude Blenke, E.; Evers, M.J.W.; Baumann, V.; Winkler, J.; Storm, G.; Mastrobattista, E. Critical evaluation of quantification methods for oligonucleotides formulated in lipid nanoparticles. *Int. J. Pharm.* **2018**, *548*, 793–802. [CrossRef]
28. Rodallec, A.; Franco, C.; Robert, S.; Sicard, G.; Giacometti, S.; Lacarelle, B.; Bouquet, F.; Savina, A.; Lacroix, R.; Dignat-George, F.; et al. Prototyping Trastuzumab Docetaxel Immunoliposomes with a New FCM-Based Method to Quantify Optimal Antibody Density on Nanoparticles. *Sci. Rep.* **2020**, *10*, 4147. [CrossRef]
29. Panke, C.; Weininger, D.; Haas, A.; Schelter, F.; Schlothauer, T.; Bader, S.; Sircar, R.; Josel, H.P.; Baer, U.; Burtscher, H.; et al. Quantification of cell surface proteins with bispecific antibodies. *Protein Eng. Des. Sel.* **2013**, *26*, 645–654. [CrossRef]
30. Fox, J.; Weisberg, S. *An R Companion to Applied Regression*, 3rd ed.; Sage Publications: Thousand Oaks, CA, USA, 2019.
31. Hothorn, T.; Bretz, F.; Westfall, P. Simultaneous inference in general parametric models. *Biom. J.* **2008**, *50*, 346–363. [CrossRef]
32. R: The R Project for Statistical Computing. Available online: https://www.r-project.org/ (accessed on 13 June 2020).
33. Gray, G.D.; Basu, S.; Wickstrom, E. Transformed and immortalized cellular uptake of oligodeoxynucleoside phosphorothioates, 3′-Alkylamino oligodeoxynucleotides, 2′-o-methyl oligoribonucleotides, oligodeoxynucleoside methylphosphonates, and peptide nucleic acids. *Biochem. Pharmacol.* **1997**, *53*, 1465–1476. [CrossRef]
34. Moreno, P.M.D.; Pêgo, A.P. Therapeutic antisense oligonucleotides against cancer: Hurdling to the clinic. *Front. Chem.* **2014**, *2*, 87. [CrossRef] [PubMed]
35. Winkler, J. Oligonucleotide conjugates for therapeutic applications. *Ther. Deliv.* **2013**, *4*, 791–809. [CrossRef] [PubMed]

36. Godeau, G.; Arnion, H.; Brun, C.; Staedel, C.; Barthélémy, P. Fluorocarbon oligonucleotide conjugates for nucleic acids delivery. *MedChemComm* **2010**, *1*, 76–78. [CrossRef]
37. Iqbal, N.; Iqbal, N. Human Epidermal Growth Factor Receptor 2 (HER2) in Cancers: Overexpression and Therapeutic Implications. *Mol. Biol. Int.* **2014**, *2014*, 1–9. [CrossRef] [PubMed]
38. Tai, S.; Sun, Y.; Squires, J.M.; Zhang, H.; Oh, W.K.; Liang, C.-Z.; Huang, J. PC3 is a cell line characteristic of prostatic small cell carcinoma. *Prostate* **2011**, *71*, 1668–1679. [CrossRef] [PubMed]
39. Bladou, F.; E Gleave, M.; Penault-Llorca, F.; Serment, G.; Lange, P.H.; Vessella, R.L. In vitro and in vivo models developed from human prostatic cancer. *Prog. Urol.* **1997**, *7*, 384–396. [PubMed]
40. Maeda, H. Polymer therapeutics and the EPR effect. *J. Drug Target.* **2017**, *25*, 781–785. [CrossRef]
41. Sharifi, N.; Salmaninejad, A.; Ferdosi, S.; Bajestani, A.N.; Khaleghiyan, M.; Estiar, M.A.; Jamali, M.; Nowroozi, M.R.; Shakoori, A. HER2 gene amplification in patients with prostate cancer: Evaluating a CISH-based method. *Oncol. Lett.* **2016**, *12*, 4651–4658. [CrossRef]
42. Andersson, J.; Rosestedt, M.; Asplund, V.; Yavari, N.; Orlova, A. In vitro modeling of HER2-targeting therapy in disseminated prostate cancer. *Int. J. Oncol.* **2014**, *45*, 2153–2158. [CrossRef]
43. Uehara, H. Angiogenesis of prostate cancer and antiangiogenic therapy. *J. Med. Investig.* **2003**, *50*, 146–153.
44. Kluetz, P.G.; Figg, W.D.; Dahut, W.L. Angiogenesis Inhibitors in the treatment of Prostate Cancer. *Expert Opin. Pharmacother.* **2010**, *11*, 233–247. [CrossRef] [PubMed]
45. Li, Y.; Cheng, Q.; Jiang, Q.; Huang, Y.; Liu, H.; Zhao, Y.; Cao, W.; Ma, G.; Dai, F.; Liang, X.-J.; et al. Enhanced endosomal/lysosomal escape by distearoyl phosphoethanolamine-polycarboxybetaine lipid for systemic delivery of siRNA. *J. Control. Release* **2014**, *176*, 104–114. [CrossRef] [PubMed]
46. Zahednezhad, F.; Saadat, M.; Valizadeh, H.; Zakeri-Milani, P.; Baradaran, B. Liposome and immune system interplay: Challenges and potentials. *J. Control. Release* **2019**, *305*, 194–209. [CrossRef] [PubMed]
47. Bennett, C.F.; Chiang, M.Y.; Chan, H.; Shoemaker, J.E.; Mirabelli, C.K. Cationic lipids enhance cellular uptake and activity of phosphorothioate antisense oligonucleotides. *Mol. Pharmacol.* **1992**, *41*, 1023–1033. [PubMed]
48. Anderson, M.; Omri, A. The Effect of Different Lipid Components on the In Vitro Stability and Release Kinetics of Liposome Formulations. *Drug Deliv.* **2004**, *11*, 33–39. [CrossRef]
49. Coderch, L.; Fonollosa, J.; De Pera, M.; Estelrich, J.; De La Maza, A.; Parra, J.L. Influence of cholesterol on liposome fluidity by EPR: Relationship with percutaneous absorption. *J. Control. Release* **2000**, *68*, 85–95. [CrossRef]
50. Mourtas, S.; Fotopoulou, S.; Duraj, S.; Sfika, V.; Tsakiroglou, C.; Antimisiaris, S.G. Liposomal drugs dispersed in hydrogels: Effect of liposome, drug and gel properties on drug release kinetics. *Colloids Surf. B Biointerfaces* **2007**, *55*, 212–221. [CrossRef]
51. Rodallec, A.; Sicard, G.; Giacometti, S.; Carré, M.; Pourroy, B.; Bouquet, F.; Savina, A.; Lacarelle, B.; Ciccolini, J.; Fanciullino, R. From 3D spheroids to tumor bearing mice: Efficacy and distribution studies of trastuzumab-docetaxel immunoliposome in breast cancer. *Int. J. Nanomed.* **2018**, *13*, 6677–6688. [CrossRef]

Publisher's Note: MDPI stays neutral with regard to jurisdictional claims in published maps and institutional affiliations.

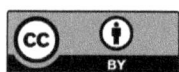

© 2020 by the authors. Licensee MDPI, Basel, Switzerland. This article is an open access article distributed under the terms and conditions of the Creative Commons Attribution (CC BY) license (http://creativecommons.org/licenses/by/4.0/).

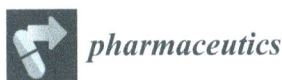

Review

Like a Rolling Stone: Sting-Cgas Pathway and Cell-Free DNA as Biomarkers for Combinatorial Immunotherapy

Guillaume Sicard [1], Frédéric Fina [2], Raphaelle Fanciullino [1], Fabrice Barlesi [3,4] and Joseph Ciccolini [1,*]

1. SMARTc Unit, CRCM Inserm U1068, Aix Marseille University, 13007 Marseille, France; guillaume.sicard@ap-hm.fr (G.S.); raphaelle.fanciullino@univ-amu.fr (R.F.)
2. Anatomo-pathology Unit, La Timone University Hospital of Marseille, 13005 Marseille, France; frederic.fina@ap-hm.fr
3. School of Medicine, Aix Marseille University, 13007 Marseille, France; Fabrice.BARLESI@gustaveroussy.fr
4. Gustave Roussy Institute, 94800 Villejuif, France
* Correspondence: joseph.ciccolini@univ-amu.fr; Tel.: +33-(0)4-9183-5509

Received: 4 July 2020; Accepted: 10 August 2020; Published: 11 August 2020

Abstract: Combining immune checkpoint inhibitors with other treatments likely to harness tumor immunity is a rising strategy in oncology. The exact modalities of such a combinatorial regimen are yet to be defined, and most attempts have relied so far on concomitant dosing, rather than sequential or phased administration. Because immunomodulating features are likely to be time-, dose-, and-schedule dependent, the need for biomarkers providing real-time information is critical to better define the optimal time-window to combine immune checkpoint inhibitors with other drugs. In this review, we present the various putative markers that have been investigated as predictive tools with immune checkpoint inhibitors and could be used to help further combining treatments. Whereas none of the current biomarkers, such as the PDL1 expression of a tumor mutational burden, is suitable to identify the best way to combine treatments, monitoring circulating tumor DNA is a promising strategy, in particular to check whether the STING-cGAS pathway has been activated by cytotoxics. As such, circulating tumor DNA could help defining the best time-window to administrate immune checkpoint inhibitors after that cytotoxics have been given.

Keywords: combinatorial immunotherapy; cytotoxics; biomarkers; precision medicine

1. Introduction: Doom and Gloom

Precision medicine is a broad generic term, generally used to describe all of the resources used to decipher the molecular and genomic profiles of tumors, primarily for selecting the drugs which are the most likely to be clinically effective in cancer patients.

For decades, improving either response rates or survival in cancer patients has been achieved in a stepwise manner. Despite the recent and growing use of bio-guided medicine in oncology, the use of targeted therapies or anti-angiogenic therapy has been considered as an incremental innovation, with a significant but moderate impact on survival eventually. Indeed, apart from rare counter-examples such as imatinib in CML or trastuzumab in HER2-positive breast cancer, it has taken decades to reach meaningful prolonged survival, beyond a rapid and spectacular increase in response rates [1].

More recently, immunotherapy has been considered as a ground-breaking innovation in oncology. Although the role of tumor immunity has been known for decades [2], the introduction of immune checkpoint inhibitors (e.g., anti-CTLA4, or PD1/PDL1 axis antagonists) as new anticancer agents quickly led to spectacular improvements in clinical outcomes, including 5 year-survival rates above

30%. Unfortunately, successful immunotherapy is restricted to a too limited, but relevant, number of cancers with once dismal prognosis, such as metastatic melanoma and advanced non-small cell lung cancer (NSCLC).

Consequently, after first years of use as single-agents, all the newly developed immune checkpoint inhibitors are to be combined with other therapeutic strategies such as chemotherapy, targeted therapy, anti-angiogenics, or radiation therapy. Importantly, most combinational trials have been designed thus far on an empirical basis, i.e., by adding novel immune checkpoint inhibitors to already existing and sometimes decade-old regimens. Still, today a rising amount of evidence suggests that to achieve a maximum efficacy while controlling toxicities, there is probably an optimal way immune checkpoint inhibitors should be combined with other anticancer drugs or with radiation therapy [3]. Of note, this kind of optimal design cannot be identified anymore with standard trial-and-error approaches, owing to the ever growing complexity and the countless possibilities of different combinations to be tested [4].

Academic clinical studies have already shown, with other anticancer agents such as anti-angiogenics and cytotoxics, that optimizing administration scheduling can help improving clinical outcomes. This, calls for new methods to administrate drugs and determine the right dosing, scheduling, and sequencing when setting up a combinatorial regimen [5].

It should be noted that clinical evidence establishing pharmacokinetic/pharmacodynamic (PK/PD) relationships (e.g., drug exposure levels predict survival and are associated with treatment-related toxicities) with anti-CTLA4 Ipilimumab have been published, as well as high inter-patient variability in pharmacokinetic profiles [6]. With other immune checkpoint inhibitors targeting the PD1/PDL1 axis, exposure–effects relationships are not fully elucidated yet since conflictual results have been published so far, such as with anti-PD1 nivolumab [7,8].

As their name suggests, immune checkpoint inhibitors inhibit the key checkpoints of immune response [9]. Tumor cells have the ability to escape from host immunity [10] and the role of immune checkpoint inhibitors is to target transmembrane proteins such as the CTLA4, PD1, and PD-L1 ligand. Currently, the 7 immune checkpoint inhibitors which have been FDA-approved are [11] anti-CTLA4 (Ipilimumab), Anti-PD1 (Nivolumab, Pembrolizumab, Cemiplimab), and Anti-PD-L1 (Avelumab, Atezolizumab, Durvalumab). Many others immune checkpoint inhibitors are currently being developed and are already in clinical testing phases [12]. Mechanisms of action of immune checkpoint inhibitors are briefly summarized in Figure 1.

Immune checkpoint inhibitors are used in current practice in oncology as single agent, and more and more frequently now in combination with chemotherapy, radiation therapy, or in association with another immune checkpoint inhibitor such as the anti-CTLA4 + anti-PD1 combo in metastatic melanoma [13].

The first FDA-approved immune checkpoint inhibitor was Ipilimumab in the early 2010's [14] in advanced melanoma. Ipilimumab is a fully human monoclonal antibody that targets and binds to cytotoxic T-lymphocyte-associated antigen 4 (CTLA4) and blocks its interaction with its ligands, i.e., CD80 and CD86. Consequently, Ipilimumab potentiates the antitumor T-cell response, resulting in unrestrained T-cell proliferation, plus it provides co-stimulatory signals (CD80/CD86) through CD28 on T lymphocytes. CTLA4 is constitutively expressed on the lymphocytes T regulatory (best known as T Regs) surface. The role of CTLA4 is an inhibitory function, which impedes acquisition of T cell effector function, thus preventing immunity from going out of control.

Anti-PD1 monoclonal antibodies Nivolumab and Pembrolizumab have been approved in 2014, and Cemiplimab in 2018. Anti-PD-L1 monoclonal antibody Atezolizumab was approved in 2016 and Avelumab and Durvalumab in 2017. Programmed cell death protein 1 (PD1) is a transmembrane protein expressed by multiple immune cells, whereas its ligand, PD-L1 is expressed by non-blood cells and overexpressed by tumor cells [15]. The PD1/PD-L1 axis is major immunosuppressive pathway, that normally helps to control immune reactions. This axis leads to the reduced proliferation of T Lymphocytes, anergy and exhaustion, apoptosis of activated T lymphocytes, diminution of T lymphocytes'

TCR-mediated activation and proliferation, plus a decrease in several cytokines such as interferon-γ (IFN-γ) and interleukin-2, as well as increase in T Regs further inhibiting immune response [16].

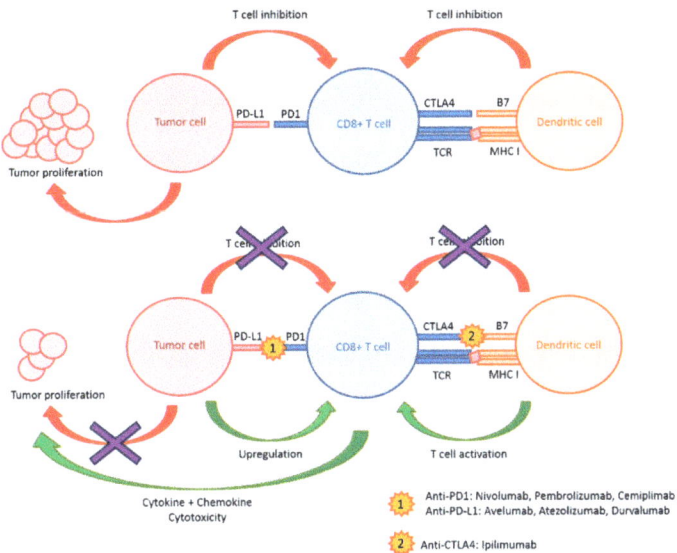

Figure 1. Schematic representation of how immune checkpoint inhibitors work.

Regarding side-effects, immune checkpoint inhibitors are generally well tolerated drugs but can trigger severe toxicities rarely seen in oncology thus far, best known as immune-related adverse events (IRAE). The most recurrent toxicities are immune events indeed, such as skin and digestive toxicities and metabolic disorders [17]. Cardiac toxicity has been also reported with immune checkpoint inhibitors, including cases of lethal myocarditis [18]. Because some of these toxicities can thus be life-threatening, optimizing the efficacy/toxicity balance is of major interest with immunotherapy.

The use of immune checkpoint inhibitors in association with conventional chemotherapies or oral targeted therapies is a promising strategy because there are no overlapping toxicities with immunotherapy, whereas a synergistic effect is expected at the tumor level. These combinations are based upon the hypothesis that sensitivity to immune checkpoint inhibitors will be increased by immunomodulating properties of the associated drugs. For instance, Cisplatin increases activated T lymphocytes as well as their intratumoral infiltration, thus acting synergistically with immune checkpoint inhibitors [19]. However, determining the optimal modalities of administration of cisplatin so that its modulating features are maximal, is yet to be determined.

2. Looking for the Ideal Biomarker in Immunotherapy: Welcome to the Jungle!

Importantly, the search for a robust, validated, and fully predictive biomarker with immunotherapy is still an ongoing story [20]. Ideally, such a biomarker could, beyond predicting clinical outcomes, help defining the best time-window for further combining treatments. This should accelerate the identification of optimal combinatorial strategies with immune checkpoint inhibitors, so as to expedite transfer to bedside practice and reduce attrition rates during clinical trials.

The ideal biomarker should be specific to tumor cells, sensitive enough to separate cancer patients from healthy individuals, translatable (i.e., not specific of one type of cancer or patient) and easy and quick to quantify in a patient-friendly way (e.g., measured in peripheral blood, and not from tumor biopsies), in addition to being robust and reproducible.

The search for predictive biomarkers with immunotherapy is challenging, as fully understanding the underlying pharmacology of these drugs is tricky. Roughly, two categories of biomarkers can be distinguished: the ones linked to the tumor or the ones linked to the host. The principal biomarker linked to the host is the gut microbiome, plus neutrophil-to-lymphocyte ratios (NLR). Regarding a tumor biomarker, molecular target expression (e.g., PD-L1), inflammation state (e.g., Myeloid-Derived Suppressive Cells, tertiary lymphoid structures, tumor-infiltrating lymphocytes), and tumor antigen expression (e.g., tumor mutational burden, microsatellite instability) are the most frequently tested markers. However, all these markers are still characterized by inconsistencies in predictive cut-off values depending on the studies, thus lowering their implementation in routine oncology as robust decision-making tools.

3. Microbiome and Immunotherapy: Everything Counts

Interest on the role gut microbiota could play in the response to immune checkpoint inhibitors is increasingly growing. Microbiota seem to play a major role on T Regs expression and in the activation of T Lymphocytes indeed [21]. One of the mechanisms of action explaining the role of microbiota is stimulating the response of T lymphocytes against microbial antigens. This response may be tumor specific or may be the source of cross-reactions against tumor specific antigens. In addition, T lymphocytes with bacterial epitopes were found in the tumor microenvironment as well [22]. In parallel, some studies demonstrated the negative impact of antibiotic treatment before starting immune checkpoint inhibitor treatment [23]. Controlling antibiotic therapy is easily feasible, even if they cannot always be easily ruled out in oncology in patients with sepsis. However, checking that the patient's microbiota is optimal for an optimal immunotherapy response remains highly challenging. Microbiota transplants are already a strategy in the treatment of *Clostridium difficile* infections, but to what extent it could be transposed to cancer patients is still currently under clinical investigation.

4. PD1 and PD-L1: Wish you Were Here

The expression of PD1 by immune cells and PD-L1 by tumor cells has been the first biomarker proposed in modern immunotherapy. The overexpression of PD-L1 confers a poorer prognosis across multiple tumor types, making therapeutic intervention on this immunomodulatory axis enticing. The quantification of PD-L1 appeared intuitively as an interesting biomarker of tumor sensitivity to immunotherapy, but the relevance of expression of PD-L1 alone remains debated today [24]. Furthermore, the cut-off for positivity of PD-L1 expression is yet be fully determined [25]. In addition, a meta-analysis in solid tumors demonstrated that immune checkpoint inhibitors decreased the risk of death by 34% to 100% in patients with positive PD-L1 and by 0% to up to 20% in PD-L1 negative patients [26], highlighting the complexity of using PD-L1 expression as a biomarker. About 10 PD-L1 immunohistochemical diagnostic assays are currently on the market or in development [27]. A study, comparing four different assays in lung cancer (i.e., two from Dako and two from Ventana medical system) highlighted differences in mean tumor cell and immune cell staining between the assays. Consequently, methods for measuring PDL1 cannot be used interchangeably in clinical practice, thus raising questions on possible technical biases and use for decision-making [28].

This discrepancy is found as well regarding the FDA approval of immune checkpoint inhibitors, because of the great heterogeneity in terms of cut-off [26]. For Nivolumab, during clinical trials different thresholds of PD-L1 expression were tested and ranged from 1% to 10% (i.e., Checkmate studies 017, 025, 057, 066, 067, and 141). All PD-L1 quantifications were performed on tumor cells, and the final choice for a positive cut-off seems to be highly tumor-type dependent.

For Pembrolizumab, during clinical trials different positivity thresholds for PD-L1 expression were tested too, ranging from >1% (Keynote 66) to >50% (Keynote 010 and 024).

All PD-L1 protein expression quantification was performed on tumor cells except for Keynote 006 where PD-L1 was quantified on both tumor cells and in tumor microenvironments. The threshold selection seems to be tumor-type dependent, i.e., high (>50%) for non-small-cell lung cancer (NSCL) and low (>1%) for the other types. For Atezolizumab, during clinical trials different positivity thresholds of PD-L1 expression were tested too, ranging from >1% to >50% [29]. For Durvalumab, a clinical trial NCT01693562 in NSCLC suggests that patient who had detectable levels of PD-L1 expression over 25% on tumor cells may have longer survival [30].

These different clinical trials highlight once again the great heterogeneity observed in terms of detectable levels of PD-L1 protein expression and tested material.

Given the lack of uniformity and positive results in patients defined as negative, the use of levels of PD-L1 protein expression seems difficult in routine practice. Moreover, PD-L1 expression is dynamic and modulated by radiation therapy or chemotherapy [31]. This PD-L1 expression modulation described with radiation therapy and alkylating agents such as platinum-based drugs, is a hope for non-responders patients to immunotherapy as monotherapy [32].

Actually, several drugs can modulate the transcriptional and post-transcriptional regulation of PD-L1. For instance, Lenalidomide, currently used in multiple myeloma patients, down-regulates PD-L1 expression [33]. An in vitro study testing six different drugs (topoisomerase-2 inhibitor, microtubulin inhibitor, CDK (cyclin dependent kinase) 4/6 inhibitor, topoisomerase-1 inhibitor, PI3K-mTOR dual inhibitor, and SRC-3 inhibitor 6) in breast cancer cells demonstrated a PD-L1 mRNA induction in an overwhelming majority of cases [34]. The use of drugs to either up- or down-regulate the expression of PD-L1 is an interesting research path, but this makes interpreting PD-L1 expression in pretreated patients (e.g., with the microtubulin inhibitor or lenalidomide) complicated because it may not reflect the basal expression level.

Technically speaking, tumor quantification of PD-L1 expression requires invasive biopsy procedures in patients. Alternatively, serum soluble PD-L1 quantification is currently being developed. However, no significant association was found between serum or plasma PD-L1 levels and tumoral PD-L1 expression [35]. Importantly, soluble PD-L1 is also present in healthy patients and increases with age [36]. Still, concentrations in soluble PD-L1 are higher in cancer patients, but without a clearly defined positive threshold, soluble PD-L1 will be difficult to interpret, as for PD-L1 expression in tumor cells.

5. Riders on the Storm: Tertiary Lymphoid Structures, Tumor-Infiltrating Lymphocyte and Tumor Microenvironment

Tertiary lymphoid structures are developed at an inflammation site, e.g., around a tumor, and from an organization angle they look like lymph nodes. Their role is essential in the adaptive tumor immune response. This inflammatory state at the peripheral of the tumor facilitates the trafficking of lymphocytes, as well as their infiltration, and can also support effective antigen presentation and lymphocyte activation [37]. The presence of tertiary lymphoid structures is associated with a favorable clinical outcome for cancer patients, regardless of the stage of the disease. More particularly, the presence of CD8+ activated T lymphocytes is correlated with a favorable prognosis. Indeed, even if their natural cytotoxic activity is not considered sufficient to be curative [38], lack of lymphocytes is associated with poor response to immunotherapy. The key issue for these lymphocytes is their intratumoral penetration, so their localization has to be close to the tumor and the normalized vasculature [39]. The tumor microenvironment is an interface that promotes tumor growth, which is usually very immunosuppressed. It is characterized by acidic extracellular pH, hypoxia, high interstitial fluid pressure, aerobic glycolysis (a.k.a. the Warburg effect), glutamine addiction, and altered choline-phospholipid metabolism [40]. The neovasculature plays an essential role in the tumorigenic and immunosuppressive capacities of the microenvironment. In fact, tumor vascular stromal cells and endothelial cells decrease the recruitment, adhesion, and activity of T lymphocytes [41]. Beyond carcinogenesis, the anarchic tumor vasculature, as well as the overexpression of pro-angiogenic factors, has been recently implicated in mechanisms of resistance, including those limiting the efficacy of clinically-approved immune checkpoint inhibitors [42]. Tumor vascular normalization seems to be essential in tumor microenvironment regarding T lymphocyte recruitment and activity, decreased inflammatory reaction, and proper drug delivery [43].

Characterization and identification of the tumor microenvironment is essentially performed by immunohistochemical or immunofluorescence detection on biopsy samples and by flow cytometry analysis [44]. It is a pivotal field of research, but the characterization of tumor microenvironments and tertiary lymphoid structures remains complex, especially because their structures are also found in many inflammatory and/or autoimmune diseases.

6. Tumor Mutational Burden and Microsatellite Instability: Born to be Wild

The two most sensitive cancer types to immunotherapy are melanoma and NSCLC, which are both characterized by a high mutational tumor burden [45]. Tumor mutational burden and microsatellite instability reflect tumor genomic instability. Production of neo-antigens is the consequence of these mutations. The immune response to these neo-antigens, mediated by CD8+ and CD4+ T lymphocytes, is the basis of immunotherapy. Immune checkpoint inhibitors are highly effective in tumors presenting microsatellite-high instability (MSIH) and DNA mismatch repair-deficient tumors [46]. Consequently in 2018, the FDA approved Pembrolizumab in any advanced solid tumors with those characteristics [47].

This agnostic decision goes in the direction of an individualized precision medicine based on the specificities of the tumor for each patient, and does not, anymore, depend on the tumor localization. In the Checkmate 227 study, the first line treatment by two immune checkpoint inhibitors (Nivolumab plus Ipilimumab) showed a significantly longer progression free survival on the tumor mutational burden positive patient (≥ 10 mutations/Mb) independent of PD-L1 expression in advanced non-small-cell lung cancer [48]. Nevertheless, once again, as with PD-L1 expression the question of defining the right positive threshold is critical with the tumor mutational burden. Some studies have defined a positivity threshold for ≥ 20 mutations/Mb, i.e., twice as much than the Checkmate 227 study [45].

7. Breakout: Cell-free DNA and STING-cGAS Pathway

Cell-free DNA (cfDNA) is an interesting biomarker already used in acute cardiovascular pathologies and as a mortality predictor in myocardial infarction [49] and in inflammatory and autoimmune disease such as severe systemic lupus erythematosus [50]. The role of cfDNA seems to be associated to the STING-cGAS pathway [51]. Discovered in 2009, the STING-cGAS pathway was first described during infection as an effector of type-I interferon (IFN) production [52]. In infectiology, pathogen DNA is first recognized by cytoplasmic cyclic GMP-AMP synthase (cGAS), then the complex binds to stimulator of interferon genes (STING), thus inducing type-I interferon (IFN) and other cytokines' production [53]. This pathway plays a major role in innate immune response against DNA pathogens. Recently, STING-cGAS role in oncology has been described with immune checkpoint inhibitors [54,55]. In cancer cells, the STING-cGAS pathway is activated by cfDNA produced by two mechanisms. First, the dysregulation of DNA replication in cancer cells by endonucleases leading to cytosolic accumulation in cancer cells. Second, during mitosis damaged DNA produces cytosolic micronuclei which trigger cGAS during their rupture [56]. Accumulation of DNA in cytoplasm is considered as a danger for living cells, thus triggering the innate immune response via the activation of STING-cGAS, regardless of the DNA origin (i.e., exogenous or endogenous), since the production of type-I IFN is a universal response [57]. Type-I IFN plays, indeed, a major role in immune cells' regulation, especially in Natural Killer (NK) cell proliferation, activation, and antitumor activity. In addition, it enhances the capacity of dentritic cells to cross-present the antigen to the activated CD8+ T lymphocytes [58]. Thus, type-I IFN strengthens innate immunity in patients and, therefore, is likely to increase the efficacy of immune checkpoint inhibitors (Figure 2).

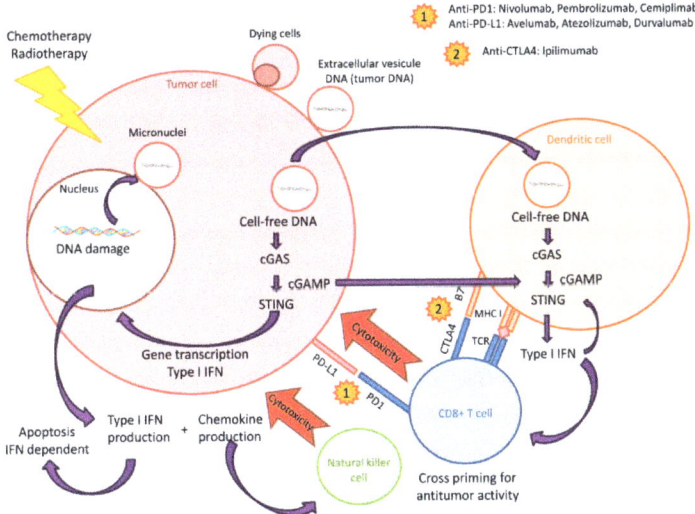

Figure 2. Sting/cGas Pathway.

STING-cGAS pathway activation is also found in the senescence phenomenon. In an aging cell, cytosolic cell-free DNA accumulates and the activated STING-cGAS pathway will increase senescence and inflammation [59]. Diagnostic use of cell-free DNA seems to be very promising in clinical oncology. The genome-wide sequencing of cfDNA for non-invasive prenatal diagnostic has been validated in over 100,000 patients, and is currently used now in a routine clinical setting [60].

Indeed, the use of cfDNA as a prognostic marker and monitoring of residual disease is increasing [61]. In addition, cell-free DNA could be used as a surrogate marker for STING-cGAS pathway activation, i.e., to determine immunogenic response to standard therapy such as cytotoxics.

In oncology, different studies showed that cfDNA length in patients are 180 bp, and are thus qualified as short [62] or between 90–150 bp [63]. A total of 180 bp fragments are characteristic for apoptotic cell death, i.e., when cellular chromatin is degraded by a caspase-activated DNase, whereas bigger, 10,000 bp fragments are rather associated with necrotic cell death [64]. The cfDNA from the tumor cell is always shorter than the cfDNA from the non-tumor cells [65]. The size is, therefore, cancer-specific and makes possible to discriminate apoptotic and non-necrotic events in cancer cells. The cfDNA length is, therefore, an important parameter to take into account for STING-cGAS pathway activation. The minimal length for triggering immune reaction is 20–40 bp, and immune optimal response is achieved between 45 and 70 bp [66]. Activation of STING-cGAS pathway and type-I IFN production are, therefore, DNA length-dependent. Otherwise, cfDNA concentration increases in advanced stages of cancer disease, as demonstrated with locally advanced cervical cancer [67] and metastatic colorectal cancer [68]. The cfDNA concentration is, therefore, a dynamic biomarker correlated to disease stage, thus allowing longitudinal monitoring of the tumor and possibly of treatment efficacy [69]. Indeed, both the size and concentrations of cfDNA are linked to IFN expression. The larger the size of the cell-free DNA length, the lower the concentration: 1.67 µg/mL for the DNA fragments of <500 bp, 0.167 µg/mL for the DNA fragments >500 bp and 0.0167 µg/mL for the DNA fragments >2000 bp [66]. For small length cfDNA fragments, concentration is critical because too low concentrations reflect primarily cellular senescence. Of note, small DNA fragments in low concentration do not trigger the STING-cGAS pathway, thus avoiding the auto-inflammation phenomenon [70]. The release from the nucleus of larger DNA fragments leads to the formation of micronuclei in cytoplasm, previously described as playing a key role in the activation of STING-cGAS.

These results suggest that STING-cGAS signaling plays a pivotal role in the intrinsic antitumor immunity and that this pathway should be activated to harness tumor immunity in patients.

As previously described with PD-L1 protein expression, chemotherapy, targeted therapy, and radiation therapy can all activate the STING-cGAS pathway [71].

For instance, radiation therapy can increase damaged DNA and cytosolic accumulation via STING-cGAS activation [72]. This could partly explain the use of radiation therapy for its ability to enhance responses to immunotherapy, since ionizing radiation-mediated tumor regression depends on type-I IFN and the adaptive immune response [73].

Regarding cytotoxics, the alkylating agent Cisplatin has been described as a powerful immunomodulating drug. Cisplatin boosts the immunogenicity of the tumor, i.e., by increasing the expression of Major Histocompatibility Complex class I (MHC I) at tumor cell surface, thus facilitating recognition by activated CD8+ T lymphocyte. Cisplatin also upregulates the STING-cGAS pathway [74]. These immunomodulatory properties could explain the synergistic effects shown between cisplatin and immune checkpoint inhibitors. Antitumor efficacy with this combination could be explained by the increased number in tumor-infiltrating CD8+ and CD4+ T lymphocytes [75]. Topoisomerase II inhibitors (e.g., doxorubicin, etoposide and epirubicin) were also described as modulating the STING-cGAS pathway and cfDNA [76]. In a study of cfDNA kinetics, the peak of DNA seems to be the highest 24 h after exposure to doxorubicin and epirubicin in breast cancer models [77]. These dynamics was also observed, in the same study, with 5-Fluorouracil. This time window could correspond to a maximum STING activation and calls for administrating immune checkpoint inhibitors 24 h after that of cytotoxics, thus suggesting a possible sequence-effect when combining drugs with immunotherapy.

Some targeted therapy, such as Poly ADP Ribose Polymerase (PARP) inhibitors seems to modulate the STING-cGAS pathway as well [78]. PARP is implicated in the DNA repair process, for which inhibition leads to an accumulation of cytosolic DNA, further activating the STING-cGAS pathway [79]. PARP inhibitors induce STING-dependent antitumor immunity [80]. This induced immunity is independent of the BRCA status of the patients [81] as demonstrated in gynecological cancers [80]. The role of PARP inhibition in cytosolic DNA accumulation was also described in prostate cancer [82]. Immunomodulating features with PARP inhibitors have been also demonstrated in NSCLC [83]. In vivo, small-cell lung cancer models showed that PARP response to damaged DNA increases PD-L1 protein expression, and increased cytotoxic T-cell infiltration [84]. These two mechanisms helped to boost antitumor effect of immune checkpoint inhibitors eventually.

Regarding immunotherapy, the STING-cGAS pathway has been identified as essential for the antitumoral effect of immune checkpoint inhibitors. For instance, STING-deficient mice are refractory to the antitumor effects of PD-L1 [85]. Conversely, direct administration of the STING or cGAS agonist shows an antiproliferative effect, and the STING agonist further reverses resistance to anti-PD1 [86]. Elsewhere, cGAS administered as nanoparticles increases production of type-I IFN, however, with no impact on tumor growth in the absence of immunotherapy [87]. This last study underlines the major role of STING-cGAS pathway on type-I IFN production and T lymphocyte activation but also the essential role of immune checkpoint inhibitors to translate this into therapeutic effect. Link between STING-cGAS pathway activation and immune checkpoint inhibitor efficacy has been demonstrated in several studies [88]. In ovarian cancer mouse models, overexpression of STING-cGAS upregulates PD-L1 protein expression [74]. This pathway appears to be an interesting target for potentiating the immunotherapy effect. Numerous clinical trials are currently underway studying agonist STING combining immune checkpoint inhibitors or in monotherapy from pre-clinical to phase 3 study [89].

Finally, as previously mentioned, the STING-cGAS pathway plays a major role in activated T lymphocytes by increasing the production of several chemokines. Among them, CCL5 and CXCL10 are known as being chemotactic for T lymphocytes, allowing tumoral accumulation and increasing tertiary lymphoid structures' formation [90]. STING further activates dendritic cells and initiates the priming of T lymphocytes [91]. Study of the STING-cGAS pathway activation by cfDNA is, therefore, an indirect way of studying the tumoral microenvironment and the tumor-infiltrating lymphocyte [92].

8. cfDNA and STING-cGAS Pathway Activation: Stairway to Heaven or Highway to Hell?

The cfDNA-mediated activation of the STING-cGAS pathway seems, therefore, to be a promising way to optimize immune checkpoint inhibitor therapy; however, this pathway is a double-edged sword [93]. Beyond the antitumoral effect of STING-cGAS, it also plays a major role in carcinogenesis, particularly via inflammation activation, autoimmune response, and direct tissue toxicity [71]. In carcinogenesis, MYD 88 (molecule myeloid differentiation factor 88) signaling seems to play a major role in cancer development via cytokine, chemokine, and growth factor production. In functional STING mice exposed to DMBA (a polyaromatic hydrocarbon known as carcinogenic agent), cutaneous skin tumors with pro-inflammatory cytokine production and phagocytic infiltration were observed [94]. Conversely, deficient STING mice did not develop such skin tumors post DMBA exposure, suggesting the role STING could play in skin cancer development [95]. Conversely, in some cancer types such as melanoma or colon cancer, the STING-cGAS pathway can be impaired by loss-of-function mutation or epigenetic silencing of the STING-cGAS promoter regions [96]. In this case, quantification of cell-free DNA could not be associated to an upregulation of STING-cGAS. Furthermore, in tongue squamous cells induced by human papillomavirus models, STING-cGAS activation eases T Regs infiltration and could, therefore, have a negative impact [97].

The cfDNA, itself, can be a confounding factor. As previously underlined, cfDNA is more important in cancer patients, and is not always synonymous of inflammatory situations. The cfDNA reflects genome plasticity, leading to a physiological and autonomous process of cells for its elimination [59]. Half-life of cfDNA should also be considered; it varies between 15 min and few hours [98], thus raising questions about appropriate sampling time for decision-making.

9. Discussion: Shine a Light

Immunotherapy and more specifically, immune checkpoint inhibitors, have fueled huge hope in oncology. However, the clinical results in terms of survival have failed to meet the initial expectations because only a minority of patients show long term survival, in a minority of cancer disease such as melanoma, NSCLC, head, neck, and kidney cancers. Consequently, combinatorial regimens now turned to as the rule, and not anymore, the exception with immunotherapy, in an attempt to harness tumor immunity prior to administrating immune checkpoint inhibitors. This strategy is expected to transform promising and breakthrough pharmaceutical innovations into meaningful survival in patients. The main difficulty when using immune checkpoint inhibitors is the complexity of their mechanisms of action which cannot be reduced to PD-L1, PD1, or CTLA4 inhibition anymore as once thought, but require as well, an adequate tumor micro-environment enriched with activated lymphocytes with little T Regs or MDSC activity. In this respect, using canonical cytotoxics is an appealing strategy to increase immunogenic cell death while down-regulating immunosuppressive cells [99]. However, achieving such immunomodulating features requires fine tuning since they are much probably drug- and dose-dependent [100]. For instance, in several non-clinical studies combining anti-PD1 or anti-PDL1 with anti CDK 4/6 or anti-OX40 drugs, it has been demonstrated that even slight changes in scheduling are likely to dramatically change the response to the combinations [101]. The same phenomenon has been observed as well when combining immune checkpoint inhibitors with radiation therapy [102]. All these studies call for a comprehensive understanding of the exact dynamics of tumor reengineering when drugs are used to harness immunity and expected to yield synergistic effect with immunotherapy. Indeed, capturing this exact dynamic is a tricky but critical issue, because it could provide valuable information on the best dosing, timing, and sequencing, especially when combining cytotoxics with immune checkpoint inhibitors. Unfortunately, as of today current combinatorial strategies remain empirical and concomitant dosing is frequent. Consequently, many clinical trials have failed to yield meaningful results in terms of prolonged survival [103]. Notably, as previously explained, baseline PDL1 expression levels cannot help determining the optimal modality of combination between immune checkpoint inhibitors and associated treatments such as chemotherapy. The same observation can be made with tumor burden, medical records, microbiota features, or any of the numerous parameters tested so far as putative predictive markers with immunotherapy. This calls for using more dynamic markers better reflecting real-time changes in the tumor micro-environment such as immunogenic cell death. Because as seen before, STING-cGAS is a critical signaling pathway associated with response to immunotherapy and that release of cfDNA, especially the shorter ones, activates this pathway, blood quantification of cfDNA could be a convenient surrogate to monitor STING-cGAS activation. This could help predicting the best timing to use immune checkpoint inhibitors next. As previously stated, cfDNA seems to be the only biomarker whose kinetics would allow to define this optimal window, especially with a combinatorial regimen. Indeed, peak of cell-free DNA is dependent upon the tumor itself but also by the concomitant use of other anticancer therapies such as chemotherapy, radiation therapy, but also oral targeted therapies. By discriminating large (i.e., >10,000 bp) cfDNA associated with necrosis from the short (i.e., 180 bp) ones associated with tumor apoptosis with immunogenic response via STING-cGAS, it paves the way for a qualitative and quantitative monitoring of cancer patients.

In addition, quantification of cfDNA is achieved by liquid biopsy, thus facilitating its implementation and allowing repeated and longitudinal measures throughout time. As a comparison, immunomonitoring provides valuable information on activated T lymphocytes or T Regs (i.e., to assess the impact of chemotherapy on the immune system,) but this can only be done after tumor biopsy, thus limiting its repeated use in routine patients.

To date, current biomarkers such as TMB, MSIH, or PD-L1 expression levels are mostly used prior to therapy in a binary, Go/No-Go, fashion. Indeed, despite the current vagueness for defining positivity threshold, PDL1 expression is a green light for using immune checkpoint inhibitors, as MSIH stats for pembrolizumab (Figure 3). Once treatment has started, monitoring these markers does not allow tuning, nor dosing, scheduling, or sequencing should combinatorial regimen be administrated, and evaluation for response is performed several cycles later.

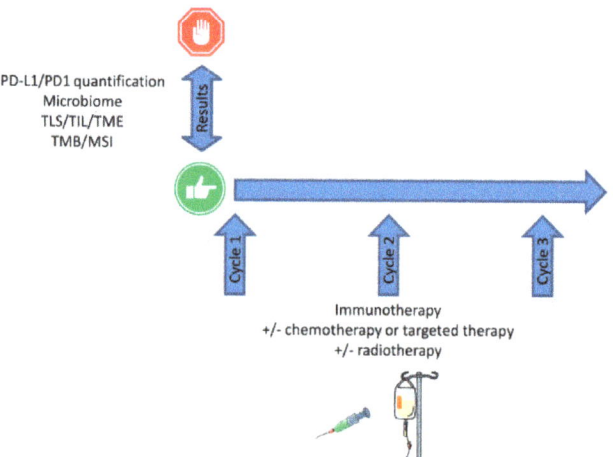

Figure 3. Current use of biomarker prior to setting up combinatorial immunotherapy. Upfront testing helps to determine the Go/No Go by predicting the odds of success. However, no longitudinal monitoring is currently feasible and basal levels have to be considered as granted.

Conversely, monitoring cfDNA is a dynamic strategy. The cfDNA can also be a Go to start immunotherapy. In case of absence of a DNA peak, this calls for starting for treatments such as neo-adjuvant chemotherapy or radiation therapy expected to trigger immunogenic cell death—monitoring cfDNA could thus help to determine the best time-window to start immunotherapy with respect to changes in tumor immunity (Figure 4). By doing so, the current concomitance of treatments should not be longer the rule as immune checkpoint inhibitors administration would be more wisely guided by a real-time biomarker. With respect to the ever-increasing drug-costs in oncology, developing novel strategies to optimize treatment efficacy and treatment cost-effectiveness is now critical. Rather than relying on a basal biomarker, longitudinal monitoring would allow fine tuning of the therapy, i.e., by stopping a therapy which is doomed to fail, before imaging reveals treatment failure. Unlike costly pan-genomic analysis of tumors or microbiota, cfDNA could be a cheap, rapid, non-invasive, and convenient way to check whether immunotherapy is likely to yield clinical benefit or not.

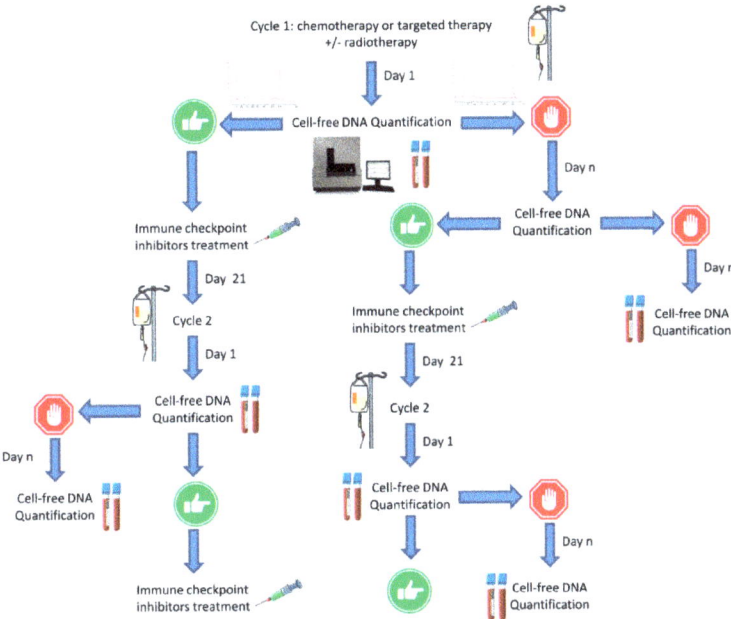

Figure 4. Proposed strategy for refining combinatorial immunotherapy. After that standard treatment is given, longitudinal monitoring of cell-free DNA helps to determine the best timing for further administering immune checkpoint inhibitors. Rather than pre-defined dosing, longitudinal monitoring allows customized treatment throughout time.

Author Contributions: G.S., F.F., R.F., F.B. and J.C. collected data and wrote the manuscript. G.S. and J.C. prepared the figures. All authors have read and agreed to the published version of the manuscript.

Funding: This work was funded by A*MIDEX grant "SMART project" (Aix Marseille Univ France) P.I.'ed by Fabrice Barlesi.

Conflicts of Interest: The authors declare no conflict of interest.

References

1. Barlési, F.; Scherpereel, A.; Rittmeyer, A.; Pazzola, A.; Tur, N.F.; Kim, J.-H.; Ahn, M.-J.; Aerts, J.G.; Gorbunova, V.; Vikström, A.; et al. Randomized Phase III Trial of Maintenance Bevacizumab with or without Pemetrexed after First-Line Induction with Bevacizumab, Cisplatin, and Pemetrexed in Advanced Nonsquamous Non–Small-Cell Lung Cancer: AVAPERL (MO22089). *J. Clin. Oncol.* **2013**, *31*, 3004–3011. [CrossRef]
2. Fitzhugh, D.J.; Lockey, R.F. History of Immunotherapy: The First 100 Years. *Immunol. Allergy Clin. N. Am.* **2011**, *31*, 149–157. [CrossRef]
3. Kaufman, H.L.; Atkins, M.B.; Subedi, P.; Wu, J.; Chambers, J.; Mattingly, T.J.; Campbell, J.D.; Allen, J.; Ferris, A.E.; Schilsky, R.L.; et al. The promise of Immuno-oncology: Implications for defining the value of cancer treatment. *J. Immunother. Cancer* **2019**, *7*, 129. [CrossRef]
4. Ledford, H. The perfect blend. *Nature* **2016**, *532*, 162–165. [CrossRef]
5. Barbolosi, D.; Ciccolini, J.; Lacarelle, B.; Barlesi, F.; Andre, N. Computational oncology—Mathematical modelling of drug regimens for precision medicine. *Nat. Rev. Clin. Oncol.* **2015**, *13*, 242–254. [CrossRef]
6. Feng, Y.; Roy, A.; Masson, E.; Chen, T.-T.; Humphrey, R.; Weber, J.S. Exposure-Response Relationships of the Efficacy and Safety of Ipilimumab in Patients with Advanced Melanoma. *Clin. Cancer Res.* **2013**, *19*, 3977–3986. [CrossRef]
7. Bellesoeur, A.; Ollier, E.; Allard, M.; Hirsch, L.; Boudou-Rouquette, P.; Arrondeau, J.; Thomas-Schoemann, A.; Tiako, M.; Khoudour, N.; Chapron, J.; et al. Is there an Exposure–Response Relationship for Nivolumab in Real-World NSCLC Patients? *Cancers* **2019**, *11*, 1784. [CrossRef] [PubMed]
8. Topalian, S.L.; Hodi, F.S.; Brahmer, J.R.; Gettinger, S.N.; Smith, D.C.; McDermott, D.F.; Powderly, J.D.; Carvajal, R.D.; Sosman, J.A.; Atkins, M.B.; et al. Safety, activity, and immune correlates of anti-PD-1 antibody in cancer. *North Engl. J. Med.* **2012**, *366*, 2443–2454. [CrossRef] [PubMed]
9. Seidel, J.A.; Otsuka, A.; Kabashima, K. Anti-PD-1 and Anti-CTLA-4 Therapies in Cancer: Mechanisms of Action, Efficacy, and Limitations. *Front. Oncol.* **2018**, *8*, 8. [CrossRef]
10. Stewart, T.J.; Abrams, S.I. How tumours escape mass destruction. *Oncogene* **2008**, *27*, 5894–5903. [CrossRef]
11. Hargadon, K.M.; Johnson, C.E.; Williams, C.J. Immune checkpoint blockade therapy for cancer: An overview of FDA-approved immune checkpoint inhibitors. *Int. Immunopharmacol.* **2018**, *62*, 29–39. [CrossRef] [PubMed]
12. Darvin, P.; Toor, S.M.; Nair, V.S.; Elkord, E. Immune checkpoint inhibitors: Recent progress and potential biomarkers. *Exp. Mol. Med.* **2018**, *50*, 1–11. [CrossRef] [PubMed]
13. Vaddepally, R.K.; Kharel, P.; Pandey, R.; Garje, R.; Chandra, A.B. Review of Indications of FDA-Approved Immune Checkpoint Inhibitors per NCCN Guidelines with the Level of Evidence. *Cancers* **2020**, *12*, 738. [CrossRef]
14. Lipson, E.J.; Drake, C.G. Ipilimumab: An anti-CTLA-4 antibody for metastatic melanoma. *Clin. Cancer Res.* **2011**, *17*, 6958–6962. [CrossRef]
15. Zheng, Y.; Fang, Y.; Li, J. PD-L1 expression levels on tumor cells affect their immunosuppressive activity. *Oncol. Lett.* **2019**, *18*, 5399–5407. [CrossRef]
16. Cai, J.; Wang, D.; Zhang, G.; Guo, X. The Role Of PD-1/PD-L1 Axis in Treg Development and Function: Implications for Cancer Immunotherapy. *Onco Targets Ther.* **2019**, *12*, 8437–8445. [CrossRef]
17. Darnell, E.P.; Mooradian, M.J.; Baruch, E.N.; Yilmaz, M.; Reynolds, K.L. Immune-Related Adverse Events (irAEs): Diagnosis, Management, and Clinical Pearls. *Curr. Oncol. Rep.* **2020**, *22*, 39. [CrossRef]
18. Palaskas, N.; Lopez-Mattei, J.; Durand, J.B.; Iliescu, C.; Deswal, A. Immune Checkpoint Inhibitor Myocarditis: Pathophysiological Characteristics, Diagnosis, and Treatment. *J. Am. Hear. Assoc.* **2020**, *9*, e013757. [CrossRef]
19. Merritt, R.E.; Mahtabifard, A.; Yamada, R.E.; Crystal, R.G.; Korst, R.J.; Bove, E.L.; De Leval, M.R.; Migliavacca, F.; Guadagni, G.; Dubini, G.; et al. Cisplatin augments cytotoxic T-lymphocyte-mediated antitumor immunity in poorly immunogenic murine lung cancer. *J. Thorac. Cardiovasc. Surg.* **2003**, *126*, 1609–1617. [CrossRef]
20. Havel, J.J.; Chowell, D.; Chan, T.A. The evolving landscape of biomarkers for checkpoint inhibitor immunotherapy. *Nat. Rev. Cancer* **2019**, *19*, 133–150. [CrossRef]
21. Brandi, G.; Frega, G. Microbiota: Overview and Implication in Immunotherapy-Based Cancer Treatments. *Int. J. Mol. Sci.* **2019**, *20*, 2699. [CrossRef] [PubMed]

22. Zitvogel, L.; Ma, Y.; Raoult, D.; Kroemer, G.; Gajewski, T.F. The microbiome in cancer immunotherapy: Diagnostic tools and therapeutic strategies. *Science* **2018**, *359*, 1366–1370. [CrossRef] [PubMed]
23. Pinato, D.J.; Gramenitskaya, D.; Altmann, D.M.; Boyton, R.J.; Mullish, B.H.; Marchesi, J.R.; Bower, M. Antibiotic therapy and outcome from immune-checkpoint inhibitors. *J. Immunother. Cancer* **2019**, *7*, 287–288. [CrossRef]
24. Gandini, S.; Massi, D.; Mandalà, M. PD-L1 expression in cancer patients receiving anti PD-1/PD-L1 antibodies: A systematic review and meta-analysis. *Crit. Rev. Oncol. Hematol.* **2016**, *100*, 88–98. [CrossRef]
25. Ribas, A.; Hu-Lieskovan, S. What does PD-L1 positive or negative mean? *J. Exp. Med.* **2016**, *213*, 2835–2840. [CrossRef]
26. Shen, X.; Zhao, B. Efficacy of PD-1 or PD-L1 inhibitors and PD-L1 expression status in cancer: Meta-analysis. *BMJ* **2018**, *362*, k3529. [CrossRef]
27. Udall, M.; Rizzo, M.; Kenny, J.; Doherty, J.; Dahm, S.; Robbins, P.; Faulkner, E. PD-L1 diagnostic tests: A systematic literature review of scoring algorithms and test-validation metrics. *Diagn. Pathol.* **2018**, *13*, 12. [CrossRef]
28. Hendry, S.; Byrne, D.J.; Wright, G.M.; Young, R.J.; Sturrock, S.; Cooper, W.; Fox, S.B. Comparison of Four PD-L1 Immunohistochemical Assays in Lung Cancer. *J. Thorac. Oncol.* **2017**, *13*, 367–376. [CrossRef]
29. Shah, N.J.; Kelly, W.J.; Liu, S.V.; Choquette, K.; Spira, A. Product review on the Anti-PD-L1 antibody atezolizumab. *Hum. Vaccines Immunother.* **2017**, *14*, 269–276. [CrossRef]
30. Syed, Y.Y. Durvalumab: First Global Approval. *Drugs* **2017**, *77*, 1369–1376. [CrossRef]
31. Wang, Y.; Kim, T.H.; Fouladdel, S.; Zhang, Z.; Soni, P.; Qin, A.; Zhao, L.; Azizi, E.; Lawrence, T.S.; Ramnath, N.; et al. PD-L1 Expression in Circulating Tumor Cells Increases during Radio(chemo)therapy and Indicates Poor Prognosis in Non-small Cell Lung Cancer. *Sci. Rep.* **2019**, *9*, 566. [CrossRef]
32. Shevtsov, M.; Sato, H.; Multhoff, G.; Shibata, A. Novel Approaches to Improve the Efficacy of Immuno-Radiotherapy. *Front. Oncol.* **2019**, *9*, 9. [CrossRef]
33. Jelinek, T.; Mihalyova, J.; Kascak, M.; Duras, J.; Hajek, R. PD-1/PD-L1 inhibitors in haematological malignancies: Update 2017. *Immunology* **2017**, *152*, 357–371. [CrossRef]
34. Gilad, Y.; Eliaz, Y.; Yu, Y.; Han, S.J.; Malley, B.W.O.; Lonard, D.M. Drug-induced PD-L1 expression and cell stress response in breast cancer cells can be balanced by drug combination. *Sci. Rep.* **2019**, *9*, 15099. [CrossRef]
35. Aghajani, M.; Roberts, T.L.; Yang, T.; McCafferty, C.; Caixeiro, N.J.; De Souza, P.; Niles, N. Elevated levels of soluble PD-L1 are associated with reduced recurrence in papillary thyroid cancer. *Endocr. Connect.* **2019**, *8*, 1040–1051. [CrossRef]
36. Chen, Y.; Wang, Q.; Shi, B.; Xu, P.; Hu, Z.; Bai, L.; Zhang, X. Development of a sandwich ELISA for evaluating soluble PD-L1 (CD274) in human sera of different ages as well as supernatants of PD-L1+ cell lines. *Cytokine* **2011**, *56*, 231–238. [CrossRef]
37. Tang, H.; Qiu, X.; Timmerman, C.; Fu, Y.-X. Targeting Tertiary Lymphoid Structures for Tumor Immunotherapy. *Adv. Struct. Saf. Stud.* **2018**, 275–286. [CrossRef]
38. Peske, J.D.; Woods, A.; Engelhard, V.H. Control of CD8 T-Cell Infiltration into Tumors by Vasculature and Microenvironment. *Adv. Breast Cancer Res.* **2015**, *128*, 263–307. [CrossRef]
39. Engelhard, V.H.; Rodriguez, A.B.; Mauldin, I.S.; Woods, A.N.; Peske, J.D.; Slingluff, C.L.; Peske, D. Immune Cell Infiltration and Tertiary Lymphoid Structures as Determinants of Antitumor Immunity. *J. Immunol.* **2018**, *200*, 432–442. [CrossRef]
40. Ramamonjisoa, N.; Ackerstaff, E. Characterization of the Tumor Microenvironment and Tumor–Stroma Interaction by Non-invasive Preclinical Imaging. *Front. Oncol.* **2017**, *7*, 7. [CrossRef]
41. Schaaf, M.B.; Garg, A.D.; Agostinis, P. Defining the role of the tumor vasculature in antitumor immunity and immunotherapy. *Cell Death Dis.* **2018**, *9*, 115. [CrossRef]
42. Siemann, D.W. The unique characteristics of tumor vasculature and preclinical evidence for its selective disruption by Tumor-Vascular Disrupting Agents. *Cancer Treat. Rev.* **2011**, *37*, 63–74. [CrossRef] [PubMed]
43. Narang, A.S.; Varia, S. Role of tumor vascular architecture in drug delivery. *Adv. Drug Deliv. Rev.* **2011**, *63*, 640–658. [CrossRef] [PubMed]
44. De Chaisemartin, L.; Goc, J.; Damotte, D.; Validire, P.; Magdeleinat, P.; Alifano, M.; Cremer, I.; Fridman, W.H.; Sautès-Fridman, C.; Dieu-Nosjean, M.-C.; et al. Characterization of Chemokines and Adhesion Molecules Associated with T cell Presence in Tertiary Lymphoid Structures in Human Lung Cancer. *Cancer Res.* **2011**, *71*, 6391–6399. [CrossRef] [PubMed]

45. Goodman, A.M.; Sokol, E.S.; Frampton, G.M.; Lippman, S.M.; Kurzrock, R. Microsatellite-Stable Tumors with High Mutational Burden Benefit from Immunotherapy. *Cancer Immunol. Res.* **2019**, *7*, 1570–1573. [CrossRef]
46. Le, D.T.; Durham, J.N.; Smith, K.N.; Wang, H.; Bartlett, B.; Aulakh, L.K.; Lu, S.; Kemberling, H.; Wilt, C.; Luber, B.S.; et al. Mismatch repair deficiency predicts response of solid tumors to PD-1 blockade. *Science* **2017**, *357*, 409–413. [CrossRef]
47. Boyiadzis, M.M.; Kirkwood, J.M.; Marshall, J.L.; Pritchard, C.C.; Azad, N.S.; Gulley, J.L. Significance and implications of FDA approval of pembrolizumab for biomarker-defined disease. *J. Immunother. Cancer* **2018**, *6*, 35. [CrossRef]
48. Hellmann, M.D.; Paz-Ares, L.; Caro, R.B.; Zurawski, B.; Kim, S.-W.; Costa, E.C.; Park, K.; Alexandru, A.; Lupinacci, L.; Jimenez, E.D.L.M.; et al. Nivolumab plus Ipilimumab in Advanced Non–Small-Cell Lung Cancer. *N. Engl. J. Med.* **2019**, *381*, 2020–2031. [CrossRef]
49. Jylhävä, J.; Lehtimäki, T.; Jula, A.; Moilanen, L.; Kesäniemi, Y.A.; Nieminen, M.S.; Kähönen, M.; Hurme, M. Circulating cell-free DNA is associated with cardiometabolic risk factors: The Health 2000 Survey. *Atherosclerosis* **2014**, *233*, 268–271. [CrossRef]
50. Ahn, J.; Ruiz, P.; Barber, G.N. Intrinsic self-DNA triggers inflammatory disease dependent on STING. *J. Immunol.* **2014**, *193*, 4634–4642. [CrossRef]
51. Sun, L.; Wu, J.; Du, F.; Chen, X.; Chen, Z.J. Cyclic GMP-AMP Synthase Is a Cytosolic DNA Sensor That Activates the Type I Interferon Pathway. *Science* **2012**, *339*, 786–791. [CrossRef] [PubMed]
52. Ishikawa, H.; Barber, G.N. STING is an endoplasmic reticulum adaptor that facilitates innate immune signalling. *Nature* **2008**, *455*, 674–678. [CrossRef] [PubMed]
53. Tao, J.; Zhou, X.; Jiang, Z. cGAS-cGAMP-STING: The three musketeers of cytosolic DNA sensing and signaling. *IUBMB Life* **2016**, *68*, 858–870. [CrossRef] [PubMed]
54. Khoo, L.T.; Chen, L.-Y. Role of the cGAS–STING pathway in cancer development and oncotherapeutic approaches. *EMBO Rep.* **2018**, *19*, e46935. [CrossRef]
55. Saeed, A.F.U.H.; Ruan, X.; Guan, H.; Su, J.; Saeed, A.F. Regulation of cGAS-Mediated Immune Responses and Immunotherapy. *Adv. Sci.* **2020**, *7*, 1902599. [CrossRef]
56. Crasta, K.C.; Ganem, N.J.; Dagher, R.; Lantermann, A.B.; Ivanova, E.V.; Pan, Y.; Nezi, L.; Protopopov, A.; Chowdhury, D.; Pellman, D. DNA breaks and chromosome pulverization from errors in mitosis. *Nature* **2012**, *482*, 53–58. [CrossRef]
57. Dhanwani, R.; Takahashi, M.; Sharma, S. Cytosolic sensing of immuno-stimulatory DNA, the enemy within. *Curr. Opin. Immunol.* **2017**, *50*, 82–87. [CrossRef]
58. Diamond, M.S.; Kinder, M.; Matsushita, H.; Mashayekhi, M.; Dunn, G.P.; Archambault, J.M.; Lee, H.; Arthur, C.D.; White, J.M.; Kalinke, U.; et al. Type I interferon is selectively required by dendritic cells for immune rejection of tumors. *J. Exp. Med.* **2011**, *208*, 1989–2003. [CrossRef]
59. Lan, Y.Y.; Heather, J.M.; Eisenhaure, T.; Garris, C.S.; Lieb, D.; Raychowdhury, R.; Hacohen, N. Extranuclear DNA accumulates in aged cells and contributes to senescence and inflammation. *Aging Cell* **2019**, *18*, e12901. [CrossRef]
60. Jensen, T.J.; Goodman, A.M.; Kato, S.; Ellison, C.K.; Daniels, G.A.; Kim, L.; Nakashe, P.; McCarthy, E.; Mazloom, A.R.; McLennan, G.; et al. Genome-Wide Sequencing of Cell-Free DNA Identifies Copy-Number Alterations That Can Be Used for Monitoring Response to Immunotherapy in Cancer Patients. *Mol. Cancer Ther.* **2018**, *18*, 448–458. [CrossRef]
61. Bronkhorst, A.J.; Ungerer, V.; Holdenrieder, S. The emerging role of cell-free DNA as a molecular marker for cancer management. *Biomol. Detect. Quantif.* **2019**, *17*, 100087. [CrossRef] [PubMed]
62. Giacona, M.B.; Ruben, G.C.; Iczkowski, K.A.; Roos, T.B.; Porter, D.M.; Sorenson, G.D. Cell-Free DNA in Human Blood Plasma. *Pancreas* **1998**, *17*, 89–97. [CrossRef] [PubMed]
63. Mouliere, F.; Chandrananda, D.; Piskorz, A.M.; Moore, E.K.; Morris, J.; Ahlborn, L.B.; Mair, R.; Goranova, T.E.; Marass, F.; Heider, K.; et al. Enhanced detection of circulating tumor DNA by fragment size analysis. *Sci. Transl. Med.* **2018**, *10*, eaat4921. [CrossRef] [PubMed]
64. Jahr, S.; Hentze, H.; Englisch, S.; Hardt, D.; Fackelmayer, F.O.; Hesch, R.D.; Knippers, R. DNA fragments in the blood plasma of cancer patients: Quantitations and evidence for their origin from apoptotic and necrotic cells. *Cancer Res.* **2001**, *61*, 1659–1665. [PubMed]
65. Jiang, P.; Lo, Y.M.D. The Long and Short of Circulating Cell-Free DNA and the Ins and Outs of Molecular Diagnostics. *Trends Genet.* **2016**, *32*, 360–371. [CrossRef]

66. Luecke, S.; Holleufer, A.; Christensen, M.H.; Jønsson, K.L.; Boni, G.A.; Sørensen, L.K.; Johannsen, M.; Jakobsen, M.R.; Hartmann, R.; Paludan, S.R. cGAS is activated by DNA in a length-dependent manner. *EMBO Rep.* **2017**, *18*, 1707–1715. [CrossRef]
67. Tian, J.; Geng, Y.; Lv, D.; Li, P.; Córdova-Delgado, M.; Liao, Y.; Tian, X.; Zhang, X.; Zhang, Q.; Zou, K.; et al. Using plasma cell-free DNA to monitor the chemoradiotherapy course of cervical cancer. *Int. J. Cancer* **2019**, *145*, 2547–2557. [CrossRef]
68. Spindler, K.-L.G.; Pallisgaard, N.; Andersen, R.F.; Brandslund, I.; Jakobsen, A. Circulating Free DNA as Biomarker and Source for Mutation Detection in Metastatic Colorectal Cancer. *PLoS ONE* **2015**, *10*, e0108247. [CrossRef]
69. Almodovar, K.; Iams, W.T.; Meador, C.B.; Zhao, Z.; York, S.; Horn, L.; Yan, Y.; Hernandez, J.; Chen, H.; Shyr, Y.; et al. Longitudinal Cell-Free DNA Analysis in Patients with Small Cell Lung Cancer Reveals Dynamic Insights into Treatment Efficacy and Disease Relapse. *J. Thorac. Oncol.* **2017**, *13*, 112–123. [CrossRef]
70. Bronkhorst, A.J.; Wentzel, J.F.; Ungerer, V.; Peters, D.L.; Aucamp, J.; Villiers, E.; Holdenrieder, S.; Pretorius, P.J. Sequence analysis of cell-free DNA derived from cultured human bone osteosarcoma (143B) cells. *Tumor Boil.* **2018**, *40*, 1010428318801190. [CrossRef]
71. Ahn, J.; Xia, T.; Konno, H.; Konno, K.; Ruiz, P.; Barber, G.N. Inflammation-driven carcinogenesis is mediated through STING. *Nat. Commun.* **2014**, *5*, 5166. [CrossRef] [PubMed]
72. Vanpouille-Box, C.; Alard, A.; Aryankalayil, M.J.; Sarfraz, Y.; Diamond, J.M.; Schneider, R.J.; Inghirami, G.; Coleman, C.N.; Formenti, S.C.; DeMaria, S. DNA exonuclease Trex1 regulates radiotherapy-induced tumour immunogenicity. *Nat. Commun.* **2017**, *8*, 15618. [CrossRef] [PubMed]
73. Deng, L.; Liang, H.; Xu, M.; Yang, X.; Burnette, B.; Arina, A.; Li, X.-D.; Mauceri, H.; Beckett, M.; Darga, T.; et al. STING-Dependent Cytosolic DNA Sensing Promotes Radiation-Induced Type I Interferon-Dependent Antitumor Immunity in Immunogenic Tumors. *Immunity* **2014**, *41*, 843–852. [CrossRef] [PubMed]
74. Grabosch, S.; Bulatovic, M.; Zeng, F.; Ma, T.; Zhang, L.; Ross, M.; Brozick, J.; Fang, Y.; Tseng, G.; Kim, E.; et al. Cisplatin-induced immune modulation in ovarian cancer mouse models with distinct inflammation profiles. *Oncogene* **2018**, *38*, 2380–2393. [CrossRef] [PubMed]
75. Wakita, D.; Iwai, T.; Harada, S.; Suzuki, M.; Yamamoto, K.; Sugimoto, M. Cisplatin Augments Antitumor T-Cell Responses Leading to a Potent Therapeutic Effect in Combination with PD-L1 Blockade. *Anticancer Res.* **2019**, *39*, 1749–1760. [CrossRef]
76. Sistigu, A.; Yamazaki, T.; Vacchelli, E.; Chaba, K.; Enot, D.P.; Adam, J.; Vitale, I.; Goubar, A.; Baracco, E.E.; Remédios, C.; et al. Cancer cell—Autonomous contribution of type I interferon signaling to the efficacy of chemotherapy. *Nat. Med.* **2014**, *20*, 1301–1309. [CrossRef]
77. Swystun, L.L.; Mukherjee, S.; Liaw, P.C. Breast cancer chemotherapy induces the release of cell-free DNA, a novel procoagulant stimulus. *J. Thromb. Haemost.* **2011**, *9*, 2313–2321. [CrossRef]
78. Chabanon, R.M.; Postel-Vinay, S. Inhibiteurs de PARP—Exploiter les défauts de réparation de l'ADN pour stimuler l'immunité anti-tumorale. *Med. Sci.* **2019**, *35*, 728–731.
79. Yélamos, J.; Moreno-Lama, L.; Jimeno, J.; Ali, S.O. Immunomodulatory Roles of PARP-1 and PARP-2: Impact on PARP-Centered Cancer Therapies. *Cancers* **2020**, *12*, 392. [CrossRef]
80. Ding, L.; Kim, H.-J.; Wang, Q.; Kearns, M.; Jiang, T.; Ohlson, C.E.; Li, B.B.; Xie, S.; Liu, J.F.; Stover, E.H.; et al. PARP Inhibition Elicits STING-Dependent Antitumor Immunity in Brca1-Deficient Ovarian Cancer. *Cell Rep.* **2018**, *25*, 2972–2980.e5. [CrossRef]
81. Reisländer, T.; Lombardi, E.P.; Groelly, F.J.; Miar, A.; Porru, M.; Di Vito, S.; Wright, B.; Lockstone, H.; Biroccio, A.; Harris, A.L.; et al. BRCA2 abrogation triggers innate immune responses potentiated by treatment with PARP inhibitors. *Nat. Commun.* **2019**, *10*, 3143. [CrossRef] [PubMed]
82. Ho, S.S.; Zhang, W.Y.; Tan, N.Y.J.; Khatoo, M.; Suter, M.A.; Tripathi, S.; Cheung, F.S.; Lim, W.K.; Tan, P.H.; Ngeow, J.; et al. The DNA Structure-Specific Endonuclease MUS81 Mediates DNA Sensor STING-Dependent Host Rejection of Prostate Cancer Cells. *Immunity* **2016**, *44*, 1177–1189. [CrossRef]
83. Chabanon, R.M.; Muirhead, G.; Krastev, D.; Adam, J.; Morel, D.; Garrido, M.; Lamb, A.; Hénon, C.; Dorvault, N.; Rouanne, M.; et al. PARP inhibition enhances tumor cell–intrinsic immunity in ERCC1-deficient non–small cell lung cancer. *J. Clin. Investig.* **2019**, *129*, 1211–1228. [CrossRef] [PubMed]
84. Sen, T.; Rodriguez, B.L.; Chen, L.; Della Corte, C.M.; Morikawa, N.; Fujimoto, J.; Cristea, S.; Nguyen, T.; Diao, L.; Li, L.; et al. Targeting DNA Damage Response Promotes Antitumor Immunity through STING-Mediated T-cell Activation in Small Cell Lung Cancer. *Cancer Discov.* **2019**, *9*, 646–661. [CrossRef] [PubMed]

85. Woo, S.-R.; Fuertes, M.B.; Corrales, L.; Spranger, S.; Furdyna, M.J.; Leung, M.Y.; Duggan, R.; Wang, Y.; Barber, G.N.; Fitzgerald, K.A.; et al. STING-dependent cytosolic DNA sensing mediates innate immune recognition of immunogenic tumors. *Immunity* **2014**, *41*, 830–842. [CrossRef]
86. Fu, J.; Kanne, D.B.; Leong, M.; Glickman, L.H.; McWhirter, S.M.; Lemmens, E.; Mechette, K.; Leong, J.J.; Lauer, P.; Liu, W.; et al. STING agonist formulated cancer vaccines can cure established tumors resistant to PD-1 blockade. *Sci. Transl. Med.* **2015**, *7*, 283ra52. [CrossRef]
87. Cheng, N.; Watkins-Schulz, R.; Junkins, R.D.; David, C.N.; Johnson, B.M.; Montgomery, S.A.; Peine, K.J.; Darr, D.B.; Yuan, H.; McKinnon, K.P.; et al. A nanoparticle-incorporated STING activator enhances antitumor immunity in PD-L1-insensitive models of triple-negative breast cancer. *JCI Insight* **2018**, *3*, 3. [CrossRef]
88. Li, A.; Yi, M.; Qin, S.; Song, Y.; Chu, Q.; Wu, K. Activating cGAS-STING pathway for the optimal effect of cancer immunotherapy. *J. Hematol. Oncol.* **2019**, *12*, 35. [CrossRef]
89. Jiang, M.; Chen, P.; Wang, L.; Li, W.; Chen, B.; Liu, Y.; Wang, H.; Zhao, S.; Ye, L.; He, Y.; et al. cGAS-STING, an important pathway in cancer immunotherapy. *J. Hematol. Oncol.* **2020**, *13*, 1–11. [CrossRef]
90. Liu, J.; Li, F.; Ping, Y.; Wang, L.; Chen, X.; Wang, D.; Cao, L.; Zhao, S.; Li, B.; Kalinski, P.; et al. Local production of the chemokines CCL5 and CXCL10 attracts CD8+ T lymphocytes into esophageal squamous cell carcinoma. *Oncotarget* **2015**, *6*, 24978–24989. [CrossRef]
91. Gajewski, T.F.; Schreiber, H.; Fu, Y.-X. Innate and adaptive immune cells in the tumor microenvironment. *Nat. Immunol.* **2013**, *14*, 1014–1022. [CrossRef] [PubMed]
92. Woo, S.-R.; Corrales, L.; Gajewski, T.F. The STING pathway and the T cell-inflamed tumor microenvironment. *Trends Immunol.* **2015**, *36*, 250–256. [CrossRef] [PubMed]
93. Bose, D. cGAS/STING Pathway in Cancer: Jekyll and Hyde Story of Cancer Immune Response. *Int. J. Mol. Sci.* **2017**, *18*, 2456. [CrossRef] [PubMed]
94. Barber, G.N. STING: Infection, inflammation and cancer. *Nat. Rev. Immunol.* **2015**, *15*, 760–770. [CrossRef] [PubMed]
95. Salcedo, R.; Cataisson, C.; Hasan, U.; Yuspa, S.H.; Trinchieri, G. MyD88 and its divergent toll in carcinogenesis. *Trends Immunol.* **2013**, *34*, 379–389. [CrossRef]
96. Konno, H.; Yamauchi, S.; Berglund, A.; Putney, R.M.; Mulé, J.J.; Barber, G.N. Suppression of STING signaling through epigenetic silencing and missense mutation impedes DNA damage mediated cytokine production. *Oncogene* **2018**, *37*, 2037–2051. [CrossRef]
97. Liang, D.; Xiao-Feng, H.; Guan-Jun, D.; Er-Ling, H.; Sheng, C.; Ting-Ting, W.; Qin-Gang, H.; Ni, Y.; Hou, Y. Activated STING enhances Tregs infiltration in the HPV-related carcinogenesis of tongue squamous cells via the c-jun/CCL22 signal. *Biochim. Biophys. Acta* **2015**, *1852*, 2494–2503. [CrossRef]
98. Fleischhacker, M.; Schmidt, B. Circulating nucleic acids (CNAs) and cancer—A survey. *Biochim. Biophys. Acta* **2007**, *1775*, 181–232. [CrossRef]
99. Vanmeerbeek, I.; Sprooten, J.; De Ruysscher, D.; Tejpar, S.; Vandenberghe, P.; Fucikova, J.; Spisek, R.; Zitvogel, L.; Kroemer, G.; Galluzzi, L.; et al. Trial watch: Chemotherapy-induced immunogenic cell death in immuno-oncology. *OncoImmunology* **2020**, *9*, 1703449. [CrossRef]
100. Kepp, O.; Galluzzi, L.; Martins, I.; Schlemmer, F.; Adjemian, S.; Michaud, M.; Sukkurwala, A.Q.; Menger, L.; Zitvogel, L.; Kroemer, G. Molecular determinants of immunogenic cell death elicited by anticancer chemotherapy. *Cancer Metastasis Rev.* **2011**, *30*, 61–69. [CrossRef]
101. Schaer, D.A.; Beckmann, R.P.; Dempsey, J.A.; Huber, L.; Forest, A.; Amaladas, N.; Li, Y.; Wang, Y.C.; Rasmussen, E.R.; Chin, D.; et al. The CDK4/6 Inhibitor Abemaciclib Induces a T Cell Inflamed Tumor Microenvironment and Enhances the Efficacy of PD-L1 Checkpoint Blockade. *Cell Rep.* **2018**, *22*, 2978–2994. [CrossRef] [PubMed]
102. Young, K.H.; Baird, J.R.; Savage, T.; Cottam, B.; Friedman, D.; Bambina, S.; Messenheimer, D.J.; Fox, B.; Newell, P.; Bahjat, K.S.; et al. Optimizing Timing of Immunotherapy Improves Control of Tumors by Hypofractionated Radiation Therapy. *PLoS ONE* **2016**, *11*, e0157164. [CrossRef] [PubMed]
103. Ciccolini, J.; Barbolosi, D.; André, N.; Benzekry, S.; Barlesi, F. Combinatorial immunotherapy strategies: Most gods throw dice, but fate plays chess. *Ann. Oncol.* **2019**, *30*, 1690–1691. [CrossRef] [PubMed]

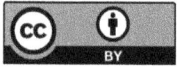

© 2020 by the authors. Licensee MDPI, Basel, Switzerland. This article is an open access article distributed under the terms and conditions of the Creative Commons Attribution (CC BY) license (http://creativecommons.org/licenses/by/4.0/).

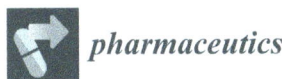

Article

A Tumor-Immune Interaction Model for Synergistic Combinations of Anti PD-L1 and Ionizing Irradiation Treatment

Jong Hyuk Byun [1,2], In-Soo Yoon [3], Yong Dam Jeong [1], Sungchan Kim [1,4] and Il Hyo Jung [1,4,*]

[1] Department of Mathematics, Pusan National University, Busan 46241, Korea; maticax@gmail.com (J.H.B.); wde0539@hanmail.net (Y.D.J.); scfrom88@daum.net (S.K.)
[2] Institute of Mathematical Sciences, Pusan National University, Busan 46241, Korea
[3] College of Pharmacy, Pusan National University, Busan 46241, Korea; insoo.yoon@pusan.ac.kr
[4] Finance Fishery Manufacture Industrial Mathematics Center on Big Data, Pusan National University, Busan 46241, Korea
* Correspondence: ilhjung@pusan.ac.kr

Received: 6 August 2020; Accepted: 29 August 2020; Published: 31 August 2020

Abstract: Combination therapy with immune checkpoint blockade and ionizing irradiation therapy (IR) generates a synergistic effect to inhibit tumor growth better than either therapy does alone. We modeled the tumor-immune interactions occurring during combined IT and IR based on the published data from Deng et al. The mathematical model considered programmed cell death protein 1 and programmed death ligand 1, to quantify data fitting and global sensitivity of critical parameters. Fitting of data from control, IR and IT samples was conducted to verify the synergistic effect of a combination therapy consisting of IR and IT. Our approach using the model showed that an increase in the expression level of PD-1 and PD-L1 was proportional to tumor growth before therapy, but not after initiating therapy. The high expression level of PD-L1 in T cells may inhibit IT efficacy. After combination therapy begins, the tumor size was also influenced by the ratio of PD-1 to PD-L1. These results highlight that the ratio of PD-1 to PD-L1 in T cells could be considered in combination therapy.

Keywords: immunotherapy; anti-PD-L1; ionizing irradiation; pharmacokinetics; tumor-immune interaction; global sensitivity; immuno-oncology; mathematical modeling

1. Introduction

Immunotherapy using immune checkpoint blockade (IT) is an anti-cancer therapy that recovers immunity by suppressing various tumor mechanisms that evade the immune response [1–4]. In particular, new ITs primarily aim to inhibit cytotoxic T-lymphocyte-associated protein 4 (CTLA-4), programmed cell death protein 1 (PD-1), and programmed death ligand 1 (PD-L1) to enable T lymphocytes to attack cancer cells [5–7]. Despite the impressive potential of these checkpoint blockade in the treatment of various cancers, this therapy strategy remains challenging because the response to a certain subgroup of IT is varied among the cancer patients [8,9]. In recent years, several studies have aimed to achieve synergistic effects through combination therapy to compensate for the shortcomings of monotherapy [10–13].

There are mathematical models of immune-tumor interactions to demonstrate the data of Deng et al. [14]. These studies [15,16] revealed the synergistic effect of anti-PD-L1 and IR combination therapy in mice. Chappell et al. [15] discussed that IT is directly involved in increasing T cell levels and indirectly stimulates tumor death via T cells. The underlying assumption considered that IR affects the death rate of both tumors and T cells. Based on this assumption, they formulated a mathematical model for the interaction between T cells and tumors. Model simulation was roughly conducted, focusing on the relationship between six compartments considering inhibition and activation. The main finding was the modeling and its equilibrium analysis; however, data fitting was not performed accurately. Additionally, the sensitivity analysis of the main parameters was relatively less investigated. Due to excessive suppression of IT and the bias of control growth, the synergistic effect of combined IR and IT was not accurately measured. Nevertheless, this model was able to explain how IT and IR affected tumors and T cells.

The other model was from Nikolopoulou et al. [16]. They considered PD-1 and PD-L1 expressed on the surface of tumors and T cells. The model was established through the assumption that tumors express PD-L1, and T cells express both PD-1 and PD-L1 on their surface. Negative feedback from the PD-1-PD-L1 complex occurs by the binding of PD-1 and PD-L1, resulting in inhibition of T cell growth. This model simplifies the binding process of PD-1 and PD-L1 by employing equilibrium assumptions. Thus, a three-compartment model was used. Anti-PD-L1 was composed of a system that reduced tumor size by suppressing the growth inhibition of T cells by inhibiting PD-L1. However, this model was less well verified by experimental data; anti-PD-L1 monotherapy was applied, but was less effective. Nevertheless, it is valuable to note the effect of immunotherapy on tumors or T cells through correlation with PD-1 and anti-PD-L1.

In this study, we proposed a mathematical model for tumor-immune interactions using anti-PD-L1 and IR in combination therapy. Here, we refer to anti-PD-L1 exclusively as IT. Deng et al. presented mice data for change in tumor size during combination therapy with anti-PD-L1 and IR. In the study, TUBO tumor cells from a spontaneous mammary tumor were injected subcutaneous injection (s.c.) into the flanks of mice. After allowing to grow for about two weeks, tumors were treated by IR with single dose and IT with administrated intraperitoneal injection to mice every three days for a total of three times. The experiment of control (without treatment), IR only, IT only and combination of IR and IT are conducted. They revealed that combination therapy had a synergistic effect that enhances host antitumor immunity and increases the efficacy of either treatment alone. Our mathematical model reproduced Deng et al.'s published data to describe tumor-T cell interaction through IT and IR, including PD-1 and PD-L1. Thus, this model enabled us to examine suppression of the tumor size by combination therapy and explore the effects of the ratio of PD-1 to PD-L1. Model simulation verified the data from combination therapy after estimating parameters using control, IT only, and IR only data. The synergistic effect was also confirmed through the model. Using global sensitivity, we measured the influence of essential parameters related to the change in PD-1 and PD-L1. Our approach showed that PD-1 or PD-L1 expression levels positively determined tumor size before therapy, but the sum of the expression level of PD-1 and PD-L1 was uncorrelated to tumor size after therapy has begun. Additionally, the high expression level of PD-L1 in T cells may inhibit IT efficacy. After combination therapy begins, the efficiency was influenced by the ratio of PD-1 to PD-L1. The model results revealed that the ratio of PD-1 to PD-L1 in T cells could be considered as one of the factors to determine the efficacy of combination therapy.

2. Materials and Methods

2.1. Assumptions

We have made the following assumptions. (i) Tumors express PD-L1 on the surface, and an increase in tumor size leads to an increase in the rate of the concentration of PD-L1. Additionally, an increase in CD8+ T cell number induces an increase in the rate of the concentration of PD-1 and PD-L1 because T cells express both PD-1 and PD-L1. (ii) The tumor grows logistically, and the natural death of the tumor is not considered. Tumor elimination depends on IT indirectly and IR directly. (iii) IT therapy is modeled using a pharmacokinetic two-compartment model that reflects administration by intraperitoneal injection (I.P.). The two-compartment model is also considered for IR therapy.

IR therapy is administered immediately, but tumor suppression by IR is relatively delayed. The extra compartment reflects the delay in tumor inhibition by the therapy. The concentration in the tissue compartment is denoted by A_T. (iv) Volume, V, in mice is assumed to be 50 µL. (v) The initial density (10^9 cells/L) of T cells is 6×10^{-4}, and the initial concentrations of PD-1 and PD-L1 are assumed to be 1×10^{-5}. This assumption indicates that the initial density of T cells is small, and their concentrations begin to increase after the tumor is implanted. A schematic diagram of tumor-immune interactions is shown in Figure 1.

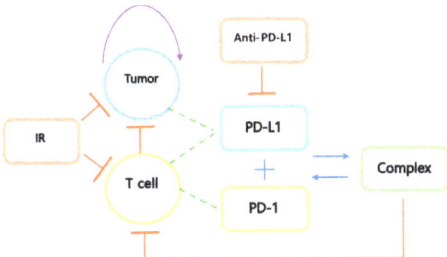

Figure 1. The tumor undergoes logistic growth, and T cells activate the cytokines interleukin 1 (IL1) and interleukin 12 (IL12). IL1 and IL12 are activated by stimulation of the tumor. The tumor expresses PD-L1 on the cell surface, and T cells express both PD-L1 and PD-1 on their surface. The binding process of PD-L1 and PD-1 results in negative feedback in T cells. IT inhibits the growth of both tumor and T cells and inhibits PD-L1 by preventing the formation of the PD-L1-PD-1 complex, which prevents the inhibition of T cell growth.

2.2. Data Derivation from the Study

Published data was obtained from the experiments of Deng et al. Their study was to verify the synergistic antitumor effects of IR and IT. A combination of IT and IR significantly enhanced the inhibition of TUBO growth in their study. The outline of the experiment process was as follows. BALB/c mice were inoculated by subcutaneous injection with 1×10^6 TUBO cells (the size 5 mm^3). After injected s.c. and waiting for 14 days (growing), tumors were locally treated with single 12 Gy of IR and 200 µg IT (antibody, clone 10F.9G2) by intraperitoneal injection every three days for a total of four doses. Tumor size was measured in mice with no therapy, IT only, IR only, and combination therapy with IT and IR. For reproducing the experimental data, the data values were extracted from the study. Adobe Illustrator is used to find the coordinates of published data. Data values, shown in Figure 2 (left top panel), are presented in Table 1. Deng et al.'s study was to verify the synergistic antitumor effects of IR and IT. A combination of IT and IR significantly enhanced the inhibition of TUBO growth in their study.

Table 1. Experimental data. Here, the control means without any therapy. IR therapy occurs on day 14 with 12 Gy, and IT therapy begins on day 14 and continues every three days for a total of four doses with 200 µg. Both indicate a combination therapy of IR and IT and each column represents time and tumor size, respectively.

Control		IR		IT (Anti-PD-L1)		Both	
0	5	0	5	0	5	0	5
13.8587	120.487	14.0761	95.8553	13.9674	135.2759	14.0761	94.2126
18.0435	202.7944	18.0435	133.8006	18.2065	206.0865	18.0977	87.8069
21.0326	289.9808	21.087	158.5662	21.3043	242.3534	21.1413	53.0777
25.0543	472.4868	24.8913	204.7183	24.9457	316.4249	25.1087	40.0989
28.0977	628.6693	28.1522	303.4149	31.1413	591.012	28.2065	27.7271
-	-	30.9783	402.0936	-	-	31.087	24.56
-	-	-	-	-	-	34.9457	17.505

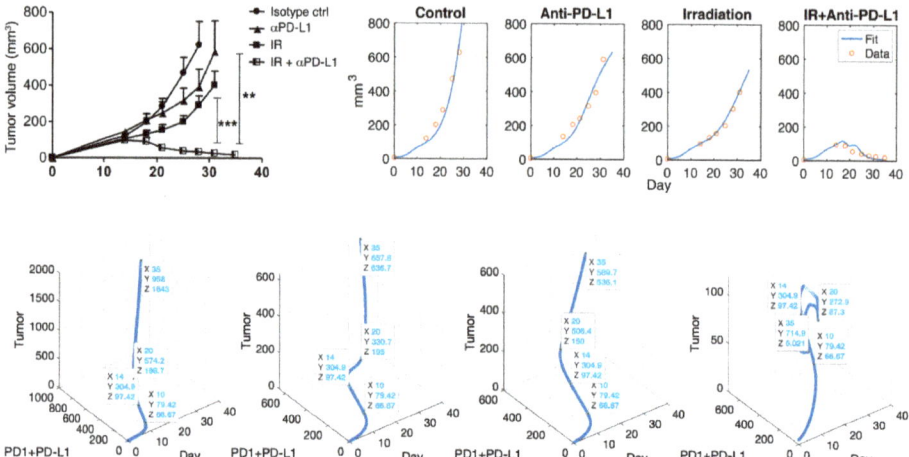

Figure 2. Note that α PD-L1 is IT (anti-PD-L1). Deng et al. showed the synergistic effect of combination therapy (top left). Simulation results (top right) after data fitting are presented through the mathematical model. This model captures the control, IT, and IR well, and this model also fits combination therapy. The blue curve indicates data fit using the Equations (1)–(6), and the red circle is experimental data. A scatter plot is shown for tumor vs. PD-1+PD-L1 vs. day (bottom). Each figure indicates control, IT, IR, and the combination of IR and IT in turn. Data tips are marked on day 10 (before therapy), 14 (beginning of IR and IT therapy), 20 (during IT therapy), and 35 (final timepoint). The sum of PD-1 and PD-L1 does not always positively correlate with tumor size after therapy. The coordinates X, Y, and Z, as shown in bottom figure, represent days, PD-1 + PD-L1 concentration and tumor size, respectively. **: $p < 0.01$; ***: $p < 0.001$.

2.3. Mathematical Modeling

Let C, T, PL, PD, S, R, and A denote tumor (volume), the density of CD8+ T cells (T cells), PD-L1, PD-1, PD-1-PD-L1 complex (µg/µL), IR (Gy), and IT (µg/µL), respectively. The tumor grows logistically, and T cells are activated by the cytokines interleukin 12 (IL12) and are proliferated by interleukin 2 (IL2). Both IL12 and IL2 are activated by stimulation of the tumor. Among the several types of immune cells playing a role against cancer, we have focused only on T cells. IL-12 and IL-2 play a significant role in the activation and differentiation of the population of T cells [17]. The tumor expresses PD-L1 on the cell surface, and T cells express both PD-L1 and PD-1 on their surface. The binding process of PD-L1 and PD-1 induces negative feedback in T cells. IT inhibits the growth of both tumor and T cells and inhibits PD-L1 by preventing the formation of the PD-L1-PD-1 complex, which indirectly prevents the inhibition of T cell growth.

2.3.1. Modeling Therapy with IR (R) and IT (A)

An exponential decay model was used to model for IR as follows:

$$\frac{dR_1}{dt} = -k_1 R_1, \quad \frac{dR}{dt} = k_1 R_1 - k_R R, \quad R_1(14) = 12 \text{ and } R_1(t) = 0 \text{ if } t < 14. \tag{1}$$

In the case of IT, a pharmacokinetic model was used with a two-compartment model as follows:

$$\frac{dA_T}{dt} = -(k_T + k_{el}) A_T, \quad \frac{dA}{dt} = k_T A_T - k_A A, \quad A_T(t) = 0, \\ \text{if } t < 14, \; A_T(14) = \frac{200}{V}. \tag{2}$$

Furthermore, 200 µg IT is administered every three days for a total of four doses in a 50 µL volume after beginning IT on day 14.

2.3.2. Compartmental Modeling of the Tumor(C), T Cell(T), PD-L1(PL), PD-1(PD), and Complex(S)

$$\frac{dC}{dt} = k_c \left(1 - \frac{C}{C_{max}}\right) \cdot C - \left(\frac{d_{TC}T}{T_{IC} + T} + \frac{d_{RC}R}{R_{IC} + R}\right) \cdot C.$$

The second term of the right-hand side (RHS) indicates tumor elimination by IT and IR therapy.

$$\frac{dT}{dt} = (k_{I12} + k_{I2}T) \frac{\kappa}{S_{IC} + k_D S} - \left(d_T + \frac{d_{RT}R}{R_{IC} + R}\right) T.$$

The first term of the RHS indicates that the PD-1-PD-L1 complex suppresses T cell growth. The second term of the RHS describes natural cell death and additional elimination by IR.

$$\frac{dPL}{dt} = \nu \cdot (\mu C + \eta T) - \frac{d_{APL}A}{A_{IC} + A} PL - k_{on} PL \cdot PD + k_{off} S - d_{PL} PL.$$

The first term of the RHS represents the increase in PD-L1 expression in tumors and T cells. The second term indicates inhibition of PD-L1 by IT. The third and fourth terms indicate the binding process of PD-1 and PD-L1. We assume that this reaction occurs according to the mass action law, indicating a one to one correspondence.

$$\frac{dPD}{dt} = \nu(1-\eta)T - k_{on} PL \cdot P + k_{off} S - d_{PD} PD.$$

In the first term of the RHS, η, $0 \leq \eta \leq 1$ determines the ratio of PD-1 to PD-L1 induced by T cells. That is, PD-L1 is more expressed as η approaches one.

$$\frac{dS}{dt} = k_{on} PL \cdot P - k_{off} S.$$

2.3.3. Model Reduction: Quasi Steady-State Approximation (QSSA)

We assume that PD-1-PD-L1 complex S is quickly saturated. Then equilibrium is reached within a short period of time, and so we may apply quasi-steady-state assumption (QSSA) and obtain $k_{on} PL \cdot P = k_{off} S$. Assume that $k_D = \frac{k_{on}}{k_{off}}$. Then the system is simplified as follows.

$$\frac{dC}{dt} = \underbrace{k_c\left(1 - \frac{C}{C_{max}}\right) \cdot C}_{\text{Tumor growth}} - \left(\underbrace{\frac{d_{TC}T}{T_{IC} + T}}_{\text{Inhibition by T cells}} + \underbrace{\frac{d_{RC}R}{R_{IC} + R}}_{\text{Inhibition by IR}}\right) \cdot C, \quad (3)$$

$$\frac{dT}{dt} = \left(\underbrace{k_{I12}}_{\text{Activation by IL12}} + \underbrace{k_{I2}T}_{\text{Growth by IL2}}\right) \underbrace{\frac{\kappa}{S_{IC} + k_D PL \cdot PD}}_{\text{Inhibition by complex}} - \left(\underbrace{d_T}_{\text{Death}} + \underbrace{\frac{d_{RT}R}{R_{IC} + R}}_{\text{Inhibition by IR}}\right) T, \quad (4)$$

$$\frac{dPL}{dt} = \underbrace{\nu(\mu C + \eta T)}_{\text{Growth by tumor and T cells}} - \underbrace{\frac{d_{APL}A}{A_{IC} + A} PL}_{\text{Inhibition by IT}} - \underbrace{d_{PL} PL}_{\text{Degradation}}, \quad (5)$$

$$\frac{dPD}{dt} = \underbrace{v \cdot (1-\eta)}_{\text{Growth and the ratio expression level of the T cells}} T - \underbrace{d_{PD} \; PD}_{\text{Degradation}}. \quad (6)$$

Descriptions or units of the estimated parameters and compartments are presented in Table 2.

Table 2. Estimated parameters and initial values used in the model are presented together with their descriptions and units.

Initial/Parameters	Description and Units	Estimated Values
$C(0)$	Tumor initial volume (mm^3)	5
$T(0)$	Initial lymphocytic density of CD8+ T cells (10^9 cells/L)	6×10^{-4} (Assumed)
$PL(0)$	Initial concentration of PD-L1 (µg/µL)	1×10^{-5} (Assumed)
$PD(0)$	Initial concentration of PD-1 (µg/µL)	1×10^{-5} (Assumed)
$A_t(14)$	Initial concentration of Anti-PD-L1 (µg/µL) in tissue	4
$A(0)$	Concentration of anti-PD-L1 (µg/µL)	0
$R_1(14)$	Irradiation (Gy)	12
k_c	Tumor growth rate (1/mm^3/day)	0.29428
C_{max}	Maximum tumor size (mm^3)	3×10^3
d_{TC}	Maximum tumor death rate by T cells (1/day)	0.53643
T_{IC}	Half maximum density of T cells (10^8 cells/L)	1×10^3
d_{RC}	Maximum tumor death rate by irradiation (1/day)	0.5
R_{IC}	Half maximum irradiation (Gy)	8
V	Volume in mice (µL)	50
k_{I12}	T cell activation rate by cytokine IL12 (10^8 cells/L/day)	10
k_{I2}	T cell proliferation rate by cytokine IL12 (1/day)	1×10^2
k_D	Equilibrium constant (1/µg/µL)	1
κ	Inhibition constant of PD-L1 and PD-1 (µg/µL)	10
η	Expression level ratio of PD-L1 to PD-1 in T cells (unitless)	0.5
S_{IC}	Half maximum inhibition of PD-L1 and PD-1 (µg/µL)	1×10^3
d_T	T cell death rate (1/day)	0.1
d_{RT}	Maximum T cell death rate by irradiation (1/day)	1
v	Expression level of PD-L1 on activated T cells (10^3 µg/cell/day)	0.1
d_{PL}	Degradation rate of PD-L1 (1/day)	1×10^{-2}
d_{PD}	Degradation rate of PD-1 (1/day)	1×10^{-2}
μ	Expression level of PD-L1 by tumor vs. T cells (cell/µL/mm^3)	0.1
d_{APL}	Maximum PD-L1 inhibition rate by anti-PD-L1 (1/day)	20
A_{IC}	Half-maximum inhibition (µg/µL)	1
k_T	Intercompartment distribution rate (1/day)	1.5×10^{-3}
k_{el}	Elimination rate of anti-PD-L1 in tissue (1/day)	0.1
k_A	Elimination rate of anti-PD-L1 (1/day)	0.05
k_1	Delay rate with the mean duration $1/k_1$ (1/day)	0.15
k_R	Elimination rate of ionizing irradiation (1/day)	0.09

3. Results

3.1. Simulation using the Cancer-Immune Model with IR and IT Therapy

Combination therapy with IT and IR significantly enhanced the inhibition of tumor growth in mice, as shown in Figure 2 (top left). The mathematical model consisting of (1)–(6) was used to fit the data, as shown in Figure 2 (top right). Data from the control (no therapy), IT only, and IR only samples were fitted. From three data fittings, we estimated parameter values, as shown in Table 2. MATLAB, MathWorks®, was used for model implementation with ODE45, and parameter estimation was conducted with the nonlinear least square method using MATLAB and Berkeley Madonna. Using the estimated parameters, the model captured the synergistic effect of the combination therapy consisting of IR and IT, as shown in Figure 2 (IR + IT). Additionally, the model failed to capture data around day 22. This is because repeated combination therapies cause a slightly overstated discrepancy in the model. However, the overall data fitting is reliable, and the model captures the efficacy of the combination therapy in mice.

In the control case, tumor size, PD-1 and PD-L1 expression were positively exponentially proportional. In this case, the regression (function) over time from day 0 to 35 was $f(t) = 11.45e^{0.0052 \cdot t}$ with $R^2 = 0.9975$. Cases were compared before and after therapy. Before therapy, the linear regression was $f(t) = 0.267t + 22.27$ with $R^2 = 0.8019$. Linearity was well followed after therapy begins (day 14) and the regression was $f(t) = 2.461t - 859.8$ with $R^2 = 0.8732$. In the case of IT, there was a positive correlation after initiating therapy. The linear regression was $f(t) = 1.451t - 315.7$ with $R^2 = 0.9891$. Although the growth rate was suppressed by IT, the relationship between IT and tumor growth still had a positive correlation. Likewise, in the case of IR, the growth rate was lower, and the linear regression was $f(t) = 1.294t - 343.4$ with $R^2 = 0.6277$, which shows positive correlation. However, there was a negative correlation after beginning combination therapy, in which the tumor size decreases due to the synergistic effect. The linear regression was $f(t) = -0.2029t + 150.7$ with $R^2 = 0.9731$.

3.2. The Expression Levels of PD-1 and PD-L1

We utilized the model to explore which parameters cause tumor suppression among PD-1 and PD-L1. That is, we analyzed the changes in tumor size vs. parameters related to the changes in PD-1 and PD-L1. From (5)–(6), expression levels v and μ determine the magnitude of the expression levels of PD-1 and PD-L1 on the surface of tumors and T cells. Given that T cells can express both PD-1 and PD-L1, the ratio η, $0 \leq \eta \leq 1$, determines the ratio of the expression levels of PD-1 and PD-L1 in T cells. That is, if η is increasing, then so is the expression level of PD-L1 in T cells. Analyzing these parameters enables us to evaluate whether the concentration is more influential in removing the tumor among the expression levels of PD-1 and PD-L1. Specifically, we investigated how the IT efficacy is maximized depending on the expression level ratio of PD-1 to PD-L1. For this analysis, we attempted local changes in parameters, as shown in Figure 3, and two of the three parameters were compared. When modulating μ and v (left panel), an increase in u and v stimulates tumor growth. This is because an increase in PD-1 and PD-L1 under a fixed η causes T cell suppression, resulting in tumor growth. When modulating v and η (middle), tumor growth depends on an increase in v and decrease in η. This change indicates that IT could be more efficient when PD-1 is more highly expressed than PD-L1. When η and μ are varied (right), tumor growth depends on decreasing η and increasing μ. Thus, in the local sense, the decrease in η and the increase in v and μ result in tumor growth. This indicates that IT efficacy is more potent when PD-1 level on T cells is smaller.

In Figure 4, we investigated tumor size vs. the sum of PD-1 and PD-L1 expression. We noticed that the total expression level of PD-1 and PD-L1 does not positively correlate tumor size when the tumor is inhibited by combination therapy, unlike IT and IR only. We inferred that this was because the balance of PD-1 and PD-L1 was broken, leading to a reduced concentration of the complex formed by PD-1 binding to PD-L1 and ultimately blocking T cell inhibition. However, these local changes in parameters could have biased influences given that these processes naturally assume that the other parameters remain constant. In particular, the change in expression levels of PD-1 and PD-L1 are simultaneously affected by various parameters.

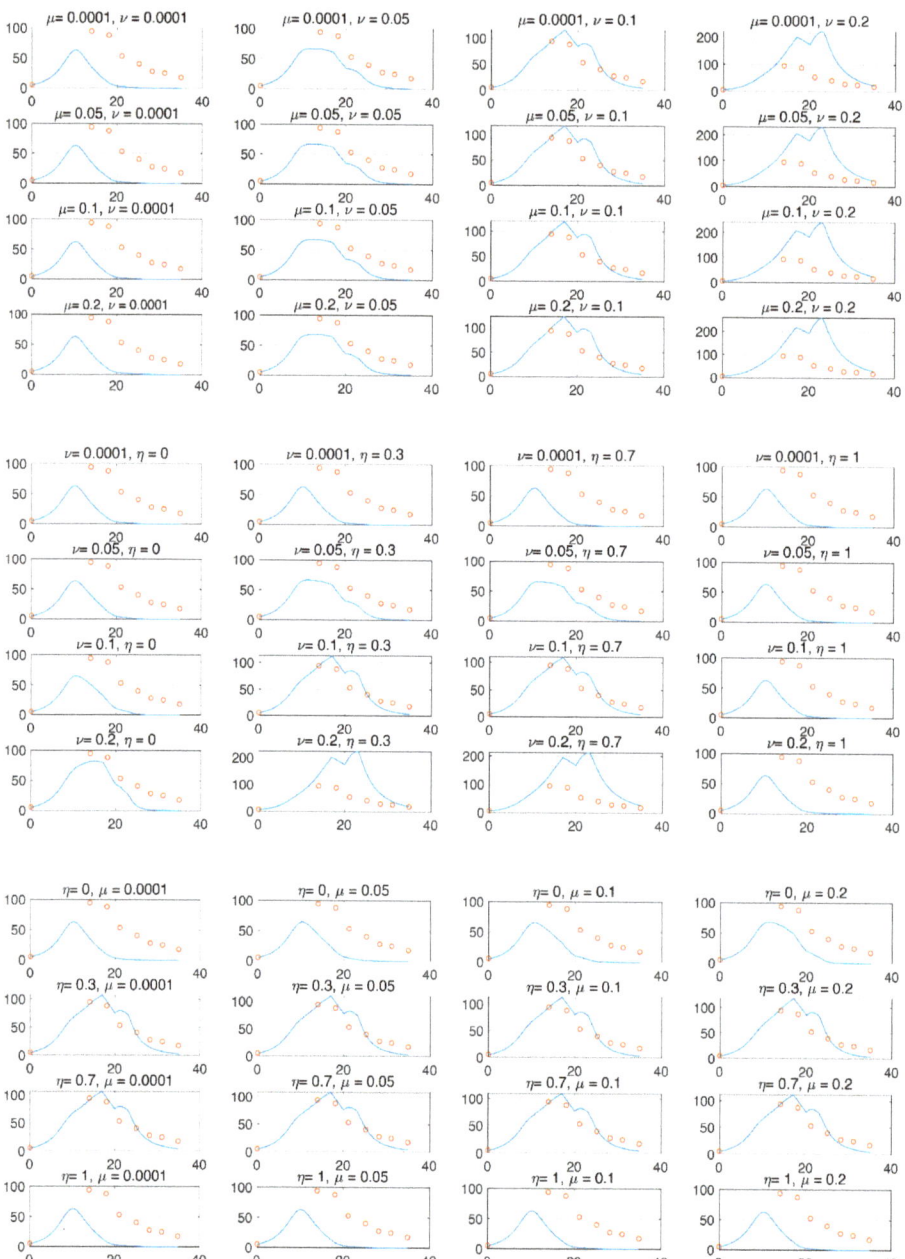

Figure 3. The x and y axes represent day and tumor size, respectively. Top panel: μ and ν are varied from $[1 \times 10^{-4}, 0.2]$ and $[1 \times 10^{-4}, 0.2]$, respectively. Center panel: μ and η are varied from $[1 \times 10^{-4}, 0.2]$ and $[0, 1]$, respectively. Bottom panel: η and μ are varied from $[0, 1]$ and $[1 \times 10^{-4}, 0.2]$, respectively. From these local changes, each parameter positively or negatively influences the change in tumor.

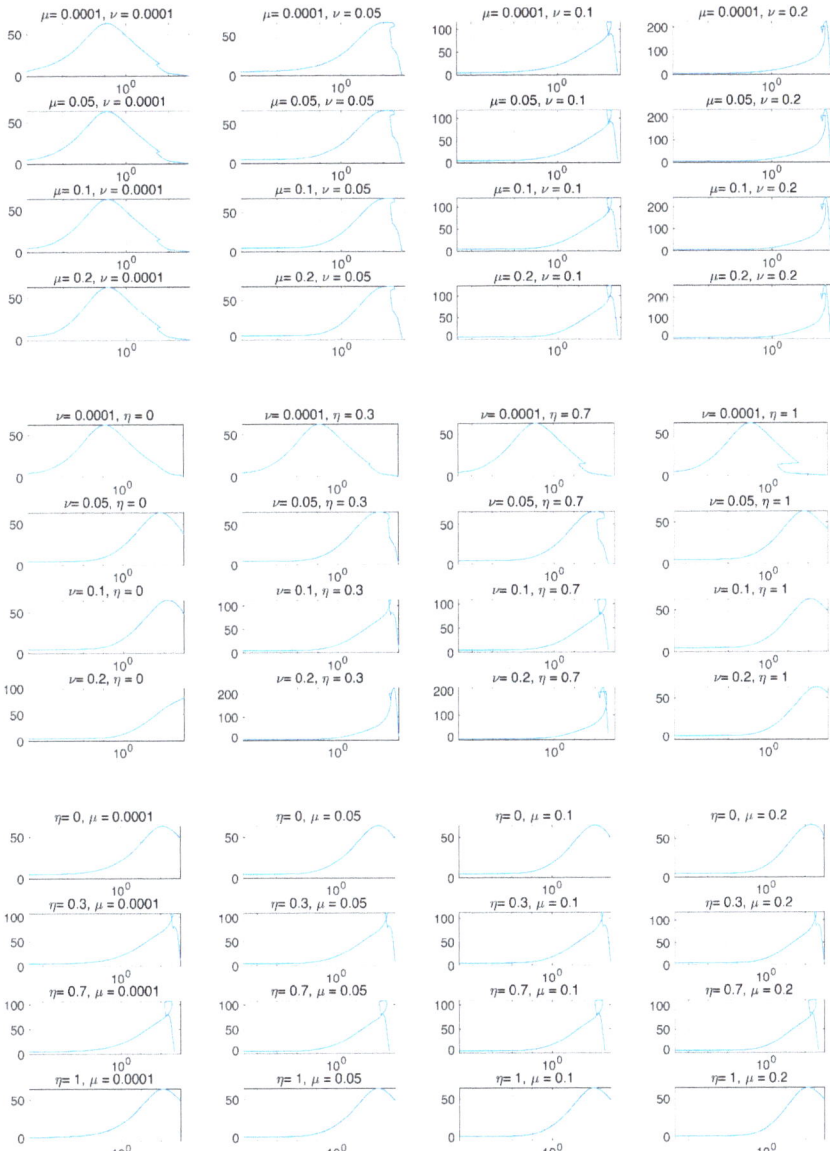

Figure 4. The x and y axes represent the sum of PD-1 and PD-L1 and tumor size, respectively. The x axis is plotted on a logarithmic scale. Each graph indicates the two parameters that are varied. μ, ν, and η are varied from $[1 \times 10^{-4}, 0.2]$, $[1 \times 10^{-4}, 0.2]$, and $[0, 1]$, respectively. After beginning combination therapy, the sum of PD-1 and PD-L1 is not positively proportional to tumor size.

Performing a two-parameter comparison could induce prediction bias. Thus, global sensitivity analysis is required to analyze how all parameters associated with the changes in PD-1 and PD-L1 are simultaneously changed.

From Figures 3 and 4, the model verified that the magnitude of tumor reduction was changed according to the change in the parameter, and the change in tumor size due to the change in the sum of PD-1 and PD-L1 expression was compared. The model showed that the concentration of the sum of PD-1 and PD-L1 was not proportional to tumor size after therapy begins, indicating that if tumor size decreases, the correlation between them is deregulated. We believe that the synergistic effect of combination therapy accelerated the dysregulation of this correlation. However, further studies on the correlation between tumor size and the sum of PD-L1 and PD-1 expression should be conducted with more data.

The challenge is to determine how uncertainty in the output of a model can be apportioned to different sources of uncertainty in the model input (factors) [18]. Local methods analyze sensitivity around some (often optimal) points in the factor space, whereas global methods attempt to analyze variability across the full factor space. Changing one factor at a time means that whatever effect is observed on the output is due solely to that factor. Conversely, a non-zero effect implies influence; i.e., it never detects uninfluential factors as relevant. Local sensitivity has the above disadvantage; therefore, we performed global sensitivity analysis and analyzed tumor changes under the influence of other variables. The elimination rate k_{el} is contained to evaluate the influence. Providing k_{el} enables comparison to the influence of a dummy-parameter not directly related to PD-1 and PD-L1.

3.3. Global Sensitivity Analysis of the Parameter Space: Latin Hypercube Sampling Partial Rank Correlation Coefficient

We evaluated the influence of the parameters on the tumor size using global sensitivity analysis. Influences of the parameters were measured at days 10, 14, 20, and 35, using the partial rank correlation coefficient (PRCC) [18,19] based on Latin hypercube sampling (LHS) [20,21]. LHS is a sampling method that provides an unbiased estimation of the output of a model while requiring fewer samples to achieve the same accuracy of simple random sampling. For parameters x_j, $j = 1, 2, \cdots, k$ and tumor y, a correlation coefficient (CC) between x_j and y is calculated as

$$r_{x_j y} = \frac{Cov(x_j, y)}{\sqrt{Var(x_j) Var(y)}},$$

where $Cov(x, y)$ is the covariance between x_j and y, and $var(x_j)$ is the variance of x_j. CC varies between −1 and 1. Pearson correlation coefficient (PCC) characterizes the linear relationship considering residuals $x_j - \hat{x}_j$ and $y - \hat{y}$, where $\hat{x}_j = c_0 + \sum_{i=1, i \neq j}^{k} c_i x_i$ and $\hat{y} = b_0 + \sum_{i=1, i \neq j}^{k} b_i x_i$. PRCC performs PCC, with x_j and y being first-rank transformed parameters and tumor size is determined by LHS, respectively.

PRCC is a robust sensitivity measure for monotonic relationships between input and output. PRCC performs a partial correlation analysis on rank-transformed data in two steps: (i) input and output data are first rank-transformed, and then (ii) the linear regression model is applied. LHS is used for parameter sampling, in which each parameter is assumed to be uniformly distributed. We explored four parameters related to the changes in PD-1 and PD-L1 stimulated by the tumor and T cells. Herein, tumor size over the parameters is plotted using LHS, as shown in Figure 5. By varying the parameters associated with the changes in PD-1 and PD-L1, tumor size increases or decreases. The number of sampling parameters was 1000, and the ranges of the parameters were as follows:

$$\nu \sim U(1 \times 10^{-5}, 0.2), k_{el} \sim U(1 \times 10^{-5}, 5), \eta \sim U(1 \times 10^{-8}, 1), \mu \sim (1 \times 10^{-5}, 0.2), \tag{7}$$

where U is uniform distribution. The resultant PRCCs with p-values are measured in Figures 6–9 using LHS. This was done at the following timepoints: day 10 (before therapy), 14 (beginning of therapy), 20 (during therapy), and 35 (after therapy). Additionally, PCC was calculated for comparison. PCC is intuitive because there is no change in parameters and tumor size, but the linear relationship of PRCC between variations in parameters and tumor size becomes more apparent compared to PCC.

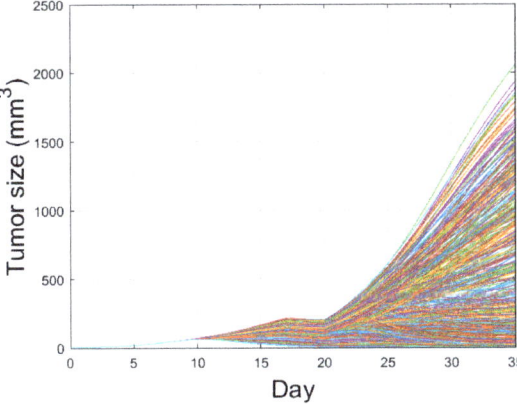

Figure 5. Tumor growth curve with combination therapy of IR and IT is plotted with the parameter variations using Latin Hypercube Sampling. One thousand cases with four parameters randomly extracted from (7) were conducted. By varying these parameters, some tumors are eliminated, some reach maximal tumor sizes, and the others are in between the two extremes. The amount of combination therapy and other parameter values were unchanged except for η, ν, μ, and k_{el}.

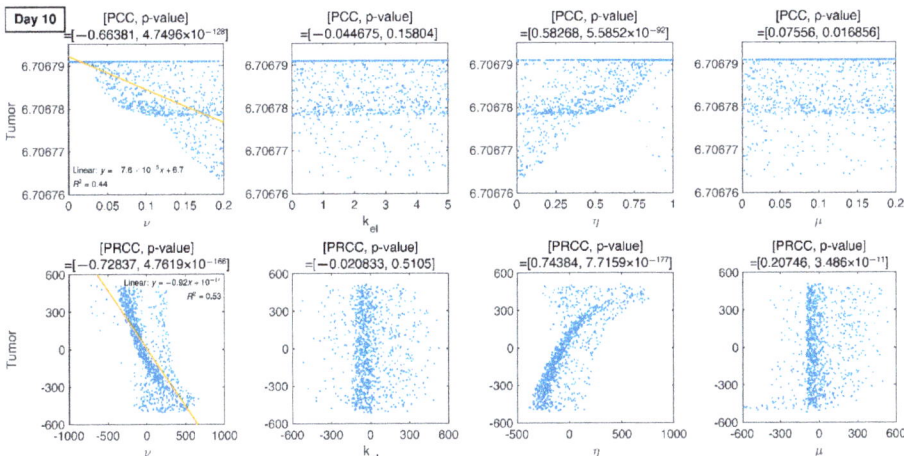

Figure 6. PCC and PRCC scatter plots of tumor size versus parameters k_{el}, μ, ν, and η on day 10. All four parameters are varied simultaneously. The sample size is 1000. The x-axis represents the parameter values in PCC or the residuals of the linear regression between the rank-transformed values of the parameters. The y-axis represents the tumor size in PCC or the residuals of the linear regression between the rank-transformed values of tumor versus the rank-transformed values of the parameters. The title of each plot represents the PRCC value with the corresponding p-value. The linear relationship between parameters and tumor variation becomes more apparent with PRCC compared to PCC.

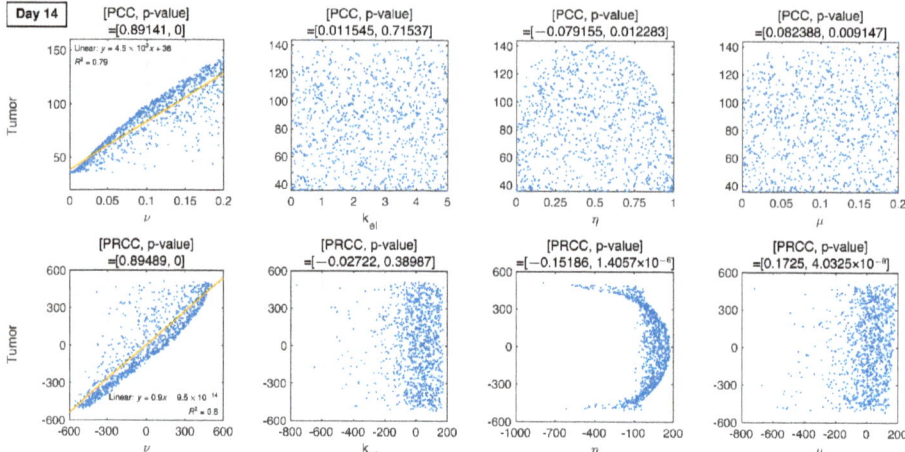

Figure 7. Dotted points indicate tumor size on day 14. Combination therapy begins on day 14. An increase in ν is proportional to tumor growth with PRCC and p-value. Other parameters are less influential.

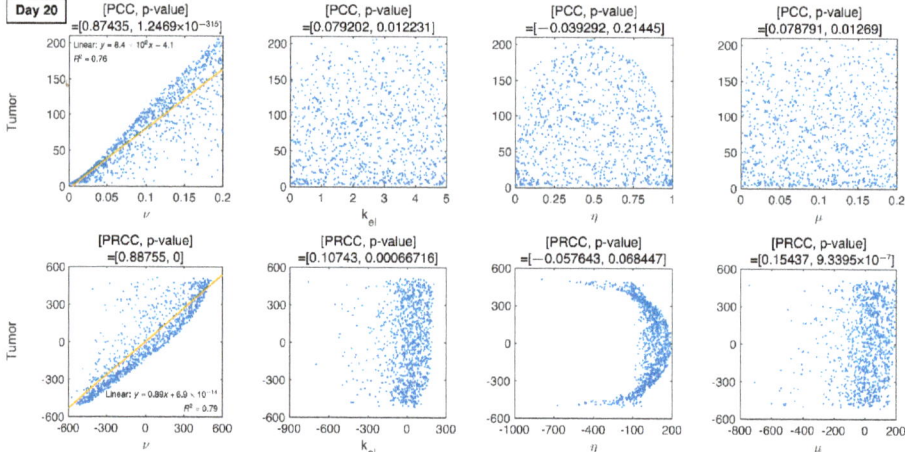

Figure 8. On day 20 (during IT therapy and after IR therapy), PRCC and p-values of four parameters are determined. An increase in ν is proportional to tumor growth, but other parameters have little influence.

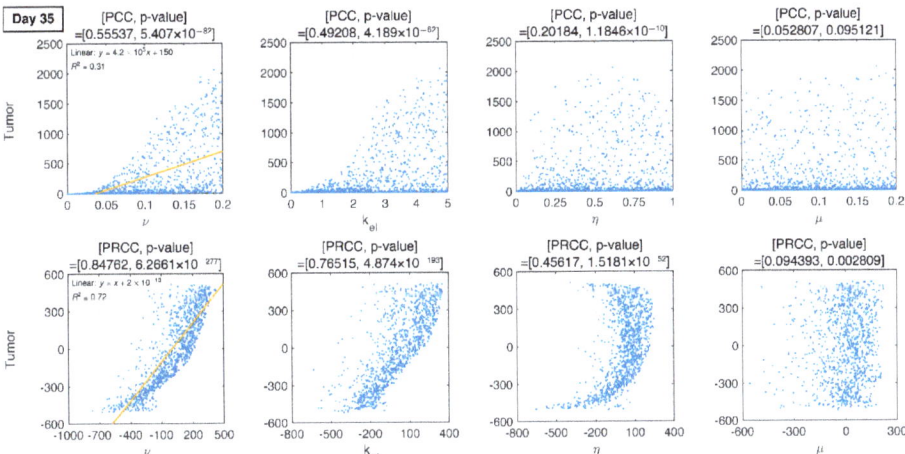

Figure 9. In the final phase, the elimination rate of IT, k_{el}, is proportional to tumor growth. v remains proportional to tumor growth.

3.4. Analysis of Changes in Parameters

We compare PCC and PRCC with *p*-values, as shown in Figures 6–9. PCC directly compares tumor size vs. parameters. While PCC is intuitive, it has a disadvantage in that the relationship between parameters and tumor size is not clearly identified. Therefore, PRCC is performed to examine the influence of parameters more clearly by transforming the value. Ultimately, the global sensitivity analysis investigates the changes in essential outputs caused by simultaneous changes in parameters. We explored the parameter influence at each critical timepoint. In particular, the change in parameters can be compared before and after therapy. The influence of k_{el} and v did not significantly affect both tumor growth and inhibition at day 10, before therapy. In the case of v, negative linearity is observed in PRCC as compared to that in PCC. In the case of η, the linearity is not observed in PCC, but PRCC captures positive linearity. When combination therapy begins on day 14 (Figure 7), k_{el}, η and μ are not correlated to the change in tumor size. Tumor size has a positive linear relationship to v, unlike before therapy. In Figure 8, which shows day 20 of IT therapy, tumor size and v have a positive relationship, which becomes more apparent compared to PCC. After therapy (day 35), v and k_{el} are positively correlated with tumor size, as shown in Figure 9. This correlation indicates that the elimination rate of IT is influential to the change in tumor size when the amount of IT is small. From global sensitivity analysis, we may conclude that parameter influence over tumor size is different before and after therapy. These levels accelerated tumor inhibition after therapy began. Particularly, η determining the ratio of PD-1 to PD-L1 does not follow the linear relationship to tumor size.

Changes in tumor size with respect to v before and after therapy were investigated. There was a negative correlation in the absence of therapy (before day 14), as shown in Figures 6–9. However, a positive correlation was observed after IT, IR, and combination therapy began. This seemingly contradictory result demonstrated that, prior to initiating therapy, PCC showed a small change in tumor size (less than 3E-5), so the negative correlation may not have a significant effect on the change in tumor size. PRCC showed this difference to be more exaggerated, indicating that it was essential to examine both PCC and PRCC. Changes in v after 14 days of therapy were positively correlated with tumor size. This relationship was due to the negative feedback by which the increase in v caused by T cells leads to an increase in PD-L1, and a decrease in T cells by increasing the amount of PD-1 and PD-L1 binding. This mechanism increased tumor size and suggested that high PD-L1 expression levels in T cells could inhibit the efficiency of IT. Likewise, an increase in expression level $v \cdot \mu$ expressed on tumor cells caused an increase in PD-L1 regardless of therapy. Additionally, an increase in $v \cdot \mu$ resulted in an increase in tumor size for similar reasons.

4. Discussion and Conclusions

Localized IR has been mediated tumor reduction in a T cell-dependent fashion. Therapeutic blockade of the T cell negative regulator PD-L1 could enhance T cell effector function when PD-L1 was expressed in tumors, as it happens in the tumor microenvironment after IR [22,23]. PD-L1 expression in the tumor microenvironment provided an opportunity for therapeutic intervention using immunotherapies such as anti PD-L1, anti PD-1 and CTLA-4 [24,25].

The purpose of this work was to obtain insight into mechanisms of the tumor-immune interactions while combination therapy of IR and IT was conducted. Notably, we considered PD-1 and PD-L1 in the model to discuss how these targets change. Mathematical modeling is one of the most important tools in analyzing the characteristics of the synergistic combinations and providing some useful insights about the dynamic of the interactions. A mathematical model for the tumor-immune interactions was developed. QSSA was used to simplify the model. Additionally, two-compartment models for treatment were considered to reflect the delay of tumor repression. The simulation was implemented for control, IT only, and IR only data. From the estimated parameters, combination therapy with IR and IT was fit. Simulations of our model are shown to be in reliable agreement with mouse experiments for all cases [14].

The model addressed how tumors and T cells were inhibited or stimulated by changes in PD-1 and PD-L1 expression. To this end, we utilized global sensitivity analysis to examine the influence of four parameters and confirmed the corresponding changes in tumor size. It was possible to employ a model to investigate how T cells and tumor growth were stimulated by PD-L1 and PD-1. The model predicted that T cells would have a significant influence on tumor growth and inhibition based on the ratio of PD-1 to PD-L1 when IT is applied. This result was explored in the global sensitivity analysis of the parameter changes, rather than with local changes. We compared PCC and PRCC from LHS among global sensitivities. PCC was intuitive, but the relationship between parameters and tumor size variation was more apparent when assessed with PRCC than PCC.

Our approach complemented Deng et al.'s experiments that combination therapy of IR and IT was likely an important part of the complex regulation in the IR tumor microenvironment that suppresses antitumor immunity. Two models can be contrasted. The model of Nikolopoulou et al. was a system of three ODEs with 19 parameters. They theoretically investigated the change in tumors against anti-PD-1. Their major contribution was to predict the general behavior of the tumor-immune response to therapy. Sensitivity analysis using PRCC via LHS and bifurcation analysis for tumor and T cells were also conducted. The model of Chappell et al. was a system of 4 ODEs with 16 parameters. Their study concerned tumor-T cell interactions with combination therapy of IR and IT. Regardless of the consideration of PD-1 and PD-L1, one of their contributions was reproducing the synergistic effects of IR and IT. Theoretical analysis such as model equilibria and stability was also conducted. Our approach reflected those models and additionally focus on the change in the expression levels of PD-1 and PD-L1. However, the proposed model has some limitations. We assumed that PD-L1 is permanently expressed on tumor cells and the expression increases with a tumor progression. However, PD-L1 is heterogeneously expressed on cancer cells and can be decreased over a period. Furthermore, we did not consider other immune checkpoint molecules upregulated on cancer cells that also have a significant impact on the cancer cell immune escape.

In Figures 6–9, the ratio rate η determined the ratio of PD-1 to PD-L1 in T cells. Before therapy, η and tumor size were positively correlated. That is, in our model, after cancer cells were implanted and before therapy, the binding of PD-1 to PD-L1 was small, and as a result, T cell suppression was small and the increase in tumor size was minimal, as shown in the experimental data (Figure 6). The linearity was deregulated after beginning combination therapy (Figures 7–9). IT depleted PD-L1 to reduce the amount of binding to PD-1, thereby reducing T cell suppression and consequently suppressing tumors. IR additionally eliminated tumors and reduced the amount of PD-L1. Therefore, tumor size was determined based on T cell decrease/increase, where a decrease was caused by IR directly or an increase was caused by inhibiting the binding of PD-1 to PD-L1 indirectly.

Interestingly, as η decreased, the tumor size variation became more severe. The smaller the differentiation by T cells to PD-L1 was, the smaller the amount of PD-L1 was, and thus tumor growth was suppressed by IT. Meanwhile, when η was small with sufficient PD-L1, T cells increased the expression level of PD-1, thereby increasing the concentration of the PD-1-PD-L1 complex. As a result, the proliferation of the T cells was suppressed, and the tumor size increased. Therefore, two opposite cases can occur. Combination therapy overcomes the challenge by inhibiting the tumor both directly and indirectly. Using this model, we examined ways to regulate PD-L1 and PD-1 to improve the efficacy of combination therapy. After reducing PD-L1 and PD-1 expression by inhibiting tumor and T cells through IR, further depletion of PD-L1 through IT resulted in a decrease in the amount of PD-1-PD-L1 complex, thereby preventing the inhibition of T cell growth. This result indicated that if PD-L1 is lowly expressed in T cells, the efficacy of IT improves. That is, the level of PD-1-PD-L1 complex can be lower by reducing η.

It was noted that when η was small (i.e., when PD-1 was highly expressed in T cells or PD-L1 expression was low in T cells) and PD-L1 expression on the tumor was high, the tumor could be less inhibited as the PD-1-PD-L1 complex concentration was increased, indicating that T cell growth may be further suppressed. Additionally, combination therapy should be considered in two cases: when PD-L1 expression is high and when PD-1 expression is low or high in T cells. The expression level of PD-L1 was determined based on combination therapy. That is, when the expression level of PD-1 in T cells is low, successful therapy can be achieved by suppressing PD-L1 alone. Still, in the case of high expression of PD-L1 in T cells, such a strategy may fail due to excessive T cell reduction, although the tumor size was also reduced.

We investigated the tumor-immune interaction through a mathematical model. Through combination therapy, we verified the synergistic effect of combined IR and IT after parameter estimation through data fitting. Our model analyzed the mechanism of tumor inhibition through the relationship between PD-1 and PD-L1. We also examined the influence of each parameter through global sensitivity analysis of crucial parameters associated with the change in PD-1 and PD-L1. However, this analysis assumed a uniform distribution considering a slight variation in the parameters. Importantly, this assumption could not suggest a feasible condition for the parameters. In the next study, we will provide the distribution of the parameter space using Bayesian inference. This study could be valuable in that the Bayesian inference may be used for consideration of multiple doses and combination therapy remains challenging in the tumor-immune system.

Author Contributions: J.H.B. conceptualized the roles, designed the studies, analyzed the data, performed modeling, and illustrated the numerical simulation. I.H.J. conceptualized and designed the roles and studies. I.-S.Y. conceptualized the roles and analyzed the data. Y.D.J. and S.K. designed the studies and analyzed the data. All authors have read and agreed to the published version of the manuscript.

Funding: This work was funded by the National Research Foundation of Korea (NRF) grant funded by the Korea government (NRF-2018H1A2A1062811, NRF-2019R1A2C2007249, and NRF-2020R1C1C1A01004631).

Conflicts of Interest: The authors declare no conflict of interest.

References

1. Shuptrine, C.W.; Surana, R.; Weiner, L.M. Monoclonal antibodies for the treatment of cancer. *Semin. Cancer Biol.* **2012**, *22*, 3–13. [CrossRef] [PubMed]
2. Chen, D.S.; Mellman, I. Oncology meets immunology: The cancer-immunity cycle. *Immunity* **2013**, *39*, 1–10. [CrossRef] [PubMed]
3. Milberg, O.; Gong, C.; Jafarnejad, M.; Bartelink, I.H.; Wang, B.; Vicini, P.; Narwal, R.; Roskos, L.; Popel, A.S. A QSP Model for Predicting Clinical Responses to Monotherapy, Combination and Sequential Therapy Following CTLA-4, PD-1, and PD-L1 Checkpoint Blockade. *Sci. Rep.* **2019**, *9*, 1–17. [CrossRef] [PubMed]

4. Valentinuzzi, D.; Simončič, U.; Uršič, K.; Vrankar, M.; Turk, M.; Jeraj, R. Predicting tumour response to anti-PD-1 immunotherapy with computational modelling. *Phys. Med. Biol.* **2019**, *64*. [CrossRef]
5. Wei, S.C.; Duffy, C.R.; Allison, J.P. Fundamental Mechanisms of Immune Checkpoint Blockade Therapy. *Cancer Discov.* **2018**, *8*, 1069–1086. [CrossRef]
6. Iwai, Y.; Hamanishi, J.; Chamoto, K.; Honjo, T. Cancer immunotherapies targeting the PD-1 signaling pathway. *J. Biomed. Sci.* **2017**, *24*, 1–11. [CrossRef] [PubMed]
7. Weiner, L.M.; Dhodapkar, M.V.; Ferrone, S. Monoclonal antibodies for cancer immunotherapy. *Lancet* **2009**, *373*, 1033–1040. [CrossRef]
8. Jiang, H.; Hegde, S.; Knolhoff, B.L.; Zhu, Y.; Herndon, J.M.; Meyer, M.A.; Nywening, T.M.; Hawkins, W.G.; Shapiro, I.M.; Weaver, D.T.; et al. Targeting focal adhesion kinase renders pancreatic cancers responsive to checkpoint immunotherapy. *Nat. Med.* **2016**, *22*, 851–860. [CrossRef]
9. Esteva, F.J.; Hubbard-Lucey, V.M.; Tang, J.; Pusztai, L. Immunotherapy and targeted therapy combinations in metastatic breast cancer. *Lancet Oncol.* **2019**, *20*, e175–e186. [CrossRef]
10. dePillis, L.G.; Eladdadi, A.; Radunskaya, A.E. Modeling cancer-immune responses to therapy. *J. Pharmacokinet. Pharmacodyn.* **2014**, *41*, 461–478. [CrossRef]
11. Serre, R.; Benzekry, S.; Padovani, L.; Meille, C.; Andre, N.; Ciccolini, J.; Barlesi, F.; Muracciole, X.; Barbolosi, D. Mathematical modeling of cancer immunotherapy and its synergy with radiotherapy. *Cancer Res.* **2016**, *76*, 4931–4940. [CrossRef] [PubMed]
12. Wei, S.C.; Anang, N.-A.A.S.; Sharma, R.; Andrews, M.C.; Reuben, A.; Levine, J.H.; Cogdill, A.P.; Mancuso, J.J.; Wargo, J.A.; Pe'er, D.; et al. Combination anti–CTLA-4 plus anti–PD-1 checkpoint blockade utilizes cellular mechanisms partially distinct from monotherapies. *Proc. Natl. Acad. Sci. USA* **2019**, *116*, 22699–22709. [CrossRef] [PubMed]
13. Yu, J.L.; Jang, S.R.J. A mathematical model of tumor-immune interactions with an immune checkpoint inhibitor. *Appl. Math. Comput.* **2019**, *362*, 124523. [CrossRef]
14. Deng, L.; Weichselbaum, R.R.; Fu, Y.; Deng, L.; Liang, H.; Burnette, B.; Beckett, M. Irradiation and anti—PD-L1 treatment synergistically promote antitumor immunity in mice Find the latest version: Irradiation and anti—PD-L1 treatment synergistically promote antitumor immunity in mice. *J. Clin. Investig.* **2014**, *124*, 687–695. [CrossRef]
15. Chappell, M.; Chelliah, V.; Cherkaoui, M.; Derks, G.; Dumortier, T.; Evans, N.; Ferrarini, M.; Fornari, C.; Ghazal, P.; Guerriero, M.L.; et al. Mathematical Modelling for Combinations of Immuno-Oncology and Anti-Cancer Therapies. *Rep. QSP UK Meet.* **2015**, 1–15. [CrossRef]
16. Nikolopoulou, E.; Johnson, L.R.; Harris, D.; Nagy, J.D.; Stites, E.C.; Kuang, Y. Tumour-immune dynamics with an immune checkpoint inhibitor. *Lett. Biomath.* **2018**, *5*, S137–S159. [CrossRef]
17. Lai, X.; Friedman, A. Combination therapy of cancer with cancer vaccine and immune checkpoint inhibitors: A mathematical model. *PLoS ONE* **2017**, *12*, e0178479. [CrossRef]
18. Saltelli, A.; Tarantola, S.; Campolongo, F.; Ratto, M. *Sensitivity Analysis in Practice: A Guide to Assessing Scientific Models*; Wiley: Chichester, UK, 2004; ISBN 0470870931.
19. Marino, S.; Hogue, I.B.; Ray, C.J.; Kirschner, D.E. A methodology for performing global uncertainty and sensitivity analysis in systems biology. *J. Theor. Biol.* **2008**, *254*, 178–196. [CrossRef]
20. Conover, W.J. A Distribution-Free Approach to Inducing Rank Correlation Among Input Variables. *Commun. Stat. Simul. Comput.* **1982**, *11*, 311–334. [CrossRef]
21. Davenport, J.M. Rank Correlation Plots for Use with Correlated Input Variables. *Commun. Stat. Simul. Comput.* **1982**, *11*, 335–360. [CrossRef]
22. Gong, J.; Le, T.Q.; Massarelli, E.; Hendifar, A.E.; Tuli, R. Radiation therapy and PD-1/PD-L1 blockade: The clinical development of an evolving anti-cancer combination. *J. Immunother. Cancer* **2018**, *6*, 1–17. [CrossRef] [PubMed]
23. Tang, C.; Welsh, J.W.; De Groot, P.; Massarelli, E.; Chang, J.Y.; Hess, K.R.; Basu, S.; Curran, M.A.; Cabanillas, M.E.; Subbiah, V.; et al. Ipilimumab with stereotactic ablative radiation therapy: Phase i results and immunologic correlates from peripheral T cells. *Clin. Cancer Res.* **2017**, *23*, 1388–1396. [CrossRef] [PubMed]

24. Park, K.J.; Lee, J.L.; Yoon, S.K.; Heo, C.; Park, B.W.; Kim, J.K. Radiomics-based prediction model for outcomes of PD-1/PD-L1 immunotherapy in metastatic urothelial carcinoma. *Eur. Radiol.* **2020**. [CrossRef]
25. Hamanishi, J.; Mandai, M.; Matsumura, N.; Abiko, K.; Baba, T.; Konishi, I. PD-1/PD-L1 blockade in cancer treatment: Perspectives and issues. *Int. J. Clin. Oncol.* **2016**, *21*, 462–473. [CrossRef] [PubMed]

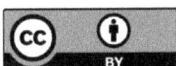

© 2020 by the authors. Licensee MDPI, Basel, Switzerland. This article is an open access article distributed under the terms and conditions of the Creative Commons Attribution (CC BY) license (http://creativecommons.org/licenses/by/4.0/).

MDPI
St. Alban-Anlage 66
4052 Basel
Switzerland
Tel. +41 61 683 77 34
Fax +41 61 302 89 18
www.mdpi.com

Pharmaceutics Editorial Office
E-mail: pharmaceutics@mdpi.com
www.mdpi.com/journal/pharmaceutics

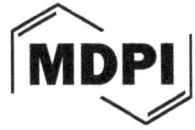

www.ingramcontent.com/pod-product-compliance
Lightning Source LLC
LaVergne TN
LVHW070247100526
838202LV00015B/2190